Diagnostic Musculoskeletal Surgical Pathology

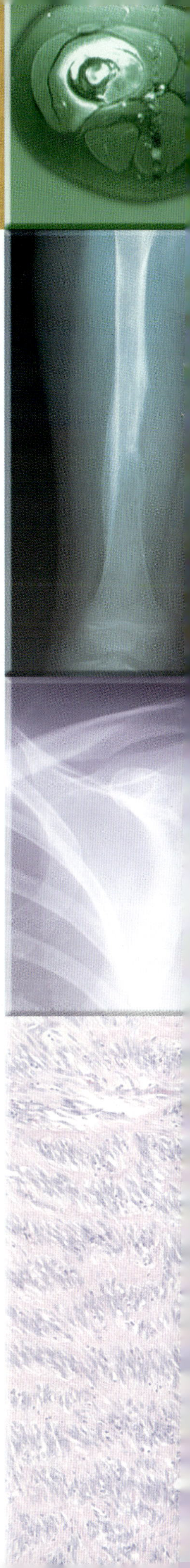

Diagnostic Musculoskeletal Surgical Pathology

CLINICORADIOLOGIC AND CYTOLOGIC CORRELATIONS

Scott E. Kilpatrick, MD
Pathologists Diagnostic Services
Forsyth Medical Center
Winston-Salem, North Carolina;
Department of Pathology and Laboratory Medicine
University of North Carolina
Chapel Hill, North Carolina

In Collaboration With:
Jordan B. Renner, MD
Department of Radiology
School of Medicine
University of North Carolina
Chapel Hill, North Carolina

Contribution By:
Andrew Creager, MD
Department of Pathology
Duke University Medical Center
Durham, North Carolina

SAUNDERS
An Imprint of Elsevier Science

SAUNDERS
An Imprint of Elsevier, Inc. (USA)

The Curtis Center
Independence Square West
Philadelphia, Pennsylvania 19106-3399

DIAGNOSTIC MUSCULOSKELETAL SURGICAL PATHOLOGY: 0-7216-9163-3
Clinicoradiologic and Cytologic Correlations

Notice

Pathology is an ever-changing field. Standard safety precautions must be followed, but as new research and clinical experience broaden our knowledge, changes in treatment and drug therapy may become necessary or appropriate. Readers are advised to check the most current product information provided by the manufacturer of each drug to be administered to verify the recommended dose, the method and duration of administration, and contraindications. It is the responsibility of the treating physician, relying on experience and knowledge of the patient, to determine dosages and the best treatment for each individual patient. Neither the Publisher nor the author assumes any liability for any injury and/or damage to persons or property arising from this publication.

The Publisher

Library of Congress Cataloging-in-Publication Data

Kilpatrick, Scott E.
Diagnostic musculoskeletal surgical pathology: clinicoradiologic and cytologic correlations / Scott E. Kilpatrick in collaboration with Jordan B. Renner.—1st ed.
p. ; cm.
ISBN 0-7216-9163-3
1. Musculoskeletal system—Pathophysiology. 2. Musculoskeletal system—Diseases—Diagnosis. 3. Pathology, Surgical. I. Renner, Jordan B. II. Title.
[DNLM: 1. Neoplasms, Connective and Soft Tissue—pathology. 2. Diagnostic Techniques, Surgical. 3. Neoplasms, Bone Tissue—pathology. QZ 340 K48d 2004]
RC925.6.K535 2004
616.7′075–dc21 2003041524

Acquisitions Editor: Natasha Andjelkovic
Developmental Editor: Agnes Byrne
Project Manager: Jodi Kaye

Printed in China.

Last digit is the print number: 9 8 7 6 5 4 3 2 1

To the memory of my wife Robyn.
You will always be my soul mate and my love.

PREFACE

The diagnosis of bone and soft tissue tumors is quite difficult. I believe most of the difficulty lies in their rarity but is further compounded by the absence of a useful diagnostic approach. Surgical pathologists have generally viewed "bone tumors" and "soft tissue tumors" as diagnostically separate categories (as emphasized by separate textbooks), despite the fact that both categories largely represent tumors of similar mesenchymal origin. Furthermore, many tumors are common to both bone and soft tissue (e.g., osteosarcoma, Ewing's sarcoma). In the clinical arena, the opposite holds true. Therapy for bone and soft tissue lesions is generally performed by orthopedic surgeons and medical oncologists who treat tumors in both anatomic compartments.

Traditionally, the most common diagnostic approach for bone and soft tissue lesions has been based mostly on histogenesis (e.g., fibrous/fibrohistiocytic, lipogenic, osteogenic). However, by itself, the use of such a classification system depends upon the recognition of the histogenetic subtype and/or differential diagnosis. The differential diagnosis often includes tumors of differing histogenesis. To render an accurate diagnosis, one must at least consider the correct diagnosis, as ancillary tests are helpful only if the *appropriate* studies are obtained. In some cases, the original histogenetic classification of a certain tumor is now considered invalid. The best example of this is malignant fibrous histiocytoma, which most experts now agree does not show true "histiocytic" differentiation. Arguably, a more useful diagnostic approach is one that emphasizes *both* the histogenesis and the predominant cytomorphologic/matrix features of the tumor in question. This classification scheme is the basis for the organization of this textbook (e.g., small round cell tumors, giant cell lesions, osseous tumors, vascular tumors). The combined classification is useful both clinically and pathologically. For example, small round cell sarcomas are observed far more commonly in children, whereas pleomorphic and myxoid sarcomas are generally observed in older adults (>50 years of age). Spindle cell and epithelioid/polygonal cell sarcomas are most commonly seen in young to middle-aged adults. As may be expected, limitations exist regarding this classification scheme. Certain sarcomas, such as embryonal rhabdomyosarcoma, may display a range of cytomorphologic features, from typical small round cell forms to predominant spindle cell morphology; a myxoid stroma is often observed in the botryoid form. In some examples, synovial sarcoma is best considered an epithelioid/polygonal cell sarcoma. For these reasons, I do not favor abandoning the traditional classification system, but rather would propose using a combination of both the traditional and cytomorphologic schemes, ensuring that all pertinent diagnoses are at least entertained. Finally, the use of a cytomorphologic classification provides a better "fit" for including fine needle aspiration biopsy results. When applicable, for the more common bone and soft tissue lesions, I have attempted to provide cytologic descriptions along with the corresponding histology.

The practice of orthopedic pathology requires correlation with radiographs. In effect, the radiologic findings represent the "gross specimen" for the anatomic pathologist. Since the trend in all of anatomic pathology has been toward rendering diagnoses with less invasive procedures and consequently less diagnostic material (e.g., core needle and fine needle aspiration biopsies), the correlation of clinical and radiologic data has become increasingly more important. Furthermore, many institutions are beginning to use preoperative chemotherapy protocols for a variety of pediatric and adult high-grade soft tissue sarcomas. Compared to a decade ago, pathologists as a group are now seeing fewer "untreated" gross resection specimens. For these reasons, I have chosen to emphasize the radiologic features, where necessary, over those of the classic gross specimen. Recognizing my own limitations, I enlisted the expertise of an orthopedic radiologist, Dr. Jordan Renner, who has graciously provided the radiologic illustrations and descriptions.

In summary, the purpose of this textbook is to provide a practical and "bench-useful" guide for the modern cytologic and histologic diagnosis of orthopedic surgical pathology. Although my plan is to be as comprehensive as necessary to illustrate the various entities, the goal is not to provide an encyclopedic text. During the writing of this book, my major focus group has always been diagnostic surgical pathologists; however, it is my hope that this textbook may be a useful adjunct for anyone involved in the diagnosis and therapy of bone and soft tissue lesions.

Scott Ethan Kilpatrick, M.D.

ACKNOWLEDGMENTS

I wish to thank those whose shoulders I have stood upon. To Dr. Christopher Fletcher, Director of Surgical Pathology at Brigham & Women's Hospital, thanks for teaching and inspiring me to pursue soft tissue pathology. I will never forget the opportunity I had to study at St. Thomas's Hospital in London. To Drs. K. Krishnan Unni and Antonio Nascimento, attending pathologists at the Mayo Clinic, thanks for patiently teaching me the basic principles of bone and soft tissue pathology. Thanks to all of you for "opening doors" of opportunity for me. I would also like to thank the University of North Carolina, Department of Pathology and Laboratory Medicine, for providing me with the chance and time to pursue this dream.

CONTENTS

CHAPTER 1

Principles of Musculoskeletal Tumor Diagnosis and Management

The diagnosis of bone and soft tissue tumors has always been difficult in part because of their absolute rarity (<1% of all malignant neoplasms), but the difficulty is compounded by the realization that a malignant diagnosis may lead to adverse consequences (e.g., amputation). Further apprehension may be related to the fact that many sarcomas (and pseudosarcomas) affect children. According to Enzinger and Weiss,[1] 15% of soft tissue sarcomas arise in patients younger than 15 years old, whereas approximately 40% occur in older adult patients (>55 years old).

Biopsy Techniques

Traditionally, at most institutions, diagnostic tissue from orthopedic tumors has been (and for the most part still is) obtained from open, incisional biopsies. Such samples usually provide the surgical pathologist with more than enough tissue to analyze morphologic architecture and to perform ancillary studies, if deemed necessary. The disadvantages include a higher rate of intraoperative and postoperative complications; the development of a scar; and the potential, especially if not carefully planned by an experienced orthopedic oncologic surgeon, to affect subsequent surgical management. Since the 1990s, greater emphasis has been placed on techniques that sample relatively smaller amounts of tissue (without compromising quality), are more readily accepted by the patient, may be performed easily in outpatient clinic settings, and are less likely to be associated with significant complications.

Core needle biopsy (CNB) and fine needle aspiration biopsy (FNAB) meet the aforementioned demands and are relatively cost-effective. In some institutions and many circumstances, FNAB is the superior technique. The argument in favor of CNB over FNAB generally is related to the fact that CNB yields actual tissue and subsequently allows assessment of architecture and provides a source for ancillary studies (e.g., immunohistochemistry). Nevertheless, practitioners of FNAB emphasize that tissue samples are obtained easily by FNAB in the form of cell blocks. Additional FNAB passes may be performed to obtain material for cytogenetic analysis, flow cytometry, and image analysis. The advantages of FNAB over CNB and open biopsy include virtually no risk of significant complications and the technical ease of the procedure.[2-4] The ability to render an immediate interpretation allows for planning of surgical intervention or neoadjuvant therapy or both at the initial presenting clinic visit, avoiding a potentially inconvenient second clinic visit. At some institutions, the practice has employed concomitant use of FNAB and CNB, allowing for the advantage of immediate interpretation in the former and the assurance of adequate tissue for ancillary studies in the latter. All of these biopsy techniques are summarized in Table 1.1.

Despite the utility of FNAB for the diagnosis of musculoskeletal diseases, there are clinical conditions and practice scenarios in which CNB or open, incisional biopsy is preferred. In the absence of on-site evaluation, FNAB for musculoskeletal lesions is not recommended. Because of the potential for sampling errors, lesions that appear predominantly fatty by imaging studies are best not evaluated by needle biopsy. Normal-appearing adipose tissue may be a component of inadvertently sampled subcutaneous fat, lipoma, or low-grade liposarcoma. Consequently, FNAB may be useful for ruling in a diagnosis of low-grade liposarcoma but is inadequate for ruling out the diagnosis, especially among deeply seated lesions. Nevertheless, we do not believe that the enrollment of patients on protocols, especially children on pediatric protocols, precludes the use of needle biopsy. Our experience and the experience of others suggest that FNAB is a highly accurate and acceptable technique for this purpose. Among 18 patients clinically eligible for these

TABLE 1.1 Comparison of Fine Needle Aspiration Biopsy, Core Needle Biopsy, and Open Biopsy

Characteristics	FNAB	CNB	Open Biopsy
Technical ease of procedure	Easily learned and applied	Easily learned and applied	Difficult; requires specialty training
Cytologic smears	Yes—recommend Diff-Quik for matrix material; Pap for nuclear detail	No	No
Histologic tissue	Yes (cell block)—usually most helpful for ancillary studies, not morphology	Yes—helpful for morphology and ancillary studies	Yes—helpful for morphology and ancillary studies
Availability of ancillary studies (e.g., immunohistochemistry, cytogenetics, flow cytometry)	Yes—requires additional FNAB passes	Yes—may require additional CNB passes	Yes—may require additional tissue
Speed of interpretation	Fast; often within minutes to hours	Tissue requires fixation and processing; 1-2 days	Tissue requires fixation and processing; 1-2 days
Risk of complications	Exceedingly low	Low, but higher than FNAB	Low, but significantly higher than either FNAB or CNB
Risk of tumor contamination of biopsy site	Exceedingly low	Low, but higher than FNAB	Low, but significantly higher than either FNAB or CNB
Accuracy rate for histologic subtyping	30-75%, histologic classification unreliable in fatty tumors and adult pleomorphic sarcomas	75-90%	>95%

CNB, core needle biopsy; FNAB, fine needle aspiration biopsy.

protocols, Kilpatrick and colleagues[5] documented an accurate diagnosis in 17 cases (94%). Overall, 12 pediatric patients were enrolled on a variety of histogenetic-specific pediatric protocols for neuroblastoma (Pediatric Oncology Group), rhabdomyosarcoma (Intergroup Rhabdomyosarcoma Study Group), osteosarcoma (Children's Cancer Group/Pediatric Oncology Group), and Ewing's sarcoma (Pediatric Oncology Group).

In most circumstances, for bone tumors to be accessible for FNAB or CNB analysis, soft tissue extension or sufficient cortical destruction or both must be present. Tumors that are predominantly sclerotic may not be adequately sampled, especially with FNAB. Bone tumors usually not amenable to needle biopsy include the following:

- Osteoma
- Osteoid osteoma
- Osteoblastoma
- Low-grade osteosarcoma
- Enchondroma
- Low-grade chondrosarcoma
- Metaphyseal fibrous defect
- Fibrous dysplasia
- Osteofibrous dysplasia
- Hemangioma

Fine Needle Aspiration Biopsy

Most cytopathologists define FNAB as the use of a 22-gauge or smaller needle; the risk of needle tract seeding is exceedingly low and appears to be between 0.003% (3/100,000) and 0.009% (9/100,000).[3] Major complications, including death, usually involve intra-abdominal and intrathoracic FNABs associated with larger bore needles (≥18 gauge).[3]

Among bone and soft tissue tumors, false-positive and false-negative rates range from less than 1% to approximately 5% and approximately 2% to 15%.[6-9] In most series, false-positive diagnoses are defined as the rendering of a malignant cytologic diagnosis for a benign (histologically confirmed) entity; conversely the definition of a false-negative diagnosis has varied depending on whether unsatisfactory or inadequate diagnoses were included. When the latter are excluded, most of these false-negative rates range between less than 1% and 5%. Bommer and colleagues[7] analyzed 450 FNABs of bone lesions, reporting only 1 (0.2%) false-positive and 10 (2.2%) false-negative results. Of the false-negative diagnoses, 8 (1.7%) were unsatisfactory or contained too few cells for diagnosis; only 2 (0.4%) were "true" false-negative "interpretive difficulties." In an analysis of 136 primary soft tissue tumors, Layfield and associates[8] documented 2 cases (an angiolipoma and a lipoma) that were incorrectly classified as malignant (liposarcoma), generating a 2% false-positive rate. An additional three cases with cytologic specimens insufficient for diagnosis had histologically confirmed malignant neoplasms at subsequent biopsy, yielding a false-negative rate of 2%.[8] Ackerman and Rydholm[10] retrospectively evaluated 517 soft tissue tumors (315, benign; 202, sarcomas) analyzed by FNAB. Of cases, 29 (6%) were considered inadequate or insufficient for diagnosis (24, benign; 5, sarcomas). There were 14 (2.7%) false-negative cases and 14 (2.7%) false-positive cases.[10] A common pitfall was lipomatous tumors. In their ongoing experience with more than 1200 benign and malignant bone and soft tissue aspirates (during the study period of 1990-1999), Kilpatrick and colleagues[11] encountered no false-positive cases. Among 145 sarcoma aspirates, they documented 7 (5%) unsatisfactory samples (4, bone; 3, soft tissue). The only example of a "true" false-negative (malignant tumor diagnosed as benign cytologically) case resulted in no adverse consequences for the patient.[11]

Although the value of FNAB in distinguishing malignancy from benignancy has been established in several studies and often approaches and exceeds 90%, its accuracy for establishing a specific histologic subtype has been far less tested. Layfield and associates[8] evaluated 51 histologically confirmed soft tissue sarcomas; an accurate histologic subtype was established by FNAB in 38 (74%) cases. FNAB from one example of well-differentiated liposarcoma was insufficient for diagnosis, and one case of rhabdomyosarcoma consisted of "fibrous tissue only."[8] Costa and coworkers[12] retrospectively reviewed 45 sarcomas, of which only approximately 21% were correctly subtyped. The authors' conclusion was "FNA usually does not provide a specific diagnosis." Among 110 soft tissue lesions (of which 23 were sarcomas), Hook and colleagues[13] documented specificity and positive predictive values for the nonspecific diagnosis of sarcoma as 98% and 91%. Subclassification of sarcomas "was possible in only 30% of cases."[13] In the series of Kilpatrick and colleagues,[14] 61 (86%) of 71 adequate samples were correctly recognized as sarcoma. An accurate histologic subtype was rendered in only 34 (48%) cases. Failure to provide a specific histologic subtype does not always preclude initiation of appropriate therapy, however. Excluding inadequate samples (three cases), Kilpatrick and colleagues[14] observed only one false-negative FNAB specimen in their series. The lesion was excised, and the patient has suffered no adverse outcome as a consequence of the misinterpretation.

Core Needle Biopsy

CNB generally involves obtaining cores of tissue using a 14-gauge to 18-gauge needle or biopsy gun. For bone lesions, 8-gauge to 11-gauge bone needles also have been used. Immediate assessment of adequacy may involve touch preparations or frozen section analysis or both. As with FNAB, complications and needle tract seeding are rare but, because of the larger bore needle, are more likely to occur with CNB than with FNAB. Compared with FNAB, CNB is probably more accurate for histologic subtyping, especially among the entire spectrum of soft tissue tumors. Bennert and Abdul-Karim[2] analyzed 37 sarcomas by FNAB and reported successful subtyping in 30 (81%) tumors. Concomitant CNB was performed in all of these cases. In their series, the main advantage of CNB over FNAB was that the former helped establish "the specific subtype of sarcoma when the fine needle aspirate was reported as sarcoma, not otherwise specified."[2] Among diagnostic FNABs, however, CNB did not contribute significantly to overall patient management. We agree with Bennert and Abdul-Karim that an unsatisfactory FNAB, especially if clinically suspicious for sarcoma, should be followed by repeat FNAB, CNB, or open biopsy. Welker and colleagues[15] evaluated 161 musculoskeletal masses in 155 patients by CNB, including 83 sarcomas, 67 benign mesenchymal tumors, and 11 metastatic epithelial malignancies. The authors documented a positive predictive value of 100%, a negative predictive value of 82%, a sensitivity of 81.8%, and a specificity of 100%. Accuracy rates for establishing benign versus malignant, histologic grade, and histologic subtype were reported as 92.4%, 88.6%, and 72.7%.[15] Twelve (of 161) masses required open biopsy for diagnosis. Two complications (1.1%) involving two patients occurred, hematoma and persistent drainage of a biopsy tract, neither of which affected subsequent patient management. Two (1.1%) false-negative diagnoses (malignant tumor diagnosed initially as benign) were reported, but no adverse effect on patient management was observed.[15] In pediatric patients, Willman and colleagues[16] analyzed 50 CNB specimens, of which 43 represented a neoplastic process. For the latter, CNB was diagnostic in 39 (91%) cases. There were no complications resulting from the procedure. Among cases of Ewing's sarcoma/primitive neuroectodermal tumor, cytogenetic results were obtained in five (of seven cases); however, in only one case was the characteristic t(11;22) observed.[16] The remainder yielded a normal karyotype, raising issues of specimen adequacy.

Understanding Sarcoma Therapy and Its Relationship to Diagnosis

With the exception of pediatric small round cell tumors and osteosarcoma, therapy for most bone and soft tissue sarcomas, especially adult forms, is based predominantly on anatomic site and stage, the latter of which incorporates histologic grade.[17] Although histologic subtyping may help determine the histologic grade (e.g., Ewing's sarcoma is high grade by definition), it is not always necessary. At most institutions, the therapy for adult pleomorphic malignant fibrous histiocytoma is similar to therapy for pleomorphic liposarcoma and pleomorphic leiomyosarcoma because all represent high-grade sarcomas. Consequently, for the evaluation of FNAB in the therapeutic management of soft tissue sarcomas, the percentage of cases in which FNAB is sufficient for the initiation of definitive therapy is more important than its accuracy rate for histologic subtyping. In a series of soft tissue sarcomas, the diagnosis rendered by FNAB was sufficient for the initiation of definitive therapy (not requiring additional open incisional biopsy) in 73 patients (of 88 patients with adequate specimens [83%]).[11] Histologic subtyping of Ewing's sarcoma, skeletal osteosarcoma, and rhabdomyosarcoma is essential because many patients are clinically eligible for histogenetic-specific protocols.

Clinical and Radiologic Correlation

Correlation with clinical and radiologic features, when available, cannot be overemphasized. Certain tumors are virtually nonexistent in children (e.g., liposarcoma), and others, for reasons not understood, occur only rarely in certain ethnic groups (e.g., Ewing's sarcoma tends to be rare in African-Americans). Radiologic studies, including computed tomographic scans and magnetic resonance imaging, provide information regarding location (e.g., visceral involvement, intramuscular), size, presence (or absence) of bone involvement (e.g., primary bone tumor with soft tissue extension versus primary soft tissue tumor), homogeneity versus heterogeneity, content (e.g., cystic versus fatty), and relationships to neurovascular structures (e.g., nerve sheath tumor). Combining clinical and radiographic information helps the pathologist provide a more accurate and definitive diagnosis. An example of such a general approach is illustrated in Figure 1.1.

For bone tumors, it is virtually always preferable to begin with conventional radiographs for several reasons. First, it is important to recognize certain benign tumors or tumor-like conditions that do not require further analysis or treatment. One example is metaphyseal fibrous defect. A radiologist experienced with bone lesions can readily identify its classic features. Unless complicated by fracture or associated with atypical features, surgical intervention is not warranted because most of these lesions resolve spontaneously. Second, when necessary, radiographs aid the surgeon in choosing the optimal site for tissue biopsy. Third, for the surgical pathologist, accurate assessment of features such as location (epiphyseal versus metaphyseal), pattern of bone destruction, matrix calcification, periosteal reaction, and associated soft tissue abnormalities usually relates to the aggressiveness of the lesion and allows for a more specific diagnosis. In this manner, radiographs serve as the "gross bone specimen" for the pathologist (Fig. 1.2).

Limitations exist regarding the interpretation of radiographs. In some cases, the radiographic appearance of a tumor can be misleading. An aneurysmal bone cyst may show aggressive and even "malignant" features on radiographs. In contrast, intraosseous osteosarcomas sometimes may appear innocuous. For these reasons, radiologic features should not supplant histologic interpretation in establishing a diagnosis. Nevertheless, the pathologic diagnosis of a bone tumor should be a multidisciplinary one, comprising clinical data, radiologic features, and optimal histology. Using this approach, the surgical pathologist can avoid potential misdiagnoses. Table 1.2 summarizes radiographic features that favor a benign versus a malignant lesion.

Among FNAB samples of orthopedic tumors, Liu and coworkers[18] found that "knowledge of clinical history improved the correct precise diagnosis for both soft tissue and bone lesions for all observers regardless of experience." The increased accuracy seemed most dramatic among bone tumors (e.g., osteosarcoma and chondrosarcoma), perhaps resulting from specific information gleaned from the radiographs.[18] Clinical history and radiographic findings tend to be more helpful for establishing a specific subtype among bone sarcomas than soft tissue sarcomas. Among 140 sarcomas (42 bone; 80 soft tissue), Kilpatrick and colleagues[11] reported greater diagnostic accuracy for bone sarcomas (82%) than for soft tissue sarcomas (54%). The number of differential diagnoses under consideration for a primary bone tumor is often significantly fewer than that considered for primary soft tissue lesions. In a 10-year-old boy, a permeative, osteoblastic lesion by radiographs and cytologic evidence of pleomorphic sarcoma is almost assuredly osteosarcoma. Conversely, in a 60-year-old man, a large soft tissue mass and cytologic evidence of pleomorphic sarcoma may represent malignant fibrous histiocytoma, liposarcoma, leiomyosarcoma, malignant peripheral nerve sheath tumor, or extraskeletal osteosarcoma. Malignant melanoma and metastatic carcinoma also must be considered sometimes. In the latter situation, clinicoradiologic correlation may help eliminate a few but, in our experience, usually not all of the choices.

Practical Approach for Diagnosis

Bone Tumors: Benign versus Malignant

In most bone tumor pathology textbooks, little attempt is made to characterize specific features of bone tumors indicative of benignancy versus malignancy. Instead the individual features or patterns of specific types of neoplasms are given and are correlated with the corresponding clinical and radiologic features of the tumor. Nevertheless, certain histologic features tend to favor a benign diagnosis, whereas others strongly support a malignant one. Table 1.3 summarizes these features.

Soft Tissue Tumors: Benign versus Malignant

Because of the enormous number of soft tissue tumors and tumor-like lesions and the often subtle pathologic differences

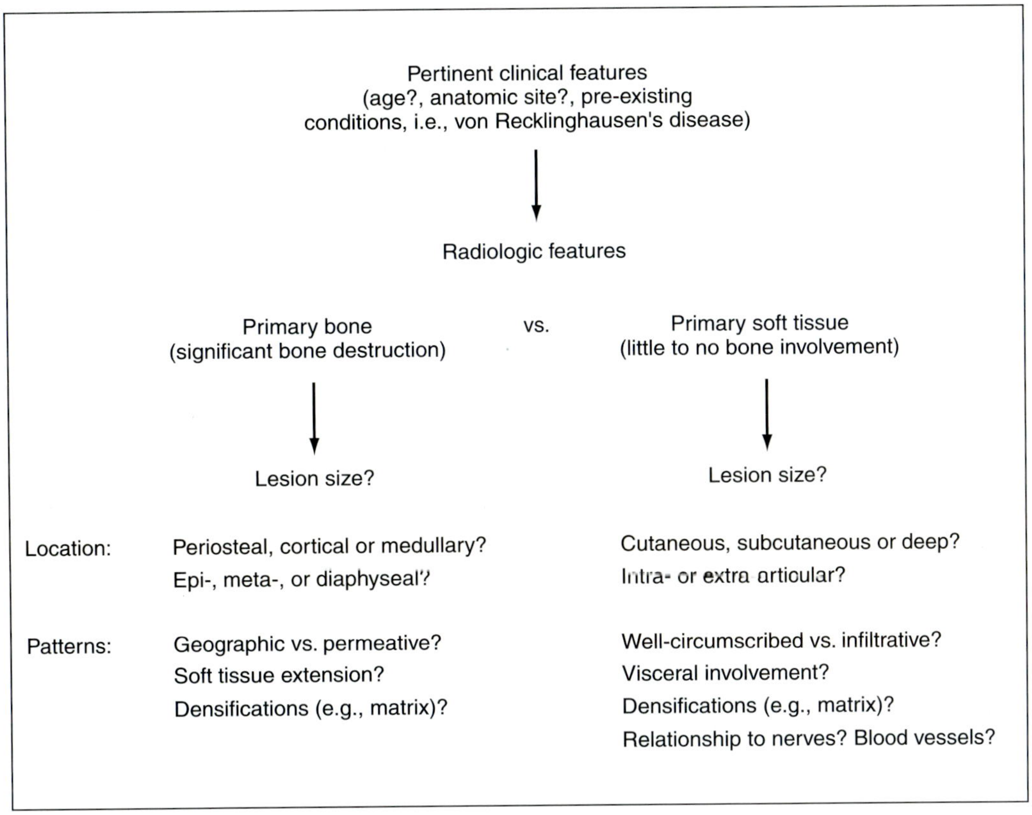

FIGURE 1.1 Initial clinical and radiologic approach to the work-up of a musculoskeletal tumor.

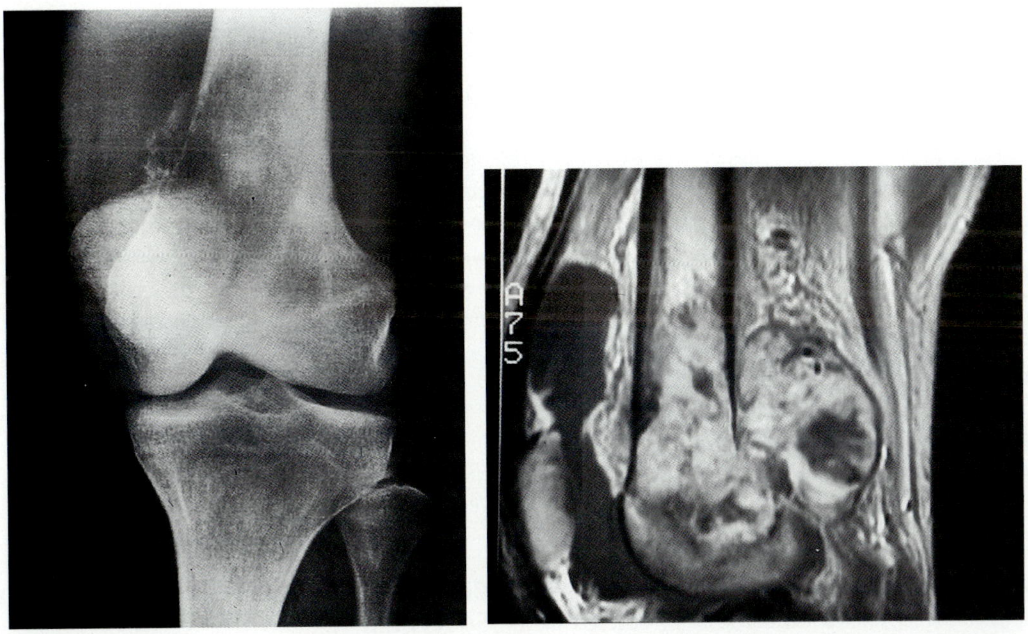

A B

FIGURE 1.2 Myxoid chondrosarcoma. An oblique view of the knee shows an ill-defined lytic lesion in the supracondylar portion of the distal femur. Cortical destruction along the medial femoral cortex is associated with irregular periosteal new bone production. The radiographic findings indicate an aggressive osseous lesion extending through cortical bone to involve adjacent soft tissue **(A).** Sagittal magnetic resonance imaging shows an extensive osseous lesion in the distal femur. The lesion's margins are poorly defined proximally, and the lesion extends distally into the condylar portion of the femur. A large, heterogeneous soft tissue mass posterior to the femur is better appreciated than on the radiograph. A large joint effusion (black) is present anterior to the femur **(B).**

TABLE 1.2 Radiographic Features Favoring Benign versus Malignant Lesions

Benign	Malignant
Geographic destruction	Moth-eaten and permeative destruction
Occasionally moth-eaten	Rarely geographic
Rarely permeative	
Nonaggressive rind of bone sclerosis	Absence of nonaggressive bone sclerosis
Periosteal reaction uncommon but, if present, usually smooth, solid, and uninterrupted	Periosteal reaction common and often interrupted, spiculated, and lamellated
Absence of soft tissue extension	Soft tissue extension common

TABLE 1.3 Histologic Features Favoring Benign versus Malignant Diagnoses in Bone Tumors

Benign	Malignant
Well-circumscribed, noninvasive	Permeation and invasive
Absence of lamellar bone trapping	Presence of lamellar bone trapping
If bone production, bone rimmed by at least a single row of osteoblasts	If bone production, absence of osteoblast rimming
Soft tissue extension rare	Soft tissue extension common
Anaplasia lacking	Anaplasia common
Mitoses, less commonly numerous and virtually never atypical	Mitoses, numerous and often atypical

TABLE 1.4 Clinicoradiologic, Histologic, and Cytologic Features of Benign versus Malignant Soft Tissue Lesions

Features	Benign Characteristics	Malignant Characteristics
Size and properties	Small, often well-circumscribed	Large, more often infiltrative
Anatomic location	Superficial and/or cutaneous	Deep and/or intramuscular
Tumor cellularity	Slightly to moderately cellular	Moderately to markedly cellular
Cellular cohesion	Tendency to form cohesive fragments	Tendency toward discohesiveness
Nuclear features	Uniform, "open" or vesicular chromatin	More commonly pleomorphic and variable coarse chromatin
Mitotic activity	Less mitotically active (often <1 mitosis/10 HPF)	More mitotically active (often >10 mitoses/10 HPF)
Necrosis	Usually absent	Often present

HPF, high-power fields.

Based partly on the results of Kilpatrick SE, Geisinger KR: Soft tissue sarcoma: The usefulness and limitations of fine-needle aspiration biopsy. Am J Clin Pathol 1998;110:50-68.

between prognostically different but related tumors, establishing a practical approach to the diagnosis of soft tissue tumors is considerably more difficult than that of bone tumors. Nevertheless, by combining clinicoradiologic data with pathology, one can make certain generalizations regarding benignancy versus malignancy. These features are summarized in Table 1.4.

Bone and Soft Tissue Tumors: Histologic Subtyping

When one has decided that a given lesion is malignant, histologic subtyping should be attempted because certain sarcomas, such as rhabdomyosarcoma, osteosarcoma, and Ewing's sarcoma, are treated with histogenetic-specific protocols.

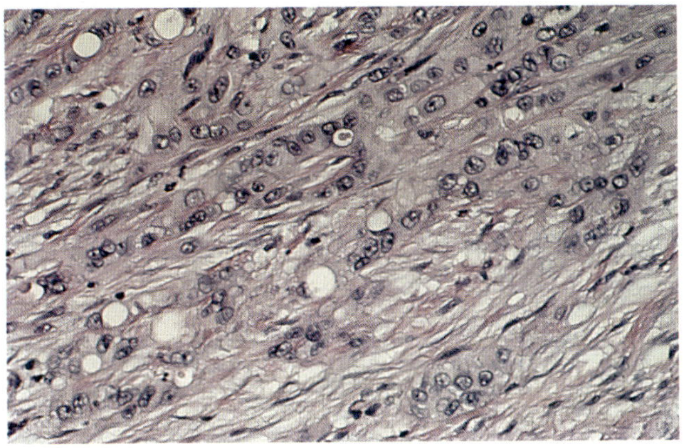

FIGURE 1.3 Epithelioid hemangioendothelioma may be confused with metastatic carcinoma, especially lobular carcinoma of the breast, particularly if the inconspicuous primitive vascular differentiation is not recognized and appropriate ancillary studies are not obtained. Additionally, keratins may be expressed in metastatic carcinoma and epithelioid hemangioendothelioma. Only epithelioid hemangioendothelioma shows staining with endothelial markers (e.g., CD31). (H&E.)

Traditionally the most common approach for histologic subtyping has been based on histogenesis (e.g., fibrous/fibrohistiocytic, lipogenic, osteogenic). By itself, the use of such a classification system depends, however, on the recognition of the histogenetic subtype or differential diagnosis or both. To render an accurate diagnosis, one at least must consider the correct diagnosis. Ancillary tests are helpful only if the appropriate studies are obtained (Fig. 1.3). A better approach is one that emphasizes the histogenesis and the predominant cytomorphologic features of the sarcoma in question, as illustrated in Table 1.5.

This combined classification is useful clinically and pathologically. Small round cell sarcomas are observed far more commonly in children, whereas pleomorphic and myxoid sarcomas generally are observed in older adults (>50 years old). Spindle cell and epithelioid/polygonal cell sarcomas are seen most commonly in young to middle-aged adults. As may be expected, limitations exist regarding this classification scheme. Certain sarcomas, such as embryonal rhabdomyosarcoma, may display a range of cytomorphologic features, from typical small round cell forms to predominant spindle cell morphology; a myxoid stroma often is observed in the botryoid form. In some examples, synovial sarcoma is best considered an epithelioid/polygonal cell sarcoma. For these reasons, we do not favor abandoning the traditional classification system, but rather would propose using a combination of the traditional and cytomorphologic schemes, ensuring that all pertinent diagnoses are at least entertained. The cytomorphologic system also proves most advantageous when attempting the diagnosis of sarcomas by FNAB. In our experience, cell blocks, although often containing perfectly adequate material for immunocytochemistry, generally lack sufficient tissue to pursue histogenetic subtyping confidently based solely on tissue architecture. Finally, one should always bear in mind that nonmesenchymal tumors can involve soft tissue, presenting as a primary soft tissue mass (e.g., metastatic carcinoma, malignant lymphoma, and malignant melanoma).

Histologic Grading of Sarcomas

Regardless of tumor type, histologic grading of malignant tumors is based predominantly on the resemblance of the tumor cells to their "histologic counterparts."[19] Histologic grade corresponds essentially to the differentiation within an individual histologic subtype. Malignant tumors composed of neoplastic cells closely resembling normal cells are considered well differentiated (low grade); conversely, tumors containing malignant cells differing from normal cells are considered poorly differentiated (high grade). From a practical point of view, histologic grading of malignant tumors is applicable only in neoplasms that show significant histologic or cytologic variation (and differentiation) from tumor to tumor. Tumors showing little to no variation or histologic differences (e.g., Ewing's sarcoma) should not be graded because such data provide no additional information.[19]

The primary purpose of histologic grading is to separate malignant tumors associated with a good prognosis (low grade) from tumors with a poor prognosis (high grade). The value of any histologic grading system is related not only to the ability to predict patient survival, but also to identify patients who may benefit from adjuvant therapy. There is no universally accepted system for the histologic grading of bone or soft tissue sarcomas. Practically speaking, histologic grading of bone tumors generally is limited to (and specific for) osteosarcoma and chondrosarcoma and is discussed in their respective chapters. Among rarer sarcoma subtypes, such as fibrosarcoma or leiomyosarcoma, histologic grading may use systems already in place for soft tissue sarcomas. When applicable, designating a soft tissue sarcoma as at least low or high grade is recommended. Among more specific grading systems, the two most commonly used grading systems for soft tissue sarcomas are the National Cancer Institute (NCI) system and the *Fédération Nationale des Centres de Lutte Contre le Cancer* (FNCLCC, also known as the French Federation of Cancer Centers sarcoma group) system.

The NCI system is summarized in Table 1.6. These authors propose a three-scale grading system largely incorporating histologic subtype and the percentage of tumor necrosis.[20] The grade 1 lesions include the following sarcoma subtypes: well-differentiated liposarcoma, myxoid liposarcoma, dermatofibrosarcoma protuberans, leiomyosarcoma, malignant hemangiopericytoma, malignant peripheral nerve

TABLE 1.5 Combined Traditional/Cytomorphologic Classification of Bone and Soft Tissue Tumors

Small Round Cell Tumors	**Spindle Cell Tumors**	**Myxoid Tumors**
Ewing's sarcoma	Nodular fasciitis	Myxoma, intramuscular
Rhabdomyosarcoma, childhood subtypes	Fibromatoses	Myxoma, juxta-articular
Neuroblastoma, olfactory	Metaphyseal fibrous defect	Aggressive angiomyxoma
Mesenchymal chondrosarcoma	Fibrosarcoma	Myxofibrosarcoma
Desmoplastic small round cell tumor	Leiomyoma/leiomyosarcoma	Myxoid liposarcoma
Melanotic neuroectodermal tumor	Benign and malignant peripheral nerve sheath tumors	Myxoid chondrosarcoma
Epithelioid/Polygonal Cell Tumors	**Pleomorphic Tumors**	**Osseous Tumors**
Epithelioid sarcoma	Malignant fibrous histiocytoma	Osteoma
Epithelioid hemangioendothelioma/angiosarcoma	Pleomorphic liposarcoma	Osteoid osteoma
Granular cell tumor	Pleomorphic leiomyosarcoma	Osteoblastoma
Alveolar soft part sarcoma	Pleomorphic rhabdomyosarcoma, adult type	Fibrous dysplasia
Clear cell sarcoma (melanoma of soft parts)	Dedifferentiated liposarcoma	Osteofibrous dysplasia
Synovial sarcoma*	**Giant Cell Tumors**	Osteosarcoma
Langerhans' cell histiocytosis	Giant cell tumor of tendon sheath	**Vascular Tumors**
Fatty Tumors	Pigmented villonodular synovitis	Hemangioma
Lipoma	Giant cell tumor	Hemangioendothelioma
Angiolipoma	Giant cell reparative granuloma	Hemangiopericytoma
Spindle cell/pleomorphic lipoma	**Cysts**	Glomus tumor
Well-differentiated liposarcoma	Ganglion cyst	
Chondroid Tumors	Simple bone cyst	
Enchondroma	Aneurysmal bone cyst	
Chondroblastoma	Subchondral cyst	
Chondromyxoid fibroma		
Chondrosarcoma, conventional		
Chondrosarcoma, clear cell		

*Synovial sarcoma may be considered in either the spindle cell or epithelioid group.

TABLE 1.6 Grading Parameters of the NCI System

Histologic Parameter	Grade
Well-differentiated LPS, myxoid LPS, well-differentiated malignant HP (<1 mitotic figure per 10 HPF), well-differentiated fibrosarcoma and LMS (<6 mitotic figures per 10 HPF), MPNST (resemble neurofibroma, <6 mitotic figures per 10 HPF), myxoid CS (no mitotic activity)	1
Any sarcoma not automatically designated as grade 3 with tumor necrosis ≤15%	2
Any sarcoma with >15% necrosis, RMS (all subtypes), extraskeletal OS and ES/PNET, mesenchymal CS, ASPS, synovial sarcoma, pleomorphic LPS	3

ASPS, alveolar soft part sarcoma; CS, chondrosarcoma; ES/PNET, Ewing's sarcoma/primitive neuroectodermal tumor; HP, hemangiopericytoma; HPF, high-power field; LMS, leiomyosarcoma; LPS, liposarcoma; MPNST, malignant peripheral nerve sheath tumor; OS, osteosarcoma; RMS, rhabdomyosarcoma.

Based on the data of Costa J, Wesley RA, Glatstein E, et al: The grading of soft tissue sarcomas: Results of a clinicohistopathologic correlation in a series of 163 cases. Cancer 1984;53:530-541.

sheath tumor, and myxoid chondrosarcoma. Liposarcomas are classified as well differentiated or myxoid only when other components (i.e., round cell or pleomorphic) do not exceed 15% to 20% of the tumor volume. Leiomyosarcoma is classified as grade 1 "when they exhibited an orderly fasciculated pattern, well differentiated cytologic features, absence of pleomorphism, absence of necrosis, and exceedingly low mitotic activity."[20] Malignant peripheral nerve sheath tumors are regarded as grade 1 when they closely resemble neurofibroma but show significant mitotic activity and areas of high cellularity. Adult hemangiopericytomas lacking significant necrosis and having only rare mitotic figures are

TABLE 1.7 Scoring and Grading Parameters of the FNCLCC System

Histologic Parameter	Score
I. Tumor Differentiation	
Sarcomas closely resembling normal adult tissue (e.g., well-differentiated LPS, fibrosarcoma, MPNST, LMS, chondrosarcoma)	1
Sarcomas of certain histologic subtype (e.g., myxoid LPS, conventional fibrosarcomaand MPNST, well-differentiated malignant HP, myxoid and storiform/pleomorphic MFH, myxoid CS, conventional AS)	2
Sarcomas of uncertain histologic subtype (e.g., poorly differentiated and epithelioid MPNST, giant cell and inflammatory MFH, RMS, SS, poorly differentiated LMS, round cell, pleomorphic and dedifferentiated LPS, ES/PNET, OS, ASPS, EPS, CCS, poorly differentiated/epithelioid AS, mesenchymal CS)	3
II. Tumor Necrosis	
None	0
≤50%	1
>50%	2
III. Mitotic Count	
0-9 mitoses per 10 HPF	1
10-19 mitoses per 10 HPF	2
>20 mitoses per 10 HPF	3
Histologic Grade	**Total Score**
1	2, 3
2	4, 5
3	6, 7, 8

AS, angiosarcoma; ASPS, alveolar soft part sarcoma; CCS, clear cell sarcoma; CS, chondrosarcoma; EPS, epithelioid sarcoma; ES/PNET, Ewing's sarcoma/primitive neuroectodermal tumor; HP, hemangiopericytoma; HPF, high-power fields; LMS, leiomyosarcoma; LPS, liposarcoma; MFH, malignant fibrous histiocytoma; MPNST, malignant peripheral nerve sheath tumor; OS, osteosarcoma; RMS, rhabdomyosarcoma; SS, synovial sarcoma.

Modified from Guillow L, Coindre JM, Bonichon JM, et al: Comparative study of the National Cancer Institute and French Federation of Cancer Centers sarcoma group grading systems in a population of 410 adult patients with soft tissue sarcomas. J Clin Oncol 1997;15:350-362.

grade 1 lesions. Extraskeletal Ewing's sarcoma, extraskeletal osteosarcoma, rhabdomyosarcoma, pleomorphic liposarcoma, synovial sarcoma, mesenchymal chondrosarcoma, and malignant triton tumor are designated as grade 3 lesions based solely on their histologic subtype. For sarcomas not qualifying as grade 1 or 3, the extent of necrosis determines the grade. Sarcomas with minimal necrosis (15%) are classified as grade 2; sarcomas with moderate-to-marked necrosis (>15%) are grade 3. In 1990, Costa[21] modified this grading system, and some sarcomas that were originally classified as grade 3 (e.g., synovial sarcoma, pleomorphic liposarcoma) currently are regarded as either grade 2 or 3.

The FNCLCC system initially was described by Trojani and associates[22] and later modified by Guillou and colleagues.[23] A summary of this grading system is provided in Table 1.7. This system uses three factors to establish histologic grade—tumor differentiation, mitotic count, and volume of tumor necrosis. For each of these parameters, a score of 0 to 3 is assigned, and a total score is obtained from the addition of the individual scores. Tumor differentiation corresponds to specific histologic subtypes. Well-differentiated liposarcoma, fibrosarcoma, malignant peripheral nerve sheath tumor, leiomyosarcoma, and chondrosarcoma are assigned a score of 1. When histologic subtype is "certain," a score of 2 is given. This group includes myxoid liposarcoma, conventional fibrosarcoma and malignant peripheral nerve sheath tumor, well-differentiated malignant hemangiopericytoma, myxoid and pleomorphic/storiform malignant fibrous histiocytomas, myxoid chondrosarcoma, and conventional angiosarcoma. A score of 3 is applied to sarcomas of uncertain type, including poorly differentiated and epithelioid malignant peripheral nerve sheath tumors; giant cell and inflammatory malignant fibrous histiocytomas; rhabdomyosarcoma; synovial sarcoma; poorly differentiated leiomyosarcoma; round cell, pleomorphic, and dedifferentiated liposarcoma; Ewing's sarcoma; osteosarcoma; alveolar soft part sarcoma; epithelioid sarcoma; clear cell sarcoma; and mesenchymal chondrosarcoma. Tumor necrosis is defined as none, 50% or less, and greater than 50% for scores of 0, 1, and 2. Mitotic counts of 0 to 9, 10 to 19, and 20 and greater per 10 high-power fields (HPF) yield scores of 1, 2, and 3. A total score of 2 or 3 is classified as grade 1; 4 or 5, grade 2; and 6, 7, or 8, grade 3.

Although these grading systems are applicable to open biopsy (histologic) specimens, their usefulness for FNAB samples is limited because features such as mitotic activity and percentage of necrosis are not evaluated easily in cytologic specimens. Nevertheless, one can make certain assumptions regarding histologic subtype and grade. As the aforementioned grading systems illustrate, many sarcoma subtypes are considered high grade based solely on their histologic classification. Ewing's sarcoma is a high-grade tumor, regardless of mitotic rate or percent necrosis. For many sarcomas, if one can establish a histologic subtype, the grade of the tumor also may be determined.[14] A summary of this approach applicable to FNAB is provided in Table 1.8. For sarcomas that may be low or high grade, one may use a combination of nuclear atypia, cellularity, and the presence (or absence) of tumor necrosis to designate a histologic grade (e.g., low versus high), if deemed clinically necessary. At our institutions, this is not always required.

TABLE 1.8 Soft Tissue Sarcoma Grading by Fine Needle Aspiration Biopsy

Cytologic Grade	Subtype or Cytomorphologic Group
Low grade (by definition)	Well-differentiated liposarcoma
	Myxoid liposarcoma*
	Extraskeletal myxoid chondrosarcoma
	Epithelioid hemangioendothelioma
	Infantile fibrosarcoma
	Kaposi's sarcoma
High grade (by definition)	Small round cell sarcomas
	Adult pleomorphic sarcomas
	Round cell liposarcoma*
	Epithelioid sarcoma
	Clear cell sarcoma
	Alveolar soft part sarcoma
	Angiosarcoma
Potentially low or high grade	Leiomyosarcoma
	Gastrointestinal stromal tumor
	MPNST
	Myxofibrosarcoma
	Hemangiopericytoma
	Malignant granular cell tumor
	Conventional fibrosarcoma

*Myxoid liposarcoma and round cell liposarcoma generally are considered to be low-grade and high-grade spectra of the same neoplasm.
MPNST, malignant peripheral nerve sheath tumor.
Based on the data of Kilpatrick SE, Ward WG, Cappellari JO, et al: Fine needle aspiration biopsy of soft tissue sarcomas: A cytomorphologic analysis with emphasis on histologic subtyping, grading, and therapeutic significance. Am J Clin Pathol 1999;112:179-188.

Relationship of Histologic Grade in Soft Tissue Sarcomas to Histologic Subtype

Because of the overall rarity of many sarcoma histologic subtypes, most studies examining histologic grade have tended to evaluate soft tissue sarcomas as an entire group. Nevertheless, soft tissue sarcomas represent an extremely wide spectrum of variable entities, differing in morphology and clinical behavior. Many experts have proposed that histologic grading in soft tissue sarcomas be based solely on individual and specific histologic types because the prognostic significance of various grading parameters often varies among different subtypes of soft tissue sarcoma.[1, 24] Even series with relatively large numbers of patients have had considerable difficulty analyzing the clinical relationship of histologic subtype to grade in all soft tissue sarcomas. Hashimoto and coworkers[25] evaluated 1116 soft tissue sarcoma patients in an attempt to examine the relationship between histologic grade, histologic subtype, and prognosis. Histologic grade had prognostic significance in malignant fibrous histiocytoma, leiomyosarcoma, and liposarcoma but showed no association with rhabdomyosarcoma, synovial sarcoma, malignant peripheral nerve sheath tumor, and fibrosarcoma. LeDoussal and colleagues[26] analyzed 216 patients with malignant fibrous histiocytoma and found histopathologic grade to be the most important prognostic factor for the development of metastasis and patient survival. LeDoussal and colleagues[26] used the FNCLCC. Gustafson and associates[27] described a prognostic study of 43 patients with liposarcoma of the extremity or trunk wall and found, by univariate analysis, a significant association between metastatic disease and increasing malignant grade, tumor necrosis, vascular invasion, mitotic count, and histologic subtype other than well differentiated. With multivariate analysis, tumor necrosis was the only independent risk factor.[27] Chang and associates[28] analyzed 127 patients with localized extremity liposarcoma and found a significant correlation between local failure and the presence of high tumor grade. The development of metastatic disease seemed to correlate strongly with histologic subtype.[28]

Regarding leiomyosarcoma of soft tissues, several authors reported an association between survival and location (e.g., retroperitoneum versus extremity) and tumor size; however, in these series, there seems to be no correlation between microscopic appearance and mitotic activity with the clinical course.[29, 30] Nevertheless, other investigators reported significant correlations between survival and tumor grade in leiomyosarcomas of pulmonary and bone origin.[31, 32] Antonescu and colleagues[32] in their series of 33 patients with primary leiomyosarcomas of bone used the FNCLCC grading system.

By univariate analysis, Mark and coworkers[33] reported histologic grade and tumor size as prognostically significant for soft tissue angiosarcoma. Survival in angiosarcoma also has been shown to correlate with histologic grade in bone and breast lesions.[19, 34] Nevertheless, anatomic site (e.g., extremities versus visceral involvement) also seems to be a strong predictor (perhaps stronger than histologic grade) of prognosis in angiosarcoma.[33, 35, 36] Maddux and Evans[37] studied 44 patients with angiosarcoma of the skin and soft tissues and found that the histologic variable that correlated most with survival was the degree of lymphocytic infiltrate admixed with and surrounding the tumor. No association was noted between mitotic activity and percentage of solid "undifferentiated areas" and prognosis.[37]

A retrospective study of 56 patients with synovial sarcoma concluded that large tumor size (≥5 cm), high nuclear grade, extensive tumor necrosis, the presence of rhabdoid cells, and a high American Joint Committee on Cancer (AJCC) stage were adverse prognostic indicators.[38] Enzinger and Weiss[39] also noted improved survival in synovial sarcomas with extensive ossification and calcification but a worse clinical outcome in poorly differentiated examples.

Ducatman and associates[40] evaluated 120 cases of malignant peripheral nerve sheath tumors and found no significant correlation between survival and either histologic grade or mitotic rate. In their series, each tumor was graded from 1 to 4 based on tumor cellularity, nuclear pleomorphism, mitotic index, and extent of necrosis. Tumor size (>5 cm) and the presence of neurofibromatosis adversely affected overall prognosis.[40] Survival also seemed improved after a total rather than a subtotal resection of the tumor.[40] Meis and coworkers[41] reported 78 cases of malignant peripheral nerve sheath tumors in children and, by multivariate analysis, found tumor size, age 7 years or older, tumor necrosis 25% or greater, and the presence of von Recklinghausen's disease to be "independent adverse prognostic factors."

Although the prognosis of primary skeletal osteosarcoma is related to histologic grade and response to adjuvant therapy,[19, 42] histologic grade does not correlate significantly with survival in patients with extraskeletal osteosarcoma. This situation may be due partly to the fact that extraskeletal osteosarcomas are almost invariably high-grade lesions.[43, 44] Chung and Enzinger[43] reported that no distinct histologic parameters seemed to correlate significantly with clinical behavior; however, extraskeletal osteosarcomas that were predominantly fibroblastic seemed to have a slightly better prognosis than osteoblastic, chondroblastic, or telangiectatic subtypes. Lee and Fetsch[44] found that patients with extraskeletal chrondroblastic osteosarcomas survived longer than patients with the osteoblastic subtype.

To date, histologic grade does not seem to be related to prognosis in Ewing's sarcoma, mesenchymal chondrosarcoma, and desmoplastic small round cell tumor.[45-48] Prognostic factors of known clinical significance in patients with rhabdomyosarcoma include primary site, histologic subtype (e.g., embryonal versus alveolar), age at presentation, and clinical group staging.[49-52] Histologic grade by conventional means generally has not been found to predict survival in patients with rhabdomyosarcoma.[25] The Intergroup Rhabdomyosarcoma Study Group has proposed a classification (grading) system for childhood rhabdomyosarcoma, however, that correlates with prognosis.[49] This classification, specifically designated as the International Classification of Rhabdomyosarcoma, is summarized in Table 1.9. The pleomorphic subtype of rhabdomyosarcoma, which represents predominately an adult tumor, is absent. The anaplastic variant of embryonal rhabdomyosarcoma has been included in the International Classification of Rhabdomyosarcoma classification.

At least some evidence suggests that histologic grading in hemangiopericytomas may be of prognostic significance. Based on an analysis of 106 cases, Enzinger and Smith[53] concluded that a malignant clinical course was associated with large tumor size (>5 cm), increased mitotic activity (≥4 mitotic figures per 10 HPF), high tumor cellularity, nuclear pleomorphism, and necrosis. McMaster and colleagues[54] reviewed 60 cases from the Mayo Clinic and found an association between malignant behavior, anaplasia, and mitotic activity.

Histologic grading does not seem to be of prognostic import in extraskeletal myxoid chondrosarcoma, clear cell sarcoma of soft tissues, epithelioid sarcoma, and alveolar soft part sarcoma.[55-60] Tumor necrosis may be an important indicator for patient survival, however, in epithelioid sarcoma and clear cell sarcoma of soft tissues.[56, 57] When tumor size and therapy (e.g., wide excision versus amputation) were taken into account, Evans and Baer[60] found no relationship in epithelioid sarcoma between mitotic rate and tumor necrosis and local recurrence and patient survival. Regarding the FNCLCC grading system, Guillou and colleagues[23] noted that the use of standard histologic grading systems in epithelioid sarcoma and alveolar soft part sarcoma should be discouraged: "In fact, experience has shown that grading of these rare tumor types does not correlate reliably with behavior, with the majority of those tumors showing a protracted clinical course despite a high or intermediate grade of malignancy using standard grading systems."

Data suggest that histologic grading may be useful in myxofibrosarcoma. Mentzel and coworkers[61] examined 75 patients with myxofibrosarcoma, dividing them into low-grade (mostly hypocellular and myxoid with only spindle

TABLE 1.9 International Classification of Rhabdomyosarcoma

Superior Prognosis
Embryonal rhabdomyosarcoma, botryoid subtype
Embryonal rhabdomyosarcoma, spindle cell subtype
Intermediate Prognosis
Embryonal rhabdomyosarcoma, not otherwise specified
Poor Prognosis
Alveolar rhabdomyosarcoma
Anaplastic rhabdomyosarcoma, diffuse
Undifferentiated sarcoma

cells), intermediate-grade (more cellular with focal solid areas), and high-grade (abundant solid areas, necrosis) types. Although the rate of local recurrence was independent of histologic grade, distant metastasis was observed only in tumors of intermediate to high grade.[61]

Although epithelioid hemangioendothelioma typically is regarded as a low-grade neoplasm, Mentzel and coworkers[62] found that more aggressive features, such as nuclear atypia, spindled cells, increased mitotic activity (>2 mitoses per 10 HPF), and focal "solid angiosarcomalike foci," tended to correlate with poor clinical outcome; however, these findings were not significant. A similar study evaluating primary epithelioid hemangioendothelioma of bone documented no histologic features that were predictive of clinical outcome.[63]

Malignant mesenchymoma generally has been defined as a sarcoma possessing at least two distinct types of mesenchymal differentiation (e.g., rhabdomyosarcoma, liposarcoma, osteosarcoma, chondrosarcoma, leiomyosarcoma). Reports regarding its prognosis have been conflicting, although it generally has been regarded as a high-grade neoplasm.[64, 65] Newman and Fletcher[64] analyzed nine cases of malignant mesenchyma and found that the biologic behavior was "not as aggressive as the histology would imply." Brady and colleagues[65] evaluated eight patients with malignant mesenchymoma. Six patients died of tumor, and two remained alive with evidence of residual disease. In neither of these studies did microscopic appearance correlate with clinical behavior, however, albeit absolute numbers of patients were small.

Soft tissue sarcoma subtypes for which some evidence exists that histologic grade may be prognostically significant are summarized in Table 1.10. Table 1.11 lists the sarcoma subtypes in which most evidence suggests that histologic grade is not prognostically important. An inherent weakness of all the data is a lack of a standardized or uniform grading system for which to analyze better the relationship between histologic grade, subtype, and clinical outcome.

TABLE 1.10 Soft Tissue Sarcoma Subtypes for Which Histologic Grading May Be Predictive of Prognosis

Malignant fibrous histiocytoma
Liposarcoma
Leiomyosarcoma
Angiosarcoma
Synovial sarcoma
Hemangiopericytoma
Myxofibrosarcoma
Fibrosarcoma

TABLE 1.11 Soft Tissue Sarcoma Subtypes for Which Histologic Grading Does Not Appear to Correlate with Prognosis

Malignant peripheral nerve sheath tumor
Epithelioid sarcoma
Clear cell sarcoma
Rhabdomyosarcoma, embryonal and alveolar
Ewing's sarcoma/primitive neuroectodermal tumor
Desmoplastic small round cell tumor
Mesenchymal chondrosarcoma
Myxoid chondrosarcoma
Alveolar soft part sarcoma
Epithelioid hemangioendothelioma
Malignant mesenchymoma
Osteosarcoma

Relationship of Histologic Grade in Sarcomas to Stage

The AJCC staging system is based on the widely recognized TNM profile, determined by size and extension of the primary tumor (T), lymph node involvement (N), and the presence or absence of metastases (M).[66] For therapeutic purposes, histologic grade (G) is best designated as *low* and *high*. The AJCC staging system is largely similar for bone and soft tissue sarcomas with the exception of the definitions for the primary tumor (T). As a result, there also are some differences in the stage grouping. The AJCC staging system is summarized in Table 1.12. The two subcategories for stage IV disease are designated A and B in bone sarcomas but remain unclassified for soft tissue sarcomas. In an analysis of 1215 soft tissue sarcoma patients, Russell and coworkers[67] noted that survival was inversely related to stage for all histopathologic types. The number of cases of epithelioid sarcoma and malignant hemangiopericytoma was insufficient, however, to draw definite conclusions. Notably absent were cases of clear cell sarcoma.

The Ennecking staging system has been adopted by the Musculoskeletal Tumor Society and is the primary staging system used by orthopedic oncologists. It has been employed for soft tissue and bone sarcomas.[68] It is based on two anatomic tumor growth patterns: T1 (or A) represents intracompartmental tumors confined within bone (bone sarcoma) or a muscle group or subcutaneous tissues (soft tissue sarcoma), and T2 (or B) represents extracompartmental neoplasms that arise within or involve extrafascial planes without anatomic boundaries. For bone sarcomas, this implies soft tissue extension. More specifically, *compartment* refers to anatomic regions bound by the natural barriers to tumor extension, such as fascial septa, joint capsule, ligaments and tendons, articular cartilage, or bony cortex. Two histologic grades are used: G1 represents low-grade lesions, and G2 represents high-grade lesions. Low-grade (G1) lesions represent lesions with histologic features of Broders' grade 1 or 2, whereas high-grade (G2) lesions equate to a grade 3 or 4 by the Broders system.[19] All data can be combined as follows: stage I—low-grade sarcomas, A—intracom-

TABLE 1.12 TNM Classification for Bone and Soft Tissue Sarcomas

	Bone Sarcomas		Soft Tissue Sarcomas
		Primary Tumor (T)	
TX		Primary tumor cannot be assessed	
T0		No evidence of primary tumor	
T1	Tumor confined within cortex		Tumor ≤5 cm in greatest dimension a. Superficial tumor* b. Deep tumor*
T2	Tumor invades beyond cortex		Tumor >5 cm in greatest dimension a. Superficial tumor* b. Deep tumor*
		Regional Lymph Nodes (N)	
NX		Regional lymph nodes cannot be assessed	
N0		No regional lymph node metastasis	
N1		Regional lymph node metastasis	
		Distant Metastasis (M)	
MX		Distant metastasis cannot be assessed	
M0		No distant metastasis	
M1		Distant metastasis	
		Histopathologic Grade (G)	
GX		Grade cannot be assessed	
G1		Well differentiated—low grade	
G2		Moderately differentiated—low grade	
G3		Poorly differentiated—high grade	
G4		Undifferentiated—high grade	
		Stage Grouping	
IA		G1,2 T1 N0 M0	
IB	G1,2 T2 N0 M0		G1,2 T2a N0 M0
IIA	G3,4 T1 N0 M0		G1,2 T2b N0 M0
IIB	G3,4 T2 N0 M0		G3,4 T1 N0 M0
IIC	Not defined		G3,4 T2a N0 M0
III	Not defined		G3,4 T2b N0 M0
IV		Any G Any T N1 M0	
		Any G Any T Any N M1	

*Regarding soft tissue sarcomas, a superficial tumor is defined as exclusively above superficial fascia without invasion of fascia. A deep tumor is defined as either beneath superficial fascia or invading superficial fascia. All retroperitoneal lesions, intraperitoneal visceral lesions, intrathoracic lesions, and lesions with major blood vessel invasion are classified as deep. Most head and neck tumors also are considered deep lesions.

partmental, B—extracompartmental with no evidence of metastases; stage II—high-grade sarcomas, A—intracompartmental, B—extracompartmental with no distant metastases; and stage III—sarcomas of any grade or compartment with metastases. The Enneking staging system is summarized in Table 1.13. According to the Enneking system, the surgical margin required for local control (e.g., wide versus radical resection) is determined by the grade of the tumor.[68] Histologic grade in the Enneking staging system is not based purely on morphology alone, but also incorporates clinical and radiologic features and the known biologic behavior of the specific tumor.

TABLE 1.13 Staging System of the Musculoskeletal Tumor Society (Enneking System) Applicable for Bone and Soft Tissue Sarcomas

Stage	Grade	Compartment	Metastasis
IA	G1 (low grade)	T1	M0
IB	G1	T2	M0
IIA	G2 (high grade)	T1	M0
IIB	G2	T2	M0
III	Any G	Any T	M1

A third soft tissue sarcoma staging system has been proposed by Hajdu[69] using a combined score, including tumor differentiation (histologic subtype), tumor cellularity, volume of background stroma, vascularity, tumor necrosis, and mitotic activity. The histologic grade is designated as low or high and evaluated along with tumor depth (superficial versus deep) and tumor size (<5 cm or >5 cm) to establish a stage.[69]

To define prognostic factors better for a staging system of soft tissue sarcomas, Tomita and coworkers[70] analyzed histologic and clinical data from 190 adult patients with localized soft tissue sarcoma involving the extremities or trunk. Histologically, tumors were graded as low, intermediate, or high and evaluated according to therapy. By multivariate analysis, histologic grade was the only significant prognostic factor for the staging of soft tissue sarcomas.[70]

Pathology Diagnostic Report

Having understood the aforementioned parameters of bone and soft tissue tumors, what should be included in the pathology report? For benign tumors, the diagnosis is often sufficient because even the adequacy of surgical margins is often of no importance therapeutically. Consequently, our recommendations apply mostly to the more commonly resected bone and soft tissue sarcomas and are not applicable to FNAB, CNB, or most incisional biopsy specimens, whose main purpose is to render a diagnosis. For resection specimens, providing the clinician with information regarding prognosis and cancer staging has become a necessity. Although such information may be incorporated readily anywhere in the surgical pathology report, it is best invested into so-called gross and light microscopy templates. Templates provide diagnostic, prognostic, and staging information in a clear and concise manner and, among various pathologists, create greater uniformity, insuring that within an individual institution (and often also referring institutions) all pertinent pathologic information is available for patient care. The American College of Surgeons in conjunction with the College of American Pathologists endorsed the use of cancer reporting templates as part of their accreditation process for cancer centers. An example of a recommended soft tissue sarcoma template is given in Figure 1.4. For bone sarcomas, templates are most useful for postchemotherapy resections of osteosarcomas and Ewing's sarcoma; an example from our institution is illustrated in Figure 1.5.

GROSS DESCRIPTION

Specimen Fixation:	*Fresh or in formalin*
Specimen Received:	*Incisional or excisional biopsy, limb-salvage resection, amputation, hemipelvectomy, intra-abdominal/thoracic resection, retroperitoneal resection, tumor debulking*
Anatomic Depth/Site:	*Dermal, subcutis, intramuscular/toe, foot, leg, arm*
Tumor Dimensions:	*3 dimensions (cm)*
Estimate of Tumor Necrosis:	___ *%, usually appear chalky yellow-white; include cystic area volume separately*
Growth Pattern:	*Infiltrative vs. well-circumscribed; encapsulated vs. nonencapsulated*
Surgical Margins:	*Positive vs. negative; anatomic site (e.g., anterior, posterior) and distance from margin (cm) if applicable*
Other Unusual Features:	*Bone involvement, extension into viscera*
Block Summary:	

LIGHT MICROSCOPY

Tumor Histologic Type:
Tumor Size (Largest Dimension):
Tumor Grade (FNCLCC System): Grade
    Tumor Differentiation Score:
    Tumor Necrosis Score:
    Mitotic Count Score:
    Total Score:
    Percent Necrosis:___ % (document whether pretherapy or post-therapy)
Lymph Nodes:
Surgical Margins:

FIGURE 1.4 Soft tissue sarcoma template.

Gross Description

The gross description should include how the specimen was received (fresh versus in formalin), and the appropriate labels and identifiers for the specimen should correspond to that documented on the surgical pathology request form. When possible, it is best to receive specimens fresh (not in formalin) because this optimizes effective use of ancillary studies (e.g., cytogenetics, flow cytometry), if deemed necessary. If not obvious, the orientation of the specimen, especially regarding margins, should be verified with the treating surgeon. The type of specimen received (or procedure performed) should be recorded accurately. A three-dimensional measurement and description of received tissues (e.g., bone, skeletal muscle) is necessary. The closest resection margin should be inked. In most cases, we do not believe that inking of the entire specimen is necessary because seepage of ink may result in "false-positive" margins. For limb salvage or amputation specimens, it is often easier, especially for primary bone tumors, to freeze the specimen solid over 24 hours followed by serial sectioning with a band saw and further examination. Tumor description should include three-dimensional size, location and depth (e.g., dermal, subcutaneous, intramuscular), appearance (e.g., color, consistency, prior biopsy site), involvement of neurovascular structures, and an estimation of the percent of necrosis. In most cases, necrosis appears chalky yellow-white. Cystic change and hemorrhage also should be documented and recorded separately from necrosis. For most specimens, six surgical margins may be present (superficial, deep, medial, lateral, proximal, and deep), and a measurement of the distance between these margins and the tumor should be recorded. Although usually not present, lymph nodes should be sought and examined in all amputation specimens.

Sampling of the tumor should include sections of all areas that appear grossly different. As a general rule, one block should be submitted per 1 cm of tumor greatest dimension (≤10 cm). For tumors greater than 10 cm, one to two blocks per every additional 10 cm is probably sufficient. According to the Association of Directors of Anatomic and Surgical Pathology, "it is rarely necessary to take more than a total of 10 to 12 blocks of tumor."[71] For marginal sampling, perpendicular sections (showing relationship of tumor to margin) are preferred over en face sampling. Each block should be labeled clearly with the appropriate patient identifiers and designated as to site and, if applicable, orientation.

Light Microscopy

Tumor Type: *Grade 3 or 4 (of 4) conventional osteosarcoma*
Grade 3 or 4 high-grade surface osteosarcoma
Grade 1 or 2 intraosseous well-differentiated osteosarcoma
Grade 1 or 2 parosteal osteosarcoma
Grade 2 or 3 periosteal osteosarcoma
Grade 4 telangiectatic osteosarcoma
Grade 4 small cell osteosarcoma
Ewing's sarcoma/primitive neuroectodermal tumor

Tumor Size: *3 dimensions (from gross unless changed by microscopic examination)*

Estimated postchemotherapy tumor necrosis: ________%, Grade ________
(grade is only applicable to osteosarcoma)

Postchemotherapy Osteosarcoma Grading:

Grade 1:	No effect
Grade 2:	Some necrosis
A	>50% viable tumor (<50% necrosis)
B	5%–50% viable tumor (50% to <95% necrosis)
Grade 3:	Scattered foci, <5% viable tumor (>95% necrosis)
Grade 4:	No viable tumor (complete necrosis)

Surgical Margins: *Examples: Both bone and circumferential soft tissue resection margins are negative for sarcoma. The bony resection margin (e.g., distal femur is positive for sarcoma). The circumferential soft tissue margin is positive for sarcoma.*

Other Significant Findings: *Skip lesions*

FIGURE 1.5 Osteosarcoma and Ewing's sarcoma postchemotherapy resection light microscopy template. (Adapted from Unni KK, Dahlin C: Grading of bone tumors. Semin Diagn Pathol 1984;1:165; and Wold LE: Practical approach to processing osteosarcomas in the surgical pathology laboratory. Pediatr Dev Pathol 1998;1:449.)

Light Microscopy

Histologic subtype should be provided, conforming to established guidelines for the specific diagnosis. After light microscopic examination and ancillary investigation, if a specific diagnosis cannot be rendered, the term *unclassified sarcoma* with an appropriate qualifier (e.g., pleomorphic, spindle cell, round cell, epithelioid/polygonal cell, or myxoid) is recommended.[71] The greatest dimension of the tumor should be documented clearly. As already mentioned, when applicable, a histologic grade should be rendered and may consist simply of low or high grade. There is no universally accepted grading system for soft tissue sarcomas, but the NCI and FNCLCC systems are widely used and accepted based on well-orchestrated studies. For histologic grading systems requiring a mitotic count, the most active or proliferative area should be examined and mitoses counted using a 40× objective.

Apart from histologic grade, tumor necrosis seems to represent an independent prognostic factor in soft tissue sarcomas.[20, 25, 38, 39, 53, 56, 57, 72] Among sarcomas in which histologic grade is probably of limited prognostic significance, tumor necrosis has been found to correlate with clinical behavior in epithelioid sarcoma and clear cell sarcoma.[56, 57] For these reasons, it is probably prudent to include the presence and extent of pretherapy tumor necrosis in the histopathology report as a separate item from histologic grade. What defines tumor necrosis is debatable. Guillou and associates[23] excluded all necrosis thought to be related to previous surgery or to ulceration and did not include necrosis related to hemorrhage or hyalinization. Similarly, Costa and associates[20] excluded necrosis related to surgery or ulceration, but "All other necrosis (inflammatory ischemic, individual cells, large geographic areas) was quantitated based on gross and microscopic findings." Evans[73] advocated that tumor necrosis is probably not significantly related to patient survival but appears strongly correlated with tumor size. We believe necrosis generally is best determined by an assessment (estimation) based on gross and microscopic features, excluding necrosis related to hemorrhage, surgery, ulceration, and hyalinization.

Specific histologic grading systems probably should not be applied to post-therapy (preoperative chemotherapy or radiation therapy or both) specimens. The percentage of necrosis should be estimated, but its significance, outside of Ewing's sarcoma and skeletal osteosarcoma, is uncertain. The status of the surgical margins should be documented as positive or negative. If negative, surgical margins less than 2 cm should be specified as to distance and location. Any lymph nodes retrieved should be recorded as positive or negative for metastatic disease.

Therapy-Associated Changes in Bone and Soft Tissue Sarcomas

Preoperative chemotherapy for some bone and soft tissue sarcomas, particularly osteosarcoma, rhabdomyosarcoma, and Ewing's sarcoma, has become a mainstay of therapeutic management, especially in children. Pathologists are required to examine such postchemotherapy specimens, often estimating the response to chemotherapy, usually related to the percentage of necrotic tumor. Specific features and grading systems for post-therapy osteosarcoma and Ewing's sarcoma specimens are discussed in their respective chapters. Although preoperative chemotherapy is now being used for some soft tissue sarcomas, its efficacy is unclear.

REFERENCES

1. Enzinger FM, Weiss SW: General considerations In: Soft Tissue Tumors, 3rd ed. St. Louis: CV Mosby, 1995, pp 1-16.
2. Bennert KW, Abdul-Karim FW: Fine needle aspiration cytology vs. needle core biopsy of soft tissue tumors: A comparison. Acta Cytol 1994;38:381.
3. The Papanicolaou Society: Guidelines of the Papanicolaou Society of Cytopathology for fine-needle aspiration procedure and reporting. Mod Pathol 1997;10:739.
4. Kilpatrick SE, Geisinger KR: Soft tissue sarcomas: The usefulness and limitations of fine-needle aspiration biopsy. Am J Clin Pathol 1998;110:50.
5. Kilpatrick SE, Ward WG, Chauvenet AR, et al: The role of fine needle aspiration biopsy in the initial diagnosis of pediatric bone and soft tissue tumors: An institutional experience. Mod Pathol 1998;11:923.
6. Akerman M, Willen H: Critical review on the role of fine needle aspiration in soft tissue tumors. Pathol Case Rev 1998;3:111.
7. Bommer KK, Ramzy I, Mody D: Fine-needle aspiration biopsy in the diagnosis and management of bone lesions: A study of 450 cases. Cancer (Cancer Cytopathol) 1997;81:148.
8. Layfield LJ, Anders KH, Glasgow BJ, et al: Fine-needle aspiration of primary soft-tissue lesions. Arch Pathol Lab Med 1986;110:420.
9. DeMay RM: Soft-tissue tumors. In: The Art and Science of Cytopathology, vol 2, Aspiration Cytology. Chicago: American Society of Clinical Pathologists Press, 1996, p 563.
10. Ackerman M, Rydholm A: Surgery based on fine needle aspiration cytology. Acta Orthop Scand 1994;65(suppl 256):69.
11. Kilpatrick SE, Cappellari JO, Bos GD, et al: Is fine needle aspiration biopsy a practical alternative to open biopsy for the primary diagnosis of sarcoma? Experience with 140 patients. Am J Clin Pathol 2001;115:59.
12. Costa MJ, Campman SC, Davis RL, et al: Fine-needle aspiration cytology of sarcoma: Retrospective review of diagnostic utility and specificity. Diagn Cytopathol 1996;15:23.
13. Hook SY, Jorda M, Mailhot S, et al: Fine needle aspiration cytology of superficial soft tissue lesions: A study of 110 cases (abstract). Acta Cytol 1998;42:1289.
14. Kilpatrick SE, Ward WG, Cappellari JO, et al: Fine needle aspiration biopsy of soft tissue sarcomas: A cytomorphologic analysis with emphasis

on histologic subtyping, grading, and therapeutic significance. Am J Clin Pathol 1999;112:179.
15. Welker JA, Henshaw RM, Jelinek J, et al: The percutaneous needle biopsy is safe and recommended in the diagnosis of musculoskeletal masses: Outcomes analysis of 155 patients at a sarcoma referral center. Cancer 2000;89:2677.
16. Willman JH, White K, Coffin CM: Pediatric core needle biopsy: Strengths and limitations in evaluation of masses. Pediatr Dev Pathol 2001;4:46.
17. Pollock RE, Karnell LH, Menck HR, et al: The National Cancer Data Base report on soft tissue sarcoma. Cancer 1996;78:2247.
18. Liu K, Layfield LJ, Coogan AC, et al: Diagnostic accuracy of fine-needle aspiration of soft tissue and bone lesions: Influence of clinical history and experience. Am J Clin Pathol 1999;111:632.
19. Unni KK, Dahlin DC: Grading of bone tumors. Semin Diagn Pathol 1984;1:165.
20. Costa J, Wesley RA, Glatstein E, et al: The grading of soft tissue sarcomas: results of a clinicohistopathologic correlation in a series of 163 cases. Cancer 1984;53:530.
21. Costa J: The grading of soft tissue sarcomas. In Fletcher CDM, McKee PH (eds): Pathobiology of Soft Tissue Tumors. Edinburgh: Churchill Livingstone, 1990, pp 221-238.
22. Trojani M, Contesso G, Coindre JM, et al: Soft tissue sarcomas of adults: Study of pathological prognostic variables and definition of a histopathologic grading system. Int J Cancer 1984;33:37.
23. Guillou L, Coindre JM, Bonichon F, et al: Comparative study of the National Cancer Institute and French Federation of Cancer Centers sarcoma group grading systems in a population of 410 adult patients with soft tissue sarcomas. J Clin Oncol 1997;15:350.
24. Angervall L, Kindblom L-G, Rydholm A, et al: The diagnosis and prognosis of soft tissue tumors. Semin Diagn Pathol 1986;3:240.
25. Hashimoto H, Daimuru Y, Takeshita S, et al: Prognostic significance of histologic parameters of soft tissue sarcomas. Cancer 1992;70:2816.
26. LeDoussal V, Coindre JM, Leroux A, et al: Prognostic factors for patients with localized primary malignant fibrous histiocytoma: A multicenter study of 216 patients with multivariate analysis. Cancer 1996;77:1823.
27. Gustafson P, Rydholm A, Willen H, et al: Liposarcoma: A population based epidemiologic and prognostic study of features of 43 patients, including DNA content. Int J Cancer 1993;55:541.
28. Chang HR, Hajdu SI, Collin C, et al: The prognostic value of histologic subtypes in primary extremity liposarcoma. Cancer 1986;64:1414.
29. Hashimoto H, Daimuru Y, Tsuneyoshi M, et al: Leiomyosarcoma of the external soft tissues: A clinicopathologic, immunohistochemical, and electron microscopic study. Cancer 1988;57:2077.
30. Wile AG, Evans HL, Romsdahl MM: Leiomyosarcoma of soft tissue: A clinicopathologic study. Cancer 1981;48:1022.
31. Moran CA, Suster S, Abbondanzo SL, et al: Primary leiomyosarcomas of the lung: A clinicopathologic and immunohistochemical study of 18 cases. Mod Pathol 1997;10:121.
32. Antonescu CR, Erlandson RA, Huvos AG: Primary leiomyosarcoma of bone: A clinicopathologic, immunohistochemical, and ultrastructural study of 33 patients and a literature review. Am J Surg Pathol 1997;21:1281.
33. Mark RJ, Poen JC, Tran LM, et al: Angiosarcoma: A report of 67 patients and a review of the literature. Cancer 1996;77:2400.
34. Donnell RM, Rosen PP, Lieberman PH, et al: Angiosarcoma and other vascular tumors of the breast. Am J Surg Pathol 1981;5:629.
35. Janigan DT, Husain A, Robinson NA: Cardiac angiosarcomas: A review and a case report. Cancer 1986;67:852.
36. Smith VC, Eisenberg BL, McDonald EC: Primary splenic angiosarcoma: A case report and literature review. Cancer 1985;55:1625.
37. Maddux JC, Evans HL: Angiosarcoma of skin and soft tissue: A study of 44 cases. Cancer 1981;48:1907.
38. Oda Y, Hashimoto H, Tsuneyoshi M, et al: Survival in synovial sarcoma: A multivariate study of prognostic factors with special emphasis on the comparison between early death and long-term survival. Am J Surg Pathol 1993;17:35.
39. Enzinger FM, Weiss SW: Synovial sarcoma In: Soft Tissue Tumors, 3rd ed. St. Louis: CV Mosby, 1995, pp 757-786.
40. Ducatman BS, Scheithauer BW, Plepgras DG, et al: Malignant peripheral nerve sheath tumors: A clinicopathologic study of 120 cases. Cancer 1986;57:2006.
41. Meis JM, Enzinger FM, Martz KL, et al: Malignant peripheral nerve sheath tumors (malignant schwannomas) in children. Am J Surg Pathol 1992;16:694.
42. Raymond AK, Chawla SP, Carrasco CH, et al: Osteosarcoma chemotherapy effect: A prognostic factor. Semin Diagn Pathol 1987;4:212.
43. Chung EB, Enzinger FM: Extraskeletal osteosarcoma. Cancer 1987;60:1132.
44. Lee JSY, Fetsch JF, Wasdahl DA, et al: A review of 40 patients with extraskeletal osteosarcoma. Cancer 1995;76:2253.
45. Angervall L, Enzinger FM: Extraskeletal neoplasm resembling Ewing's sarcoma. Cancer 1975;36:240.
46. Kissane JM, Askin FB, Foukes M, et al: Ewing's sarcoma of bone: Clinicopathologic aspects of 303 cases from the Intergroup Ewing's Sarcoma study. Hum Pathol 1983;14:773.
47. Nakashima Y, Unni KK, Shives TC, et al: Mesenchymal chondrosarcoma of bone and soft tissue: A review of 111 cases. Cancer 1986;57:2244.
48. Leuschner I, Radig K, Harms D: Desmoplastic small round cell tumor. Semin Diagn Pathol 1996;13:204.
49. Newton WA Jr, Gethan EA, Webber BL, et al: Classification of rhabdomyosarcomas and related sarcomas: Pathologic aspects and proposal for a new classification—an Intergroup Rhabdomyosarcoma Study. Cancer 1995;76:1073.
50. LaQuaglia MP, Gharimi F, Penenberg D, et al: Factors predictive of mortality in pediatric extremity rhabdomyosarcoma. J Pediatr Surg 1990;25:238.
51. Kilpatrick SE, Teot LA, Geisinger KR, et al: Relationship of DNA ploidy to histology and prognosis in rhabdomyosarcoma: Comparison of flow cytometry and image analysis. Cancer 1994;74:3227.
52. Lawrence W Jr, Anderson JR, Gehan EA, et al: Pretreatment TNM staging of childhood rhabdomyosarcoma: A report of the Intergroup Rhabdomyosarcoma Study Group. Cancer 1997;80:1165.
53. Enzinger FM, Smith BH: Hemangiopericytoma: An analysis of 106 cases. Hum Pathol 1976;7:61.
54. McMaster MJ, Soule EH, Ivins JC: Hemangiopericytoma: A clinicopathologic study and long-term follow-up of 60 patients. Cancer 1975;36:2232.
55. Meis-Kindblom JM, Kindblom LG, Bergh P, et al: Prognostic factors in extraskeletal myxoid chondrosarcoma (abstract). Mod Pathol 1996;9:10A.
56. Lucas DR, Nascimento AG, Sim FH: Clear cell sarcoma of soft tissues: Mayo Clinic experience with 35 cases. Am J Surg Pathol 1992;16:1197.
57. Chase DR, Enzinger FM: Epithelioid sarcoma: Diagnosis, prognosis, and treatment. Am J Surg Pathol 1985;9:241.
58. Evans HL: Alveolar soft-part sarcoma: A study of 13 examples and one with a histologically atypical component. Cancer 1985;55:912.

59. Lieberman PH, Brennan MF, Kimmel M, et al: Alveolar soft part sarcoma: A clinicopathologic study of half a century. Cancer 1989;63:1.
60. Evans HL, Baer SC: Epithelioid sarcoma: A clinicopathologic and prognostic study of 26 cases. Semin Diagn Pathol 1993;10:286.
61. Mentzel T, Calonje E, Wadden C, et al: Myxofibrosarcoma: Clinicopathologic analysis of 75 cases with emphasis on the low-grade variant. Am J Surg Pathol 1996;20:391.
62. Mentzel T, Beham A, Calonje E, et al: Epithelioid hemangioendothelioma of skin and soft tissues: Clinicopathologic and immunohistochemical study of 30 cases. Am J Surg Pathol 1997;21:363.
63. Kleer CG, Unni KK, McLeod RA: Epithelioid hemangioendothelioma of bone. Am J Surg Pathol 1996;20:1301.
64. Newman PL, Fletcher CDM: Malignant mesenchymoma: Clinicopathologic analysis of a series with evidence of low-grade behavior. Am J Surg Pathol 1991;15:607.
65. Brady MS, Perino G, Tallini G, et al: Malignant mesenchymoma. Cancer 1996;77:457.
66. Fleming ID, Cooper JS, Henson DE, et al: AJCC Cancer Staging Manual, 5th ed. Philadelphia: JB Lippincott, 1998, pp 133-146.
67. Russell WD, Cohen J, Enzinger F, et al: A clinical and pathological staging system for soft tissue sarcomas. Cancer 1977;40:1562.
68. Ennecking WF, Spanier SS, Malawar MM: The effect of the anatomic setting on the results of surgical procedures for soft parts sarcoma of the thigh. Cancer 1981;47:1005.
69. Hajdu SI: Pathology of Soft Tissue Tumors. Philadelphia, Lea & Febiger, 1979, pp 44-47.
70. Tomita Y, Kuratsu S, Naka N, et al: A staging system for soft tissue sarcoma and its evaluation in relation to treatment. Int J Cancer 1994;58:168.
71. Association of Directors of Anatomic and Surgical Pathology: Recommendations for the reporting of soft tissue sarcomas. Am J Clin Pathol 1999;111:594.
72. Kilpatrick SE, Doyon J, Choong PFM, et al: The clinicopathologic spectrum of myxoid and round cell liposarcoma: A study of 95 cases. Cancer 1996;77:1450.
73. Evans HL: Classification and grading of soft-tissue sarcomas: A comment. Hematol Oncol Clin N Am 1995;9:653.

CHAPTER 2

Immunohistochemical, Molecular, and Cytogenetic Analysis of Bone and Soft Tissue Tumors

ANDREW CREAGER

Importance of Ancillary Studies

Immunohistochemical, molecular, and genetic studies have revealed many novel, relatively sensitive (but not always specific) immunohistochemical markers, chromosomal translocations, and molecular mutations in bone and soft tissue tumors (Table 2.1). The detection of these chromosomal and molecular aberrations has involved many established and relatively new techniques, including immunohistochemistry, conventional cytogenetic analysis, polymerase chain reaction (PCR), in situ hybridization, and Southern and Northern blotting.[1,2] Of special interest is the frequency of morphologically, immunohistochemically, and clinically distinct soft tissue sarcomas harboring translocations and fusion genes involving the *EWS* gene (22q12). In addition to Ewing's sarcoma, abnormalities associated with the *EWS* gene are observed in intra-abdominal desmoplastic small round cell tumor, myxoid chondrosarcoma, and clear cell sarcoma. In this chapter, emphasis is on a variety of immunohistochemical markers, cytogenetic abnormalities, and molecular studies, applicable to the diagnosis of bone and soft tissue tumors. These studies also are discussed with specific histologic subtypes in other chapters when applicable.

Words of Caution Regarding Ancillary Studies

After intensive scientific investigation, a more realistic perspective virtually always replaces the initial enthusiasm associated with the discovery of specific immunohistochemical and molecular markers. The immunohistochemical marker CD99, initially reported as specific for Ewing's sarcoma, now has been documented convincingly in most cases of mesenchymal chondrosarcoma and synovial sarcoma and a few examples of small cell osteosarcoma, rhabdomyosarcoma, and desmoplastic small round cell tumor.[3-6] Cytokeratin positivity is observed sometimes in rhabdomyosarcoma.[7] Desmin, an immunohistochemical marker usually associated with rhabdomyosarcoma, often is expressed by the blastemal portion of Wilms' tumor.[8]

Cytogenetic and molecular analyses have yielded similar surprisingly nonspecific results. The most frequent Ewing's sarcoma translocation, t(11;22)(q24;q12) with the EWS-FLI1 fusion product, has been reported in phenotypically classic examples of mesenchymal chondrosarcoma, embryonal and alveolar rhabdomyosarcoma, polyphenotypic tumor of childhood, and neuroblastoma.[9-12] The EWS-FLI1 and the EWS-ERG fusion transcripts have been described in cases of intra-abdominal desmoplastic small round cell tumor.[13,14] The t(X;18), although present in a large portion of synovial sarcomas, may be observed in occasional malignant peripheral nerve sheath tumors. For these reasons, immunohistochemical and molecular studies should be considered ancillary, not definitive, tests. The gold standard for diagnosis is light microscopy. Knowledge and application of these ancillary tests are helpful for the pathologist faced with a difficult soft tissue sarcoma, but these data should be interpreted only with the complete knowledge of the pertinent clinical and microscopic features.

In the modern age of molecular genetics, histologic features are often underemphasized. Clinicians tend to view molecular

TABLE 2.1 Bone and Soft Tissue Sarcoma Subtypes with Associated Immunohistochemical Markers and Molecular and Cytogenetic Abnormalities

Histologic Subtype	IHC Markers	Cytogenetic Abnormalities	Molecular Events	Estimated Frequency of Events (%)
Ewing's sarcoma/primitive neuroectodermal tumor	CD99	t(11;22)(q24;q12) t(21;22)(q22;q12) t(7;22)(p22;q12) Others	FLI1-EWS fusion ERG-EWS fusion ETV1-EWS fusion	>85 5-10 <5 1-5
Alveolar rhabdomyosarcoma	Myogenin Myo-D1	t(2;13)(q35;q14) t(1;13)(p36;q14)	PAX3-FKHR fusion PAX7-FKHR fusion	80 10-20
Embryonal rhabdomyosarcoma	Myogenin Myo-D1	+2q, +8, +20		70-80
Desmoplastic small round cell tumor	Cytokeratin Desmin NSE	t(11;22)(p13;q12)	WT1-EWS fusion	>80
Clear cell sarcoma (melanoma of soft parts)	S-100 HMB 45	t(12;22)(q13;q12)	ATF1-EWS fusion	>80
Myxoid chondrosarcoma (chordoid sarcoma)	Vimentin	t(9;22)(q21-31; q12)	EWS-CHN (TEC) fusion	>50
Myxoid/round cell liposarcoma	Vimentin	t(12;16)(q13;p11)	CHOP-TLS fusion	>80
Atypical lipomatous tumor/ well-differentiated liposarcoma	Vimentin	Supernumerary ring chromosomes and giant marker chromosomes	MDM2 amplification	>60
Synovial sarcoma	Cytokeratin EMA CD99	t(X;18)(p11;q11)	SYT-SSX1 or SSX2	>90
Extrarenal rhabdoid tumor	Cytokeratin	22q11 deletion	SMARCB1 inactivation	? >90
Alveolar soft part sarcoma	Vimentin Desmin	t(X;17)(p11;q25)	ASPL-TFE3 fusion	>90
Epithelioid hemangioendothelioma	CD31 CD34	t(1;3)(p36;q25)	?	?
Infantile fibrosarcoma	Vimentin	t(12;15)(p13;q26) +8,+11, +17, +20	ETV6-NTRK3	? >90

EMA, epithelial membrane antigen; IHC markers, immunohistochemical markers that are positive in most cases; NSE, neuron-specific enolase; SYN, synaptophysin.

and immunohistochemical tests as absolute and foolproof. Many pathologists give in to their clinicians' demands, losing the opportunity to educate them regarding the realities of the ancillary tests. Advances in molecular genetics and immunohistochemistry have been extraordinarily helpful, especially in the differential diagnosis of small round cell tumors, but they are not absolute. In a timely article, Dehner[6] warned of the inherent dangers in defining diagnoses by ancillary tests. The subject of the article is a lawsuit against a pathologist for rendering a diagnosis of Ewing's sarcoma without supportive evidence of CD99 positivity. At least three other consultants who reviewed the case decided that the tumor could not be Ewing's sarcoma, favoring a diagnosis of lymphoma, solely based on the absence of CD99 positivity (and despite ultrastructural evidence of intercellular junctions). Although the jury concluded that the primary pathologist was likely correct in his diagnosis of Ewing's sarcoma, they decided that he did not meet "the standard of care" because he did not order a CD99 test.[6] The gold standard for pathologic diagnoses is light microscopy with clinicoradiologic correlation. Immunohistochemistry, cytogenetics, and molecular studies are ancillary tests. All of these entities initially were described *solely* based on their light microscopic features. To the credit of these pioneers in pathology, more recent investigators since have proved that their classifications were largely correct. In this book, we emphasize the morphologic and clinicoradiologic features of the various subtypes of small round cell tumors as most crucial for establishing a diagnosis, with immunohistochemistry and molecular genetics playing an important but supportive role. It is essential that pathologists realize, for a variety of reasons, antigen expression may be absent, and the phenotypic presentation of a tumor may be the result of one of several different molecular pathways. As summarized by Dehner:[6]

[T]he gold standard for pathologic diagnosis is predicated on the microscopic features of the tumor. Once the results of an ancillary method like immunohistochemistry become disconnected from the clinical and pathologic findings, we find ourselves separated from the first principles of diagnostic pathology that have served as one of the fundamental pillars in the practice of medicine.

Immunohistochemistry

Immunohistochemical analysis of bone and soft tissue tumors is an established and practical means of providing supportive assistance to the pathologist, especially when morphologic and clinical features are equivocal. As alluded to previously, it is crucial to recognize that immunohistochemical analysis always should be used as a secondary supplement to morphology. In this capacity, immunohistochemistry should never supplant the morphologic impression, but rather should complement the findings. The reliance on immunohistochemical findings in the absence of concrete morphologic findings has been the cause of many an incorrect diagnosis. It is accepted that tumors exist that defy conventional classification schemes even after immunohistochemistry is applied in conjunction with thorough histologic sampling. In these cases, other ancillary studies, such as molecular genetic, cytogenetic, and electron microscopic studies, may be useful, and some of these are discussed later in this chapter. This section focuses on the more common applications of immunohistochemistry, emphasizing patterns of expression, sensitivity, and specificity for the diagnosis of bone and soft tissue tumors. Table 2.2 lists many of the immunohistochemical markers used more frequently for histologic subtyping.

TABLE 2.2 Routinely Applied Immunohistochemical Markers in the Work-up of Bone and Soft Tissue Tumors

Vimentin
Cytokeratin
Epithelial membrane antigen
Desmin
Smooth muscle actin
Muscle-specific actin
Myogenic nuclear regulatory proteins (Myo-D1, myogenin)
S-100 protein
HMB 45
Melan A
Factor 8
CD31
CD34
CD45 (leukocyte common antigen)
CD30 (Ki-1)
CD99
Fli-1
WT-1
CD117 (c-kit)

Intermediate Filaments

Intermediate filament proteins are integral components of the cytoskeleton. Numerous filament types are present in different cell types throughout the body. Although many different groups/types of intermediate filaments exist, only the five major categories—cytokeratins, vimentin, desmin, neurofilament, and glial fibrillary acidic protein—are used in routine diagnostic pathology.

Cytokeratins

Cytokeratins are a heterogeneous group of intermediate filaments that include a variety of different proteins. Basic biochemical categorization of cytokeratins is based on the electrophoretic properties of these proteins, including molecular weight and pH. In practice, cytokeratins generally are subdivided into high-molecular-weight or low-molecular-weight categories. Alternatively, cytokeratins may be classified based on their expression properties in either simple or complex epithelium. Cytokeratin is an extremely sensitive marker for the distinction of epithelial malignancies from nonepithelial (mesenchymal and hematopoietic) processes. Because many different types of cytokeratins exist, differential expression patterns are observed in epithelia from varying anatomic locations; these relatively specific expression patterns may be exploited in an attempt to reveal evidence of the anatomic origin of metastases from unknown primaries (see Chapter 15 for further discussion of cytokeratins 7 and 20). Despite high sensitivity in epithelial malignancies, cytokeratin expression is not limited to epithelial tumors. Table 2.3 lists bone and soft tissue tumors that commonly (>50% of routine cases) show cytokeratin positivity (Fig. 2.1). Cytokeratin expression, as measured by immunohistochemical studies with molecular biologic confirmation, also has been observed in benign and malignant smooth muscle, melanoma (particularly metastases), and endothelial-derived tumors with and without epithelioid differentiation.[15-19] Cytokeratin expression in these tumors may be difficult to detect on routinely processed tissue specimens and may require the use of specific epitope retrieval methods and/or frozen sections. In addition, rarely, apparently aberrant cytokeratin expression is observed in other nonepithelioid sarcomas, such as malignant fibrous histiocytoma and osteosarcoma, potentially confounding the diagnosis.[20,21] Cytokeratins typically are expressed in synovial sarcoma, and the specific expression patterns in this tumor are well described in Chapter 4.

TABLE 2.3 Bone and Soft Tissue Sarcomas Commonly (>50% of Cases) Expressing Cytokeratin

Synovial sarcoma
Epithelioid sarcoma
Desmoplastic small round cell tumor
Extrarenal rhabdoid tumor
Melanotic neuroectodermal tumor of infancy
Adamantinoma

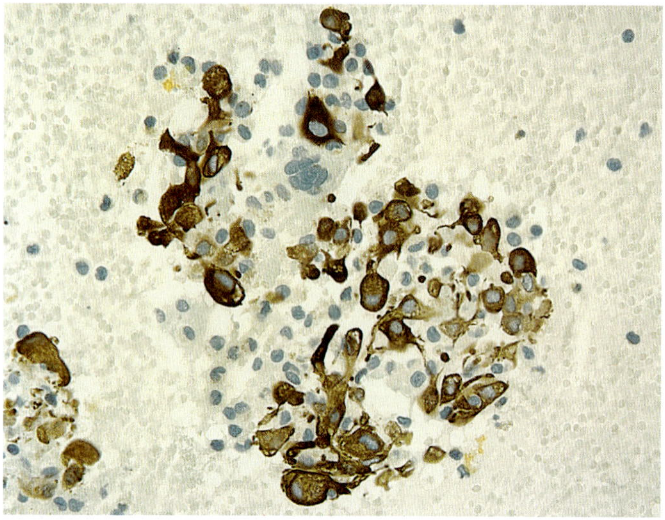

FIGURE 2.1 Strong cytoplasmic positivity for cytokeratin is typical for epithelioid sarcoma. This specimen represents cell block material from a fine needle aspiration biopsy.

Vimentin

Vimentin is a 54-kd, ubiquitously expressed intermediate filament that functions as a major cytoskeletal component, particularly during embryogenesis. As cells differentiate, and expression of more specialized intermediate filaments ensues, vimentin expression is gradually lost in many major cell lines, with the exception of mesenchymal cells. Many pathologists continue to evaluate vimentin immunoreactivity as a surrogate marker of global antigen preservation in tissue specimens. Proponents of this practice use vimentin positivity as an indicator that the tissue has been processed and preserved adequately. Others argue that this practice is of little value because vimentin is more robust than other antigens and, similar to many other intermediate filaments, may be the only remaining immunoreactive protein in largely necrotic specimens.[22] Consequently, the presence of vimentin expression alone does not indicate that other antigens have not been lost.

For diagnostic purposes, vimentin is largely nonspecific, and its utility is limited. Although virtually all mesenchymal cells express vimentin, its coexpression with other more specific intermediate filaments may be seen in some epithelial neoplasms, particularly thyroid gland, salivary gland, kidney, and adrenal gland. In the setting of metastatic carcinoma of unknown primary, coexpression of vimentin and other intermediate filaments, such as cytokeratins, may be exploited and helps narrow the differential diagnosis.[23,24] Some carcinomas may acquire the ability to express vimentin, particularly carcinomas undergoing spindle cell or "sarcomatoid" transformation.[25-30] Finally, vimentin expression commonly is observed in small round blue cell tumors and lacks diagnostic specificity in this setting.

Smooth and Skeletal Muscle Markers

Actin

Actin is an intracytoplasmic contractile protein that is found ubiquitously in all cell types throughout the body and has many isoforms, some of which are specific to smooth muscle (smooth muscle α and γ), whereas others are more specific for striated muscle (skeletal muscle α, cardiac muscle α). The α and γ isoforms also may be observed in myofibroblasts and myoepithelial cells. The ability to extrapolate differences in these isoforms and the relatively high concentrations of actin proteins within myoid cells make the use of antibodies directed against actin diagnostically helpful. In practice, two different antibodies with distinct affinities commonly are used. The first antibody, muscle-specific actin (HHF35), shows reactivity for all muscle actins, skeletal and smooth muscle, while excluding nonmuscle actins. In this general capacity, muscle-specific actin is not especially useful for distinguishing tumors of smooth muscle from those of skeletal muscle origin. The second antibody, smooth muscle actin (1A4), has greater specificity and affinity for smooth muscle actins. Tumors derived from skeletal muscle generally can be distinguished from smooth muscle tumors using this antibody.

Myofibroblasts commonly express smooth muscle actins and may show positive staining with muscle-specific actin and smooth muscle actin. This immunoexpression often is observed in tumors of myofibroblastic origin and frequently in "myofibroblastic" desmoplastic responses to invading carcinomas. Typically, myofibroblasts expressing smooth muscle actins show strong cytoplasmic margination of actin filaments; smooth muscle cells and tumors with smooth muscle differentiation tend to show a more homogeneous staining pattern (Fig. 2.2). In practice, these staining patterns overlap considerably, making reliable distinction between myofibroblasts and smooth muscle cells solely based on immunohistochemical properties difficult to impossible. The separation of myofibroblastic lesions from smooth muscle tumors should be based on morphologic grounds.

Desmin

Desmin is an intermediate intracytoplasmic filament expressed by smooth and skeletal muscle cells. In smooth muscle cells, desmin is associated with intracytoplasmic dense bodies and subplasmalemmal plaques; in skeletal

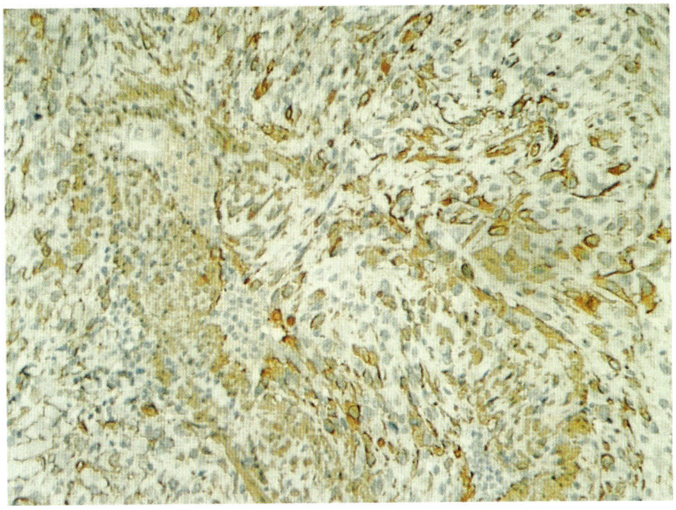

FIGURE 2.2 Leiomyosarcoma of soft tissues generally shows diffuse and strong cytoplasmic positivity for smooth muscle actin.

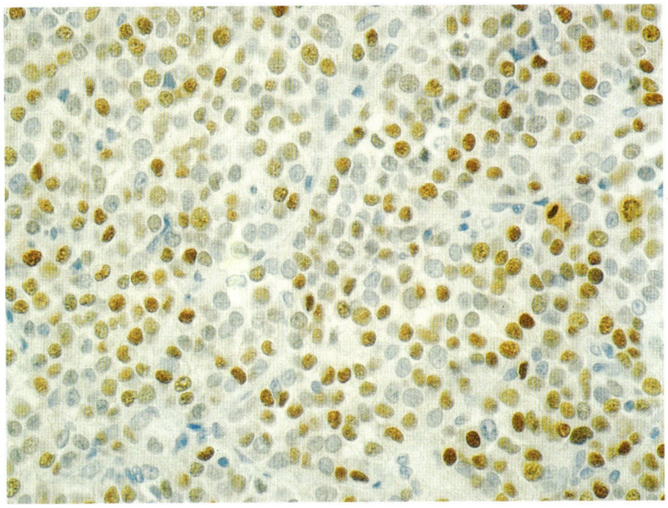

FIGURE 2.3 Myogenin is a highly specific marker for skeletal muscle differentiation and useful for confirming the diagnosis of rhabdomyosarcoma. Note the strong and diffuse nuclear staining in this alveolar rhabdomyosarcoma.

muscle, desmin is linked to the sarcomere Z-disks. It is one of the earliest expressed muscle proteins during embryogenesis and serves as part of the contractile apparatus in muscle cells. Compared with actin staining, desmin is expressed far less frequently by myofibroblasts. Other nonmyogenic cells, including mesothelial cells, endometrial stromal cells, lymph node fibroblastic reticulum cells, and submesothelial fibroblasts, may be positive for desmin.[31-34] Positive immunoexpression for desmin has been reported in tumors without true muscle differentiation, including localized tenosynovial giant cell tumor, angiomatoid fibrous histiocytoma, desmoplastic small round cell tumor, neuroblastoma, blastemal component of Wilms' tumor, and primitive neuroectodermal tumors.[35-38] Myoepithelial cells are typically negative for desmin. What desmin lacks in specificity is made up for by its great sensitivity in detecting tumors of myoid origin, especially skeletal muscle. The expression of muscle structural proteins correlates with the degree of cell differentiation in normal embryologic development and tumor cell differentiation. Because desmin and actin are expressed early during embryogenesis, their presence in smooth and skeletal muscle neoplasms, including poorly differentiated ones, is almost uniform. Myogenic transcription factors (discussed next) may be used to increase the specificity of an immunohistochemical panel in this setting.

Myogenic Transcription Factors

Myogenin and MyoD1 are two members of a family of DNA binding nuclear regulatory proteins that play a crucial role in functioning as transcription factors for the myogenic determination (MyoD) family of proteins. As such, they play a vital role in mesenchymal progenitor cell skeletal muscle differentiation and subsequent preservation of this phenotype. Transcription factors of this type are expressed early in embryologic development and, by contributing to the expression of cytoskeletal proteins such as desmin, actin, and myosin, induce the skeletal muscle phenotype. Consequently, myogenin and MyoD1 have relatively high sensitivity and specificity for skeletal muscle tumors, and antibodies against myogenin and MyoD1 are used widely to confirm the diagnosis of rhabdomyosarcoma.[39,40] It is crucial to understand that myogenin and MyoD1 are localized to the nucleus of the cell and should be interpreted as positive only in this setting (Fig. 2.3). Nonspecific cytoplasmic staining, more commonly observed with Myo-D1, is a recognized phenomenon that may be seen sometimes as a result of antigen retrieval methods.[41]

Myoglobin

Myoglobin, an oxygen-binding heme protein, is found exclusively in skeletal muscle. In contrast to the myogenic transcription factors, it is usually not present in early embryologic development. As a result, more primitive-appearing childhood rhabdomyosarcomas often do not express myoglobin, limiting its usefulness among the small round cell sarcomas. Myoglobin is detected frequently in adult pleomorphic rhabdomyosarcomas and rhabdomyomas.[39]

Endothelial Markers

CD31 (Platelet Endothelial Cell Adhesion Molecule-1)

CD31 is a 130-kd transmembrane glycoprotein expressed by endothelial cells, platelets, granulocytes, and some lymphocytes and plasma cells. Antibodies against CD31 have a high sensitivity and specificity for confirming tumors with endothelial differentiation because CD31 is expressed in virtually all benign and malignant endothelial cell proliferations, including hemangiomas, hemangioendotheliomas, and

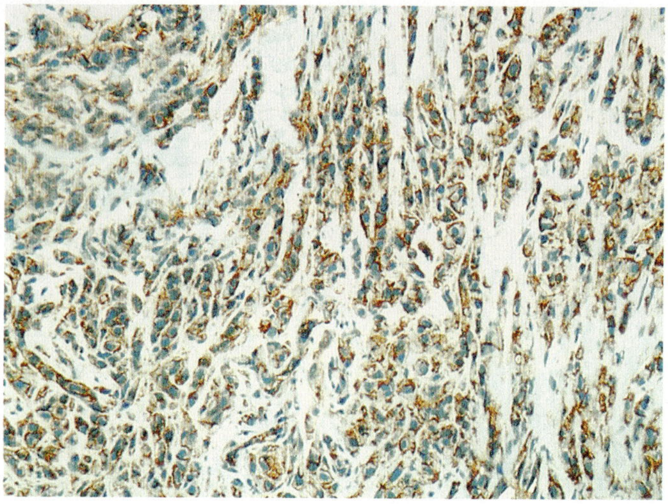

A

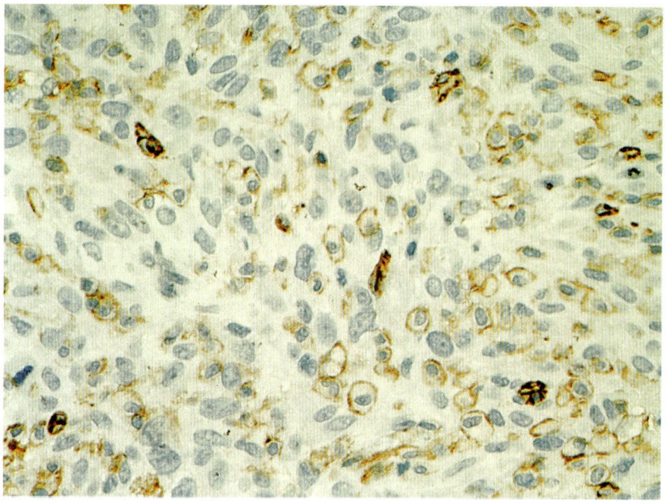

B

FIGURE 2.4 Epithelioid hemangioendothelioma showing strong and diffuse membranous staining for CD31 **(A)**. CD31 also may be expressed by histiocytes in nonendothelial sarcomas **(B)**.

angiosarcomas. It is especially useful for diagnosing poorly differentiated angiosarcomas with epithelioid cytology or poorly formed vascular channels in which nearly 90% show positivity for CD31.[42] In our practice, CD31 is the preferred marker for helping to confirm (or exclude) endothelial cell differentiation among poorly differentiated tumors (Fig. 2.4). Because CD31 is expressed by vascular and lymphatic endothelium, it is of no value in separating hemangiomas from lymphangiomas. Slone and coworkers[43] reported positivity for CD31 in the histiocytes of sinus histiocytosis with massive lymphadenopathy and Langerhans' cell histiocytosis.

CD34 (Human Hematopoietic Progenitor Cell Antigen)

CD34 is a heavily glycosylated, 110-kd transmembrane protein first identified in a myeloid leukemia cell line; the function of CD34 is unclear. Although CD34, similar to CD31, is expressed in endothelial cells, it is much less specific for endothelium. It is expressed in a variety of other cell types and tumors, including hematopoietic stem cells, interstitial cells of Cajal, cutaneous dendritic cells, smooth muscle cells, and neural elements.[44] As a result, immunoreactivity with anti-CD34 antibodies also is encountered in a histologically diverse subset of nonhematolymphoid neoplasms, including vascular tumors, solitary fibrous tumors, epithelioid sarcomas, spindle cell lipomas, dermatofibrosarcoma protuberans, myofibroblastomas, phyllodes tumor, fibroadenomas, pseudoangiomatous stromal hyperplasia of the breast, solitary fibrous tumor, and gastrointestinal stromal tumors (Table 2.4).[45-48] Despite its wide range of expression among many cell types, we have found CD34 diagnostically useful in the differential diagnoses of solitary fibrous tumor/hemangiopericytoma versus other mesenchymal lesions, spindle cell lipoma versus other fatty tumors, dermatofibrosarcoma protuberans (positive) versus dermatofibromas, epithelioid sarcoma (positive) versus metastatic carcinoma, and gastrointestinal stromal tumor (positive) versus leiomyoma/leiomyosarcoma. In all of these tumors, the cytoplasmic expression of CD34 is typically strong and diffuse (Fig. 2.5). Approximately 52% of epithelioid sarcomas express CD34, and coexpression of CD34 and cytokeratin may be helpful in ruling out carcinoma in the appropriate clinical setting.[48] Although CD34 is expressed

TABLE 2.4 Nonendothelial Soft Tissue Tumors that Commonly Show Diffuse and Strong CD34 Positivity

Spindle cell lipoma
Solitary fibrous tumor/hemangiopericytoma
Dermatofibrosarcoma protuberans
Gastrointestinal stromal tumor

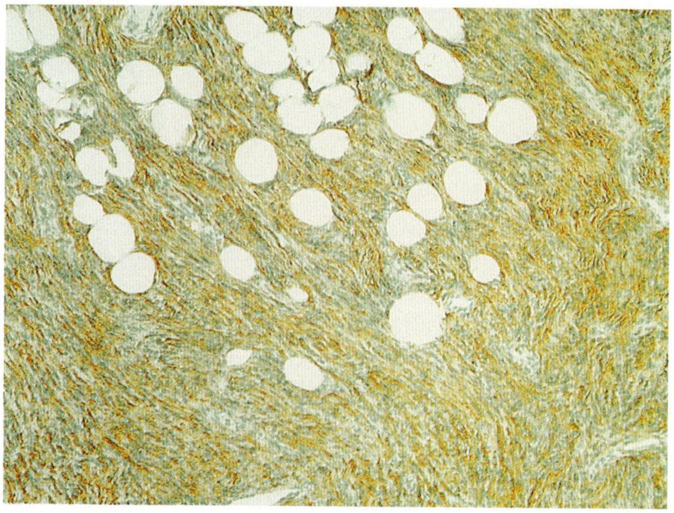

FIGURE 2.5 CD34 is a relatively nonspecific immunohistochemical marker. It may be useful in specific morphologic differential diagnostic scenarios, however, such as the distinction between dermatofibroma and dermatofibrosarcoma protuberans. The latter usually shows strong and diffuse CD34 positivity.

in greater than 90% of vascular (endothelial) tumors, it is of limited value in the diagnosis of vascular lesions because of its low specificity, particularly with regard to the aforementioned spindle cell tumors.[47] Epithelioid vascular neoplasms may express cytokeratins, and the coexpression of CD34 should prompt the use of more specific vascular markers, such as CD31 and factor VIII, to confirm (or exclude) the presence of endothelial differentiation.

Factor VIII (von Willebrand Factor)

Factor VIII–related antigen, also called *von Willebrand factor,* is a specific vascular marker expressed exclusively by endothelial cells. The value of factor VIII is limited owing to its low sensitivity, especially compared with CD31 and CD34, and the technical difficulties with immunohistochemical applications of antibodies against factor VIII. Factor VIII is a large polymeric protein that is packaged within Weibel-Palade bodies within endothelial cells. Because Weibel-Palade bodies rarely are observed in poorly differentiated angiosarcomas, the expression of factor VIII also is seen less commonly.[49] Consequently, in our laboratories, the use of factor VIII has been largely replaced by CD31.

Melanocytic Markers

HMB-45

HMB-45 is a monoclonal antibody that recognizes an epitope on the melanosome-specific oxidoreductive enzyme gp100. In this respect, HMB-45 is not specific to melanoma, but rather recognizes tumors that contain melanosomes. Because only melanosomes need to be present for its expression, HMB-45 immunoreactivity often is observed in clear cell sarcoma, psammomatous melanotic schwannoma, angiomyolipoma, clear cell tumors of the lung, and lymphangioleiomyomatosis. For this reason, HMB-45 may be diagnostically useful in some soft tissue tumors, and care should be taken not to consider HMB-45 as an absolutely specific melanoma marker. HMB-45 positivity is more specific than S-100 protein for melanoma but tends to be less sensitive, especially among spindle cell variants.[50] Most cases of desmoplastic melanoma do not show immunoexpression for HMB-45.[51,52]

Melan-A/MART-1

Melan-A, the product of the *MART-1* gene, is a component of the premelanosomal membrane and a cytoplasmic protein. Melan-A is a melanocytic differentiation antigen recognized by cytotoxic T cells; its expression first was described in the skin, retina, and melanocytic cell lines. Similar to HMB-45, Melan-A is a marker associated with the presence of melanosomes; however, Melan-A also stains normal melanocytes and benign nevi. Melan-A is positive in most cases of primary and metastatic malignant melanoma and some desmoplastic melanomas, but it is not absolutely specific for melanoma and may be observed in some angiomyolipomas, clear cell tumors of lung, clear cell sarcomas, adrenal cortical tumors, and sex-cord stromal tumors.[53]

Microphthalmia Transcription Factor

The microphthalmia transcription factor gene encodes a transcription factor that is involved in the development of melanocytes. Microphthalmia transcription factor is crucial for the embryonic development of melanocytes, providing for prolonged survival of melanocytes by transcriptional regulation of the pigmentation enzyme tyrosinase. It is expressed in resting melanocytes, benign nevi, and melanoma. Overall, microphthalmia transcription factor is a sensitive marker of melanoma and may be positive in some melanomas in which other markers are negative, such as desmoplastic melanoma. Microphthalmia transcription factor typically shows strong nuclear staining and variable cytoplasmic staining. Other tumors that frequently show microphthalmia transcription factor expression include clear cell sarcoma, melanotic schwannoma, and angiomyolipoma.[54]

Epithelial Membrane Antigen

Epithelial membrane antigen is a partially characterized antigen present on a glycoprotein expressed on the cell surface of a plethora of native epithelial cells, including breast, respiratory tract, salivary glands, pancreas, and urinary tract. Its staining pattern is typically membranous and only in this pattern (not diffuse cytoplasmic staining) is the antibody considered specific for epithelial differentiation. Epithelia not generally expressing epithelial membrane antigen include hepatocytes, adrenal cortical cells, prostatic acinar cells, follicular thyroid epithelium, germ cells, and the surface epithelium of the gastrointestinal tract. In soft tissue and nonepithelial elements, its expression is limited to the meninges, notochord, perineurial fibroblasts, and plasma cells. In practice, epithelial membrane antigen positivity may be seen in a broad range of sarcomas and sarcoma mimics, including the so-called sarcomatoid variant of anaplastic large cell lymphoma, mesothelioma, spindle cell hemangioma, meningioma, sclerosing perineurioma, malignant peripheral nerve sheath tumor, sarcomatoid variant of renal cell carcinoma, synovial sarcoma, and epithelioid sarcoma. In the appropriate clinical setting, the coexpression of epithelial membrane antigen and vimentin coupled with cytokeratin negativity helps confirm the diagnosis of ectopic meningioma.[55] Finally, it has been suggested that epithelial membrane antigen is more sensitive than cytokeratin for the diagnosis of synovial sarcoma, especially the poorly differentiated form.[56] For this reason, our immunohistochemical work-up for suspected cases of synovial sarcoma includes cytokeratin and epithelial membrane antigen.

S-100 Protein

S-100 protein is so named because of its solubility in 100% saturated ammonium sulfate. It is an acidic calcium-binding protein composed of two subunits, α and β. The combinations of these subunits define isotypes that have different tissue-specific distributions. The α-α isotype is present in skeletal muscle, myocardium, and neurons; the α-β isotype is present in chondrocytes, glial cells, melanocytes, and cutaneous adnexa; and the β-β isotype is present in Schwann's cells and Langerhans' cells. These tissue distributions are extensive and reflect the fact that S-100 protein expression can be observed in an extremely broad range of native cells and tumors. Overall, S-100 protein immunohistochemistry has a restricted role for the diagnosis of soft tissue tumors. It is probably best used for the differential diagnoses of cellular schwannoma versus malignant peripheral nerve sheath tumor and spindle cell or desmoplastic melanoma versus sarcoma. In our experience and that of others, schwannomas, including the cellular variant, express S-100 protein strongly and diffusely. In contrast, malignant peripheral nerve sheath tumors usually show patchy and focal S-100 protein expression and may be altogether negative in 50% of cases.[57,58] These immunohistochemical properties may be especially helpful in small biopsy specimens. As a general rule, one should avoid the diagnosis of malignancy in any cellular spindle cell lesion that is not obviously malignant (or anaplastic) and shows strong and diffuse S-100 protein positivity. Most of these cases are schwannomas. In an adult patient, an obviously malignant tumor that is diffusely and strongly S-100 protein positive should be considered malignant melanoma until proved otherwise. Because S-100 protein immunoreactivity is relatively nonspecific for the diagnosis of melanoma, the use of additional (more specific) melanocytic markers, such as HMB-45 or Melan-A, may help to confirm the diagnosis. In addition to melanoma and nerve sheath tumors, S-100 immunoreactivity commonly is observed in granular cell tumors, mixed tumors and myoepitheliomas/parachordomas, ossifying fibromyxoid tumor, adipocytic tumors, chondroid tumors, chordoma, and Langerhans' cell histiocytosis; focal positivity may be seen in synovial sarcoma, rhabdomyosarcoma, and leiomyosarcoma.[59-62] Cytoplasmic staining alone is considered nonspecific. To be diagnostically relevant, nuclear positivity with or without cytoplasmic expression should be present (Fig. 2.6).

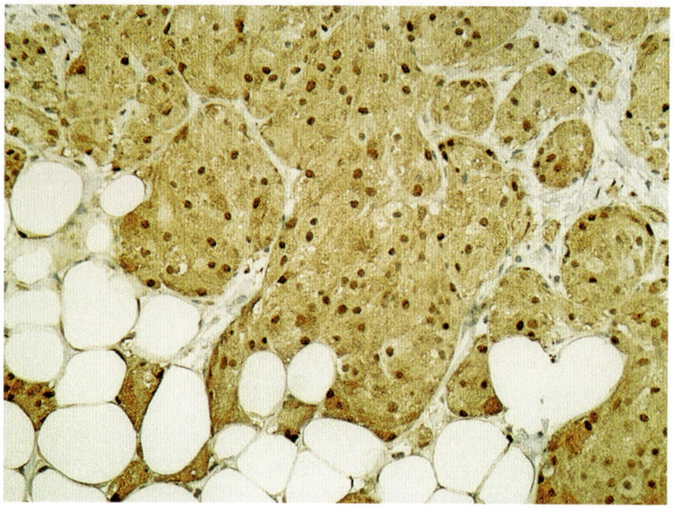

FIGURE 2.6 Granular cell tumors exhibit strong and diffuse, nuclear and cytoplasmic S-100 positivity.

Synaptophysin and Chromogranin

Synaptophysin and chromogranin are widely used "panendocrine" markers, and nearly all types of neuroendocrine tumors react with these antibodies. The chromogranin family of glycoproteins consists of three major categories, types A through C, which are located in the soluble fraction of neurosecretory granules. As such, chromogranin staining is observed in the cytoplasm of cells and usually in a granular-to-chunky pattern. Synaptophysin is a glycosylated transmembrane protein that is present in neuronal presynaptic vesicles. It is present in a broad variety of tumors of neuroectodermal and neuroendocrine derivation. When used among a panel of other immunohistochemical markers, chromogranin and synaptophysin may complement the histopathologic features and help support a more specific diagnosis. We use these markers most commonly for the separation of neuroblastoma (usually positive) from other pediatric small round cell tumors.

CD99

CD99 is the product of the *MIC2* gene and is a transmembrane glycoprotein expressed in varying degrees in almost all human tissues.[63] CD99 is expressed strongly and diffusely in greater than 90% of Ewing's sarcomas/primitive neuroectodermal tumors and typically shows prominent and characteristic membranous staining (Fig. 2.7). Although originally considered highly specific for the diagnosis of Ewing's sarcoma, CD99 since has been shown convincingly in a wide variety of tumors, including other small round cell sarcomas.[3-6] CD99 expression may be seen in more than 90% of lymphoblastic lymphomas and approximately 75% of mesenchymal chondrosarcomas.[3,4] One third of cases of desmoplastic small round cell tumor appear positive.[64] In the Intergroup Rhabdomyosarcoma Study Group data, approximately 14% of rhabdomyosarcomas expressed CD99.[65] Positivity for CD99 also has been documented in rare cases of small cell osteosarcoma.[3]

In the spindle cell tumor group, more than 75% of synovial sarcomas, including the poorly differentiated variant, express CD99, a finding that may be helpful in the distinction between synovial sarcoma and malignant peripheral nerve sheath tumor, which is almost always negative for this marker.[5,66] Most solitary fibrous tumors also appear positive for CD99.[67]

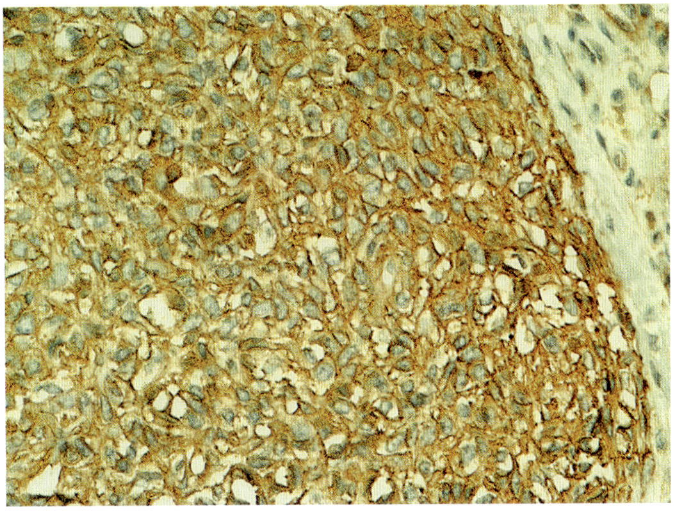

FIGURE 2.7 Most cases of Ewing's sarcoma/primitive neuroectodermal tumor exhibit strong and diffuse membranous CD99 positivity.

FLI-1

FLI-1 protein, a member of the erythroblastosis virus–associated transforming sequences family of DNA binding transcription factors, is involved in cellular proliferation and tumor genesis. Approximately 85% of Ewing's sarcoma/primitive neuroectodermal tumors have a relatively specific translocation, t(11;22)(q24;q12), involving the *EWS* gene on chromosome 22 and the *FLI-1* gene on chromosome 11, resulting in expression of the EWS-FLI-1 fusion protein. FLI-1 normally is expressed in endothelial cells and hematopoietic cells, including T lymphocytes. The chimeric EWS/FLI-1 fusion protein localizes to the nucleus, is a more powerful transcription activator than normal FLI-1, and is capable of transforming NIH 3T3 cells (fibroblasts). Although the gold standard for detecting this mutation is cytogenetic evaluation or molecular genetic studies, in practice, it is frequently difficult to obtain sufficient tissue, particularly in small biopsy specimens. Most community hospitals are not equipped to perform these tests, and most rely on reference laboratories to perform these studies. For these reasons, immunohistochemical analysis of FLI-1 expression may be a viable alternative to cytogenetics and molecular genetic analyses in the appropriate clinical context. Immunohistochemistry for the carboxy-terminus of FLI-1 protein has been shown to have a sensitivity of 71% and specificity of 92% for Ewing's sarcoma.[68] Among small round blue cell tumors, FLI-1 is frequently positive in lymphoblastic lymphoma, a potential pitfall because many cases of lymphoblastic lymphoma also may be negative for routine hematopoietic markers. Rare cases of desmoplastic small round cell tumor may show focal nuclear positivity. Although FLI-1 immunohistochemistry may be useful in the setting of small round cell tumors, it is not limited to this differential diagnosis. As mentioned previously, FLI-1 is expressed in vascular endothelium, and its sensitivity at detecting vascular neoplasms, including angiosarcoma, hemangioendotheliomas, hemangiomas, and Kaposi's sarcoma, approaches CD31 and likely exceeds CD34 and factor VIII.[69] Because FLI-1 is expressed in the nucleus, its interpretation is less likely to be hampered by potential artifacts caused by endogenous cytoplasmic peroxidase and biotin.

WT1

The *WT1* gene encodes a transcription factor that expresses at least eight protein isoforms that originally were recognized as tumor suppressors. *WT1* normally is expressed in the nuclei of mesothelial cells, glomerular podocytes, and CD34-positive stem cells.[70-72] Numerous human malignancies have been identified that express *WT1*, including hematologic tumors, mesothelial tumors, breast carcinomas, genitourinary tumors, and small round blue cell tumors.[73-78] More specifically, the antibody 6F-H2 derived from the N-terminus of *WT1* has been used mostly in the evaluation of small round blue cell tumors. Other antibodies directed against the C-terminus (C-19) have been reported and may have different staining characteristics.[78] Most (60% to 100%) desmoplastic small round cell tumors and most cases of Wilms' tumor show strong nuclear staining.[78,79] Conversely, *WT1* has shown a high sensitivity in rhabdomyosarcoma, in which it typically shows strong cytoplasmic staining in nearly all cases; nuclear staining is observed less commonly and tends to be focal in rhabdomyosarcoma.[77,78] Wilms' tumors typically stain in the nucleus or the cytoplasm of the epithelial, blastemal, or stromal cellular components. Nuclear staining seems to be confined to the blastemal and epithelial component in more than 50% of cases, whereas the cytoplasmic pattern is often confined to the stromal component, where it is expressed weakly in approximately 75% of cases. When heterologous (e.g., skeletal muscle) differentiation is observed in Wilms' tumor, strong cytoplasmic staining of *WT1* almost always is observed in these areas.[77] Lymphoblastic lymphomas also are frequently positive for *WT1*, exhibiting strong nuclear staining. In addition, other small round blue cell tumors rarely show weak positivity using 6F-H2 and include neuroblastoma, Burkitt's lymphoma, and anaplastic large cell lymphoma.[77] Ewing's sarcomas/primitive neuroectodermal tumors are uniformly negative.[78,79]

CD117

CD117, the c-kit proto-oncogene product, has a role in the development of mast cells, melanocytes, germ cells, and interstitial cells of Cajal. The last-mentioned cells are involved with regulating gut motility and coexpress CD34 and CD117. Consequently, CD117 has been found to be useful for the diagnosis of gastrointestinal stromal tumor and its separation from smooth muscle tumors of the gastrointestinal tract. Most (but not all) gastrointestinal stromal tumors appear positive for CD117 (cytoplasmic staining),

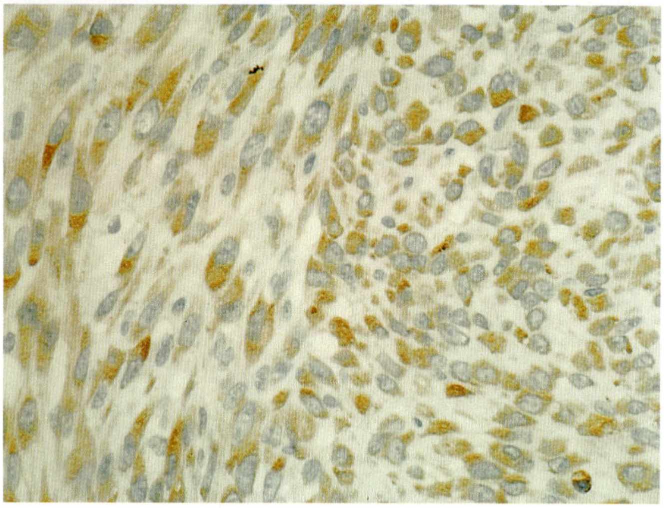

FIGURE 2.8 Strong and diffuse membranous-to-cytoplasmic CD117 (c-kit) expression is seen in most gastrointestinal stromal tumors.

and activating mutations of c-kit are usually present.[80,81] The expression of this marker has therapeutic implications. Imatinib mesylate (Gleevec) blocks the receptor tyrosine kinase function of c-kit and appears effective in the treatment of gastrointestinal stromal tumors. The diagnostic usefulness of CD117 is limited because most angiosarcomas, intra-abdominal fibromatoses, angiomyolipomas, and many melanomas also express CD117.[82-84] Kaposi's sarcoma shows positive staining in occasional examples. Smooth muscle tumors and schwannomas are generally negative. The therapeutic implications of positive staining in mesenchymal neoplasias outside of the setting of gastrointestinal stromal tumor are unclear. Gastrointestinal stromal tumor is not discussed in this book and may best be considered in specific gastrointestinal pathology texts. Because the diagnosis of gastrointestinal stromal tumor often is considered in the differential diagnosis of other mesenchymal neoplasms, however, we believe the topic of CD117 should be addressed. For suspected cases of gastrointestinal stromal tumor, we perform CD117, CD34, smooth muscle actin, and desmin immunohistochemistry (Fig. 2.8). The latter two markers are generally negative in gastrointestinal stromal tumors but usually expressed by smooth muscle neoplasms.

Prognostic and Cell Cycle Markers

Numerous cell cycle markers have been studied in an attempt to identify the usefulness of these markers for the diagnosis and prognostication of sarcomas. Among other functions, p53 arrests cells in the G_1 phase of the cell cycle after DNA damage has occurred. Mutations in the p53 gene result in loss of normal protein function in conjunction with an increased protein half-life and subsequent detectable levels of accumulated p53 protein in the nucleus. Many studies have examined expression patterns of p53 in sarcomas, and overexpression has been observed in 57% of sarcomas.[85] p53 overexpression has been associated with increased tumor grade and, independent of tumor grade, does not seem to correlate with poor survival. In difficult cases, p53 overexpression may be a useful adjunct to distinguish neurofibroma from malignant peripheral nerve sheath tumor. Nuclear immunopositivity for p53 is usually not observed in neurofibromas. Conversely, most malignant peripheral nerve sheath tumors, especially high-grade forms, appear positive for p53 (>20% nuclear staining).[86]

Proliferating cell nuclear antigen (PCNA), Ki-67, is expressed in the nucleus during the active phases of the cell cycle but is absent in the resting phase (G_0). MIB-1 is the most commonly used antibody for the detection of Ki-67 nuclear antigen expression in formalin-fixed tissue and reflects the proliferative activity of tumors. Because Ki-67 is a general marker for cell proliferation, it is not useful for the classification of bone and soft tissue tumors. It may be helpful, however, for histologic grading. A reproducible grading scheme using a modified version of the French Federation of Cancer Centers Sarcoma Group grading system, in which the mitotic count is replaced with a MIB-1 labeling index, has been proposed.[87] Using this grading system, univariate analysis showed statistically significant differences in overall survival when MIB-1 labeling indices of 0% to 9%, 10% to 29%, and 30% or greater were used to separate mitotic grades 1, 2, and 3.[88] Although this grading system may not replace the conventional FNCLCC system, it does illustrate the potential application of Ki-67.

Numerous other markers, including p16, $p21^{WAF1}$, $p27^{kip}$, MDM2, and cyclin D1, have been evaluated in bone and soft tissue tumors. As of yet, no prognostic significance has been correlated with these markers.[85,89,90]

Conventional Cytogenetics and Molecular Genetics

Ewing's Sarcoma/Primitive Neuroectodermal Tumor

Ewing's sarcoma/primitive neuroectodermal tumor is associated with two common and several rare reciprocal translocations that have in common the presence of the *EWS* gene on chromosome band 22q12 combined with genes from different members of the ETS family of transcription factors. The most common of these, t(11;22)(q24;q12), is present in nearly 85% of cases and results in a fusion protein composed of the 5′ end of the *EWS* gene and the 3′ end of the ETF family gene *FLI1* (EWS-FLI1) (Fig. 2.9). The second most common is t(21;22)(q22;q12), which involves the same segment of the *EWS* gene combined with the 3′ end of the ETF family gene *ERG*. Finally, in a few cases, t(7;22), t(17;22), t(2;22), and inv(22) have been described, in which the *EWS* gene combines with ETS family genes *ETV1*,

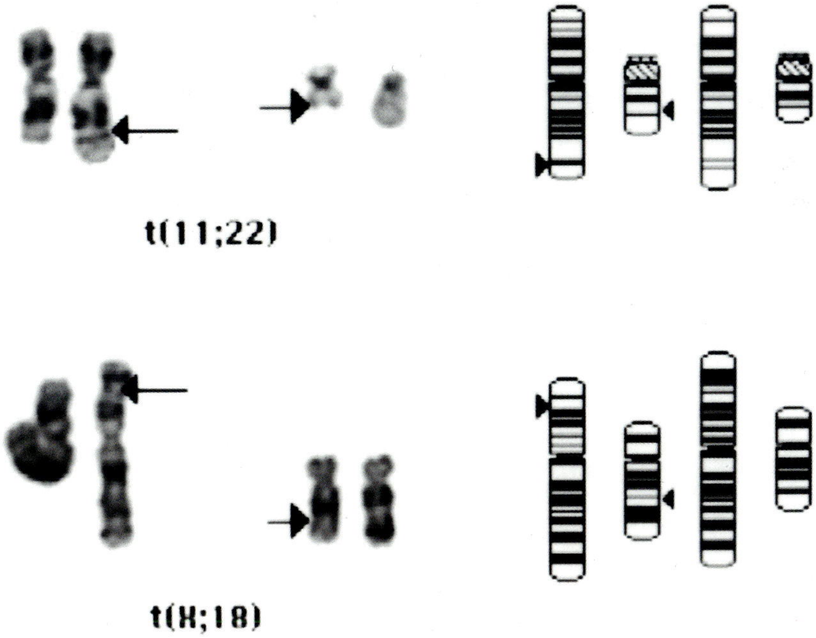

FIGURE 2.9 Cytogenetic analysis showing t(11;22)(q24;q12) in a Ewing's sarcoma *(top)* and t(X;18)(p11;q11) in a synovial sarcoma. Both of these confirmatory karyotypes were obtained from fine needle aspiration biopsy specimens. (From Kilpatrick SE, et al: The role of fine needle aspiration biopsy in the initial diagnosis of pediatric bone and soft tissue tumors: An institutional experience. Mod Pathol 1998;11:923.)

E1AF, FEV, and *ZSG*.[91,92] In addition, secondary chromosomal aberrations involving gains in 1q and chromosomes 8 and 12 may be seen in 50% of cases of Ewing's sarcoma.[93] Despite these aberrations, it is clear that the driving force behind Ewing's sarcoma is the presence of a fusion gene between *EWS* and one of several ETS family genes. It is not clear how the chimeric fusion proteins result in tumorigenesis. It has been suggested that increased transcription activation by EWS may result in down-regulation of the putative tumor suppressor transforming growth factor-β type II, providing Ewing's sarcoma cells a means to avoid programmed cell death.[91,92] Other putative targets include inactivation of INK4, a locus that encodes the cell cycle inhibitor CDKN2A. As previously mentioned, the most frequent Ewing's sarcoma translocation, t(11;22)(q24;q12) with the EWS-FLI1 fusion product, has been reported in phenotypically classic examples of mesenchymal chondrosarcoma, embryonal and alveolar rhabdomyosarcoma, polyphenotypic tumor of childhood, and neuroblastoma.[9-12]

Rhabdomyosarcoma

Alveolar Rhabdomyosarcoma

Alveolar rhabdomyosarcoma is associated with two common and highly specific reciprocal translocations, both of which involve the *FKHR* gene on chromosome 13. The most common cytogenetic abnormality is the t(2;13)(q35;q14) that juxtaposes the *PAX3* gene with the *FKHR* gene. Less frequently, t(1;13)(p36;q14) is observed and involves fusion of the *PAX7* gene with the *FKHR* gene. These translocations create chimeric genes that combine the *PAX3/PAX7* DNA binding domain and the *FKHR* transcriptional activation domain.[94,95] The resulting fusion products function as powerful transcriptional activators and, through complex mechanisms, may impose additional oncogenic effects by deregulating cell proliferation, apoptosis, and cell differentiation. In addition to the reciprocal translocations mentioned previously, other more complex molecular aberrations resulting in genetic amplification have been discovered by comparative genomic hybridization studies in alveolar rhabdomyosarcoma.[96] Investigators have focused on the prognostic significance of these fusion products; among patients presenting with metastatic alveolar rhabdomyosarcoma, PAX3-FKHR and PAX7-FKHR fusion transcripts seem to represent high-risk subgroups (worse survival) and favorable outcome subgroups, respectively.[97] Finally, although demonstration of these specific molecular alterations can be performed by conventional cytogenetics or reverse transcriptase (RT)–PCR, a subset (approximately 20%) of alveolar rhabdomyosarcomas do not contain either of these translocations and may harbor other less well characterized molecular alterations.[97]

Embryonal Rhabdomyosarcoma

Complex (but nonspecific) genetic, structural, and numerical alterations have been identified in embryonal rhabdomyosarcoma by conventional cytogenetics and commonly include gains in chromosomes 2, 8, and 20 and rare rearrangements involving 1p11-q11 and 12q13. The application of comparative genomic hybridization has confirmed these findings in addition to showing numerous additional chromosomal gains and losses.[98] Molecular genetic studies have identified alterations in known tumor-suppressor genes and oncogenes and genomic amplification in certain subsets of embryonal rhabdomyosarcoma. Furthermore, loss of chromosomal material in the 11p15 region may be observed in embryonal rhabdomyosarcoma. The significance of this finding is supported by the fact that introduction of chromosomal material from this region into embryonal rhabdomyosarcoma cell lines may result in growth inhibition.[99] Several putative tumor suppressors have been identified in the 11p15 region and may contribute to tumorigenesis through a complex mechanism involving parental allelic inactivation "imprinting" coupled with mechanical loss of the active allele.[100] Although these findings may provide insight into the biology of embryonal rhabdomyosarcoma, there exist no specific and diagnostically useful chromosomal aberrations or translocations.

Desmoplastic Small Round Cell Tumor

Desmoplastic small round cell tumor is associated with a highly specific reciprocal translocation t(11;22)(p13;q12), resulting in juxtaposition of the *EWS* gene on 22q12 with the *WT1* gene on 11p13.[101] Most commonly, an in-frame fusion of *EWS* exons 1 through 7 with *WT1* exons 8 through 10 is observed, although several different breakpoints have been described. The common resulting fusion gene encodes the putative transcription modulation domain of *EWS* and three *WT1* zinc-finger binding domains. The role of this fusion protein in the tumorigenesis of desmoplastic small round cell tumor is not disputed; t(11;22)(p13;q12) is a sensitive and specific marker for desmoplastic small round cell tumor and is identified easily by conventional cytogenetics.[102] The fusion transcripts can be identified in tumors using any of a number of molecular biologic techniques. Detection of these transcripts in ascites fluid by RT-PCR also has been described.[103]

Clear Cell Sarcoma (Melanoma of Soft Parts)

Clear cell sarcoma has a characteristic reciprocal translocation t(12;22)(q13;q12), present in most cases. This translocation juxtaposes the *EWS* (22q12) and *ATF* (12q13) genes and results in a fusion protein composed of the N-terminal domain of *EWS* and the *ATF1* bZIP domain. This most commonly creates an in-frame fusion of *EWS* exon 8 to *ATF1* codon 65.[104] *ATF1* is an active transcription factor that binds to cAMP inducible promoters, and the EWS/ATF fusion alters the function of *ATF1* such that it serves as a constitutive transcriptional activator that represses TP53/CBP-mediated transactivation.[105,106] Additional nonspecific chromosomal aberrations may occur in clear cell sarcoma and include gains in chromosomes 7 and 8 and alterations in chromosome 22 that do not include t(12;22). Because there is considerable overlap between the histologic features and immunophenotype of clear cell sarcoma and cutaneous malignant melanoma, demonstration of t(12;22) and its associated fusion transcript by conventional cytogenetics or molecular genetic studies can be valuable for confirming the diagnosis of clear cell sarcoma. To our knowledge, t(12;22) has never been shown in cutaneous melanoma. Demonstration of the melanocyte-specific splice form of microphthalmia transcription factor in clear cell sarcoma has been identified using RT-PCR.[104] Although microphthalmia transcription factor transcripts support the melanocytic differentiation of clear cell sarcoma, they do not aid in its distinction from melanoma.

Extraskeletal Myxoid Chondrosarcoma

Although bona fide examples of primary skeletal forms with cytogenetic confirmation exist, extraskeletal myxoid chondrosarcoma appears to be a separate entity from conventional "myxoid" skeletal chondrosarcomas as evidenced by a relatively specific translocation, t(9;22)(q22;q12) in more than 50% of cases.[107,108] The translocation t(9;22)(q22;q12) results in a fusion transcript involving the *CHN* (or *TEC*) gene on 9q22 and the *EWS* gene on 22q12. The resulting chimeric gene activates transcription of target genes that are linked to cellular proliferation.[109] In addition, multiple other complex chromosomal aberrations have been described in extraskeletal myxoid chondrosarcoma, either independent or in addition to t(9;22). Less commonly, another apparently unique reciprocal translocation t(9;17)(q22;q11) is observed in extraskeletal myxoid chondrosarcoma. The translocation t(9;17)(q22;q11) results in fusion of *NR4A3* (9q22) with *RBP56* (17q11).[110,111] The resultant fusion proteins from both of these translocations seem to have a similar degree of oncogenicity when *EWS* and *RBP56* are combined with their respective transcription factors. A single case report of t(9;15)(q22;q21) resulting in fusion of *TCF12* (9q22) and *NR4A3* (15q21) has been described in an extraskeletal myxoid chondrosarcoma.[112]

Myxoid and Round Cell Liposarcoma

Myxoid and round cell liposarcomas are associated with a reciprocal translocation t(12;16)(q13;p11) that is present in more than 90% of cases, providing further evidence that these tumors likely represent a spectrum of a similar neoplasm. The translocation results in a fusion product consisting of the *CHOP* (12q13) and the *FUS* (16p11) genes.[113,114] Three common breakpoints in the *FUS* gene (exons 5, 7, and 8) may combine with the *CHOP* (exon 2) breakpoint, resulting in three possible in-frame fusion genes depending on the breakpoint in the *FUS* gene. Demonstration of FUS/CHOP by conventional cytogenetic analysis or molecular biologic techniques is highly sensitive and specific for the diagnosis of myxoid/round cell liposarcoma. Rarely, translocations involving chromosomes 12 and 22, t(12;22)(q13;q12), may be observed in myxoid/round cell liposarcoma.[115]

Well-Differentiated Liposarcoma (Atypical Lipoma)

Well-differentiated liposarcoma (atypical lipoma) has been shown to contain supernumerary ring (circular) or giant (rod) marker chromosomes in more than 60% of cases and frequently shows amplification of 12q15-21, 12q13-15, and 12q21.[116,117] The *MDM2* and *CDK4* genes are housed in the 12q14-15 region and frequently are amplified in well-differentiated liposarcoma.[118] To our knowledge, the cytogenetic structural abnormalities with the 12q15-21, 12q13-15, or 12q21 amplifications have not been reported in benign adipocytic tumors, and demonstrations of their presence may be helpful in distinguishing lipoma from well-differentiated liposarcoma.

Synovial Sarcoma

Synovial sarcoma shows the reciprocal translocation t(X;18)(p11;q11) in more than 90% of cases (see Fig. 2.9). This translocation may be the only identifiable cytogenetic aberration, or it may be seen in conjunction with other chromosomal aberrations, including gains in chromosomes 7, 8, and 12 and with monosomy chromosome 3. The t(X;18) results in fusion of the *SYT* gene (18q11) with one of three related but distinct X-chromosomal gene subsets, including *SSX1*, *SSX2*, or, rarely, *SSX4*.[119-121] Kawai and colleagues[122] documented an association between synovial sarcoma subtype (biphasic versus monophasic) and the SYT-SSX subtype; biphasic tumors exclusively harbored the SYT-SSX1 rearrangement, whereas monophasic fibrous types predominantly had the SYT-SSX2 rearrangement. Other investigators have not shown such a relationship, however.[123] O'Sullivan and colleagues[124] at Washington University Medical Center evaluated RNA extracted from 34 synovial sarcoma specimens and 20 malignant peripheral nerve sheath tumors for the presence of the t(X;18) by RT-PCR. Approximately 85% of synovial sarcomas and 75% of malignant peripheral nerve sheath tumors showed the translocations. Of the 15 cases of malignant peripheral nerve sheath tumors bearing the translocation, 3 represented malignant Triton tumors, and 6 arose in patients with neurofibromatosis. The results could not be attributed to diagnostic inaccuracies because "diagnoses were based on well-established morphologic, immunohistochemical, and EM [electron microscopy] criteria, and were carefully scrutinized because synovial sarcoma, especially the monophasic variant, and MPNST [malignant peripheral nerve sheath tumor] have substantial morphologic and immunophenotypic overlap."[124]

Synovial sarcomas containing the SYT-SSX1-type fusion may be associated with a worse prognosis than sarcomas harboring the SYT-SSX2 subtype.[122,123] Inagaki and coworkers[123] documented a statistically significant relationship between the SYT-SSX1 fusion and high Ki-67 expression and a high mitotic rate, suggesting that the SYT-SSX fusion subtype is associated with the tumor cell proliferative activity. A more recent multi-institutional study of 182 cases of synovial sarcoma found no correlation between SYT-SSX subtype and patient outcome.[125]

Extrarenal Rhabdoid Tumor

Extrarenal rhabdoid tumor is associated with aberrations of chromosome 22q11.2, most commonly deletions. In addition, reciprocal translocations occasionally may be seen involving 22q11.2 and numerous other chromosomes. Homozygous deletions and mutations in the *SMARCB1* (hSNF5, INI1) gene, located at 22q11.2, have been identified in most extrarenal rhabdoid tumors.[126-128] *SMARCB1* is a tumor-suppressor gene that frequently shows homozygous deletions in extrarenal rhabdoid tumors, particularly those associated with additional chromosomal translocations. *SMARCB1* deletions and mutations are not specific for extrarenal soft tissue rhabdoid tumors, however, and may be observed in renal and central nervous system rhabdoid tumors, medulloblastoma, choroid plexus carcinoma, glioblastoma, and occasionally rhabdomyosarcomas.[129,130]

Alveolar Soft Part Sarcoma

Alveolar soft part sarcoma is associated with a specific unbalanced cytogenetic aberration, der(17)t(X;17)(p11;q25).[131] It has been shown that this cytogenetic translocation results in fusion of the *TFE3* (Xp11) gene, a member of the microphthalmia transcription factor family, with a novel gene, *ASPL* (17q25).[132] It has been postulated that this fusion product promotes oncogenesis by transcriptional deregulation, and the fusion proteins' nuclear localization tends to support this hypothesis. Although the presence of the ASPL/TFE3 fusion product has high sensitivity and specificity for the diagnosis of alveolar soft part sarcoma, rare renal cell neoplasms also may show these aberrations, and care always should be taken to interpret these findings in the appropriate clinical context.[133]

Epithelioid Hemangioendothelioma

Epithelioid hemangioendothelioma has been associated with a reciprocal translocation, t(1;3)(p36.3;q25), in two cases.[134] Although the potential for this to represent a specific molecular alteration in epithelioid hemangioendothelioma must be considered, larger studies are needed to confirm these findings, and specific genetic fusion products have yet to be characterized. In addition, Boudousquie and colleagues[135] described an epithelioid hemangioendothelioma arising in the back of a 45-year-old man with pulmonary and bone marrow metastases and a karyotype that revealed clonal abnormalities: a complex unbalanced t(7;22) involving multiple breakpoints, a robertsonian t(14;14), and loss of the Y chromosome.

Infantile Fibrosarcoma

Infantile fibrosarcomas are associated with a reciprocal translocation t(12;15)(p13;q26) that appears fairly specific for this tumor. The translocation results in juxtaposition of the tyrosine kinase receptor gene, *NTRK3* (15q26), with the *ETV6* (12p13) gene. The resultant fusion protein, ETV6/NTRK3, contains the N-terminal *ETV6* and the kinase domain of *NTRK3* and has active tyrosine kinase activity that results in oncogenic activation. The fusion transcripts can be detected by RT-PCR, fluorescence in situ hybridization, and conventional cytogenetic analysis, although it has been reported that the translocation may be difficult to detect using conventional cytogenetic banding techniques because the regions exchanged between chromosomes 12 and 15 are similar in size and banding characteristics.[136,137] In addition to this characteristic translocation, gains in chromosomes 8, 11, 17, and 20 commonly are observed in infantile fibrosarcoma and likely represent later events.[136]

REFERENCES

1. Ladanyi M: The emerging molecular genetics of sarcoma translocation. Diagn Mol Pathol 1995;4:162.
2. Fletcher JA: Cytogenetics and molecular biology of soft tissue tumors. In Weiss SW, Brooks JSJ (eds): Soft Tissue Tumors. Monographs in Pathology; No. 38. Philadelphia: Williams & Wilkins, 1996, pp 37-64.
3. Stevenson AJ, Chatten J, Bertoni F, et al: CD99 (p30/32^{MIC2}) neuroectodermal/Ewing's sarcoma antigen as an immunohistochemical marker: Review of more than 600 tumors and the literature experience. Appl Immunohistochem 1994;2:231.
4. Granter SR, Renshaw AA, Fletcher CD, et al: CD99 reactivity in mesenchymal chondrosarcoma. Hum Pathol 1996;27:1273.
5. Dei Tos AP, Wadden C, Calonje E, et al: Immunohistochemical demonstration of glycoprotein p30/32 MIC2 (CD99) in synovial sarcoma: A potential cause of diagnostic confusion. Appl Immunohistochem 1995;3:168.
6. Dehner LP: On trial: A malignant small cell tumor in a child: Four wrongs do not make a right. Am J Clin Pathol 1998;109:662.
7. Miettinen M, Rapola J: Immunohistochemical spectrum of rhabdomyosarcoma and rhabdomyosarcoma-like tumors: Expression of cytokeratin and the 68-kD neurofilament protein. Am J Surg Pathol 1989;13:120.
8. Folpe AL, Patterson K, Gown AM: Antibodies to desmin identify the blastemal component of nephroblastoma. Mod Pathol 1997;10:895.
9. Thorner P, Squire J, Chilton-McNeill S, et al: Is the EWS/FLI-1 fusion transcript specific for Ewing's sarcoma and peripheral primitive neuroectodermal tumor? A report of four cases showing this transcript in a wider range of tumor types. Am J Pathol 1996;148:1577.
10. Sorenson PHB, Shimada H, Liu XF, et al: Biphenotypic sarcomas with myogenic and neural differentiation express the Ewing's sarcoma EWS/FLI1 fusion gene. Cancer Res 1995;55:1385.
11. Burchill SA, Wheeldon J, Cullinane C, et al: EWS-FLI-1 fusion transcripts identified in patients with typical neuroblastoma. Eur J Cancer 1997;33:239.
12. Sainati L, Scapinello A, Montaldi A, et al: A mesenchymal chondrosarcoma of a child with the reciprocal translocation (11;22)(q24;q12). Cancer Genet Cytogenet 1993;71:144.
13. Ordi J, de Alava E, Torne A, et al: Intraabdominal desmoplastic small round cell tumor with the EWS/ERG fusion transcript. Am J Surg Pathol 1998;22:1026.
14. Katz RL, Quezado M, Senderowicz AM, et al: An intra-abdominal small round cell neoplasm with features of primitive neuroectodermal and desmoplastic round cell tumor and a EWS/FLI-1 fusion transcript. Hum Pathol 1997;28:502.
15. Gown AM, Boyd HC, Chang Y, et al: Smooth muscle cells can express cytokeratins of "simple" epithelium: Immunocytochemical and biochemical studies in vitro and in vivo. Am J Pathol 1988;132:223.
16. Ramaekers FC, Pruszczynski M, Smedts F: Cytokeratins in smooth muscle cells and smooth muscle tumours. Histopathology 1988;12:558.
17. Tauchi K, Tsutsumi Y, Yoshimura S, et al: Immunohistochemical and immunoblotting detections of cytokeratin in smooth muscle tumors. Acta Pathol Jpn 1990;40:574.
18. Zarbo RJ, Gown AM, Nagle RB, et al: Anomalous cytokeratin expression in malignant melanoma: One- and two-dimensional Western blot analysis and immunohistochemical survey of 100 melanomas. Mod Pathol 1990;3:494.
19. Meis-Kindblom JM, Kindblom LG: Angiosarcoma of soft tissue: A study of 80 cases. Am J Surg Pathol 1998;22:683.
20. Rosenberg AE, O'Connel JX, Dickersin GR, et al: Expression of epithelial markers in malignant fibrous histiocytoma of the musculoskeletal system: An immunohistochemical and electron microscopic study. Hum Pathol 1993;24:284.
21. Dardick I, Schatz JE, Colgan TJ: Osteogenic sarcoma with epithelial differentiation. Ultrastruct Pathol 1992;16:463.
22. Judkins AR, Montone KT, LiVolsi VA, et al: Sensitivity and specificity of antibodies on necrotic tumor tissue. Am J Clin Pathol 1998;110:641.
23. Viale G, Dell'Orto R, Coggi G, et al: Co-expression of cytokeratins and vimentin in normal and diseased thyroid glands: Lack of diagnostic utility of vimentin immunostaining. Am J Surg Pathol 1989;13:1034.
24. Azumi N, Battifora H: The distribution of vimentin and keratin in epithelial and nonepithelial neoplasms: A comprehensive immunohistochemical study on formalin and alcohol-fixed tumors. Am J Clin Pathol 1987;88:286.
25. Thompson LDR, Wieneke JA, Miettinen M, et al: Spindle cell (sarcomatous) carcinomas of the larynx: Clinicopathologic study of 187 cases. Am J Surg Pathol 2002;26:153.
26. Jones EC, Young RH: Myxoid and sclerosing sarcomatoid transitional cell carcinoma of the urinary bladder: A clinicopathologic and immunohistochemical study of 25 cases. Mod Pathol 1997;10:908.
27. Iczkowski JA, Shanks JH, Gadaleanu V, et al: Inflammatory pseudotumor and sarcoma of urinary bladder: Differential diagnosis and outcome in thirty-eight spindle cell neoplasms. Mod Pathol 2001;14:1043.
28. Gobbi H, Simpson JF, Borowsky A, et al: Metaplastic breast tumors with a dominant fibromatosis-like phenotype have a high risk of local recurrence. Cancer 1999;85:2170.
29. Lewis JE, Olsen KD, Sebo TJ: Spindle cell carcinoma of the larynx: Review of 26 cases including DNA content and immunohistochemistry. Hum Pathol 1997;28:664.
30. Nishihara K, Tsuneyoshi M: Undifferentiated spindle cell carcinoma of the gallbladder: A clinicopathologic, immunohistochemical, and flow cytometric study of 11 cases. Hum Pathol 1993;24:1298.
31. Hurliman J: Desmin and neural marker expression in mesothelial cells and mesotheliomas. Hum Pathol 1994;25:753.
32. Franquemont DW, Frierson HF Jr, Mills SE: An immunohistochemical study of normal endometrial stroma and endometrial stromal neoplasms: Evidence for smooth muscle differentiation. Am J Surg Pathol 1991;15:861.
33. Andriko JW, Kaldjian EP, Tsokos M, et al: Reticulum cell neoplasms of lymph nodes: A clinicopathologic study of 11 cases with recognition of a new subtype derived from fibroblastic reticular cells. Am J Surg Pathol 1998;22:1048.
34. Van Muijen GN, Rulter DJ, Wamaar SO: Co-expression of intermediate filament polypeptides in human fetal and adult tissues. Lab Invest 1987;57:359.

35. Folpe AL, Weiss SW, Fletcher CDM, et al: Tenosynovial giant cell tumors: Evidence for desmin-positive dendritic cell subpopulation. Mod Pathol 1998;11:939.
36. Ordonez NG: Desmoplastic small round cell tumor: II. An ultrastructural and immunohistochemical study with emphasis on new immunohistochemical markers. Am J Surg Pathol 1998;22:1314.
37. Sugimoto T, Mine H, Horii Y, et al: Neuroblastoma cell lines showing smooth muscle cell phenotypes. Diagn Mol Pathol 2000;9:221.
38. Parham DM, Dias P, Kelly DR, et al: Desmin positivity in primitive neuroectodermal tumors of childhood. Am J Surg Pathol 1992;16:483.
39. Furlong MA, Mentzel T, Fanburg-Smith JC: Pleomorphic rhabdomyosarcoma in adults: Clinicopathologic study of 38 cases with emphasis on morphologic variants and recent skeletal muscle-specific markers. Mod Pathol 2001;14:595.
40. Cessna MH, Zhou H, Perkins SL, et al: Are myogenin and myoD1 expression specific for rhabdomyosarcoma? A study of 150 cases, with emphasis on spindle cell mimics. Am J Surg Pathol 2001;25:1150.
41. Wang NP, Marx J, McNutt MA, et al: Expression of myogenic regulatory proteins (myogenin and myoD1) in small blue round cell tumors of childhood. Am J Pathol 1995;147:1799.
42. De Young BR, Frierson HF, Ly MN, et al: CD31 immunoreactivity in carcinomas and mesotheliomas. Am J Clin Pathol 1988;110:374.
43. Slone SP, Fleming DR, Buchino JJ: Sinus histiocytosis with massive lymphadenopathy and Langerhans cell histiocytosis express the cellular adhesion molecule CD31. Arch Pathol Lab Med 2003;127:341.
44. van de Rijn M, Rouse R: CD34: A review. Appl Immunhistochem 1994;2:71.
45. Natkunam Y, Rouse RV, Zhu S, et al: Immunoblot analysis of CD34 expression in histologically diverse neoplasms. Am J Pathol 2000;156:21.
46. Suster S, Fisher C: Immunoreactivity for the human hematopoietic progenitor cell antigen (CD34) in lipomatous tumors. Am J Surg Pathol 1997;21:195.
47. Miettinen M, Lindenmeyer AE, Chaubal A: Endothelial cell markers CD31, CD34, and BNH9 antibody to H- and Y-antigens: Their specificity and sensitivity in the diagnosis of vascular tumors and comparison with von Willebrand factor. Mod Pathol 1994;7:82.
48. Miettinen M, Fanburg-Smith JC, Virolainen M, et al: Epithelioid sarcoma: An immunohistochemical analysis of 112 classical and variant cases and a discussion of the differential diagnosis. Hum Pathol 1999;30:934.
49. Swanson PE, Wick MR: Immunohistochemical evaluation of vascular neoplasms. Clin Dermatol 1991;9:243.
50. Gown AM, Vogel AM, Hoak D, et al: Monoclonal antibodies specific for melanocytic tumors distinguishing subpopulations of melanocytes. Am J Pathol 1986;123:195.
51. Carlson JA, Dickersin GR, Sober AJ, et al: Desmoplastic neurotropic melanoma: A clinicopathologic analysis of 28 cases. Cancer 1995;75:478.
52. Anstey A, Cerio R, Ramnarain N, et al: Desmoplastic malignant melanoma: An immunocytochemical study of 25 cases. Am J Dermatopathol 1994;16:14.
53. Busam KJ, Jungbluth AA: Melan-A, a new melanocytic differentiation marker. Adv Anat Pathol 1999;6:12.
54. Chang KL, Folpe AL: Diagnostic utility of microphthalmia transcription factor in malignant melanoma and other tumors. Adv Anat Pathol 2001;8:273.
55. Schnitt SJ, Vogel H: Meningiomas: Diagnostic value of immunoperoxidase staining for epithelial membrane antigen. Am J Surg Pathol 1986;10:640.
56. Folpe AL, Schmidt RA, Chapman D, et al: Poorly differentiated synovial sarcoma: Immunohistochemical distinctions from primitive neuroectodermal tumors and high grade malignant peripheral nerve sheath tumors. Am J Surg Pathol 1998;22:673.
57. Weiss SL, Langloss JM, Ezinger FM: Value of S-100 protein in the diagnosis of soft tissue tumors with particular reference to benign and malignant Schwann cell tumors. Lab Invest 1983;49:299.
58. White W, Shiu MH, Rosenblum MK, et al: Cellular schwannoma: A clinicopathologic study of 57 patients and 58 tumors. Cancer 1990;66:1266.
59. Guillou L, Wadden C, Kraus MD, et al: S-100 protein reactivity in synovial sarcomas: A potentially frequent diagnostic pitfall; immunohistochemical analysis of 100 cases. Appl Immunohistochem 1996;4:167.
60. Kilpatrick SE, Hitchcock MG, Kraus MD, et al: Mixed tumors and myoepitheliomas of soft tissue: A clinicopathologic study of 19 cases with a unifying concept. Am J Surg Pathol 1997;21:13.
61. Coindre JM, de Mascarel A, Trojani M, et al: Immunohistochemical study of rhabdomyosarcoma: Unexpected staining with S100 protein and cytokeratin. J Pathol 1988;155:127.
62. Kaddu S, Beham A, Cerroni L, et al: Cutaneous leiomyosarcoma. Am J Surg Pathol 1997;21:979.
63. Ambros IM, Ambros PF, Strehl S, et al: MIC2 is a specific marker for Ewing's sarcoma and peripheral primitive neuroectodermal tumors: Evidence for a common histogenesis of Ewing's sarcoma and peripheral primitive neuroectodermal tumors from MIC2 expression and specific chromosome aberration. Cancer 1991;67:1886.
64. Ordonez NG: Desmoplastic small round cell tumor: An ultrastructural and immunohistochemical study with emphasis on new immunohistochemical markers. Am J Surg Pathol 1998;22:1314.
65. Qualman SJ, Coffin CM, Newton WA, et al: Intergroup Rhabdomyosarcoma Study: Update for pathologists. Pediatr Dev Pathol 1998;1:550.
66. Van de Rijn M, Barr FG, Xiong QB, et al: Poorly differentiated synovial sarcoma: An analysis of clinical, pathologic, and molecular genetic features. Am J Surg Pathol 1999;23:106.
67. Alawi F, Stratton D, Freedman PD: Solitary fibrous tumor of the oral soft tissues: A clinicopathologic and immunohistochemical study of 16 cases. Am J Surg Pathol 2001;25:900.
68. Folpe AL, Hill CE, Parham DM, et al: Immunohistochemical detection of Fli-1 protein expression: A study of 132 round cell tumors with emphasis on CD99-positive mimics of Ewing's sarcoma/primitive neuroectodermal tumor. Am J Surg Pathol 2000;24:1657.
69. Folpe AL, Chand EM, Goldblum JR, et al: Expression of Fli-1, a nuclear transcription factor, distinguishes vascular neoplasms from potential mimics. Am J Surg Pathol 2001;25:1061.
70. Gessler M, Konig A, Bruns GAP: The genomic organization and expression of the WT1 gene. Genomics 1996;27:453.
71. Baird PN, Simmons PJ: Expression of the Wilms' tumor gene (WT1) in normal hematopoeisis. Exp Hematol 1997;25:312.
72. Hastie ND: The genetics of Wilms' tumor a case of disrupted development. Annu Rev Genet 1994;28:523.
73. Menssen HD, Renkl HJ, Rodeck U, et al: Presence of Wilms' tumor gene (WT1) transcripts and the WT1 nuclear protein in the majority of human acute leukemias. Leukemia 1995;9:1060.
74. Amin KM, Litzky LA, Smythe WR, et al: Wilms' tumor 1 susceptibility (WT1) gene products are selectively expressed in malignant mesothelioma. Am J Surg Pathol 1995;146:344.
75. Silberstein GB, Van Horn K, Strickland P, et al: Altered expression of the WT1 Wilms tumor suppressor gene in human breast cancer. Proc Natl Acad Sci U S A 1997;94:8132.
76. Goldstein NS, Bassi D, Usieblo A: WT1 is an integral component of an antibody panel to distinguish pancreatobiliary and some ovarian epithelial neoplasms. Am J Clin Pathol 2001;116:246.
77. Carpentieri DF, Nichols K, Chou PM, et al: The expression of WT1 in the differentiation of rhabdomyosarcoma from other small round blue cell tumors. Mod Pathol 2002;15:1080.
78. Barnoud R, Sabourin J-C, Pasquier D, et al: Immunohistochemical expression of WT1 by desmoplastic small round cell tumor: A comparative study with other small round cell tumors. Am J Surg Pathol 2000;24:830.
79. Hill DA, Pfeifer JD, Marley EF: WT1 staining reliably differentiates desmoplastic small round cell tumor from Ewing sarcoma/primitive neuroectodermal tumor. Am J Clin Pathol 2000;114:345.

80. Hirota S, Isozak K, Moriyama Y, et al: Gain-of-function mutations of c-Kit in human gastrointestinal stromal tumors. Science 1998;279:577.
81. Rubin BP, Singer S, Tsao C, et al: KIT activation is a ubiquitous feature of gastrointestinal stromal tumors. Cancer Res 2001;156:791.
82. Sarlomon-Rikala M, Kovatich AJ, Barusevicius A, et al: CD117: A sensitive marker for gastrointestinal stromal tumors that is more specific than CD34. Mod Pathol 1998;11:728.
83. Makhlouf HR, Remotti HE, Ishak KG: Expression of KIT (CD117) in angiomyolipoma. Am J Surg Pathol 2002;26:493.
84. Yantiss RK, Spiro IJ, Compton CC, et al: Gastrointestinal stromal tumor versus intra-abdominal fibromatosis of the bowel wall: A clinically important differential diagnosis. Am J Surg Pathol 2000;24:947.
85. Creager AJ, Cohen JA, Geradts J: Aberrant expression of cell-cycle regulatory proteins in human mesenchymal neoplasia. Cancer Detect Prev 2001;25:123.
86. Halling KC, Scheithauer BW, Halling AC, et al: p53 expression in neurofibroma and malignant peripheral nerve sheath tumor: An immunohistochemical study of sporadic and NF1-associated tumors. Am J Clin Pathol 1996;106:282.
87. Hasegawa T, Yokoyama R, Lee YH, et al: Prognostic relevance of a histologic grading system using MIB-1 for adult soft tissue sarcoma. Oncology 2000;58:66.
88. Hasegawa T, Yamamoto S, Yokoyama R, et al: Prognostic significance of grading and staging systems using MIB-1 score in adult patients with soft tissue sarcoma of the extremities and trunk. Cancer 2002;95:843.
89. Inagaki H, Nagasaka T, Otsuka T, et al: Association of SYT-SSX fusion types with proliferative activity and prognosis in synovial sarcoma. Mod Pathol 2000;13:482.
90. Lonardo F, Ueda T, Huvos AG, et al: p53 and MDM2 alterations in osteosarcomas: Correlation with clinicopathologic features and proliferative rate. Cancer 1997;79:1541.
91. May WA, Lessnick SL, Braun BS, et al: The Ewing's sarcoma EWS/FLI-1 fusion gene encodes a more potent transcription activator and is a more powerful transforming gene than FLI-1. Mol Cell Biol 1993;13:7393.
92. Im YH, Kim HT, Lee C, et al: EWS-FLI-1, EWS-ERG, and EWS-ETV-1 oncoproteins of Ewing tumor family all suppress transcription of transforming growth factor beta type II receptor gene. Cancer Res 2000;60:1536.
93. Zielenska M, Zhang ZM, Ng K, et al: Acquistion of secondary structural chromosomal changes in pediatric Ewing sarcoma is a probable prognostic factor for tumor response and clinical outcome. Cancer 2001;91:2156.
94. Benicelli JL, Advani S, Schafer BW, et al: PAX3 and PAX7 exhibit conserved cis-acting transcription repression domains and utilize a common gain of function mechanism in alveolar rhabdomyosarcoma. Oncogene 1999;18:4348.
95. Benicelli JL, Edwards RH, Barr FG: Mechanism for transcriptional gain of function resulting from chromosomal translocation in alveolar rhabdomyosarcoma. Proc Natl Acad Sci U S A 1996;93:5455.
96. Gordon AT, Brinkschmidt C, Anderson J, et al: A novel and consistent amplicon at 13q31 associated with alveolar rhabdomyosarcoma. Genes Chromosomes Cancer 2000;28:220.
97. Sorensen PH, Lynch JC, Qualman SJ, et al: PAX3-FKHR and PAX7-FKHR gene fusions are prognostic indicators in alveolar rhabdomyosarcoma: A report from the Children's Oncology Group. J Clin Oncol 2002;20:2672.
98. Bridge JA, Liu J, Weibolt V, et al: Novel genomic imbalances in embryonal rhabdomyosarcoma revealed by comparative genomic hybridization and fluorescence in situ hybridization: An intergroup rhabdomyosarcoma study. Genes Chromosomes Cancer 2000;27:337.
99. Koi M, Johnson LA, Kalikin LM, et al: Tumor cell growth arrest caused by subchromosomal transferable DNA fragment from chromosome 11. Science 1993;260:361.
100. Scrable H, Cavenee W, Ghavimi F, et al: A model for embryonal rhabdomyosarcoma tumorigenesis that involves genome imprinting. Proc Natl Acad Sci U S A 1989;86:7480.
101. Gerald WL, Rosai J, Ladanyi M: Characterization of the genomic breakpoint and chimeric transcripts in the EWS-WT1 gene fusion of desmoplastic small round cell tumor. Proc Natl Acad Sci U S A 1995;92:1028.
102. Gerald WL, Ladanyi M, de Alava E, et al: Clinical, pathologic, and molecular spectrum of tumors associated with t(11;22)(p13;q12): Desmoplastic small round cell tumor and its variants. J Clin Oncol 1998;16:3028.
103. Perez RP, Zhang PJ: Detection of EWS-WT1 fusion mRNA in ascites of a patient with desmoplastic small round cell tumor by RT-PCR. Hum Pathol 1999;30:239.
104. Antonescu CR, Tschernyavsky SJ, Woodruff JM, et al: Molecular diagnosis of clear cell sarcoma: Detection of EWS-ATF1 and MITF-M transcripts and histopathological and ultrustructual analysis of 12 cases. J Mol Diagn 2002;4:44.
105. Fujimura Y, Ohno T, Siddique H, et al: The EWS-ATF-1 gene involved in malignant melanoma of soft parts with t(12;22) chromosome translocation, encodes a constitutive transcriptional activator. Oncogene 1996;12:159.
106. Fujimura Y, Siddique H, Lee L, et al. EWS-ATF-1 chimeric protein in soft tissue clear cell sarcoma associates with CREB-binding protein and interferes with p53-mediated trans-activation function. Oncogene 2001;20:6653.
107. Antonescu CR, Argani P, Erlandson RA, et al: Skeletal and extraskeletal myxoid chondrosarcoma: A comparative clinicopathologic, ultrastructural, and molecular study. Cancer 1998;83:1504.
108. Kilpatrick SE, Inwards CY, Fletcher CD, et al: Myxoid chondrosarcoma (chordoid sarcoma) of bone: A report of two cases and review of the literature. Cancer 1997;79:1903.
109. Labelle Y, Bussieres J, Courjal F, et al: The EWS/TEC fusion protein encoded by the t(9;22) chromosomal translocation in human chondrosarcomas is a highly potent transcriptional activator. Oncogene 1999;18:3303.
110. Bjerkehagen B, Dietrich C, Reed W, et al: Extraskeletal myxoid chondrosarcoma: Multimodality diagnosis and identification of a new cytogenetic subgroup characterized by t(9;17)(q22;q11). Virchows Arch 1999;435:524.
111. Panagopoulos I, Mencinger M, Dietrich CU, et al: Fusion of the RBP56 and CHN genes in extraskeletal myxoid chondrosarcomas with translocation t(9;17)(q22;q11). Oncogene 1999;18:7594.
112. Sjogren H, Wedell B, Kindblom JM, et al: Fusion of the NH2-terminal domain of the basic helix-loop-helix protein TCF12 to TEC in extraskeletal myxoid chondrosarcoma with translocation t(9;15)(q22;q21). Cancer Res 2000;60:6832.
113. Antonescu CR, Tschernyavsky SJ, Decuseara R, et al: Prognostic impact of P53 status, TLS-CHOP fusion transcript structure, and histological grade in myxoid liposarcoma: A molecular and clinicopathologic study of 82 cases. Clin Cancer Res 2001;7:3977.
114. Tallini G, Akerman M, Dal Cin P, et al: Combined morphologic and karyotypic study of 28 myxoid liposarcomas: Implications for a revised morphologic typing (a report from the CHAMP Group). Am J Surg Pathol 1996;20:1047.
115. Dal Cin P, Sciot R, Panagopoulos I, et al: Additional evidence of a variant translocation t(12;22) with EWS/CHOP fusion in myxoid liposarcoma: Clinicopathologic features. J Pathol 1997;182:437.
116. Rosai J, Akerman M, Dal Cin P, et al: Combined morphologic and karyotypic study of 59 atypical lipomatous tumors: Evaluation of their relationship and differential diagnosis with other adipose tumors (a report of the CHAMP study group). Am J Surg Pathol 1996;20:1182.
117. Micci F, Teixeira MR, Bjerkehagen B, et al: Characterization of supernumerary rings and giant marker chromosomes in well-differentiated lipomatous tumors by a combination of G-banding, CGH, M-FISH, and chromosome- and locus-specific FISH. Cytogenet Genome Res 2002;97:13.
118. Forus A, Bjerkehagen B, Sirvent N, et al: The expression of MDM2/CDK4 gene product in the differential diagnosis of well differentiated liposarcoma and large deep-seated lipoma. Br J Cancer 2000;82:1271.

119. De Leeuw B, Balemans M, Olde Weghuis D, et al: Identification of two alternative fusion genes, SYT-SSX1 and SYT-SSX2, in t(X;18) (p11.2;q11.2)-positive synovial sarcoma. Hum Mol Genet 1995;4:1097.
120. Crew AJ, Clark J, Fisher C, et al: Fusion of SYT to two genes, SSX1 and SSX2, encoding proteins with homology to the Kruppel-associated box in human synovial sarcoma. EMBO J 1995;14:2333.
121. Skytting B, Nilsson G, Brodin B, et al: A novel fusion gene, SYT-SSX4, in synovial sarcoma (letter). J Natl Cancer Inst 1999;91:974.
122. Kawai A, Woodruff J, Healey JH, et al: SYT-SSX gene fusion as a determinant of morphology and prognosis in synovial sarcoma. N Engl J Med 1998;338:153.
123. Inagaki H, Nagasaka T, Otsuka T, et al: Association of SYT-SSX fusion types with proliferative activity and prognosis in synovial sarcoma. Mod Pathol 2000;13:482.
124. O'Sullivan MJ, Kyriakos M, Zhu X, et al: Malignant peripheral nerve sheath tumors with t(X;18): A pathologic and molecular genetic study. Mod Pathol 2000;13:1336.
125. Guillou L, Benhatter J, Terrier P, et al: SYT-SSX fusion type is not a prognostic factor in synovial sarcoma patients: A multi-institutional study of 182 cases (abstract). Mod Pathol 2003;16:13A.
126. Biegel JA, Zhou JY, Rorke LB, et al: Germ-line and acquired mutations in INI1 in atypical teratoid and rhabdoid tumors. Cancer Res 1999;59:74.
127. Sevenet N, Lellouch-Tubiana A, Schofield D, et al: Spectrum of hSNF5/INI1 somatic mutations in human cancer and genotype-phenotype correlations. Hum Mol Genet 1999;8:2359.
128. Versteege I, Sevenet N, Lange J, et al: Truncating mutations of hSNF5/INI1 in aggressive paediatric cancer. Nature 1999;394:203.
129. Sevenet N, Sheridan E, Amram D, et al: Constitutional mutations of the hSNF5/INI1 gene predispose to a variety of cancers Am J Hum Genet 1999;65:1342.
130. DeCristofaro MF, Betz BL, Wang W, et al: Alteration of hSNF5/BAF47 detected in rhabdoid cell lines and primary rhabdomyosarcomas but not Wilms' tumors. Oncogene 1999;18:7559.
131. Sandberg AA, Bridge JA: Updates on the cytogenetics and molecular genetics of bone and soft tissue tumors: Alveolar soft part sarcoma. Cancer Gen Cytogenet 2002;136:1.
132. Ladanyi M, Lui MY, Antonescu CR, et al: The der(17)t(X;17) (p11;q25) of human alveolar soft part sarcoma fuses the TFE3 transcription factor gene to ASPL, a novel gene at 17q25. Oncogene 2001;20:48.
133. Argani P, Antonescu CR, Illei PB, et al: Primary renal cell neoplasms with the ASPL-TFE3 gene fusion of alveolar soft part sarcoma: A distinctive tumor entity previously included among renal cell carcinomas of children and adolescents. Am J Pathol 2001;159:179.
134. Mendlick MR, Nelson M, Pickering D, et al: Translocation t(1;3)(p36.3;q25) is a nonrandom aberration in epithelioid hemangioendothelioma. Am J Surg Pathol 2001;25:684.
135. Boudousquie AC, Lawce HJ, Sherman R, et al: Complex translocation (7;22) identified in an epithelioid hemangioendothelioma. Cancer Genet Cytogenet 1996;92:116.
136. Rubin BP, Chen CJ, Morgan TW, et al: Congenital mesoblastic nephroma t(12;15) is associated with ETV6-NTRK3 gene fusion: Cytogenetic and molecular relationship to congenital (infantile) fibrosarcoma. Am J Pathol 1999;153:1451.
137. Adem C, Gisselsson D, Dal Cin P, et al: ETV6 rearrangements in patients with infantile fibrosarcomas and congenital mesoblastic nephromas by fluorescence in situ hybridization. Mod Pathol 2001;14:1246.

CHAPTER 3

Small Round Cell Tumors of Bone and Soft Tissue

Through advances in immunohistochemistry and molecular genetics, the diagnosis of small round cell or small blue cell tumors of bone and soft tissue has become progressively easier. Difficult diagnostic challenges still exist; however, the pathologist now has at his or her disposal relatively sensitive and specific markers for correctly identifying and subtyping most cases. First, let us begin with a standard definition of a small round cell tumor. Strictly defined, *small round cell tumors* represent a heterogeneous group of neoplasms treated by divergent therapies that share a similar morphology—uniform, round-to-ovoid, often hyperchromatic nuclei with high nuclear-to-cytoplasmic ratios and only scant rims of cytoplasm. The nuclei are not necessarily small but are characteristically uniform. Nuclear pleomorphism is not usually a feature of this group of tumors. Nucleoli may be prominent but are often inconspicuous. The latter feature coupled with nuclear hyperchromasia and high nuclear-to-cytoplasmic ratios imparts a dark blue to gray color to the cells by hematoxylin and eosin staining (thus the designation *small blue cell* tumor). Although these tumors may be observed at any age, a high proportion occur in children and adolescents. Consequently, awareness of the clinical setting helps narrow the differential diagnosis and avoids unnecessary ancillary studies. Table 3.1 summarizes the various histologic subtypes included in the small round cell tumor category and the typical age ranges at which these histologic subtypes tend to occur.

Other tumors, not discussed in this chapter, occasionally exhibit round cell morphology and rarely may be included in the differential diagnosis. Examples of such tumors are listed in Table 3.2. In our experience, rhabdomyomas, especially the fetal type, are more likely to cause diagnostic confusion with rhabdomyosarcoma and are discussed in this chapter.

Knowledge of the anatomic location, including whether the tumor is primarily osseous or soft tissue, is crucial for rendering a specific diagnosis. As we have already alluded, extensive bone destruction almost always indicates primary osseous origin and excludes tumors from the differential that exclusively arise in extraskeletal soft tissues. Table 3.3 illustrates the histologic subtypes virtually exclusively of soft tissue origin and subtypes capable of arising in either location.

From a therapeutic perspective, the most important distinction among small round cell tumors is between a hematopoietic process and a solid tumor (e.g., metastatic carcinoma, sarcoma). In histologic sections, lymphomas and leukemias are usually widely infiltrative, lacking any definable organized pattern (Fig. 3.1). Solid tumors tend to display more organization among the neoplastic cells, often

TABLE 3.1 Small Round Cell Tumors with Typical Age Ranges

Histologic Type	Usual Age Range (yr)
Neuroblastoma	Birth-5
Melanotic neuroectodermal tumor	Birth-1
Ewing's sarcoma/PNET	5-25
Rhabdomyosarcoma	Birth-25
Embryonal subtype	Birth-15
Alveolar subtype	10-25
Desmoplastic small round cell tumor	15-35
Mesenchymal chondrosarcoma	10-40
Olfactory neuroblastoma	10-60
Small cell carcinoma	>50
Merkel cell carcinoma	>50
Malignant lymphoma	Any age
Acute leukemia	Birth-60
Lymphocytic	Birth-15
Granulocytic	15-60

PNET, primitive neuroectodermal tumor.

TABLE 3.2 Non–Small Round Cell Tumors that Occasionally May Exhibit Small Round Cell Morphology

Malignant peripheral nerve sheath tumor
Synovial sarcoma
Fibrosarcoma
Myxoid and round cell liposarcoma
Osteosarcoma

TABLE 3.3 Origin of Primary Musculoskeletal Small Round Cell Tumors (Bone versus Soft Tissue)

Bone Origin	Soft Tissue Origin
Ewing's sarcoma/PNET	Ewing's sarcoma/PNET
Mesenchymal chondrosarcoma	Mesenchymal chondrosarcoma
Lymphoma/leukemia	Lymphoma/leukemia
Melanotic neuroectodermal tumor	Melanotic neuroectodermal tumor
	Neuroblastoma*
	Esthesioneuroblastoma
	Desmoplastic small round cell tumor
	Rhabdomyosarcoma

*Neuroblastoma usually arises from the adrenal gland and sympathetic ganglia. Although not a primary bone neoplasm, its initial presentation may be as a bone metastasis.

PNET, primitive neuroectodermal tumor.

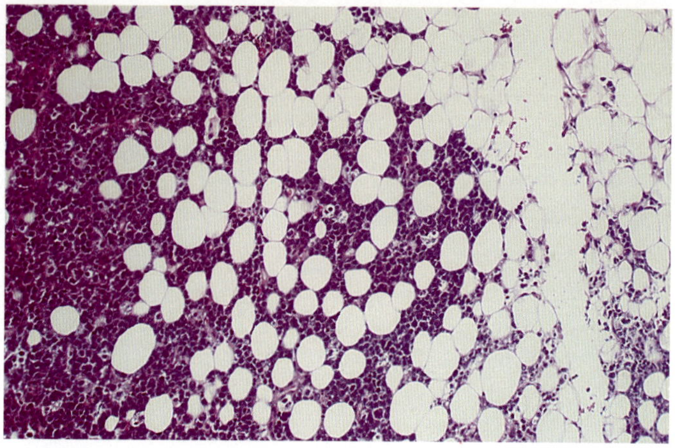

FIGURE 3.1 Malignant lymphoma characterized by a nonorganoid pattern of infiltration of adipose tissue. (H&E.)

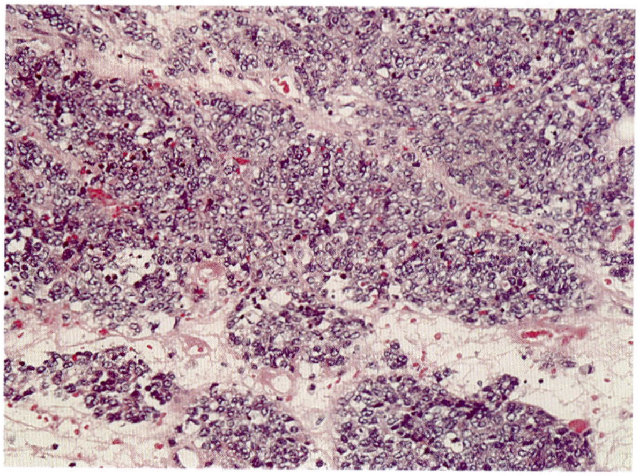

FIGURE 3.2 Ewing's sarcoma characterized by a cohesive, organoid pattern of infiltration. (H&E.)

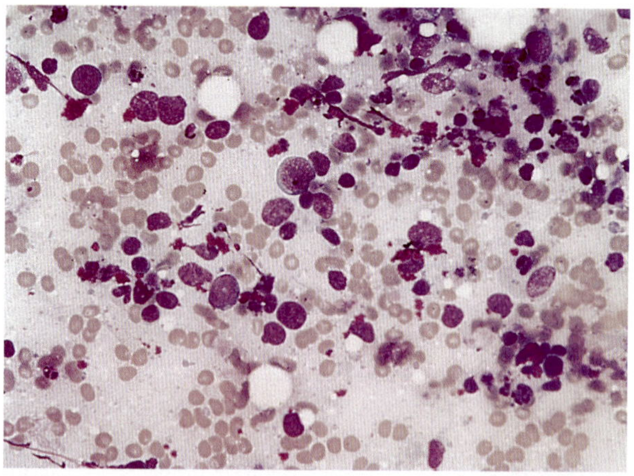

FIGURE 3.3 Fine needle aspiration biopsy of malignant lymphoma with a relatively cellular smear and numerous discohesive, ovoid-to-round tumor cells. (Diff-Quik.)

forming cohesive nests or cords (Fig. 3.2). This distinction also is well illustrated in cytologic preparations (e.g., fine needle aspiration biopsy [FNAB] or touch preparation specimens) in which hematopoietic processes are easily recognizable by their absence of cohesive clusters of tumor cells (Fig. 3.3). Mesenchymal chondrosarcoma and small cell osteosarcoma may contain hyaline cartilage or osteoid/bone or both. The occasional subtle distinctions between the two are discussed in detail later in the chapter. Neuroblastomas virtually always have at least focal neural differentiation and never originate outside of the adrenal gland and sympathetic ganglia of the thorax and abdomen. Clinical correlation and meticulous attention to pathologic features are sufficient to exclude the diagnosis in all but a few cases.[1] Although we include neuroblastoma in the differential diagnosis of small round cell tumors, the entity is better discussed within general surgical and pediatric pathology textbooks.

In the event that the morphologic features are not specific, highly sensitive and relatively specific immunohistochemical, cytogenetic, and molecular features exist among the small round cell tumors and help the pathologist arrive at a specific diagnosis.[1,2] Table 3.4 summarizes these features, which are discussed in more detail with their respective histologic subtypes.

Although underemphasized in the current molecular age, electron microscopy still merits consideration. Mierau and colleagues[3] conducted an "observer blinded" study of 50 diagnostically difficult small round cell tumors, examined by

TABLE 3.4 Specific Histologic Subtypes of Small Round Cell Tumors with Immunohistochemical Markers and Molecular and Cytogenetic Abnormalities

Histologic Subtype	IHC Markers	Cytogenetic Abnormalities	Molecular Events	Estimated Frequency of Events (%)
Ewing's sarcoma	CD99	t(11;22)(q24;q12)	FLI1-EWS	>85
	FLI-1	t(21;22)(q22;q12)	ERG-EWS	5-10
		t(7;22)(p22;q12)	ETV1-EWS	>5
		Others		1-5
Alveolar rhabdomyosarcoma	Myogenin	t(2;13)(q35;q14)	PAX3-FKHR	80
	Myo-D1	t(1;13)(p36;q14)	PAX7-FKHR	10-20
	Desmin			
	Actin			
Embryonal rhabdomyosarcoma	Myogenin	+2q, +8q, +20		70-80
	Myo-D1			
	Desmin			
	Actin			
DSRCT	Cytokeratin	t(11;22)(p13;q12)	WT1-EWS	>80
	Desmin			
	NSE			
	WT1			

DSRCT, desmoplastic small round cell tumor; IHC, immunohistochemical markers; NSE, neuron-specific enolase.

immunohistochemistry and electron microscopy. For establishing a diagnosis, electron microscopy was found to be superior to immunohistochemistry.[3] For small round cell tumors, electron microscopy generally relies on the finding of intercellular junctions to exclude fully a hematopoietic process.[1]

The small round cell sarcomas are easily diagnosable by FNAB. In our experience, accuracy rates with FNAB are the highest of all sarcoma cytomorphologic groups, exceeding 90% in pediatric patients.[4] As a group, small round cell tumors usually yield abundant cellular material by aspiration biopsy, allowing for numerous ancillary tests, if deemed clinically necessary. Because most of these ancillary studies are highly sensitive and, in the appropriate clinical context, specific, a histologic subtype is easily rendered in most cases.[4,5] Incorporating a multidisciplinary approach, Figure 3.4 illustrates a theoretical scenario for the clinicopathologic work-up of the unknown small round cell tumor, applicable to histologic or cytologic specimens.

Ewing's Sarcoma

Ewing's sarcoma and primitive neuroectodermal tumor (PNET) represent a spectrum of similar-appearing bone and soft tissue sarcomas that usually share the same cytogenetic abnormality, t(11;22)(q24;q12).[6] In the past, the distinction between these two entities rested largely on the finding of an arbitrary number of rosettes, generally seen in PNET but less obvious in Ewing's sarcoma. Evidence suggests that demographic features and biologic behavior are also similar for Ewing's sarcoma and PNET.[7,8] Most investigators now consider these tumors to form points along a continuous spectrum of the same neoplasm, with classic, mostly undifferentiated Ewing's sarcoma at one end and more neural-differentiated PNET at the opposite end.[6,7]

Clinical Features

Most Ewing's sarcomas affect children, adolescents, and young adults between 5 and 25 years old; rarely, Ewing's sarcoma also may arise in infants and toddlers.[9,10] Males are affected more commonly than females. For reasons not understood, Ewing's sarcoma is rare in African-Americans.[9] Pain and soft tissue swelling are frequent presenting symptoms, but pathologic fracture is less commonly observed. Occasionally, patients with Ewing's sarcoma may develop fever associated with an elevated erythrocyte sedimentation rate, mimicking infection.

Clinically, Ewing's sarcoma arises far more commonly as a primary bone tumor than an extraskeletal neoplasm. Most cases involve the extremities, principally the lower extremities. More specifically, the pelvic bones and metaphyseal regions of the long bones, especially the femur, tibia, and humerus, are most commonly involved. Nevertheless, compared with other primary malignancies of bone, Ewing's sarcoma more frequently arises in the diaphysis (shaft). Ewing's sarcoma characteristically presents as an aggressive and permeative, lytic lesion radiologically. A large soft tissue component is generally present, sometimes initially suggesting extraskeletal origin. Periosteal reaction may manifest as multiple layers of subperiosteal new bone formation, producing the so-called onionskin appearance (Fig. 3.5). Frequently, conventional radiographs underestimate the tumor burden because Ewing's sarcoma may involve virtually the entire length of a long bone. When arising in extraskeletal soft tissues, Ewing's sarcoma most commonly occurs in the trunk (chest wall and paravertebral region), lower extremities, and retroperitoneum.[11]

Pathologic Findings

Histology

Regardless of anatomic site of origin, the histologic and cytomorphologic characteristics are similar. At low power, Ewing's sarcoma cells may be arranged in diffuse "fields," variably sized nests, or fascicles separated by fibrovascular

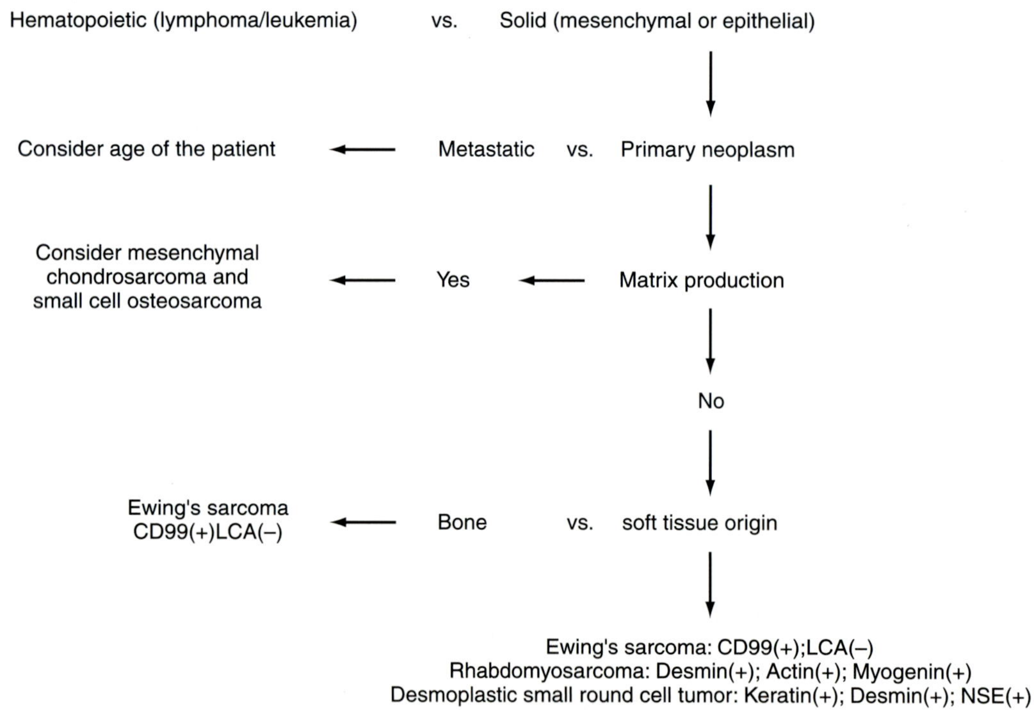

FIGURE 3.4 Work-up of a small round cell tumor.

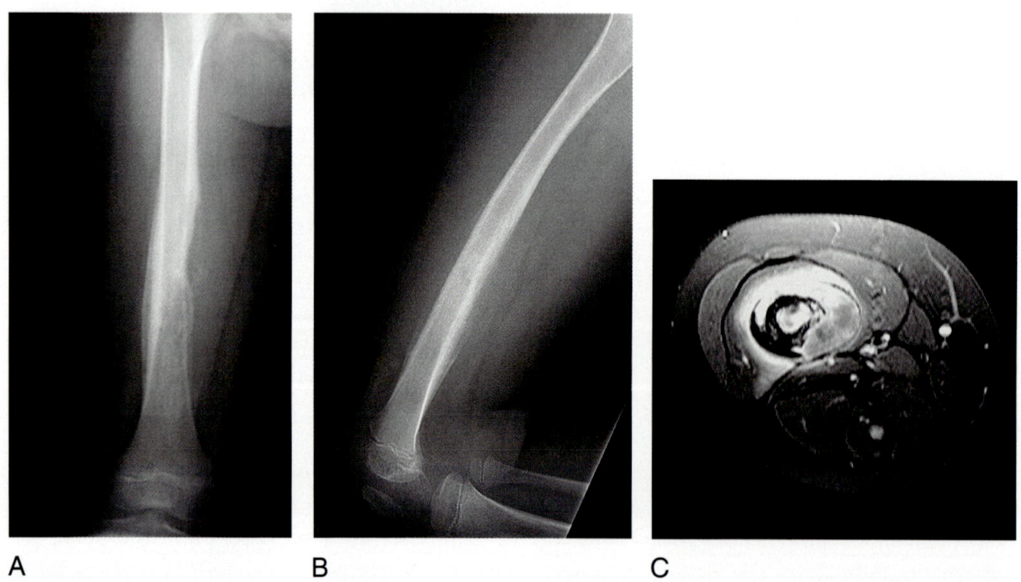

FIGURE 3.5 Ewing's sarcoma. Anteroposterior **(A)** and lateral **(B)** radiographs of the femur show a lytic, permeative lesion centered in the femoral shaft. There is extensive, circumferential, lamellated (onionskin) periosteal new bone production about the femoral shaft. Medially the femoral cortex and periosteal new bone production are breached by tumor extending into the adjacent soft tissues. A T1-weighted, fat-suppressed magnetic resonance image, obtained after the intravenous administration of gadolinium, shows intense but heterogeneous enhancement of the tumor within the femoral medullary canal and in the surrounding musculature in the quadriceps compartment **(C)**.

septa.[9] The nuclei tend to be uniform with hyperchromasia, inconspicuous nucleoli, and scant rims of esoinophilic-to-clear cytoplasm (Fig. 3.6). Rarely, Ewing's sarcoma may contain a population of larger tumor cells with vesicular nuclei, more irregular nuclear membranes, and obvious nucleoli, the so-called atypical large cell variant (Fig. 3.7).[12] Multinucleated giant cells are never present. Variable numbers of rosettes may be observed, especially in the more differentiated PNET (Fig. 3.8). Most commonly, the rosettes resemble those of neuroblastoma, exhibiting an eosinophilic core of neurofibrillary material surrounded by the tumor cells (Homer-Wright rosettes). Mitotic activity tends to be variable, and mitoses may be surprisingly sparse. Spontaneous tumor necrosis is frequently present, sometimes leaving residual viable-appearing tumor cells forming collars around blood vessels (Fig. 3.9).

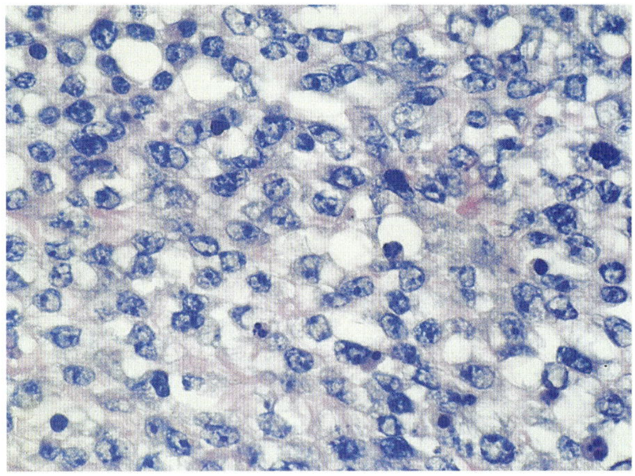

FIGURE 3.7 Atypical large cell Ewing's sarcoma with larger, more vesicular nuclei, prominent nucleoli, and significant nuclear atypia. (H&E.)

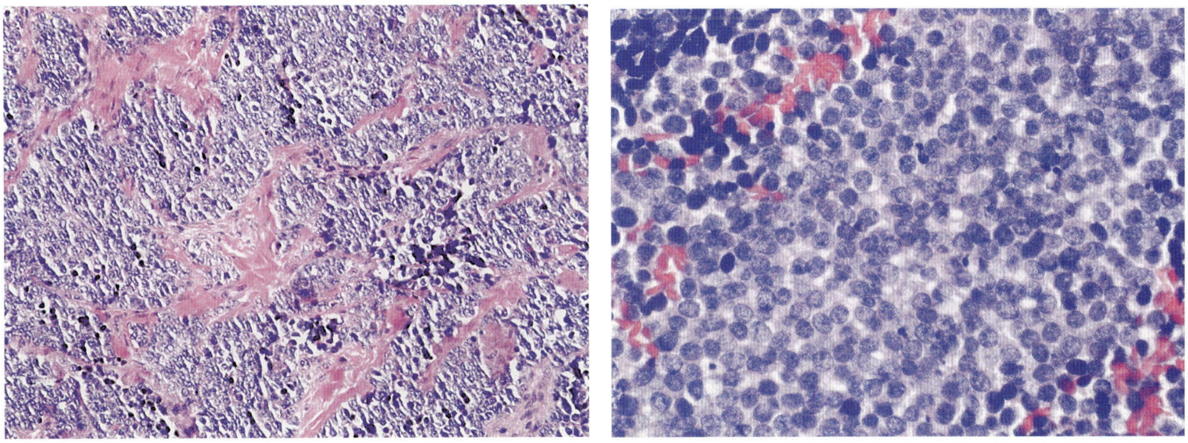

A B

FIGURE 3.6 Ewing's sarcoma with an organoid pattern of infiltration. Individual cells appear remarkably uniform with mostly round hyperchromatic nuclei, inconspicuous nucleoli, and scant amounts of cytoplasm **(A** and **B). (A,** low power; **B,** high power, H&E.)

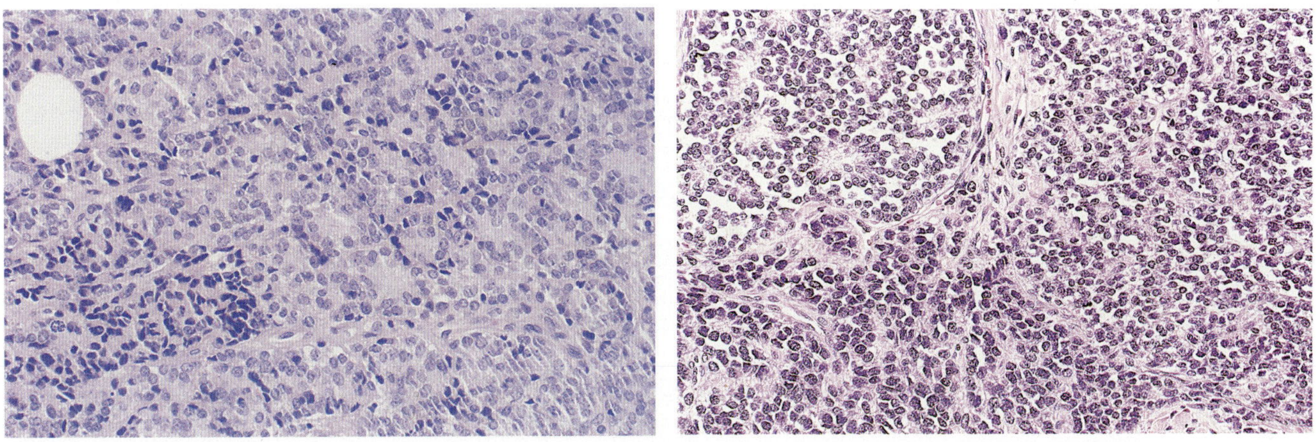

A B

FIGURE 3.8 Primitive neuroectodermal tumor, a form of Ewing's sarcoma characterized by greater neuroendocrine differentiation and the presence of obvious rosettes **(A** and **B).** Also note the presence of a pseudoalveolar pattern in **B,** mimicking alveolar rhabdomyosarcoma. **(A** and **B,** H&E.)

Fine Needle Aspiration Biopsy

The diagnosis of Ewing's sarcoma is easily established, especially if sufficient material is obtained for ancillary techniques. Cytologic specimens are markedly cellular and composed of mostly individually dispersed cells and scattered small cohesive cell clusters.[13] The tumor cells are remarkably uniform, possessing a solitary, round hyperchromatic nucleus, an extraordinarily high nuclear-to-cytoplasmic ratio, and a thin rim of cytoplasm, sometimes containing small vacuoles indicating intracytoplasmic glycogen. Nucleoli are generally inconspicuous to absent (Fig. 3.10). Rare forms of the so-called atypical (large cell) Ewing's sarcoma may exhibit more uniformly enlarged nuclei, irregular nuclear membranes, and prominent nucleoli (Fig. 3.11).[13] Binucleated and multinucleated tumor cells are not observed. Background matrix material (e.g., cartilage or osteoid) is distinctly absent. Rarely, tumor rosettes may be evident (Fig. 3.12).[14]

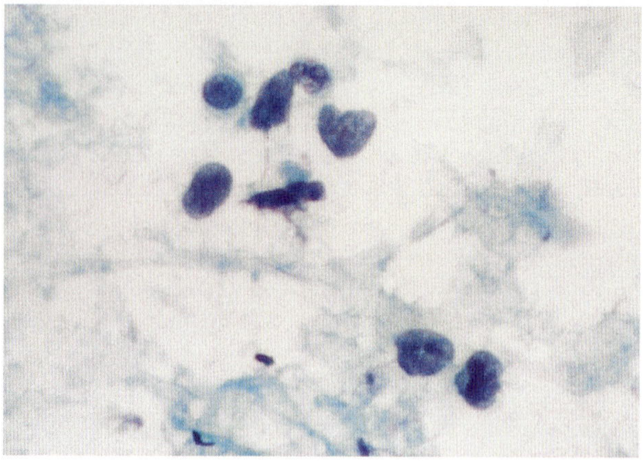

FIGURE 3.11 Atypical large cell Ewing's sarcoma with discohesive, markedly atypical tumor cells with irregular nuclear membranes and absence of uniformity in size and shape of individual tumor cells. (Papanicolaou.)

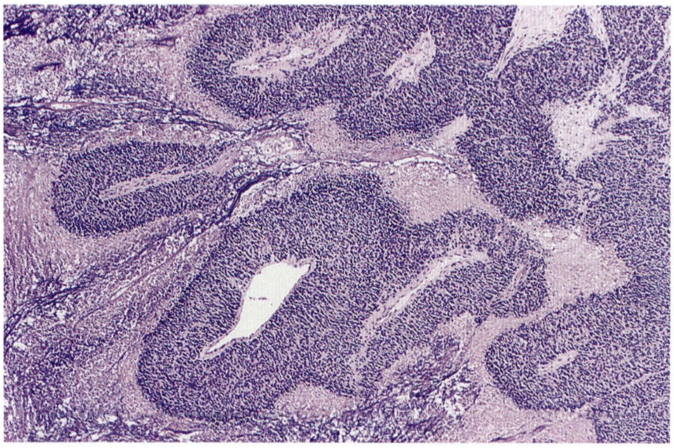

FIGURE 3.9 Ewing's sarcoma with collars of preserved tumor cells hugging blood vessels. Elsewhere, necrotic tumor is evident. (H&E.)

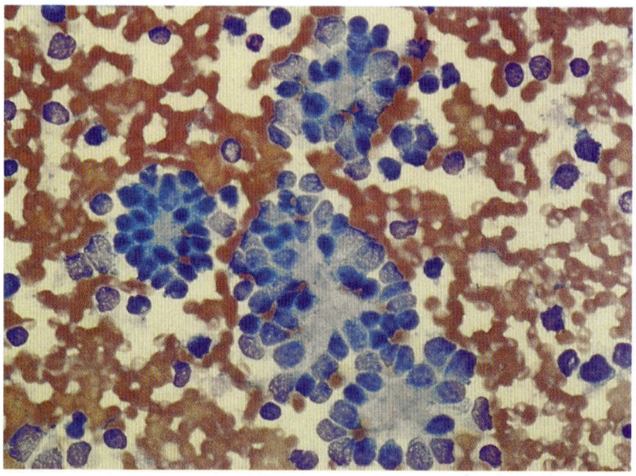

FIGURE 3.12 Rosettes, as illustrated here, are observed rarely in fine needle aspiration biopsy specimens of Ewing's sarcoma/primitive neuroectodermal tumors. (Diff-Quik.)

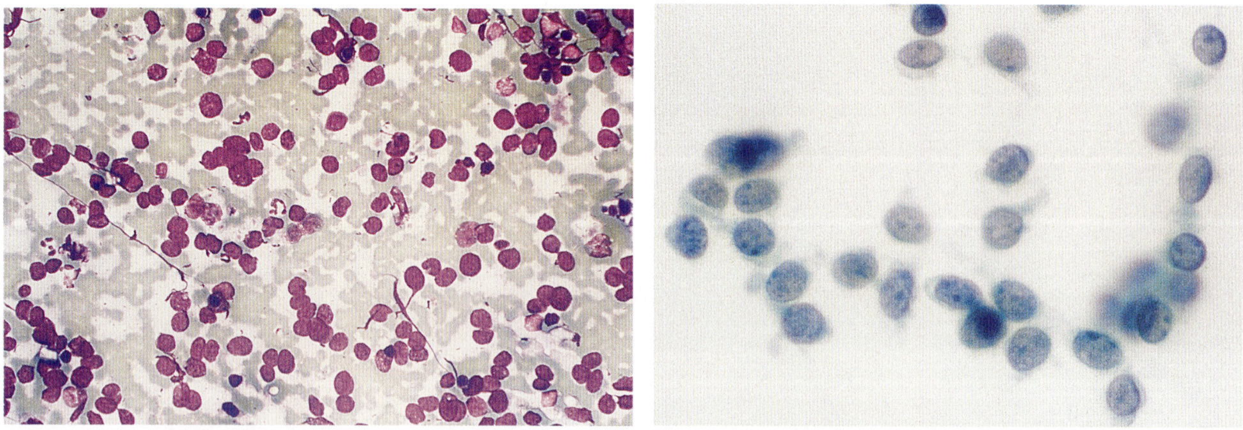

A B

FIGURE 3.10 Fine needle aspiration biopsy of Ewing's sarcoma generally yields hypercellular smears with numerous small, cohesive tumor cell clusters and solitary tumor cells. Significant nuclear pleomorphism is absent; cells have high nuclear-to-cytoplasmic ratios, ovoid-to-round nuclei, and inconspicuous nucleoli **(A** and **B). (A,** Diff-Quik; **B,** Papanicolaou.)

Ancillary Studies

Ultrastructural examination generally reveals primitive, undifferentiated tumor cells with mostly uniform, round nuclei; smooth, regular nuclear membranes; and a finely granular chromatin pattern. At least one small nucleolus usually is observed. The cytoplasm contains abundant glycogen but relatively few organelles. Neighboring cells often are joined together by intercellular junctions, a finding that completely excludes a hematopoietic process. Intracytoplasmic myofilaments and extracellular collagen are not seen in Ewing's sarcoma.

Immunocytochemically, 90% to 95% of cases of Ewing's sarcoma possess the mic-2 glycoprotein product shown by positive cytoplasmic, membranous staining for CD99.[15] The staining pattern is generally diffuse (involving virtually all cells) and strong. Although CD99 expression is a highly sensitive marker for Ewing's sarcoma, it is not entirely specific and may be observed in synovial sarcoma, small cell osteosarcoma, desmoplastic small round cell tumor, and mesenchymal chondrosarcoma.[16,17] The evaluation of other immunohistochemical stains in Ewing's sarcoma has produced conflicting results, probably related to the fact that some investigators consider Ewing's sarcoma and PNET distinct entities, rather than a spectrum of similar neoplasm. In classic Ewing's sarcoma, neuroendocrine markers (neuron-specific enolase, synaptophysin) and S-100 protein are infrequently observed. Conversely, among tumors with more neuroectodermal differentiation (e.g., PNET), Cavazzana and colleagues[18] documented neuron-specific enolase positivity in 95% of cases, synaptophysin in 73%, S-100 protein in 67%, and neurofilament protein in 38%.[18] Folpe and colleagues[19] examined 132 round cell tumors for FLI-1 nuclear expression. Of 41 cases of Ewing's sarcoma/PNET, 29 (71%) were positive. Seven (of eight) lymphoblastic lymphomas and one desmoplastic small round cell tumor also showed immunoexpression of FLI-1. Thirty-two rhabdomyosarcomas, 30 neuroblastomas, and 8 esthesioneuroblastomas were uniformly negative.[19] The immunohistochemical profile for the spectrum of the Ewing's family of tumors is summarized in Table 3.5.

TABLE 3.5 Immunohistochemical Profile for the Spectrum of Ewing's Sarcoma and Primitive Neuroectodermal Tumor

	Ewing's Sarcoma	PNET
Vimentin	+	+
CD99	+	+
FLI-1	+	+
Neuron-specific enolase	+/–	+
Synaptophysin	–	+
Neurofilament	–	+
S-100 protein	–	+
Cytokeratin	+/–	+/–
Desmin	–	+/–
Muscle-specific actin	–	+/–
Myogenin	–	–

PNET, primitive neuroectodermal tumor.

The Ewing's sarcoma gene on chromosome 22 may be associated with several translocations, including, in decreasing order of frequency, t(11;22)(q24;q12), t(21;22)(q12;q12), and t(7;22)(p22;q12).[20] The t(11;22) or EWS/FLI-1 fusion transcript is not entirely specific for Ewing's sarcoma and has been documented in rare cases of embryonal and alveolar rhabdomyosarcoma, polyphenotypic tumor of childhood, neuroblastoma, small cell osteosarcoma, intra-abdominal desmoplastic small round cell tumor, and mesenchymal chondrosarcoma.[21-25]

Prognosis and Therapy

Combination multimodality therapy has improved drastically the 5-year overall survival and disease-free survival rates, ranging, at present, from 40% to 60% and 30% to 55%. Adverse prognostic factors include older age of the patient at diagnosis, localization proximally (especially the pelvis), large tumor size, and inadequacy of surgical resection.[7,9,11,26-28] Although absolute numbers of reported patients are limited, Ewing's sarcoma arising in cutaneous (solitary dermal nodule) locations seems to be associated with a favorable clinical course.[29] Perhaps the most significant prognostic factor is the histologic response to chemotherapy, defined by the extent or volume (expressed as a percentage) of tumor necrosis.[26,27] In the Memorial series, the extent of tumor necrosis was defined specifically as follows: grade I, 50% or less necrosis; grade II, greater than 50% but less than 90% necrosis; grade III, 90% to 99% necrosis; and grade IV, 100% necrosis.[26] Among 74 patients with Ewing's sarcoma, the 5-year event-free survival rate was 6 (20%) of 30 patients with a grade I or II response and 37 (84%) of 44 patients with a grade III or IV response.[26] This histologic response to chemotherapy may have a molecular basis. de Alava and colleagues[30] documented a better prognosis for patients with Ewing's sarcomas containing the EWS-FLI1 type 1 fusion compared with cases with other EWS-FLI1 fusion types or the EWS-ERG fusion.[30] Favorable chemotherapeutic response (as measured by percent of postchemotherapy tumor necrosis) correlated with the finding of the EWS-FLI1 type 1 fusion transcript.[30]

Rhabdomyosarcoma

Rhabdomyosarcoma is the most common soft tissue sarcoma of childhood. By convention, rhabdomyosarcoma is defined as a malignant mesenchymal neoplasm showing only skeletal muscle differentiation by morphologic or ancillary techniques. The most recent International Classification of

Rhabdomyosarcoma (ICR) recognizes five prognostically significant subtypes—spindle cell and botryoid embryonal rhabdomyosarcoma (superior prognosis), embryonal rhabdomyosarcoma (intermediate prognosis), and alveolar rhabdomyosarcoma and undifferentiated sarcoma (poor prognosis).[31] The Intergroup Rhabdomyosarcoma Study Group (IRSG) added the diffuse anaplastic variant of rhabdomyosarcoma to the list of unfavorable subtypes.[32] This categorization is summarized in Table 3.6. The adult pleomorphic subtype of rhabdomyosarcoma is not discussed here but is included in a separate chapter with other pleomorphic sarcomas of adulthood.

Clinical Features

Despite having skeletal myogenic differentiation, rhabdomyosarcoma often arises in anatomic sites devoid of skeletal muscle. Although not usually considered in the differential diagnosis of primary bone tumors, extraordinarily rare examples of embryonal rhabdomyosarcoma have been described arising in bone.[33]

TABLE 3.6 ICR Classification of Rhabdomyosarcoma

	Incidence (%)*	5-Year Survival Rate (%)*
Superior Prognosis		
Embryonal rhabdomyosarcoma, botryoid subtype	6	95
Embryonal rhabdomyosarcoma, spindle cell subtype	3	88
Intermediate Prognosis		
Embryonal rhabdomyosarcoma, not otherwise specified	49	66
Poor Prognosis		
Alveolar rhabdomyosarcoma	31	53
Anaplastic rhabdomyosarcoma, diffuse	2	45
Undifferentiated sarcoma	3	44

*Percentages based on IRSG data. Total number of cases is only 94% because at least 6% of cases were interpreted as "sarcoma, not otherwise specified" owing to insufficient diagnostic material.

Qualman SJ, Coffin CM, Newton WA, et al: Intergroup Rhabdomyosarcoma Study: Update for pathologists. Pediatr Dev Pathol 1998;1:550.

Various subtypes tend to arise in specific age groups and anatomic sites. Symptoms most often are related to the site of origin but most commonly manifest as a soft tissue mass or swelling. The botryoid form of embryonal rhabdomyosarcoma generally arises in the submucosa and tends to occur in mucosa-lined hollow organs, such as the bladder, vagina, rectum, nasal cavity, and nasopharynx. Most patients are younger than 10 years old at diagnosis. The spindle cell subtype of embryonal rhabdomyosarcoma also is observed more commonly in children younger than 10 years old but most frequently arises in the paratesticular and, less commonly, head and neck regions.[34] Rubin and coworkers[35] described two examples of spindle cell rhabdomyosarcoma arising in adult patients. Conventional embryonal rhabdomyosarcoma is the most common subtype, usually seen in children younger than 10 years old but occasionally observed in adolescents and young adults. Common anatomic sites include the genitourinary tract, head and neck, and retroperitoneum. In contrast to most other subtypes, alveolar rhabdomyosarcoma is observed more frequently in adolescent patients involving, in decreasing frequency, the extremities, paranasal sinuses, and retroperitoneum.

Pathologic Findings

Conventional Embryonal Rhabdomyosarcoma (Not Otherwise Specified)

Conventional or classic embryonal rhabdomyosarcoma consists of mainly poorly differentiated tumor cells arranged in diffuse aggregates and nests. Alternating hypocellular and hypercellular regions are frequently present, sometimes creating a "pulmonary edema" pattern (Fig. 3.13). The background stroma ranges from myxoid to partly hyalinized. Individual tumor cells are ovoid to slightly spindled with round-to-ovoid, hyperchromatic nuclei; inconspicuous-to-prominent nuclei; and scant-to-abundant tapering cytoplasm (Fig. 3.14). The cytoplasm may display clearly identifiable cross striations (Fig. 3.15). Large, polygonal-appearing rhabdomyoblasts often are scattered among the more undifferentiated cells but tend to be more abundant and frequently observed in postchemotherapy specimens (Fig. 3.16). Conventional embryonal rhabdomyosarcoma lacks the features (or criteria) necessary for the diagnosis of the various specific subtypes, such as botryoid or spindle cell.

Botryoid Embryonal Rhabdomyosarcoma

The current ICR/IRSG classification requires the presence of an intact epithelium overlying a condensed tumor layer of rhabdomyoblasts (cambium layer) in at least one microscopic field.[31] The presence of a grape-like cluster of tumor cells visualized grossly or in the intraoperative setting is not enough by itself to establish the diagnosis of botryoid embry-

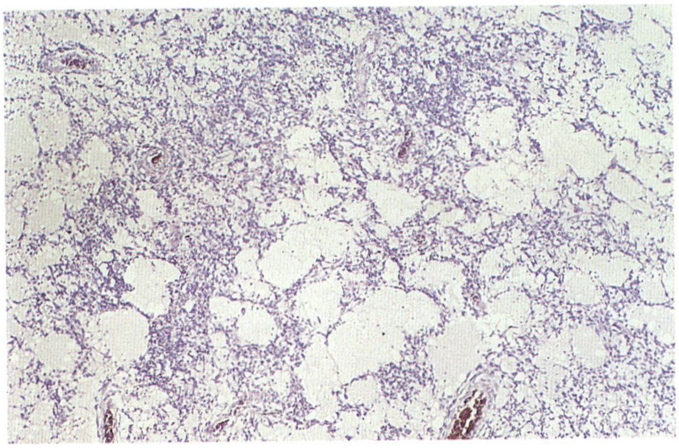

FIGURE 3.13 Low-power view of embryonal rhabdomyosarcoma with alternating hypercellular and hypocellular regions, creating a pulmonary edema–type pattern. (H&E.)

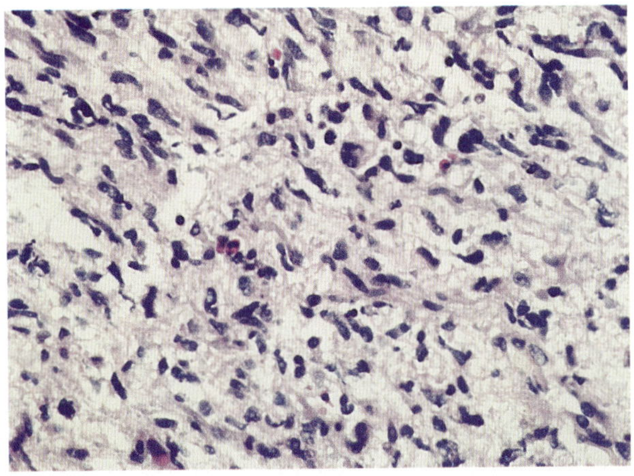

FIGURE 3.14 Poorly differentiated embryonal rhabdomyosarcoma with ovoid to slightly spindled tumor cells with hyperchromatic nuclei but lacking obvious myogenic differentiation. (H&E.)

onal rhabdomyosarcoma. The diagnosis must be confirmed microscopically. Variable amounts of rhabdomyoblastic differentiation may be evident, ranging from more undifferentiated tumor cells to diagnostic spindled-to-stellate rhabdomyoblasts with definite cross striations. The background stroma is frequently myxoid (Fig. 3.17).

Spindle Cell Embryonal Rhabdomyosarcoma

Spindle cell rhabdomyosarcoma is a relatively recently described entity, having been documented clearly in the literature only since 1993.[34] By definition, spindle cell morphology must predominate; more rounded rhabdomyoblasts or multinucleated cells are rarely observed. Most commonly, the spindle cells contain ovoid nuclei and prominent nucleoli and are arranged in whorls and storiform patterns. Cellularity is generally slight, and definite cross striations are rarely identified. Occupying the intercellular spaces is abundant collagen. This variant of spindle cell rhabdomyosarcoma sometimes is referred to as *collagen rich* (Fig. 3.18).

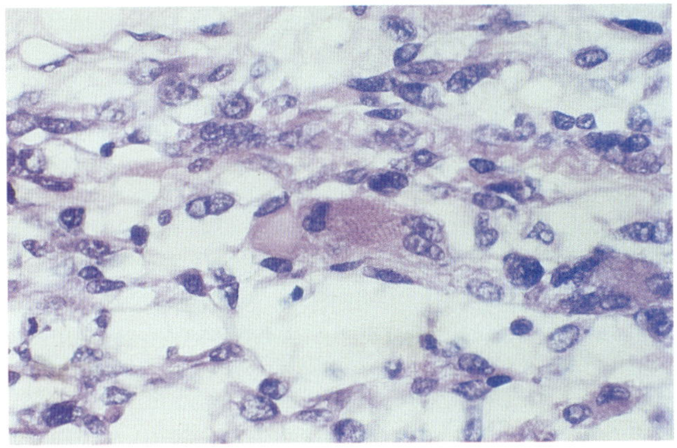

FIGURE 3.15 Embryonal rhabdomyosarcoma with a diagnostic "strap" cell with obvious cross striations. (H&E.)

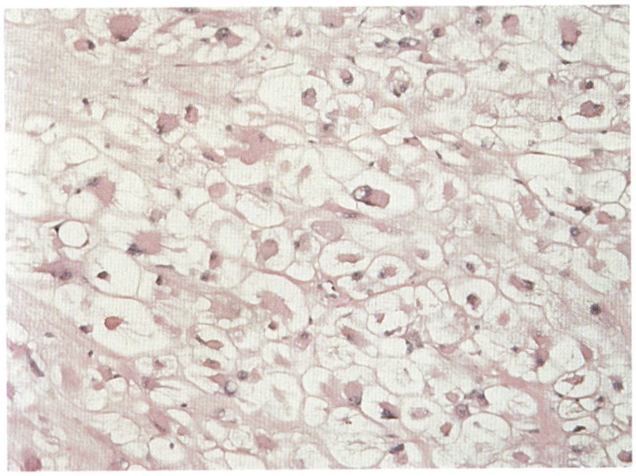

FIGURE 3.16 Diffuse cellular maturation is seen often as a response to chemotherapy and is especially common in the embryonal and botryoid forms of rhabdomyosarcoma. (H&E.)

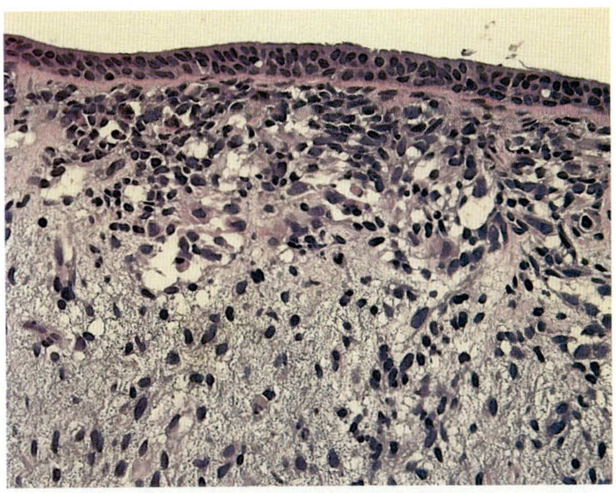

FIGURE 3.17 Botryoid rhabdomyosarcoma with an overlying intact epithelial cell layer, an underlying cambium cellular layer of tumor cells, and a myxoid stroma. (H&E.)

Less frequently, spindle cell rhabdomyosarcoma comprises more elongated tumor cells with cigar-shaped nuclei, prominent nucleoli, and tapering eosinophilic cytoplasm. The tumor cells are arranged in intersecting bundles or fascicles resembling leiomyosarcoma. Scant amounts of intercellular collagen are present. This variant sometimes is referred to as *collagen poor* (Fig. 3.19).[34]

Alveolar Rhabdomyosarcoma

In the past, the diagnosis of alveolar rhabdomyosarcoma was restricted to tumors exhibiting the classic fibrovascular septa outlining cleft-like spaces, lined by a population of mostly round tumor cells. Cytologically the tumor cells are mostly uniform, round to slightly ovoid with round, hyperchromatic-to-vesicular nuclei and one or more prominent nucleoli, surrounded by a thin rim of eosinophilic cytoplasm. Multinucleated tumor giant cells are usually present (Fig. 3.20). Definite myogenesis and so-called strap cells are not generally features of alveolar rhabdomyosarcoma. Less commonly, the neoplastic cells may be vacuolated and have more abundant, clear cytoplasm, presumably as a result of the presence of glycogen (Fig. 3.21). In 1992, Tsokos and colleagues[36] described a "solid" form of alveolar rhabdomyosarcoma, characterized as having the cytologic features of alveolar rhabdomyosarcoma but appearing more compact, lacking the "alveolar" architecture (Fig. 3.22). There was no difference in survival between the classic appearing alveolar and the more "solid" variant.[36] In addition to the solid nested pattern of alveolar rhabdomyosarcoma, we have encountered examples with tumor cells arranged in infiltrative, double-layered to single-file cords, resembling lobular carcinoma of the breast (Fig. 3.23). In our experience, it is common to encounter two or more of these patterns within the same neoplasm.

One may observe occasionally examples of rhabdomyosarcoma with elements of embryonal and alveolar differentiation. According to the current ICR classification, these

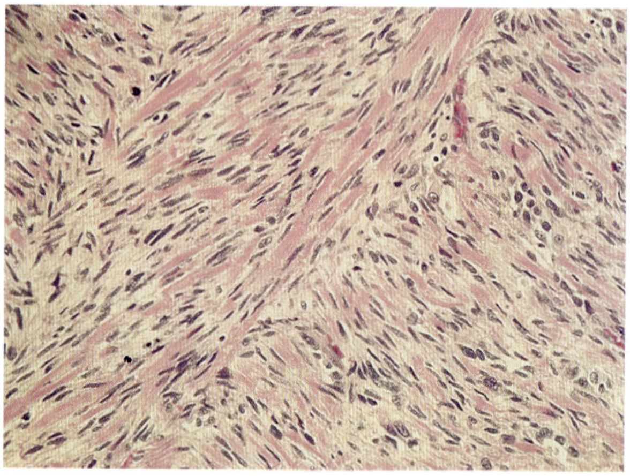

FIGURE 3.18 Spindle cell rhabdomyosarcoma exhibiting intersecting fascicles of mostly uniform-appearing spindle tumor cells and abundant collagen deposition. (H&E.)

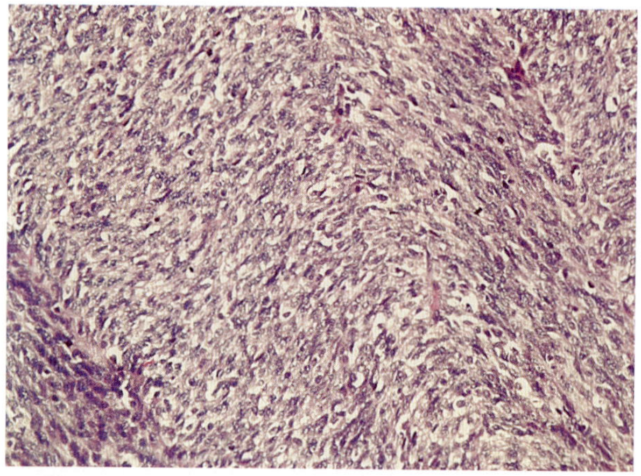

FIGURE 3.19 More cellular forms of spindle cell rhabdomyosarcoma may display intersecting fascicles of tumor cells, resembling fibrosarcoma or leiomyosarcoma of soft tissues. (H&E.)

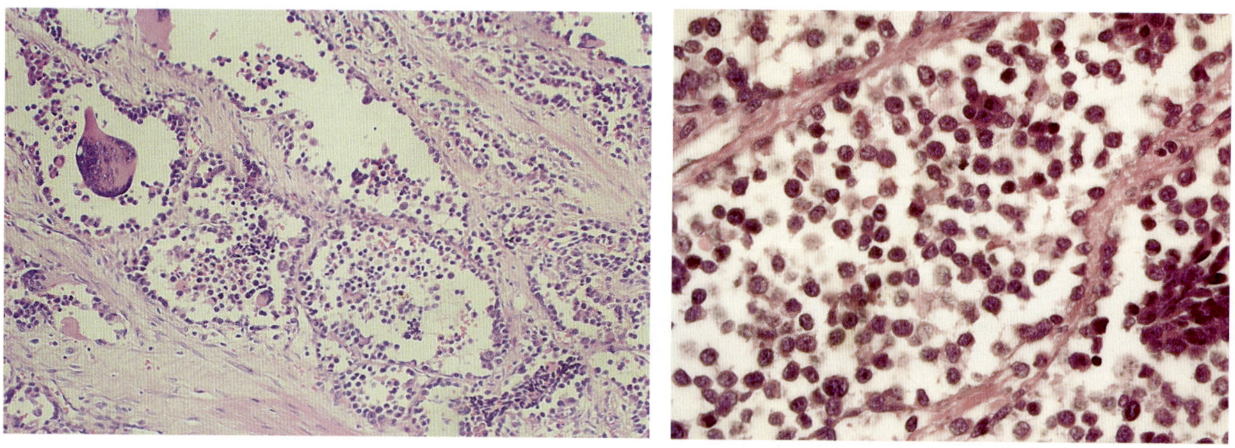

A B

FIGURE 3.20 Classic alveolar rhabdomyosarcoma with variably sized, alveolar-like spaces separated by variably thickened fibrous tissue septa. Tumor cells are observed within the alveolar spaces and hugging the fibrous tissue septa. Multinucleated tumor giant cells often are observed. Cytologically, individual tumor cells appear relatively large but mostly uniform and round to ovoid with high nuclear-to-cytoplasmic ratios **(A** and **B)**. **(A,** low power; **B,** high power, H&E.)

tumors should be considered alveolar rhabdomyosarcoma for therapeutic purposes.[31]

Anaplastic Rhabdomyosarcoma

The anaplastic subtype of rhabdomyosarcoma is synonymous with the older category of childhood pleomorphic rhabdomyosarcoma.[37] Although the concept of anaplasia in rhabdomyosarcoma has been known for some time, only recently has anaplastic rhabdomyosarcoma been recognized as a distinct entity. By definition, anaplasia in rhabdomyosarcoma is defined by the presence of large tumor cells with multilobated nuclei, three times or more the size of adjacent nuclei, and the presence of atypical and multipolar mitotic figures (Fig. 3.24).[32] The distribution of the anaplastic cells may range from focal and scattered, single cells to more diffuse, consisting of large nests or a sheet-like growth pattern. The presence of the diffuse pattern is independently and prognostically significant, associated with a considerably worse prognosis, rivaling that of the alveolar subtype.[38] Although anaplasia may be observed in either embryonal or alveolar subtypes, it is seen more commonly in embryonal rhabdomyosarcoma.

Undifferentiated Sarcoma

The IRSG includes this category of sarcoma because of its similar response rate to multimodality rhabdomyosarcoma therapy.[32] Undifferentiated sarcoma is typically characterized by sheets of mostly uniform-appearing, ovoid tumor cells lacking distinct architectural features. Mitotic activity is usually high, exceeding 10 mitoses per 10 high-power fields. At present, the diagnosis of undifferentiated sarcoma is one of exclusion. Immunohistochemical studies usually reveal positive reactivity only for vimentin. Although data are limited, most examples seem to arise in the extremities.

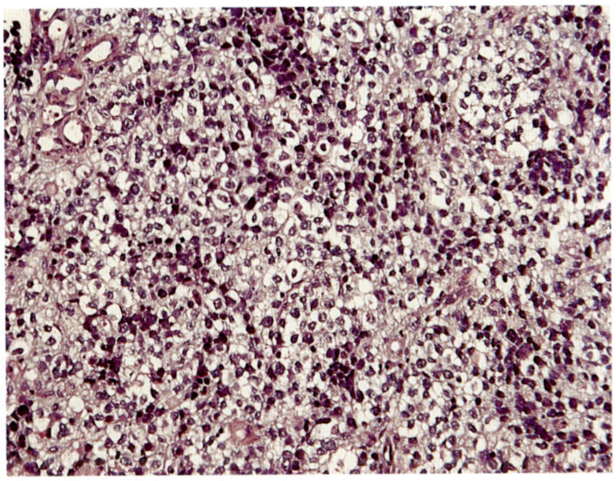

FIGURE 3.21 Alveolar rhabdomyosarcoma with clear cell features. (H&E.)

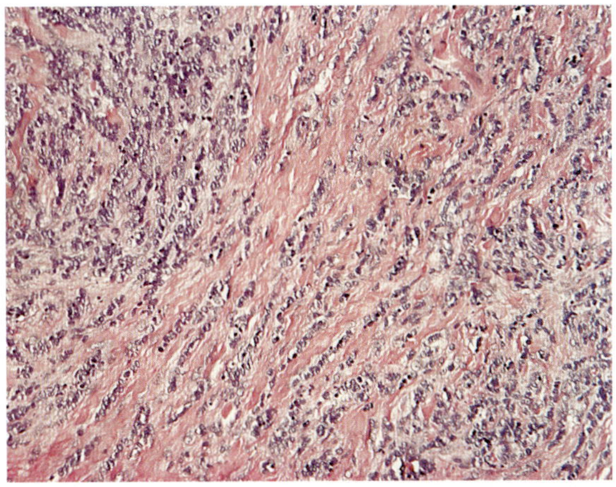

FIGURE 3.23 Solid alveolar rhabdomyosarcoma exhibiting a single-file infiltration pattern, resembling lobular carcinoma of the breast. (H&E.)

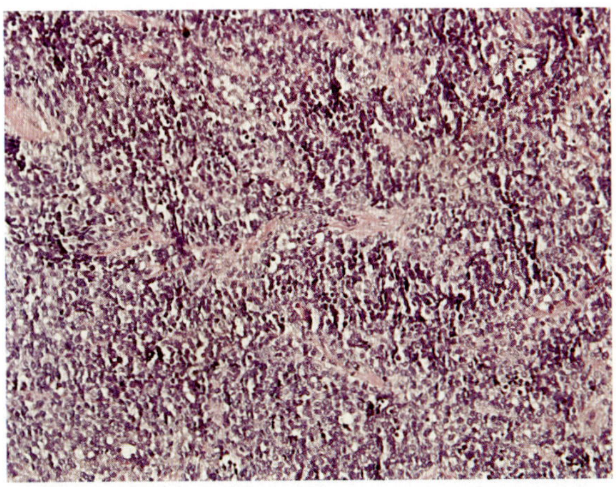

FIGURE 3.22 Solid form of alveolar rhabdomyosarcoma without the obvious alveolar spaces but maintaining the same cytomorphology as the classic variant. (H&E.)

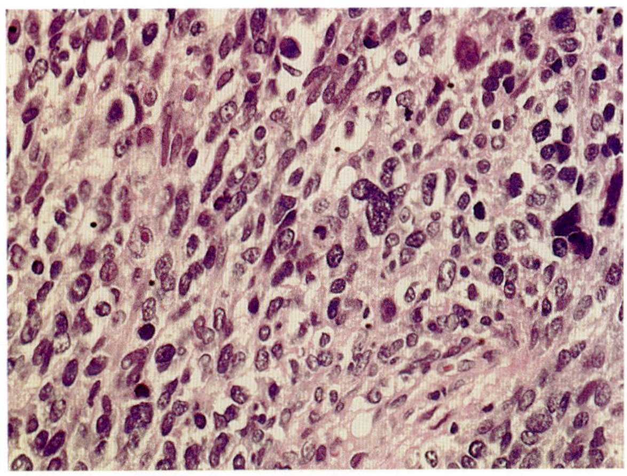

FIGURE 3.24 Anaplastic rhabdomyosarcoma with marked nuclear pleomorphism (greater than three to four times the size of adjacent cell nuclei) and multilobated nuclei. (H&E.)

Miscellaneous Tumors

Rhabdomyoblastic elements may occur in other musculoskeletal tumors, including malignant mesenchymoma (discussed with the pleomorphic sarcomas), ganglioneuroma (ectomesenchymoma), and, rarely, within malignant peripheral nerve sheath tumors (malignant triton tumor) (Fig. 3.25).

Fine Needle Aspiration Biopsy

Given the range of histologic subtypes in rhabdomyosarcoma, it is not surprising that there exists a range in cytomorphology as well. In general, the degree of cytomorphologic variability tends to exceed that observed in other small round cell sarcomas. Regardless of subtype, FNA cytologic smears of rhabdomyosarcomas are highly cellular and comprise mostly discohesive neoplastic cells and small clusters (Fig. 3.26).[40] More specifically, the embryonal subtype is composed of small to intermediate-sized cells with round and polygonal-to-spindled cell contours. Nuclei are round to ovoid and hyperchromatic and may have one or more prominent nucleoli. Scant to abundant amounts of dense to stringy cytoplasm rarely associated with cross striations may be present, depending on the degree of differentiation (Fig. 3.27). Well-differentiated rhabdomyoblasts are observed more frequently in postchemotherapy specimens. Myxoid stromal tumor fragments occasionally may be seen (Fig. 3.28). Despite the distinct histologic (and seemingly distinct cytologic) differences between the embryonal and alveolar forms of rhabdomyosarcoma, in the past, absolute distinction was not always possible. Changes in the classification of rhabdomyosarcoma—the recognition of the solid pattern of alveolar rhabdomyosarcoma—have rendered the distinction of embryonal from alveolar rhabdomyosarcoma easier, however.[36] The diagnosis of alveolar rhabdomyosarcoma now is based predominantly on cytologic features. Compared with embryonal rhabdomyosarcoma, the tumor cells in the alveolar form are larger and more uni-

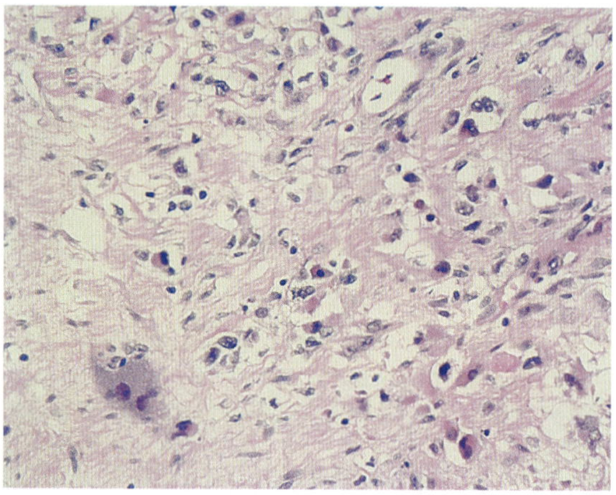

FIGURE 3.25 Ectomesenchymoma with components of embryonal rhabdomyosarcoma and ganglion cell differentiation (ganglion cell, *lower left*). (H&E.)

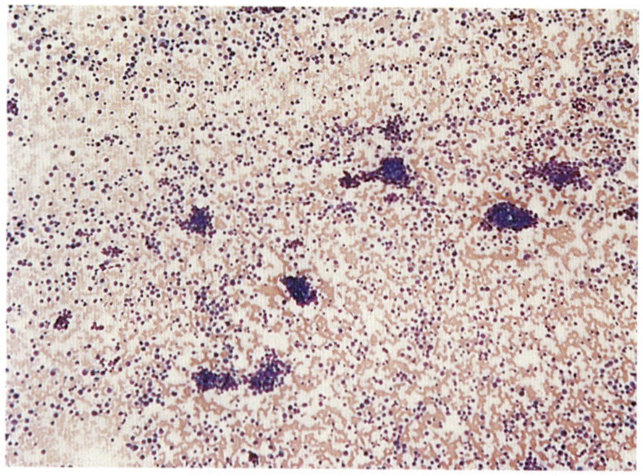

FIGURE 3.26 Fine needle aspiration biopsies of rhabdomyosarcomas typically show hypercellular smears with scattered cohesive tumor cell clusters and solitary tumor cells. (Diff-Quik.)

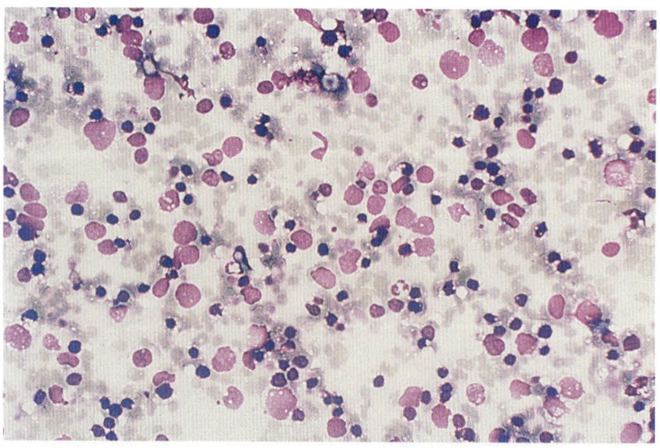

A

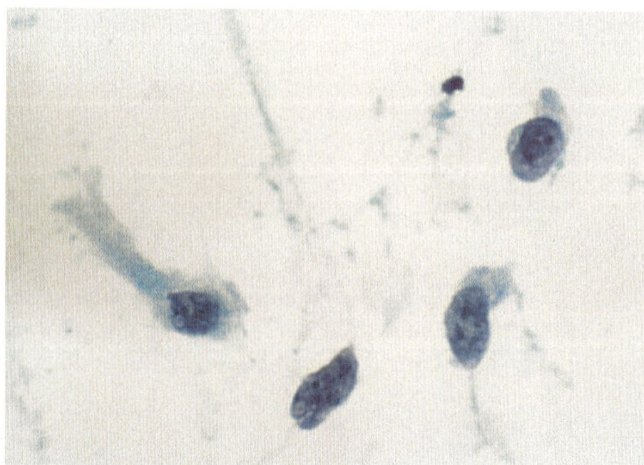

B

FIGURE 3.27 Embryonal rhabdomyosarcoma in cytologic specimen shows tumor cells ranging from small round cell forms to more spindled, irregular shapes with stringy cytoplasm (**A** and **B**). (**A,** Diff-Quik; **B,** Papanicolaou.)

formly round to polygonal with high nuclear-to-cytoplasmic ratios; round, hyperchromatic-to-vesicular nuclei; and one or more nucleoli and are surrounded by a thin rim of dense cytoplasm. A helpful diagnostic feature of alveolar rhabdomyosarcoma is the presence of multinucleated tumor giant cells (Fig. 3.29). Although uncommon, embryonal and alveolar rhabdomyosarcoma may exhibit a frothy background (tigroid appearance) resembling that seen in aspirates of germinomas (Fig. 3.30).[41]

Ancillary Studies

Ultrastructurally, most cases exhibit, at least focally, rudimentary skeletal muscle differentiation, confirmed by the presence of intracytoplasmic thick and thin filaments arranged as sarcomeres with Z-bands or large tangled aggregates.

Immunocytochemical positivity for vimentin, desmin, and muscle-specific actin is observed in more than 90% of cases.[32,42] Focally scattered, small numbers of tumor cells may express cytokeratin, especially the alveolar form.[42] In the IRSG data, approximately 14% of rhabdomyosarcomas show positivity for CD99, generally described as "weak and granular intracytoplasmic" reactivity.[32] More specific immunohistochemical markers have become available for use in paraffin-embedded tissues. The MyoD (myogenic determination) family includes a group of genes that encode DNA-binding proteins that serve as myogenic regulators, helping to maintain the skeletal muscle phenotype. Although not absolutely sensitive, antibodies to two of these regulatory factors, MyoD1 and myogenin, have been found to be useful and highly sensitive in the diagnosis of rhabdomyosarcoma.[43-45] Evidence suggests that strong expression of myogenin may be linked to the alveolar subtype.[45] Kumar and colleagues[45] noted a greater percentage of myogenin positivity in the alveolar subtype compared with the embryonal form. In contrast to the cytoplasmic reactivity observed with desmin and actin, the myogenic proteins generally are expressed by the nucleus. Rare examples of rhabdomyosar-

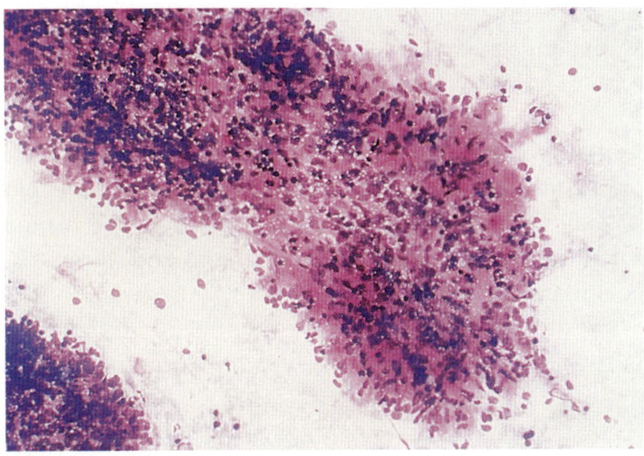

FIGURE 3.28 Embryonal rhabdomyosarcoma with a myxoid stromal tumor fragment. (Diff-Quik.)

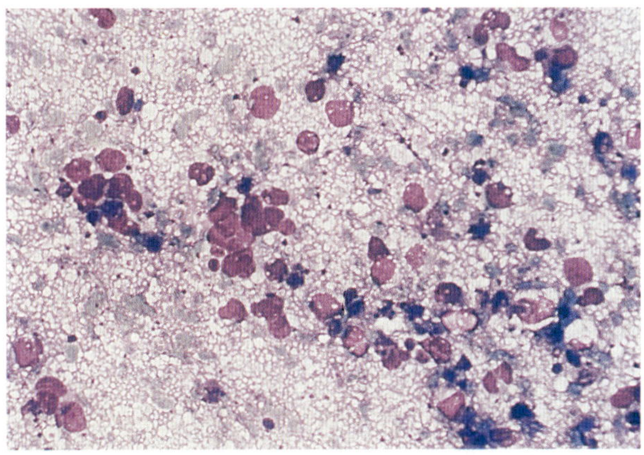

FIGURE 3.30 Rare examples of rhabdomyosarcoma may exhibit a frothy to bubbly background. (Diff-Quik.)

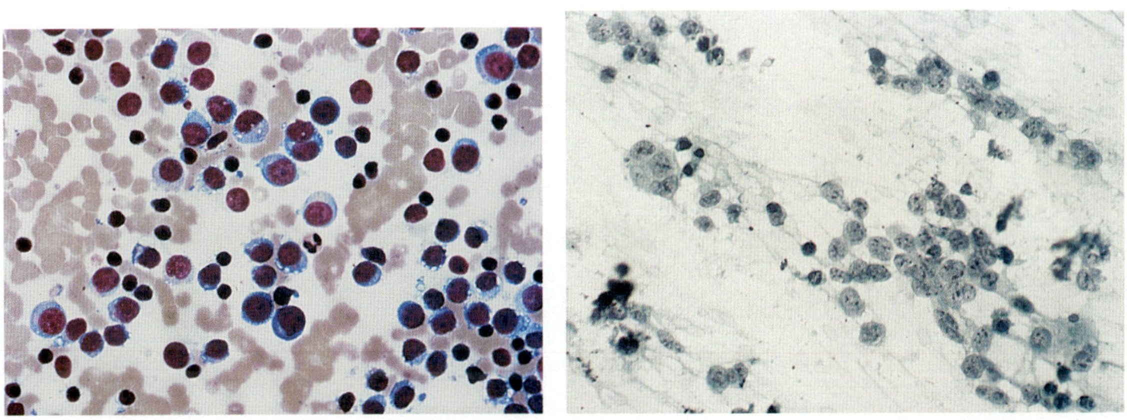

A B

FIGURE 3.29 Alveolar rhabdomyosarcoma displays a population of more uniform and round tumor cells with round nuclei, inconspicuous-to-prominent nucleoli, and high nuclear-to-cytoplasmic ratios. Note the presence of binucleated and multinucleated tumor cells, a feature never observed in Ewing's sarcoma (**A** and **B**). (**A,** Diff-Quik; **B,** Papanicolaou.)

coma also may express hematolymphoid markers. Pinto and colleagues[46] documented three alveolar rhabdomyosarcomas with variable expression of CD10, CD19, and CD20. Two of the tumors had the characteristic translocation of alveolar rhabdomyosarcoma; two also expressed MyoD1.[46] The immunohistochemical properties of rhabdomyosarcoma are summarized in Table 3.7.

Although most rhabdomyosarcomas appear aneuploid, determination of DNA ploidy may be a helpful diagnostic adjunct. Most cases of embryonal rhabdomyosarcoma appear hyperdiploid, whereas alveolar rhabdomyosarcoma frequently is tetraploid.[47] Cytogenetic analysis also may be useful because most cases of alveolar rhabdomyosarcoma, including the so-called solid subtype, have a specific translocation, either the t(2;13)(q35;q14) with the PAX3/FKHR fusion or the t(1;13)(p36;q14) with the PAX7/FKHR fusion.[48] To date, no diagnostically useful, specific translocation has been identified in embryonal rhabdomyosarcoma.

TABLE 3.7 Immunohistochemical Profile of Rhabdomyosarcoma

Immunohistochemical Antibody	Estimated Incidence of Cases That Are Positive (%)
Vimentin	100
Desmin	70-90
Muscle-specific actin	70-90
Myogenin	50-100
MyoD1	60-90
Myoglobin	75
CD99	10-25
Neuron-specific enolase	5-10
Cytokeratin	10-50

Prognosis and Therapy

Adverse prognostic factors include high tumor stage or clinical grouping, older age, and, as we have already considered, histologic subtype. Multimodality therapy, including surgery, chemotherapy, and often radiation therapy, is the preferred form of treatment. Currently the specific form of therapy given depends on the histologic subtype and the stage. To understand fully therapy in childhood rhabdomyosarcoma, it is important to have an appreciation for the complex, specific staging systems employed. These staging systems and classifications are not applicable to other sarcomas and require mention in this chapter. For childhood rhabdomyosarcoma, a traditional site-based pretreatment (T = tumor, N = node, M = metastasis) staging system and a unique, clinical group staging system are used. The TNM pretreatment staging system, summarized in Table 3.8, intimately incorporates anatomic site, is useful for therapeutic planning, and appears at least partly predictive for outcome.[49] Lymph node involvement is defined clinically. The clinical group system, summarized in Table 3.9, is based on similar clinical and pathologic parameters but also accounts for adequacy of surgical resection. Consequently, it requires pathologic examination to determine whether the tumor is confined to the anatomic site of origin and status of the surgical margins.

Until more recently, therapy among all rhabdomyosarcoma subtypes was similar, largely depending on the stage or

TABLE 3.8 TNM Pretreatment Staging for Childhood Rhabdomyosarcoma

Stage	Anatomic Sites	Extension	Size	Regional Nodes	Mets
I	Head and neck (excluding parameningeal)	T1 or T2	a or b	N0, N1, or NX	M0
	Orbit	T1 or T2	a or b	N0, N1, or NX	M0
	Genitourinary (nonbladder/nonprostate)	T1 or T2	a or b	N0, N1, or NX	M0
II	Bladder/prostate	T1 or T2	a	N0 or NX	M0
	Extremities	T1 or T2	a	N0 or NX	M0
	Cranial parameningeal	T1 or T2	a	N0 or NX	M0
	Trunk	T1 or T2	a	N0 or NX	M0
	Retroperitoneum	T1 or T2	a	N0 or NX	M0
III	Bladder/prostate	T1 or T2	a	N1	M0
	Extremities	T1 or T2	b	N0, N1, or NX	M0
	Cranial parameningeal	T1 or T2	b	N0, N1, or NX	M0
	Trunk	T1 or T2	b	N0, N1, or NX	M0
	Retroperitoneum	T1 or T2	b	N0, N1, or NX	M0
IV	All anatomic sites	T1 or T2	a or b	N0 or NX	M1

T1, tumor confined to anatomic site of origin; T2, tumor extending beyond anatomic site of origin; a, <5 cm in greatest dimension; b, >5 cm in greatest dimension; N0, regional nodes not clinically involved by tumor; N1, regional nodes clinically involved by tumor; NX, regional node status not clinically known; Mets, metastasis; M0, no distant metastasis; M1, distant metastasis is present.

extent of disease. IRSG protocols for low-risk and low-stage patients call for the addition of an alkylating agent (cyclophosphamide) to the usual regimen (vincristine and actinomycin D) if the rhabdomyosarcoma subtype is unfavorable (e.g., alveolar). Adolescent patients with metastatic disease at presentation (group IV) are treated similarly, however, regardless of subtype. For these reasons, close communication of the pathologist with the pediatrician is recommended in difficult cases to avoid unnecessary tests and additional biopsies. In some circumstances, a diagnosis of simply rhabdomyosarcoma suffices for initial treatment purposes.

As we have already mentioned, cytodifferentiation after chemotherapy has been recognized for some time. Coffin and colleagues[50] concluded that such findings were observed more frequently in botryoid and conventional embryonal subtypes than in the alveolar form. Cytodifferentiation associated with decreased proliferative activity (measured by immunohistochemistry, MIB-1, and topoisomerase II-α) in botryoid rhabdomyosarcoma correlated with improved survival. Conversely, in conventional embryonal and alveolar subtypes, unchanged or increased proliferative activity after therapy suggests more aggressive behavior.[50]

As in Ewing's sarcoma, there is some evidence to suggest that the molecular genotype may influence prognosis. Early evidence suggests that alveolar rhabdomyosarcoma with the t(1;13)(p36;q14) and PAX7/FKHR fusion may be associated with less aggressive behavior and longer disease-free survival than the more common t(2;13)(q35;q14) with the PAX3/FKHR fusion.[32]

Extracardiac Rhabdomyoma

Rhabdomyomas, benign tumors with skeletal muscle differentiation, are exceedingly rare, far less common than their malignant counterparts, rhabdomyosarcomas. Whether some or all forms of rhabdomyoma represent neoplasms or hamartomas is unclear. Table 3.10 summarizes the clinicopathologic features of the various rhabdomyoma subtypes.

Adult Rhabdomyoma

Adult rhabdomyoma is the most common form of extracardiac rhabdomyoma, occurring almost exclusively in the head and neck region of middle-aged to older adults. More specifically, the oropharynx frequently is involved and men are affected more commonly than women.[51,52] Although most examples present as solitary masses, 20% are multifocal. Histologically, adult rhabdomyomas are classically well-

TABLE 3.9 Clinical Group Staging System for Childhood Rhabdomyosarcoma

Clinical Stage	Group Stage	Extent of Disease
I	A	Localized and confined to anatomic site of origin, completely resected
	B	Localized but infiltrating beyond anatomic site of origin, completely resected
II	A	Localized with gross total resection but microscopic residual disease
	B	Completely resected but spread to regional lymph nodes (locally extensive tumor)
	C	Gross total resection but microscopic residual disease and spread to regional lymph nodes (locally extensive tumor)
III	A	Localized or spread to regional lymph nodes; gross residual disease after biopsy only
	B	Localized or spread to regional lymph nodes; gross residual disease after resection or debulking (>50% tumor volume debulking)
IV		Any clinical or group stage with distant metastasis

TABLE 3.10 Clinicopathologic Features of Rhabdomyoma Subtypes

	Adult	Fetal	Genital	Rhabdomyomatous Mesenchymal Hamartoma
Peak Age	>40 yr	Children	20-40 yr	Neonates and infants
Gender Predilection	M, F	M, F	F	M
Anatomic Sites*	Head and neck	Head and neck	Vagina, vulva, cervix	Head and neck
Multifocal	Yes	No	No	Rare

*Most common.

circumscribed, encapsulated lesions, usually less than 5 cm in greatest dimension, and comprise sheets of polygonal eosinophilic cells with granular cytoplasm; frequent cross striations; and round-to-ovoid, peripherally placed nuclei (Fig. 3.31). In cytologic preparations, the cells usually are individually dispersed and arranged in small clusters (Fig. 3.32).[52,53] The differential diagnosis is usually among the epithelioid/polygonal cell tumors, especially granular cell tumor, and hibernoma. Meticulous attention to morphology and immunohistochemistry (e.g., desmin) resolves this dilemma. Local recurrence occasionally occurs after excision.

Fetal Rhabdomyoma

Although fetal rhabdomyoma may arise at any age, most examples present in infants and children. Similar to adult rhabdomyoma, the head and neck region is the favored location, especially the preauricular and postauricular regions; these are typically slow-growing lesions.[52,54,55] Morphologically, fetal rhabdomyomas exhibit a "zoned" appearance, with more obviously mature rhabdomyoblasts peripherally and less mature mesenchymal cells centrally. The matrix is often myxoid. The presence of circumscription, lack of significant nuclear atypia, and scarce mitotic activity help exclude embryonal rhabdomyosarcoma. More cellular forms of fetal rhabdomyoma have been reported, but their existence is controversial.[56] Fetal rhabdomyoma has been reported as a component of nevoid basal cell carcinoma syndrome, albeit rarely.[57] Surgical excision is virtually always curative.

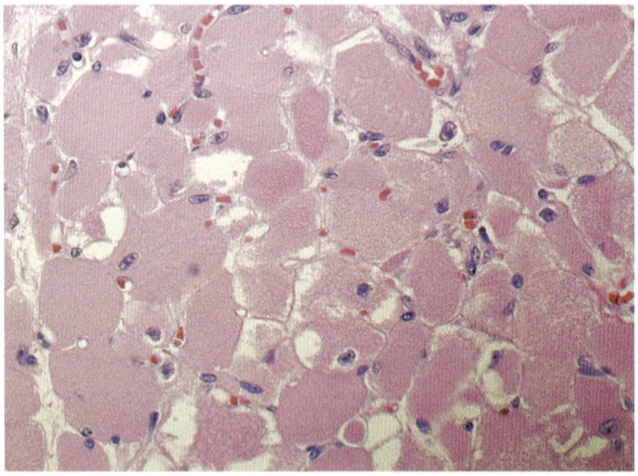

FIGURE 3.31 Adult rhabdomyoma characterized by sheets of eosinophilic, polygonal-shaped rhabdomyoblasts with ovoid, peripherally placed nuclei. (H&E.)

Genital Rhabdomyoma

Genital rhabdomyoma arises as a slow-growing, less than 3 cm, solitary polypoid lesion in the vagina, vulva, or cervix of young to middle-aged women. Most tumors are asymptomatic and found incidentally on routine physical examination.[52,58] Morphologically the polypoid mass generally is covered by epithelium, lacks a distinctive cambium layer, and consists of haphazardly arranged, elongated rhabdomyoblasts within a variably collagenous-to-myxoid matrix. Cross striations are readily apparent, but mitoses are absent (Fig. 3.33). Surgical excision is curative, and local recurrence does not occur.

Rhabdomyomatous Mesenchymal Hamartoma

Rhabdomyomatous mesenchymal hamartoma is an extremely rare congenital lesion, principally arising as one or more cutaneous polyps on the head and neck of male newborns.[59] More specifically, the most common location seems to be the chin. Histologically, mature skeletal muscle fibers are irregularly distributed and admixed with collagen, mature adipose tissue, and adnexal structures within the dermis. Local excision is curative, and recurrence has not been reported.

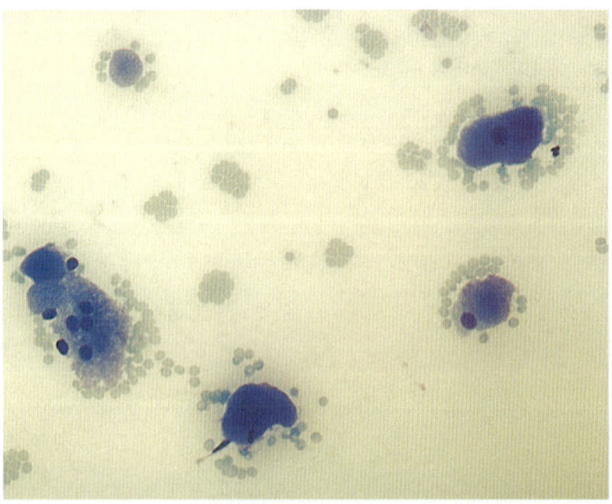

A

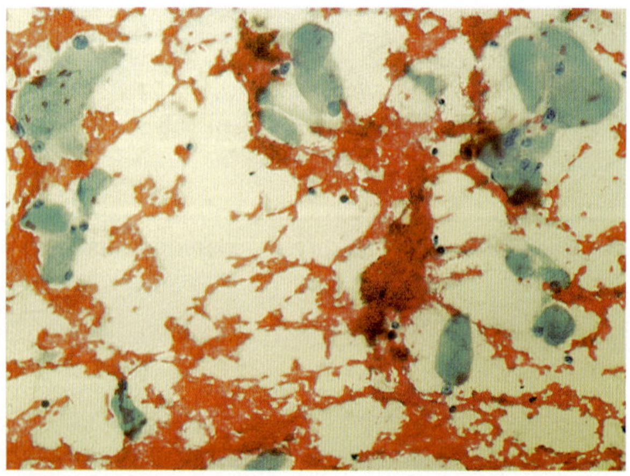

B

FIGURE 3.32 Fine needle aspiration biopsy of adult rhabdomyoma consisting of scattered, mature rhabdomyoblasts with abundant, slightly granular cytoplasm and peripherally placed but uniform-appearing nuclei **(A** and **B). (A,** Diff-Quik; **B,** Papanicolaou.)

Mesenchymal Chondrosarcoma

Clinical Features

Mesenchymal chondrosarcoma is an unusual, high-grade, bimorphic sarcoma that generally arises in bone but far less commonly in soft tissues. Although the tumor may arise at any age, most occur in patients between 10 and 30 years old, similar to that observed in skeletal osteosarcoma.[60,61] Males and females seem equally affected. Common skeletal sites include the skull and craniofacial region (especially the mandible), ribs, spine, and pelvis and lower extremities.[60]

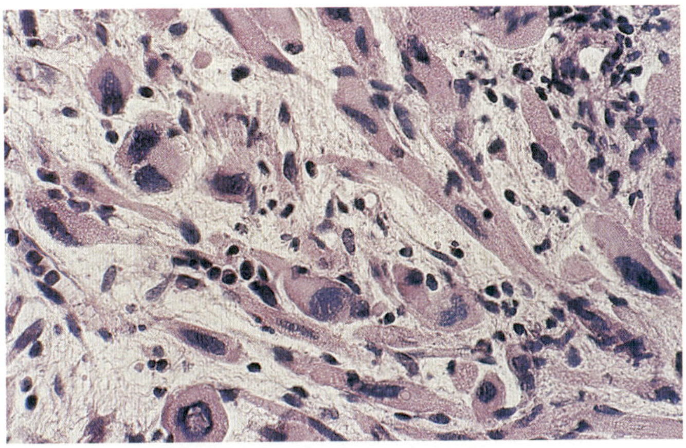

FIGURE 3.33 Haphazardly arranged, elongated rhabdomyoblasts are characteristic of genital rhabdomyoma. (H&E.) (Courtesy of Dr. Robboy, Duke University Medical Center.)

When arising in extraskeletal soft tissues, mesenchymal chondrosarcoma more commonly involves the meninges followed by the lower extremities and soft tissues of the head and neck.[60] Pain is the most common presenting symptom, often accompanied by soft tissue swelling or mass.

Radiologically, most skeletal examples are permeative and lytic with ill-defined borders and usually contain calcifications. Extraskeletal soft tissue extension is common in primary bone lesions. In contrast to Ewing's sarcoma, periosteal reaction tends to occur less frequently. Pathologic fracture also is observed less commonly.[60] Mesenchymal chondrosarcomas arising in extraskeletal sites almost always form a nonspecific soft tissue mass that, similar to its skeletal counterpart, exhibits stippled-to-flocculent calcified densities (Fig. 3.34).[60]

Pathologic Findings

Histology

Histologically the neoplasm has a characteristic bimorphic pattern consisting of undifferentiated small tumor cells, resembling Ewing's sarcoma, alternating with areas of cartilaginous differentiation, exhibiting a benign to low-grade appearance (Fig. 3.35).[62] In the more cellular regions, the undifferentiated cells are arranged in sheets and alveolar patterns. Additionally, a hemangiopericytoma-like vascular pattern characterized by angulated to staghorn-like blood vessels is common in these more cellular regions (Fig. 3.36). Occasionally, spindling of the tumor cells may be the dominant pattern. In less cellular areas, when the stroma becomes

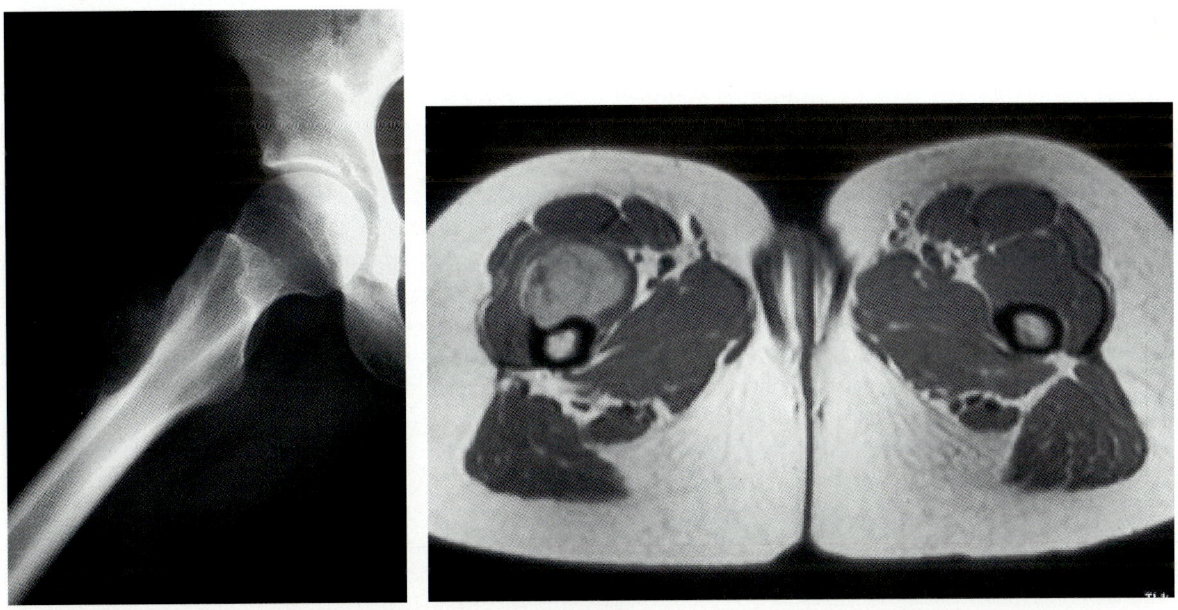

A B

FIGURE 3.34 Mesenchymal chondrosarcoma. Lateral radiograph of the proximal femur reveals an erosion of the anterior femoral cortex with irregular, flocculent soft tissue calcifications **(A).** A proton density axial magnetic resonance image shows a large soft tissue mass abutting the anterior right proximal femur, deep to the musculature and lateral to the neurovascular bundle **(B).**

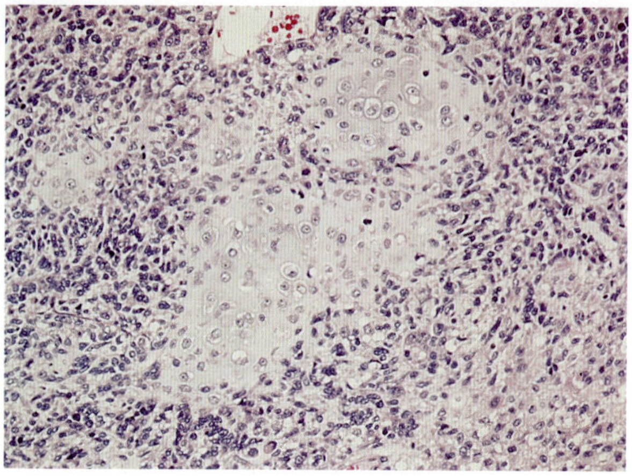

FIGURE 3.35 Bimorphic appearance of mesenchymal chondrosarcoma with nodules of well-differentiated cartilage intimately associated with a small blue round cell population of tumor cells. (H&E.)

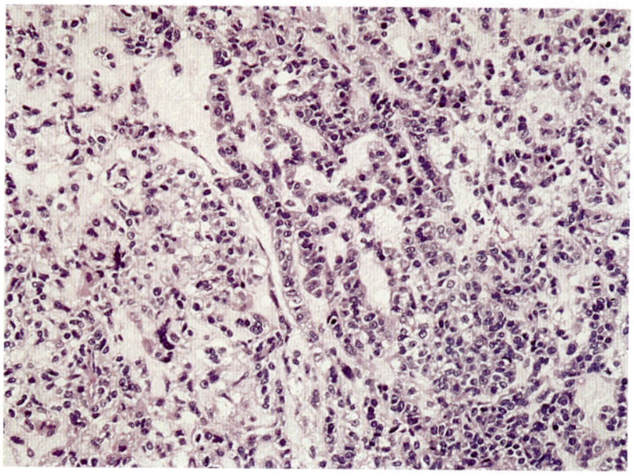

FIGURE 3.37 Mesenchymal chondrosarcoma with infiltrating tumor cells arranged in small nests and cords. (H&E.)

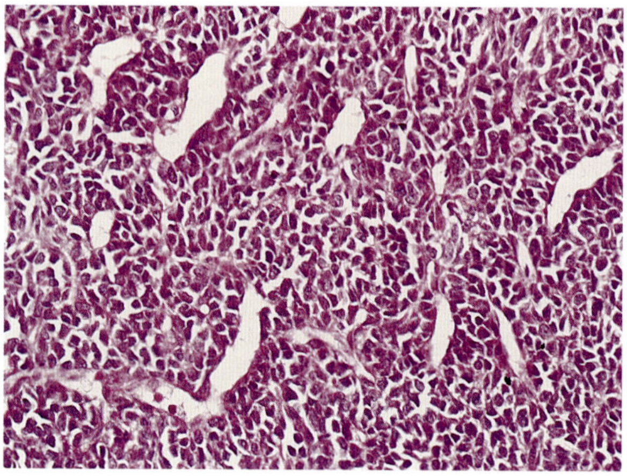

FIGURE 3.36 Mesenchymal chondrosarcoma with sheets of small round cells and a background of hemangiopericytoma-like vascular pattern. (H&E.)

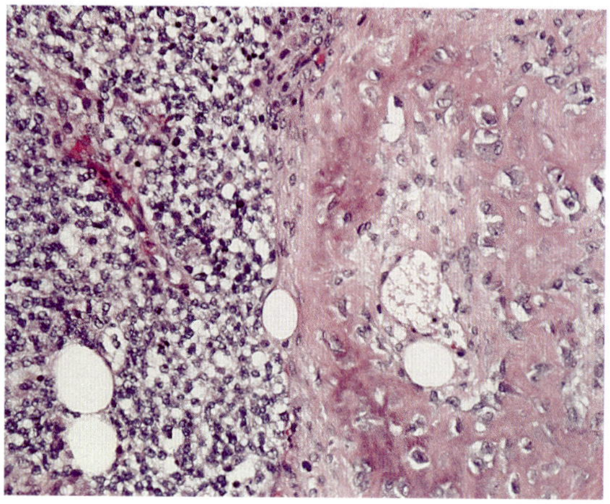

FIGURE 3.38 Mesenchymal chondrosarcoma with osteoid/woven bone formation. (H&E.)

more hyalinized to myxoid, the tumor cells may be arranged in cords and single file arrangements (Fig. 3.37). Eosinophilic material, resembling osteoid, and bone formation may be present, mimicking small cell osteosarcoma (Fig. 3.38).[60] Nevertheless, lace-like pericellular osteoid deposition should be absent. Rarely, especially in small biopsy specimens, the volume of cartilage may be so extensive as to mask the undifferentiated small cell component (Fig. 3.39). Extensive necrosis is usually not seen in primary untreated tumors.[62] Cytologically the tumor cells are mostly uniform, round to ovoid, with high nuclear-to-cytoplasmic ratios, hyperchromasia, and scant amounts of clear to slightly eosinophilic cytoplasm (Fig. 3.40). Mitotic activity is often unusually low, averaging less than one mitotic figure per 10 high-power fields.[60,62]

Fine Needle Aspiration Biopsy

Our experience with FNAB is limited in these lesions. In most cases, the undifferentiated cellular portion is sampled, and the cytologic features closely resemble those of Ewing's sarcoma but tend to show slightly more variability. It is doubtful that the cellular portion of mesenchymal chondrosarcoma can be distinguished reliably from Ewing's sarcoma based on cytology alone. Only the presence of definite matrix material can establish the diagnosis. Cytologic smears are generally highly cellular and composed of solitary cells and cohesive tumor aggregates. At high power, the tumor cells are characteristically uniform, round to ovoid with round nuclei and fairly regular membranes, inconspicuous nucleoli, and scant-to-moderate cytoplasm (Fig. 3.41).[63]

Ancillary Studies

Electon microscopy usually reveals mostly nonspecific features with the more immature cells closely resembling Ewing's sarcoma, including relatively few organelles and the occasional presence of glycogen.[64] Immunohistochemically the small blue cell component of mesenchymal chrondrosar-

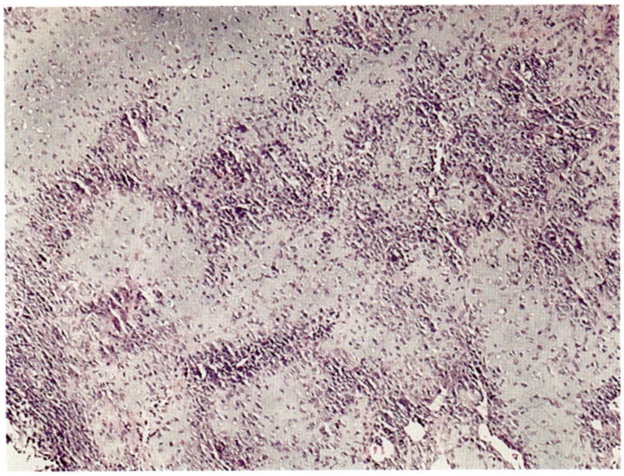

FIGURE 3.39 In occasional examples of mesenchymal chondrosarcoma, the nodules of cartilage may predominate, obscuring the underlying small round cell component. (H&E.)

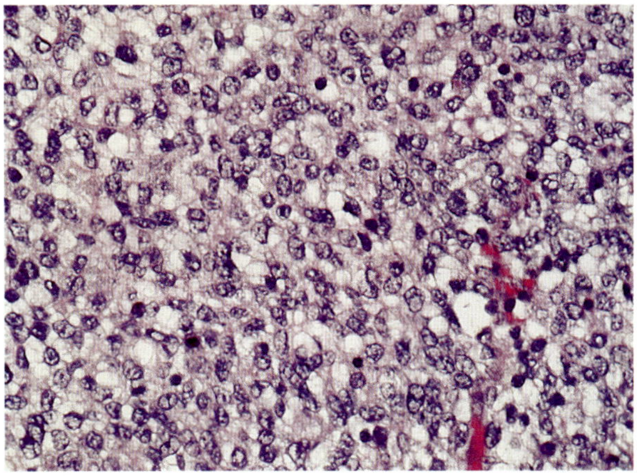

FIGURE 3.40 Individual tumor cells in mesenchymal chondrosarcoma are generally quite uniform, round to ovoid, with vesicular nuclei, a small nucleolus, and scant to abundant and clear to eosinophilic cytoplasm. (H&E.)

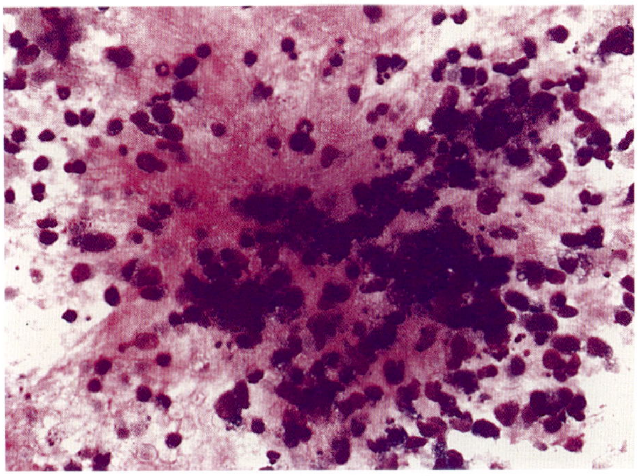

FIGURE 3.41 Fine needle aspiration biopsy of mesenchymal chondrosarcoma with clusters and solitary, small round tumor cells resembling Ewing's sarcoma but intimately associated with metachromatic matrix material. (Diff-Quik.)

TABLE 3.11 Immunohistochemical Profile of Mesenchymal Chondrosarcoma

Immunohistochemical Antibody	Reaction Pattern
Vimentin	+
S-100	+ (cartilaginous component)
CD99	+/−
Neuron-specific enolase	+/−
CD57 (Leu-7)	+/−
Cytokeratin	+/−
Desmin	+/−
MyoD1	+/−
Myoglobin	−
Muscle-specific actin	−
HMB 45	−

coma is virtually always positive for vimentin and frequently shows a divergent phenotype. A strong and diffuse, membranous reactivity for CD99 is observed in more than 75% of cases.[65,66] Consequently the undifferentiated small cell component of mesenchymal chondrosarcoma cannot be distinguished from Ewing's sarcoma based solely on CD99 immunoreactivity.[65] Neuron-specific enolase also usually is expressed. Cytokeratin positivity may be observed in 25% of cases. Less commonly, immunopositivity for desmin and MyoD1 may be seen.[66] S-100 protein is expressed in the cartilaginous component of the tumor but observed rarely in the more cellular, undifferentiated portion.[67] The immunohistochemical profile of mesenchymal chondrosarcoma is summarized in Table 3.11.

No definite and reliable cytogenetic abnormality has been observed in mesenchymal chondrosarcoma. Naumann and colleagues[68] described two tumors with "an identical Robertsonian translocation involving chromosomes 13 and 21 [der(13;21)(q10;q10)]." Rare examples also have been described harboring the t(11;22)(q24;q12), usually associated with Ewing's sarcoma.[69]

Prognosis and Treatment

The prognosis of mesenchymal chrondrosarcoma is generally poor with 5-year survival rates of 40% to 55% and 10-year survival rates of approximately 27% to 29%.[60,61] Mesenchymal chondrosarcoma involving the jaw bones seems to have a better prognosis than tumors occurring in extragnathic sites, with 5- and 10-year survival rates of 82% and 56%.[62] The mainstay of treatment is radical surgery. The role of radiation therapy and chemotherapy is unclear. Because mesenchymal chondrosarcoma clearly represents a high-grade sarcoma, however, some have advocated a combined modality treatment, similar to that of osteosarcoma.[61]

Desmoplastic Small Round Cell Tumor

Clinical Features

Desmoplastic small round cell tumor is a more recently described, usually intra-abdominal malignancy, with characteristic pathologic and molecular features. Most patients are between 15 and 35 years old; males are affected more commonly than females.[70] Abdominal distention or mass, often associated with pain, is the most frequent presenting complaint. Intestinal or urinary obstruction, resulting in constipation or difficulty voiding, also may accompany these symptoms.[70] Radiologically and at exploratory laparotomy, the typical findings include a large intra-abdominal mass usually accompanied by widespread dissemination of tumor implants on the peritoneal surface with minimal to no secondary visceral involvement. Rare examples also have been described involving the pleura, ovary, paratesticular region and scrotum, brain, and soft tissues and bone of the hand.[71-75]

Pathologic Findings

Histology

The characteristic histologic feature of desmoplastic small round cell tumor is the presence of sharply circumscribed nests and clusters of small round tumor cells within a densely fibrotic to fibromyxoid stroma.[70] The neoplastic cells are usually uniform, small, and round to ovoid with high nuclear-to-cytoplasmic ratios, hyperchromasia, and inconspicuous nucleoli. Cytoplasm is typically scant and eosinophilic but may be abundant and clear to vacuolated (Fig. 3.42). Rarely a signet ring cell–like morphology may be observed.[70] As with many small round cell tumors of childhood, a rhabdoid phenotype is a rare but potentially confounding problem.[76] Uncommon histologic features include cells with spindle-like morphology, insular growth patterns, glandular differentiation, and tumor rosettes (Fig. 3.43).

Fine Needle Aspiration Biopsy

Although data are limited, most FNAB samples are variably cellular, probably depending on the amount of desmoplastic stroma within the tumor. The neoplastic cells are mostly small, uniformly round to ovoid, and dispersed individually and in small aggregates (Fig. 3.44).[77] Nuclei exhibit a finely granular chromatin pattern and inconspicuous-to-small nucleoli. As expected, the tumor cells share a close resemblance to Ewing's sarcoma. The presence of variably cellular collagenous stromal fragments, a feature not observed in

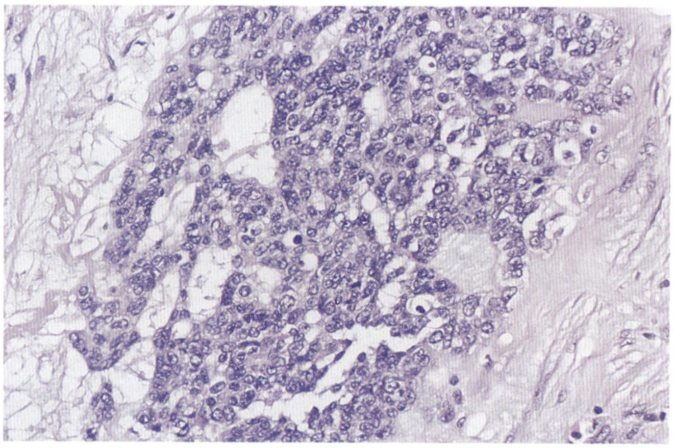

FIGURE 3.43 Desmoplastic small round cell tumor exhibits glandular differentiation and extracellular mucin. (H&E.)

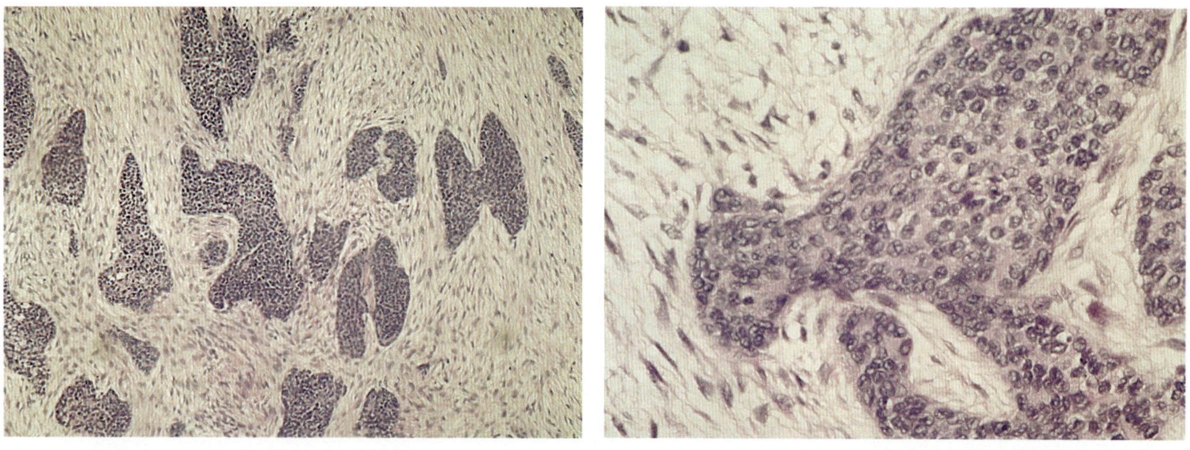

A B

FIGURE 3.42 Classic findings in desmoplastic small round cell tumor are variably sized nests of infiltrating tumor cells within a richly fibroblastic stroma. Individual tumor cells appear mostly uniform with ovoid-to-round nuclei, inconspicuous-to-small nucleoli, and high nuclear-to-cytoplasmic ratios (**A** and **B**). (**A,** low power; **B,** high power, H&E.)

Ewing's sarcoma, is a useful finding, supporting the diagnosis of desmoplastic small round cell tumor.[77] Although a difficult diagnosis to establish by cytomorphology alone, if sufficient material is obtained for cell block or ancillary studies, the polyphenotypic nature of the tumor usually can be confirmed.

Ancillary Studies

Ultrastructural findings tend to be relatively nonspecific showing intermediate filaments. Z-band-like material suggesting smooth muscle or skeletal muscle differentiation is absent.[78] Dense core granules and dendritic-like processes associated with microtubules are observed occasionally and seem to correspond to neural differentiation immunohistochemically.[78] Abundant intracytoplasmic glycogen also is seen sometimes.

Immunohistochemically, desmoplastic small round cell tumors are usually positive for pan-keratins, epithelial membrane antigen, vimentin, neuron-specific enolase, CD15 (Leu-M1), and CD57 (Leu-7). Virtually all cases express desmin, at least focally. Despite positivity for the latter, myogenin and MyoD1 generally are not expressed in these tumors.[78] Cytokeratin 20 and cytokeratin 5/6 appear negative in desmoplastic small round cell tumors, arguing against a mesothelial origin. One third of cases show positive expression for CD99 and CA-125.[78] NB84, a highly sensitive (but relatively nonspecific) marker for neuroblastoma, is positive in 50% of cases.[79] Immunohistochemical stains have been developed targeting the WT1 part of the chimeric protein resulting from the characteristic translocation. It seems that most but not all desmoplastic small round cell tumors show nuclear expression of WT1.[80-82] As expected, WT1 immunoexpression also may be observed in Wilms' tumor but is not expressed by Ewing's sarcoma/PNET. Rare cases of rhabdomyosarcoma have shown positivity for WT1.[81] The immunohistochemical profile of desmoplastic small round cell tumors is summarized in Table 3.12.

In the event that immunohistochemical stains are equivocal, determination of DNA ploidy may be useful because most examples of desmoplastic small round cell tumors are diploid, whereas rhabdomyosarcomas are typically aneuploid.[83,84]

In 75% of cases, cytogenetic analysis reveals a characteristic translocation involving the Ewing's sarcoma gene, t(11;22)(p13;q12), with the formation of the WT1/EWS fusion gene product.[85,86] Rare examples also have been described associated with the t(11;22)(q24;q12) and the

TABLE 3.12 Immunohistochemical Profile of Desmoplastic Small Round Cell Tumor

Immunohistochemical Antibody	Estimated Incidence of Cases That Are Positive (%)
Vimentin	80-100
WT1	90-100
Cytokeratin	80-100
Epithelial membrane antigen	>95
Desmin	100
Neuron-specific enolase	70-85
CD57 (Leu-7)	60-70
CD15 (Leu-M1)	60-70
CD99	10-35
CA-125	40-50
Muscle-specific actin	10-50
Myogenin	Negative
MyoD1	Negative
S-100	Negative
HMB-45	Negative
Carcinoembryonic antigen	Negative

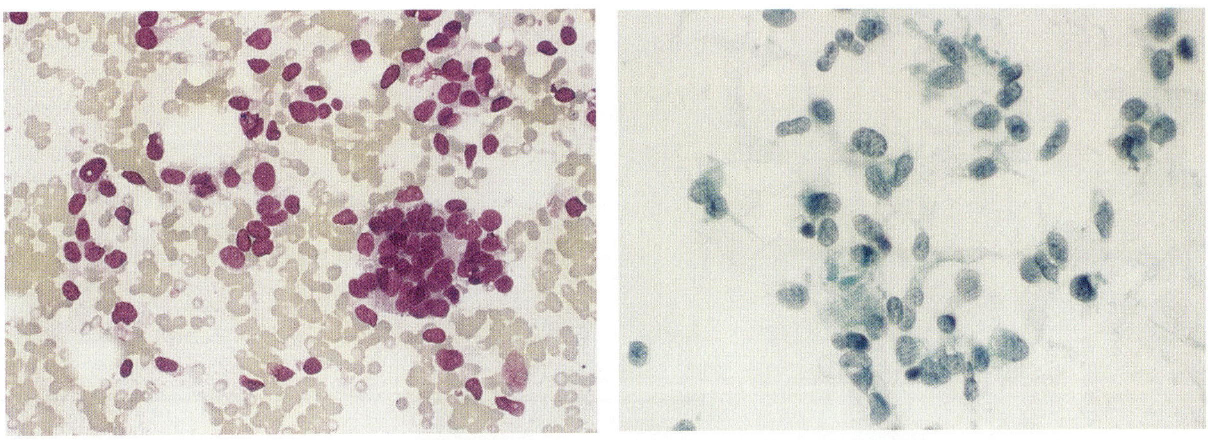

A B

FIGURE 3.44 Fine needle aspiration biopsy of desmoplastic small round cell tumor generally resembles Ewing's sarcoma, with moderately to highly cellular smears and small cohesive clusters and solitary tumor cells. Significant nuclear pleomorphism is absent **(A** and **B). (A,** Diff-Quik; **B,** Papanicolaou.)

EWS/FLI-1 fusion and the t(21;22)(q22;q12) and the EWS/ERG fusion, both of which are usually characteristic of Ewing's sarcoma.[87,88]

Prognosis and Therapy

Despite at least partial responses to multimodality therapy, virtually all patients with intra-abdominal desmoplastic small round cell tumors die of the disease.[70,89] Aggressive surgical and medical therapy is the treatment of choice in most patients; most are not cured, however. Nevertheless, combination chemotherapy seems to offer some palliation, allowing for a longer survival in isolated cases.[89]

Olfactory Neuroblastoma

Olfactory neuroblastoma, also known as esthesioneuroblastoma, is a relatively rare but site-specific neoplasm believed to arise from primitive basal cells of the olfactory membrane. Consequently, its preferential localization is within the upper nasal vault.

Clinical Features

In contrast to typical neuroblastoma, olfactory neuroblastomas rarely arise during early childhood. Most cases occur in patients older than age 20.[90,91] The tumor occurs almost exclusively high in the nasal cavity adjacent to the olfactory bulb. Localized, unilateral lesions present with nasal obstruction or epistaxis or both but also may be associated with anosmia and rhinorrhea. Larger, more destructive lesions extending to adjacent sinuses may present with headache and visual disturbances. Radiologically the lesions are destructive and may contain calcifications (Fig. 3.45).

Pathologic Findings

Histology

Histologically the tumors closely resemble childhood neuroblastoma, chiefly composed of primitive neuroepithelial cells. The degree of differentiation may range from well-differentiated lesions forming classic rosettes with central lumina (Flexner type) or pseudorosettes with a neurofibrillar core (Homer-Wright type) to poorly differentiated tumors exhibiting moderate nuclear pleomorphism and a diffuse, patternless architecture (Fig. 3.46).[91,92] At low power, the tumor usually appears as aggregates or nests within a fibrovascular stroma. In the absence of rosettes, probably the most helpful diagnostic feature is the presence of a neuropil fibrillary background.[91] In contrast to childhood neuroblastoma, ganglion cells tend to be rare but are of diagnostic value if observed. At high power, the neoplastic cells are uniform and round with round, hyperchromatic nuclei; inconspicuous nucleoli; and scant rims of slightly eosinophilic-to-vacuolated cytoplasm. Mitotic activity is variable. Rare examples have been described with foci of divergent epithelial differentiation, such as adenocarcinoma.[93]

Fine Needle Aspiration Biopsy

Cytologic specimens from these tumors are rarely obtained but show similar features of other small round cell tumors, including highly cellular smears, discohesive tumor cells with occasional small clusters, and uniformly round tumor cells with high nuclear-to-cytoplasmic ratios. The nuclei

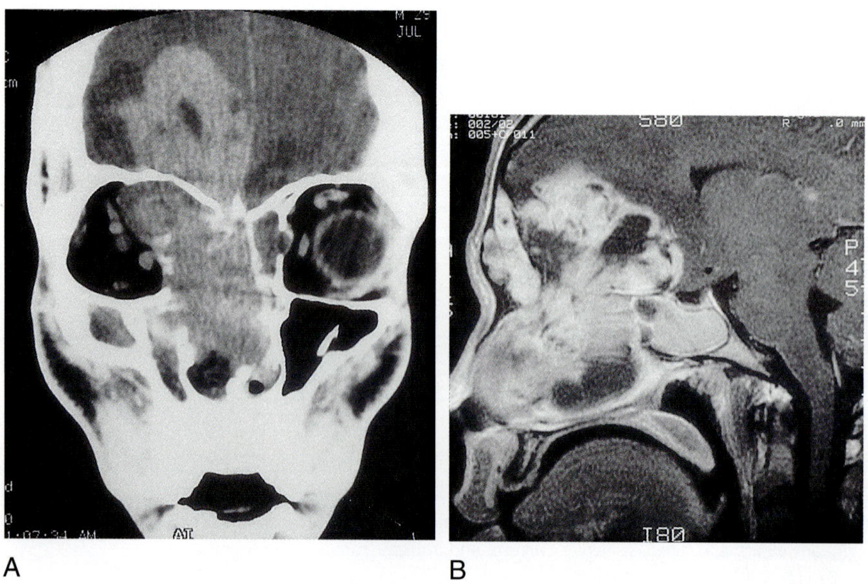

FIGURE 3.45 Olfactory neuroblastoma. A coronal computed tomographic scan shows a soft tissue mass centered in the right ethmoid sinus extending into the right orbit, right maxillary sinus, and nasal passages and across the planum sphenoidale into the anterior cranial fossa **(A)**. A sagittal magnetic resonance image in another patient shows a heterogeneous mass involving the anterior cranial fossa and nasal passages **(B)**. (**A** and **B** courtesy of Dr. M. Castillo, University of North Carolina.)

typically display a finely granular chromatin pattern with inconspicuous nucleoli and scant rims of cytoplasm.[94,95] As in histology preparations, the most useful cytologic feature is the presence of a backgound neuropil matrix, best observed in Romanowsky stained smears.

Ancillary Studies

Ultrastructurally, most tumors display typical findings of primitive neuroepithelia, including intracytoplasmic dense core granules, neuritic processes, and, less commonly, neurotubules and cilia.[95,96]

Immunohistochemical stains for neuron-specific enolase and other more specific neuroendocrine markers (e.g., chromogranin and synaptophysin) are usually positive. S-100 protein typically decorates a population of dendritic, sustentacular cells at the periphery of the tumor lobules.[97,98] Cytokeratins and epithelial membrane antigen are infrequently positive. Aiding in the distinction from Ewing's sarcoma, the tumor cells are uniformly negative for CD99.[97] The immunohistochemical characteristics of olfactory neuroblastoma are summarized in Table 3.13.

Cytogenetic and molecular studies have been conflicting. Earlier reports suggested that olfactory neuroblastoma shared a kinship with Ewing's sarcoma/PNET, owing to genetic evidence of a t(11;22) translocation.[99] More recent studies have documented an absence of the EWS-FLI1 gene fusion in olfactory neuroblastoma.[97]

Prognosis and Treatment

Prognosis generally is related to the Kadish stage, as summarized in Table 3.14.[90,100] Approximately half of patients present with stage B disease.[91] Patients with disease extending outside of the nasal cavity and paranasal sinuses have survival rates of less than 50%. The strongest prognostic indicator may be the adequacy of surgical resection.[91] Consequently, complete surgical resection coupled with adjuvant radiation therapy or chemotherapy probably offers the best chance for cure.[91,101,102] Despite a wide range in morphologic differentiation, histologic features do not seem to correlate significantly with prognosis.[92]

TABLE 3.13 Immunohistochemical Profile of Olfactory Neuroblastoma

Immunohistochemical Antibody	Estimated Incidence of Cases That Are Positive
S-100	80-90 (cells surrounding tumor lobules)
Neuron-specific enolase	90-100
Chromogranin	70-80
Synaptophysin	70-80
Neurofilament	30-40
Cytokeratin	20-25
Epithelial membrane antigen	<10
CD99	Negative

TABLE 3.14 Kadish Staging System for Olfactory Neuroblastoma

Clinical Stage	Definition	5-Year Survival Rates (%)*
A	Disease confined to nasal cavity	75
B	Disease confined to nasal cavity and paranasal sinuses	68
C	Local or distant spread beyond the nasal cavity or sinuses	41

*Survival data are based on the results of Elkon and colleagues.[90]

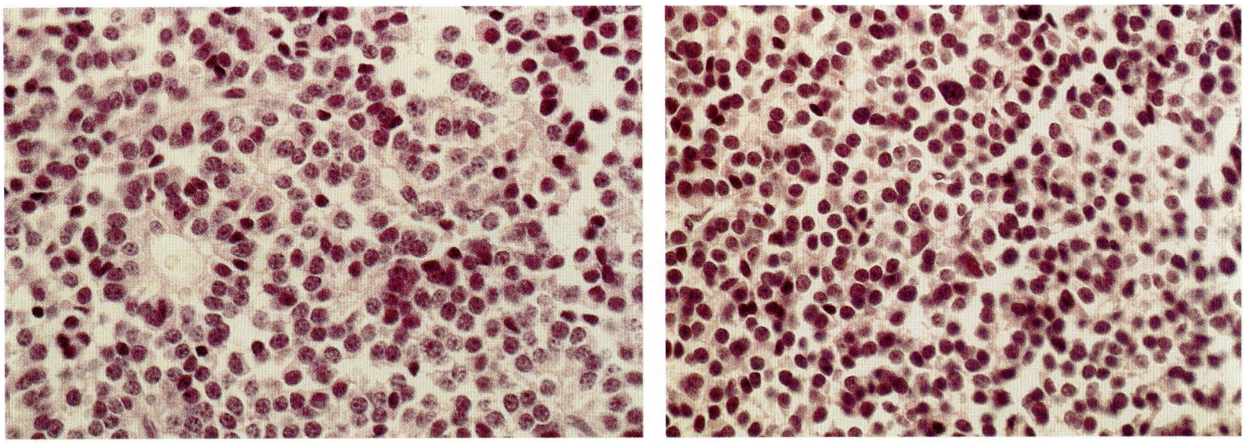

A B

FIGURE 3.46 Olfactory neuroblastoma with a uniform, small round tumor cell population and rosettes **(A).** Occasional examples may show more significant nuclear pleomorphism and atypia, lacking obvious rosettes **(B).** (**A** and **B,** H&E.)

Melanotic Neuroectodermal Tumor of Infancy

Melanotic neuroectodermal tumor of infancy, also known as congenital melanocarcinoma, retinal anlage tumor, and melanotic progonoma, is an extraordinarily rare tumor of neural crest origin that typically develops during infancy.

Clinical Features

Virtually all patients are younger than 1 year old at presentation. Most cases involve the bones of the skull and cranial facial region, principally the jaw.[103,104] Preferential sites in decreasing order of frequency include the maxilla, mandible, skull, and dura/brain. Less commonly, extraskeletal localization may occur within the soft tissues of the head and neck and the epididymis.[103,105] Radiographically, skeletal lesions generally present as radiolucent, lytic processes, frequently associated with destruction of developing teeth.

Pathologic Findings

Histology

Histologic specimens generally show two cell populations. Small round, undifferentiated tumor cells, closely resembling neuroblastoma, are within isolated nests and alveolar-like spaces. Lining the alveolar spaces is a second population of larger, more cuboidal-shaped to polygonal-shaped tumor cells containing intracytoplasmic melanin pigment (Fig. 3.47).[103,104] Less frequently, glial tissue may be associated with the small undifferentiated tumor cells.

Fine Needle Aspiration Biopsy

The diagnosis of melanotic neuroectodermal tumor of infancy by FNAB is limited to a few isolated case reports.[106,107] The cytologic findings seem to parallel those seen in tissue biopsy specimens. Smears are composed of a "bimodal" population of small neuroblastoma-like undifferentiated tumor cells

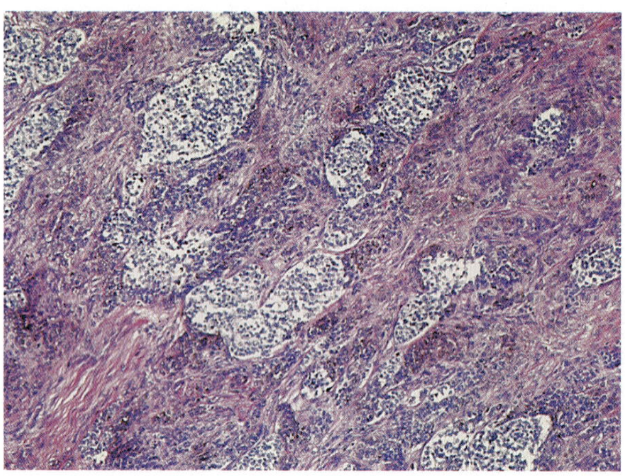

A

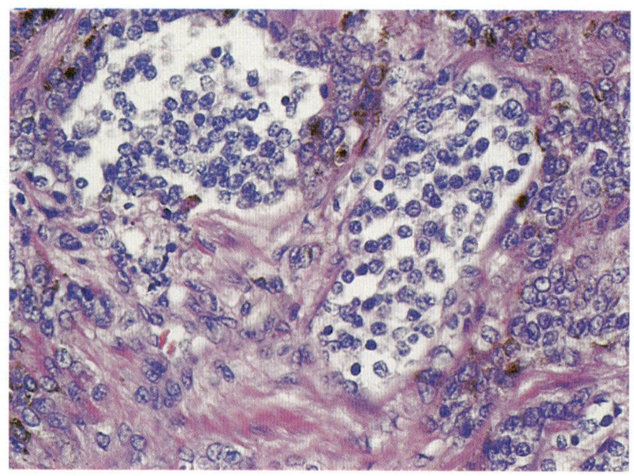

B

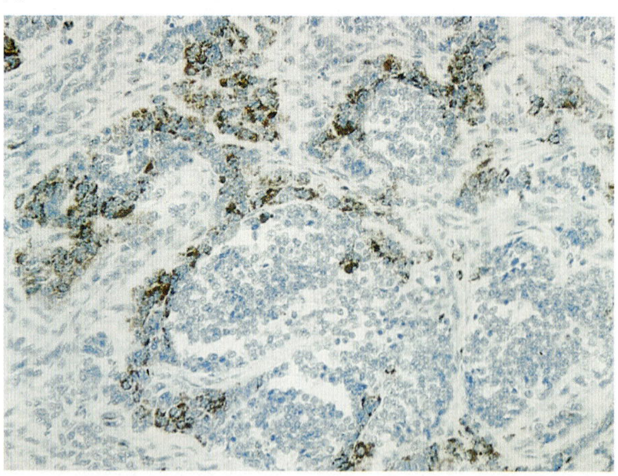

C

FIGURE 3.47 Melanotic neuroectodermal tumor with nests of neuroblastic small round blue cells rimmed by a population of pigmented cells with melanocytic differentiation. The latter are shown more easily by melanocytic markers, such as HMB 45 **(A-C)**. (**A,** low power, H&E; **B,** high power, H&E; **C,** immunoperoxidase stain for HMB 45.)

admixed with larger, epithelioid-appearing tumor cells containing intracytoplasmic melanin granules. It is likely that if adequate material is available from ancillary studies, the diagnosis may be established easily by FNAB.

Ancillary Studies

Ultrastructurally the small undifferentiated tumor cells contain relatively few organelles but may have dense core vesicles and elongated cell processes.[103] The larger cuboidal cells contain intracytoplasmic immature and mature melanosomes, virtually identical to melanosomes observed in cutaneous melanocytes. Elaborate cell junctions and basal laminae also are seen.

Immunohistochemically, virtually all cases reveal HMB-45, cytokeratin, and vimentin positivity within the large cell population (see Fig. 3.47). Immunoreactivity for neuron-specific enolase, synaptophysin, and CD57 (Leu 7) often is observed in small and large cell populations. Chromogranin and desmin are usually negative.[103,104] The immunohistochemical profile of melanotic neuroectodermal tumor of infancy is summarized in Table 3.15.

Currently, no reproducible, specific cytogenetic abnormality has been linked to melanotic neuroectodermal tumor of infancy. There is no evidence at present linking melanotic neuroectodermal tumor of infancy to other malignant small round cell tumors of infancy, including neuroblastoma and Ewing's sarcoma.[108]

TABLE 3.15 Immunohistochemical Profile of Melanotic Neuroectodermal Tumor of Infancy

Immunohistochemical Antibody	Estimated Incidence of Cases That Are Positive (%)
HMB 45 (large cells)	100
Cytokeratin (large cells)	100
Vimentin (large cells)	90-100
Epithelial membrane antigen (large cells)	30-45
Neuron-specific enolase (small and large cells)	60-90
CD57 (Leu 7) (small and large cells)	50-70
Synaptophysin (small and large cells)	40-80
Glial fibrillary acidic protein (small and large cells)	20-35
Chromogranin	<10
Desmin	<10
S-100 protein	<10
Carcinoembryonic antigen	Negative

Prognosis and Therapy

Local recurrence may occur in 50% of cases. For this reason, wide surgical resection is the preferred choice of therapy.[109] The role of radiation therapy and chemotherapy at present is unclear. Approximately 5% of cases develop metastases resulting in the death of the patient. Currently, there seems to be no histologic factor predictive of clinical behavior.

Malignant Lymphoma and Hodgkin's Disease

When malignant lymphoma or Hodgkin's disease involves bone or soft tissue, most are "secondary" lymphomas, usually associated with concomitant regional lymph node or visceral involvement or both.[110,111] Non-Hodgkin's lymphoma or malignant lymphoma is more common as a primary osseous or soft tissue malignancy than Hodgkin's disease.

Clinical Features

Primary osseous and soft tissue malignant lymphoma may affect patients at any age; however, most arise in patients older than age 30. They are seen uncommonly in children.[110,112] Symptoms usually are related to pain, especially for tumors arising in osseous sites, and/or the presence of a palpable mass. Systemic signs, such as malaise and fever, are generally absent. These symptoms (including the so-called B-symptoms) are observed frequently in patients with concurrent osseous and nonosseous disease, however.

Radiologically, when arising in bone, malignant lymphoma tends to be quite destructive with extensive permeation and frequent soft tissue extension. Osteosclerotic, osteolytic, and mixed osteolytic/osteosclerotic patterns may be present (Fig. 3.48).[110,113] The degree of bone involvement often is underestimated in radiographs. Although any bone may be involved, osseous malignant lymphoma shows a predilection for the lower extremities, especially the femur and pelvic bones. As a general rule, primary osseous malignant lymphoma more commonly afflicts the appendicular skeleton, whereas secondary involvement by malignant lymphoma more commonly involves the axial skeleton. Similar to its osseous counterpart, primary soft tissue malignant lymphoma also is seen more often within the lower extremities, especially the buttock, thigh, and leg, followed by the trunk and upper extremities.[114]

Because of its rarity, clinicoradiologic data for primary osseous Hodgkin's disease is limited, especially when compared with what is known about primary osseous malignant lymphoma. As in malignant lymphoma, most patients with osseous Hodgkin's disease have, on further investigation,

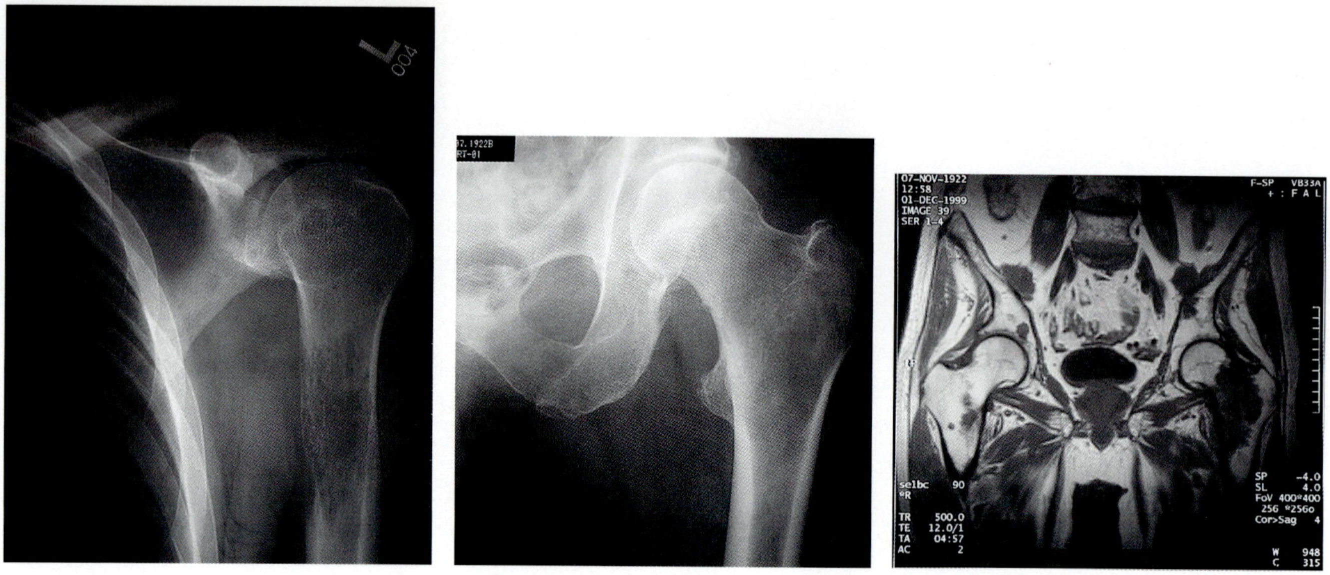

A B C

FIGURE 3.48 Malignant lymphoma. Anteroposterior radiograph of the proximal humerus shows a permeative lytic lesion in the humeral shaft **(A)**. Anteroposterior radiograph of the proximal femur shows a focal area of decreased bone density centered at the level of the lesser trochanter **(B)**. A coronal T1-weighted magnetic resonance image in the same patient shows the lesion extending into the femoral neck. A smaller lesion is present on the right **(C)**.

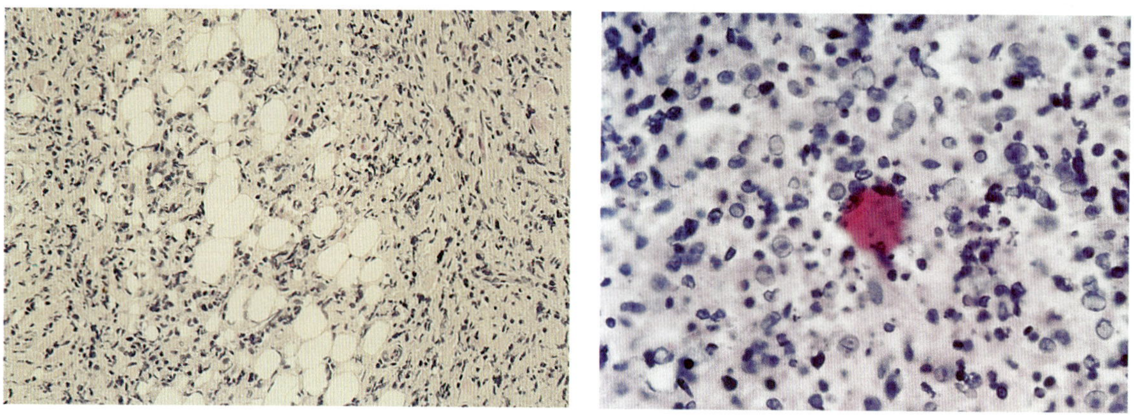

A B

FIGURE 3.49 Malignant lymphoma with marked infiltration of connective tissue. Note the absence of obvious nests and organoid patterns **(A)**. At high power, large, obviously malignant lymphoid cells are admixed with a smaller, probably reactive population of lymphocytes **(B)**. **(A,** low power, H&E; **B,** high power, H&E.)

nonosseous involvement as well. Most patients are adults.[111] The axial skeleton tends to be involved more often than the appendicular skeleton. Among cases involving the extremities, the lower limb is affected more commonly than the upper limb. Radiologically, most examples present as destructive masses with associated soft tissue extension.[111]

Pathologic Findings

Histology

As expected, most primary and soft tissue malignant lymphomas are large cell, B-cell proliferations. They typically are manifested as a diffuse infiltrative pattern of large, sometimes histiocytic-appearing lymphoid cells, admixed with a variable population of smaller, mature-appearing T cells (Fig. 3.49).[110] Compared with other small round cell tumors, the nuclei of the larger lymphoid cells show substantial variability in size and shape, including irregular nuclear membranes, polylobations, prominent grooves, and folds.[110,112] The chromatin pattern is typically vesicular, and nucleoli are often prominent. The background stroma frequently is richly fibroblastic, containing abundant collagen and reactive-appearing fibroblasts, sometimes mimicking a primary sarcoma (Fig. 3.50). Lanham and colleagues[114] reported a study of 75 cases of malignant lymphoma presenting in soft tissue. Approximately 44% of the cases were incorrectly identified. The most

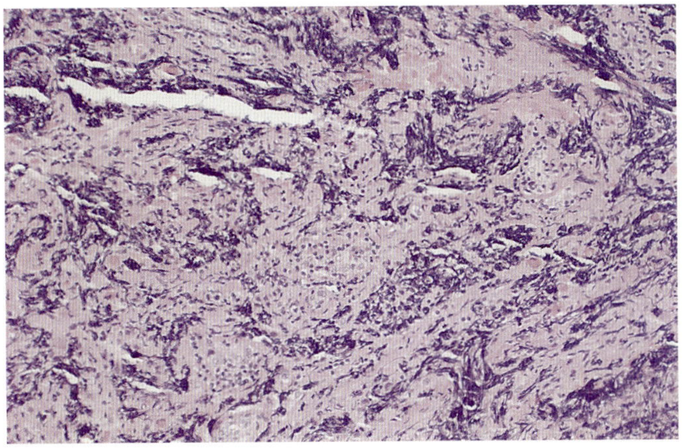

FIGURE 3.50 When present in bone, malignant lymphoma is often associated with abundant crush artifact and a richly fibroblastic stroma. (H&E.)

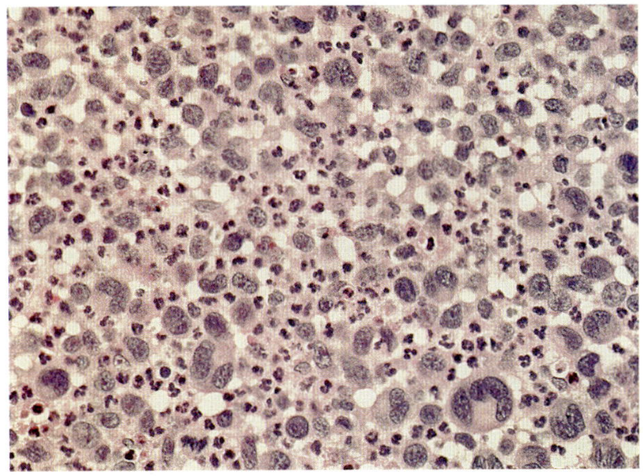

FIGURE 3.51 Anaplastic malignant lymphoma shows significant nuclear pleomorphism, often exhibiting multinucleated tumor giant cells. Background inflammatory cells, such as neutrophils, are not unusual. (H&E.)

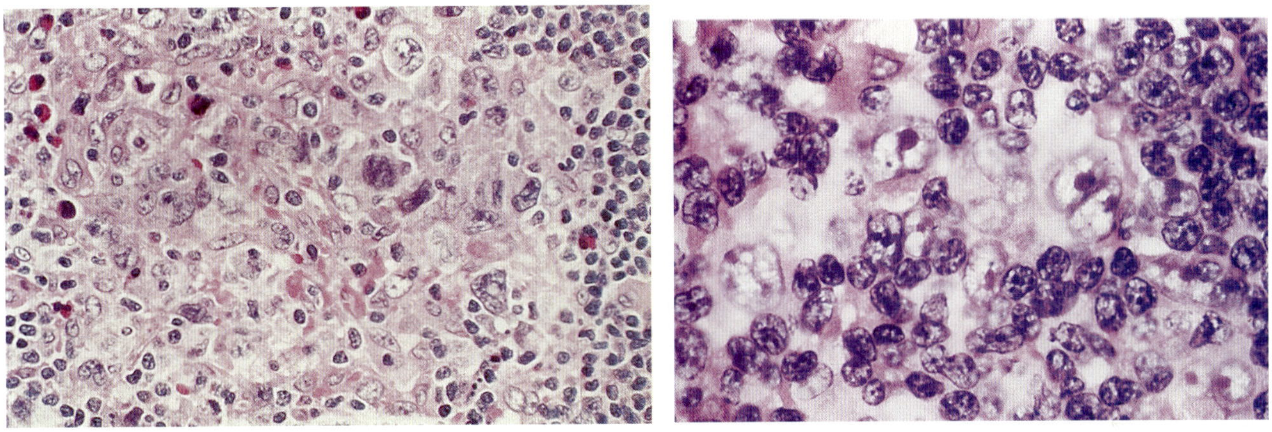

A B

FIGURE 3.52 Typical features of Hodgkin's disease include the presence of diagnostic obvious uninucleated-to-binucleated Reed-Sternberg cells with inclusion-like nucleoli and a heterogeneous background of lymphocytes, eosinophils, and histiocytes. **(A,** low power; **B,** high power, H&E.) (Courtesy of Dr. Maygarden, University of North Carolina.)

common misinterpretation was that of a pleomorphic sarcoma (e.g., pleomorphic rhabdomyosarcoma, malignant fibrous histiocytoma, or pleomorphic liposarcoma).[114] Marked nuclear pleomorphism is observed most often with anaplastic variant of malignant lymphoma (Fig. 3.51). Spontaneous tumor necrosis, especially in the osseous form, is observed commonly.

The histologic findings in osseous Hodgkin's disease differ little from the findings observed in nonosseous locations. Typically an intertrabecular infiltrate contains an admixture of lymphocytes, eosinophils, plasma cells, and histiocytes associated with scattered, randomly distributed Reed-Sternberg cells (Fig. 3.52).[111] Variable amounts of stromal fibrosis and tumor necrosis may be observed. Subtyping generally is not possible or recommended. The most likely misinterpretation is acute osteomyelitis, especially if the diagnostic Reed-Sternberg cells are sparse or not recognized.

Fine Needle Aspiration Biopsy

Because of the fibroblastic background, FNAB of malignant lymphoma may yield unsatisfactory results (i.e., too few cells for diagnosis).[115] Adequate specimens frequently are characterized by moderately cellular smears consisting of discohesive, round tumor cells with high nuclear-to-cytoplasmic ratios and a thin rim of basophilic cytoplasm (Fig. 3.53). Among large cell types, the nuclei are usually vesicular with prominent nucleoli and irregular nuclear membranes, often folded or displaying obvious grooves (Fig. 3.54). Tiny, detached pieces of cytoplasm (lymphoglandular bodies) are often numerous and randomly scattered among the lymphoid cells. Among the more common large cell malignant lymphoma, the diagnosis is generally easily established based on cytomorphology alone. For the rare examples of small cell malignant lymphoma involving bone or soft tissue, however, ancillary studies generally are required for a definitive diagnosis.

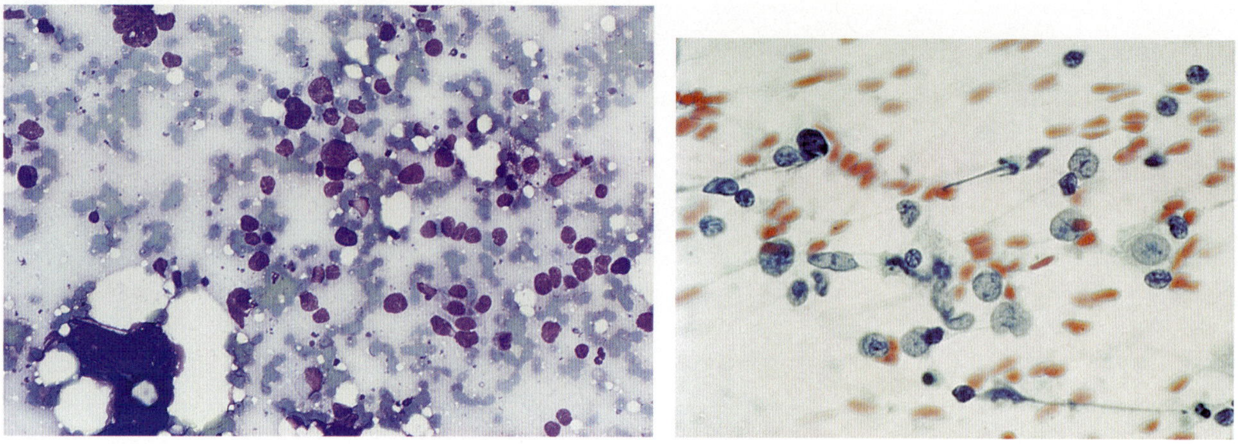

A B

FIGURE 3.53 Fine needle aspiration biopsy specimens of malignant lymphomas range from scant to highly cellular specimens with a mostly discohesive population of lymphoid cells. Note the variation in size and shape of the individual tumor cells **(A** and **B). (A,** Diff-Quik; **B,** Papanicolaou.)

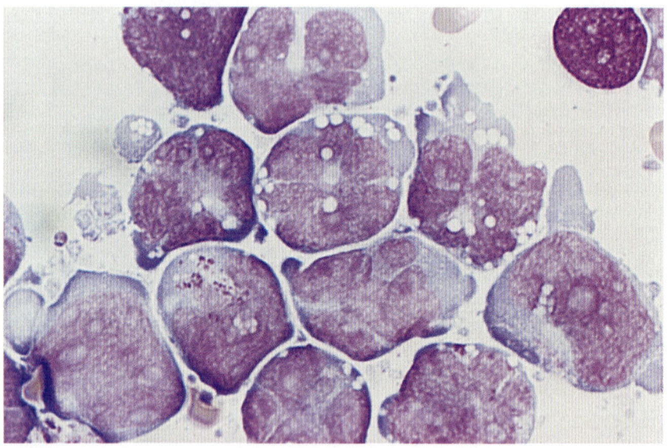

FIGURE 3.54 Large cell malignant lymphoma with markedly irregular nuclear membranes, nuclear cleaves, folds, and clover leaf-shaped forms. (Diff-Quik.)

FNAB of Hodgkin's disease is not generally problematic if the characteristic Reed-Sternberg cells can be shown in cytologic smears. The latter generally are dominated by a numerous, mostly mature-appearing lymphocytes accompanied by variable amounts of histiocytes, neutrophils, and eosinophils (Fig. 3.55).[116]

Ancillary Studies

Immunohistochemically, most large cell malignant lymphomas express B-cell markers (CD20).[110,112] As already mentioned, randomly distributed, probably reactive small lymphocytes are frequently admixed and generally express T-cell markers (CD3). Some malignant lymphomas of bone show features consistent with the "anaplastic" variant and consequently may express CD30 and ALK kinase.[112] The Reed-Sternberg cells of Hodgkin's disease usually coexpress CD15 (Leu M1) and CD30 (Ki-1) but should be negative for CD45 and B-cell and T-cell markers.[111]

In most cases, cytogenetic analysis is not helpful. Rare examples of anaplastic large cell lymphoma contain the t(2;5)(p23;q35) and the NPM/ALK fusion, however.

Prognosis and Therapy

The prognosis for primary osseous malignant lymphoma is usually better than for other similar-appearing, small round cell mesenchymal malignancies.[110] Surgery usually is not indicated unless the process is complicated by pathologic fracture. Standard therapy generally consists of radiation and adjunct chemotherapy. Patients with multifocal osseous disease tend to have a worse prognosis than do patients with solitary bone involvement. Ostrowski and colleagues[113] documented a 10-year survival rate of 53% for patients with a solitary lesion compared with a 10-year survival rate of 35% for patients with multifocal osseous disease.

The presence of osseous involvement in Hodgkin's disease does not seem to alter the overall prognosis.[111] Using standard chemotherapeutic regimens, the overall prognosis is good. As in osseous malignant lymphoma, surgery is generally not indicated for osseous Hodgkin's disease.

Plasmacytoma

Plasmacytoma (or plasma cell myeloma) is the most common primary malignancy of bone. It may present initially as a solitary lesion or manifest as a disseminated, multifocal, and systemic form, commonly referred to as *multiple myeloma.*

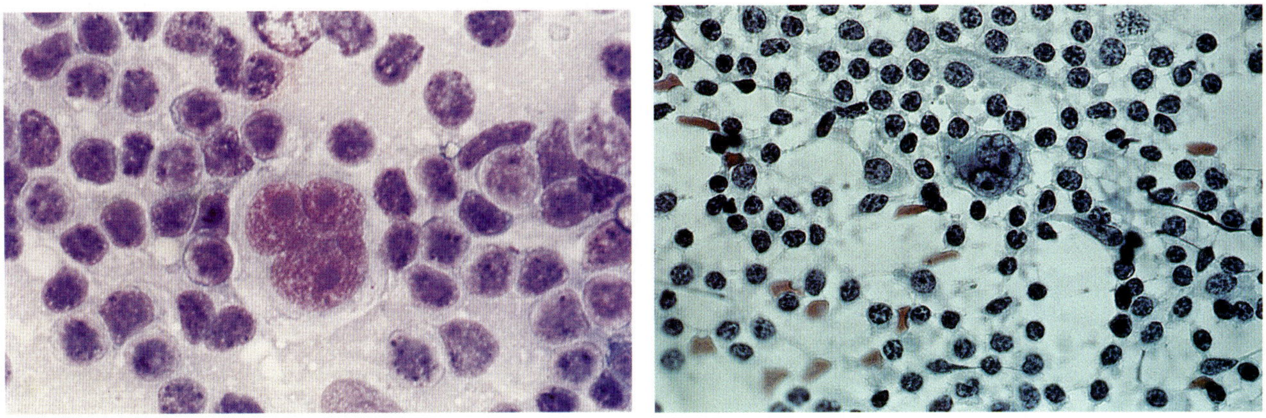

A B

FIGURE 3.55 The diagnosis of Hodgkin's disease by fine needle aspiration biopsy rests on the finding of classic and diagnostic Reed-Sternberg cells **(A** and **B). (A,** Diff-Quik; **B,** Papanicolaou.) (Courtesy of Dr. Maygarden, University of North Carolina.)

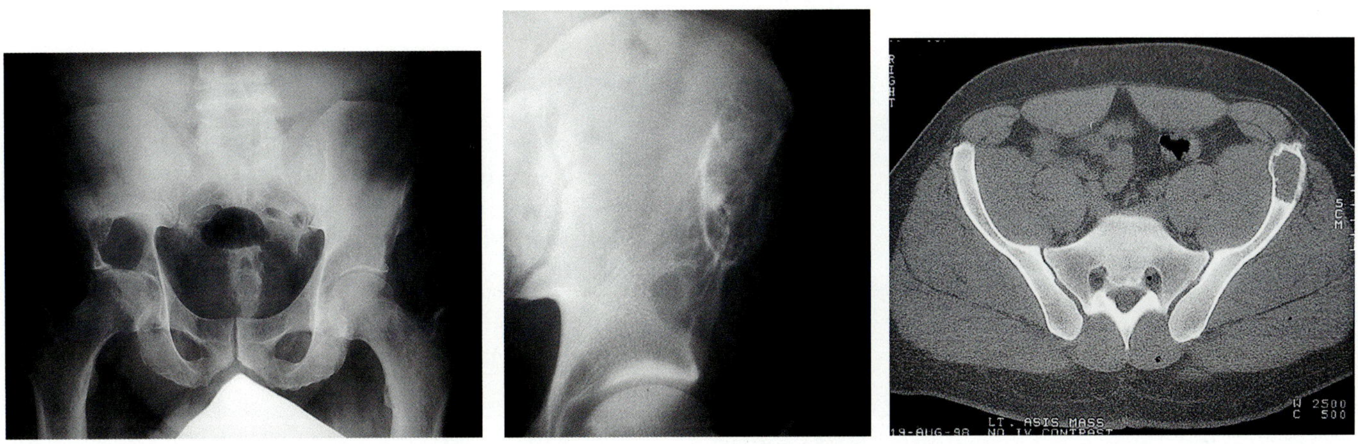

A B C

FIGURE 3.56 Plasmacytoma. Anteroposterior radiograph of the pelvis shows a lytic lesion in the right ilium extending down to the subchondral bone. The margins are well defined, and no matrix calcification is evident **(A).** Anteroposterior radiograph of the left ilium shows a well-defined lytic lesion with sclerotic margins and slight enlargement of the bone **(B).** Computed tomographic scan in the same patient shows the left iliac lesion without soft tissue involvement **(C).**

Clinical Findings

Whether solitary or multiple, most cases of multiple myeloma involve patients older than age 40; there seems to be a slight male predominance. For unknown reasons, the disorder is more common in African-Americans than in whites and tends to arise in families with prior histories of leukemia or lymphoma.[117] The most common presenting symptom is pain. Patients with the disseminated form of the disease may manifest additional systemic symptoms, including malaise and fatigue (usually secondary to anemia), fever, hypercalcemia, and renal failure. Serum protein and urine protein electrophoresis frequently reveal increased levels of monoclonal immunoglobulin in the serum and urine.[118] The most commonly detected monoclonal serum protein is IgG followed by IgA, IgM, IgD, and IgE. One fifth of affected patients may manifest only elevated light-chain immunoglobulins (Bence Jones proteinuria).

Radiographically, plasmacytomas usually form sharply circumscribed "punched-out" areas of bone destruction, generally not associated with a rim of bony sclerosis (Fig. 3.56). In the flat bones, such as the ribs or pelvis, bone expansion may be observed. Despite extensive bone destruction, bone scans are typically negative. Common anatomic sites of involvement include the skull, vertebral spine, ribs, pelvic bones, and scapula.[119] In general, the axial skeleton is involved more often than the appendicular skeleton.

Pathologic Findings

Histologically, plasmacytomas usually are recognized easily, being composed of nests and sheets of plasma cells, sometimes associated with abundant amyloid deposition. The latter may be so prominent as to obscure the underlying neoplastic process.[120] At high power, the plasma cells range from mature, easily identified forms to more blast-like, immature cells containing prominent nucleoli. An intracytoplasmic perinuclear halo is readily identified in at least more mature-appearing plasma cells. Binucleated and multinucleated forms are commonly observed (Fig. 3.57). Mitotic figures are rare.

Fine Needle Aspiration Biopsy

FNAB samples are variably cellular, containing individually dispersed, often readily identified plasma cells (Fig. 3.58). Occasionally the more differentiated plasma cells may be obscured by a population of larger, more blast-like cells, sometimes consisting of bare (naked) nuclei and prominent nucleoli.[121] Additionally, in our experience, smears rarely may contain aggregates of plasma cells in so-called pseudoclusters, suggesting a nonhematopoietic process.

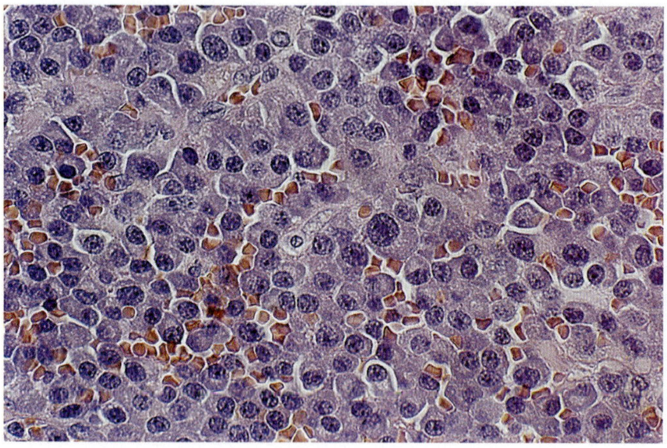

FIGURE 3.57 Plasmacytoma with sheets of plasma cells exhibiting moderate nuclear atypia. (H&E.)

Ancillary Studies

In most cases, ancillary studies are not needed for the diagnosis. Immunoperoxidase stains for λ and κ light chains may be useful in difficult cases, however. Although keratins generally are not expressed in plasma cells, epithelial membrane antigen is usually positive.

Prognosis and Therapy

The prognosis and therapy primarily correlate with the stage of the disease at initial presentation. Patients with solitary tumors without accompanying systemic signs often are treated with radiation alone, occasionally accompanied by adjunct chemotherapy. Of patients with solitary disease, 30% to 50% progress to multiple myeloma within 10 years after the original diagnosis.[122] Disseminated disease requires chemotherapy. Despite remissions in 70% of patients, the median survival for multiple myeloma is less than 3 years. Most patients succumb to renal failure or infections.

REFERENCES

1. Dehner LP: On trial: A malignant small cell tumor in a child: Four wrongs do not make a right. Am J Clin Pathol 1998;109:662.
2. Fletcher JA: Cytogenetics and molecular biology of soft tissue tumors. In Weiss SW, Brooks JSJ (eds): Soft Tissue Tumors. Monographs in Pathology, No. 38. Philadelphia: Williams & Wilkins, 1996, pp 37-64.

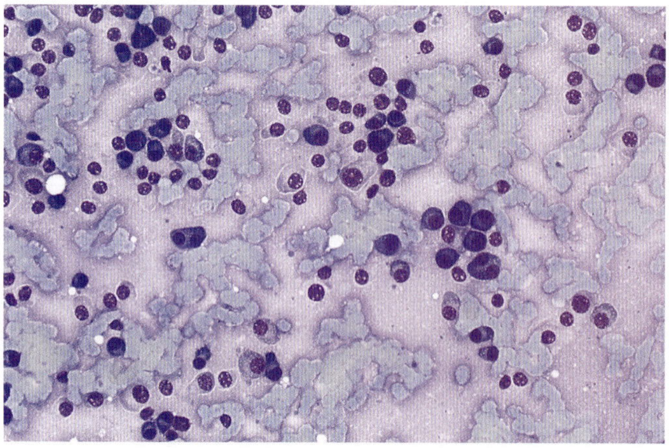

A

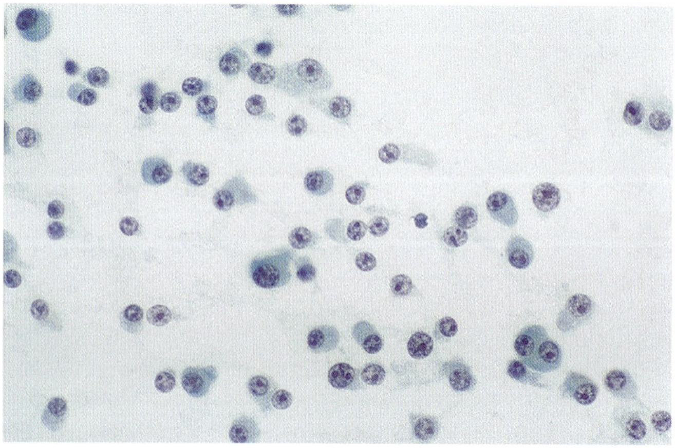

B

FIGURE 3.58 Fine needle aspiration biopsy of plasmacytoma with a mostly discohesive population of plasma cells, some of which appear stripped of their cytoplasm. Note the occasional binucleated forms. **(A,** Diff-Quik; **B,** Papanicolaou.)

3. Mierau GW, Berry PJ, et al: Appraisal of the comparative utility of immunohistochemistry and electron microscopy in the diagnosis of childhood round cell tumors. Ultrastruct Pathol 1996;20:507.
4. Kilpatrick SE, Ward WG, Chauvenet AR, et al: The role of fine-needle aspiration biopsy in the initial diagnosis of pediatric bone and soft tissue tumors: An institutional experience. Mod Pathol 1998;11:923.
5. Halliday BE, Slagel DD, Elsheikh TE, et al: Diagnostic utility of MIC-2 immunocytochemical staining in the differential diagnosis of small blue cell tumors. Diagn Cytopathol 1998;19:410.

Ewing's Sarcoma

6. Dehner LP: Primitive neuroectodermal tumor and Ewing's sarcoma. Am J Surg Pathol 1993;17:1.
7. Sidenrock KA, Nascimento AG, Rock MG: Comparison of soft tissue Ewing's sarcoma and peripheral neuroectodermal tumor. Clin Orthop 1996;329:288.
8. Parham DM, Hijazi Y, Steinberg SM, et al: Neuroectodermal differentiation in Ewing's sarcoma family of tumors does not predict tumor behavior. Hum Pathol 1999;30:911.
9. Kissane JM, Askin FB, Foulkes M, et al: Ewing's sarcoma of bone: Clinicopathologic aspects of 303 cases from the intergroup Ewing's sarcoma study. Hum Pathol 1993;14:773.
10. Maygarden SJ, Askin FB, Siegal GP, et al: Ewing sarcoma of bone in infants and toddlers: A clinicopathologic report from the Intergroup Ewing's Study. Cancer 1993;71:2109.
11. Ahmad R, Mayol BR, Davis M, et al: Extraskeletal Ewing's sarcoma. Cancer 1999;85:725.
12. Nascimento AG, Cooper KL, Unni KK, et al: A clinicopathologic study of 20 cases of large-cell (atypical) Ewing's sarcoma of bone. Am J Surg Pathol 1980;4:29.
13. Renshaw AA, Perez-Atayde AR, Fletcher JA, et al: Cytology of typical and atypical Ewing's sarcoma/PNET. Am J Clin Pathol 1996;106:620.
14. Kilpatrick SE, Geisinger KR: Soft tissue sarcomas: The usefulness and limitations of fine needle aspiration biopsy. Am J Clin Pathol 1998;110:50.
15. Perlman EJ, Dickman PS, Askin FB, et al: Ewing's sarcoma—routine diagnostic utilization of MIC2 analysis: A Pediatric Oncology Group/Children's Cancer Group Intergroup Study. Hum Pathol 1994;25:304.
16. Stevenson AJ, Chatten J, Bertoni F, et al: CD99(p30/32 MIC2) neuroectodermal/Ewing's sarcoma antigen as an immunohistochemical marker: Review of more than 600 tumors and the literature experience. Appl Immunohistochem 1994;2:231.
17. Granter SR, Renshaw AA, Fletcher CD, et al: CD99 reactivity in mesenchymal chondrosarcoma. Hum Pathol 1996;27:1273.
18. Cavazzana AO, Ninfo V, Roberts J, et al: Peripheral neuroepithelioma: A light microscopic, immunocytochemistry, and ultrastructural study. Mod Pathol 1992;5:71.
19. Folpe AL, Hill CE, Parham DM, et al: Immunohistochemical detection of FLI-1 protein expression: A study of 132 round cell tumors wit emphasis on CD-99-positive mimics of Ewing's sarcoma/primitive neuroectodermal tumor. Am J Surg Pathol 2000;24:1657.
20. Fletcher JA: Cytogenetics and molecular biology of soft tissue tumors. In Weiss SW, Brooks JSJ (eds): Soft Tissue Tumors. Monographs in Pathology, No. 38. Philadelphia: Williams & Wilkins, 1996, pp 37-64.
21. Thorner P, Squire J, Chilton-McNeill S, et al: Is the EWS/FLI-1 fusion transcript specific for Ewing's sarcoma and peripheral primitive neuroectodermal tumor? A report of four cases showing this transcript in a wider range of tumor types. Am J Pathol 1996;148:1125.
22. Sorenson PHB, Shimada H, Liu XF, et al: Biphenotypic sarcomas with myogenic and neural differentiation express the Ewing's sarcoma EWS/FLI1 fusion gene. Cancer Res 1995;55:1385.
23. Burchill SA, Wheeldon J, Cullinane C, et al: EWS-FLI-1 fusion transcripts identified in patients with typical neuroblastoma. Eur J Cancer 1997;33:239.
24. Sainati L, Scapinello A, Montaldi A, et al: A mesenchymal chondrosarcoma of a child with the reciprocal translocation (11;22)(q24;q12). Cancer Genet Cytogenet 1993;71:144.
25. Katz Rl, Quezado M, Senderowicz AM, et al: An intra-abdominal small round cell neoplasm with features of primitive neuroectodermal and desmoplastic round cell tumor and a EWS/FLI-1 fusion transcript. Hum Pathol 1997;28:502.
26. Wunder JS, Paulian G, Huvos AG, et al: The histological response to chemotherapy as a predictor of oncological outcome of operative treatment of Ewing sarcoma. J Bone Joint Surg Am 1998;80:1020.
27. Rosito P, Mancini AF, Rondelli R, et al: Italian Cooperative Study for the treatment of children and young adults with localized Ewing sarcoma of bone: A preliminary report of 6 years experience. Cancer 1999;86:421.
28. Hoffman C, Ahrens S, Dunst J, et al: Pelvic Ewing sarcoma: A retropective analysis of 241 cases. Cancer 1999;85:869.
29. Hasegawa SL. Davison JM, Rutten A, et al: Primary cutaneous Ewing's sarcoma: Immunophenotypic and molecular cytogenetic evaluation of five cases. Am J Surg Pathol 1998;22:310.
30. de Alava E, Kawai A, Healey JH, et al: EWS-FLI1 fusion transcript structure is an independent determinant of prognosis in Ewing's sarcoma. J Clin Oncol 1998;16:1248.

Rhabdomyosarcoma

31. Newton WA Jr, Gehan EA, Webber BL, et al: Classification of rhabdomyosarcomas and related sarcomas, pathologic aspects and proposal for a new classification—an Intergroup Rhabdomyosarcoma Study. Cancer 1995;76:1073.
32. Qualman SJ, Coffin CM, Newton WA, et al: Intergroup Rhabdomyosarcoma Study: Update for pathologists. Pediatr Dev Pathol 1998;1:550.
33. Lucas DR, Ryan JR, Zapulski MM, et al: Primary rhabdomyosarcoma of long bone: Case report and review of the literature. Am J Surg Pathol 1996;20:239.
34. Leuschner I, Newton WA, Schmidt D, et al: Spindle cell variants of embryonal rhabdomyosarcoma in the paratesticular region: A report of the Intergroup Rhabdomyosarcoma Study. Am J Surg Pathol 1993;17:221.
35. Rubin BP, Hasserjian RP, Singer S, et al: Spindle cell rhabdomyosarcoma (so-called) in adults: Report of two cases with emphasis on differential diagnosis. Am J Surg Pathol 1998;22:459.
36. Tsokos M, Webber BL, Parham DM, et al: Rhabdomyosarcoma: A new classification scheme related to prognosis. Arch Pathol Lab Med 1992;116:847.
37. Horn RC, Enterline HT: Rhabdomyosarcoma: A clinicopathologic study and classification of 39 cases. Cancer 1958;11:181.
38. Kodet R, Newton WA Jr, Hamoudi A, et al: Childhood rhabdomyosarcoma with anaplastic (pleomorphic) features: A report of the Intergroup Rhabdomyosarcoma Study. Am J Surg Pathol 1993;17:443.
39. Pawel BR, Hamoudi AB, Asmar L, et al: Undifferentiated sarcomas of children: Pathology and clinical behavior—an Intergroup Rhabdomyosarcoma Study. Med Pediatr Oncol 1997;29:170.
40. Ahktar M, Ali MA, Bakry M, et al: Fine needle aspiration biopsy diagnosis of rhabdomyosarcoma: Cytology, histologic, and ultrastructural correlations. Diagn Cytopathol 1992;8:465.
41. Kilpatrick SE, Geisinger KR: Soft tissue sarcomas: The usefulness and limitations of fine needle aspiration biopsy. Am J Clin Pathol 1998;110:50.
42. Miettinen M, Rapola J: Immunohistochemical spectrum of rhabdomyosarcoma and rhabdomyosarcoma-like tumors: Expression of cytokeratin and the 68-kD neurofilament protein. Am J Surg Pathol 1989;13:120.

43. Wang NP, Marx J, McNutt MA, et al: Expression of myogenic regulatory proteins (myogenin and MyoD1) in small blue cell tumors of childhood. Am J Pathol 1995;147:1799.
44. Alaggio R, d'Amore ESG, Dall'Igna P, et al: Pediatric rhabdomyosarcoma: An immunohistochemical study (abstract). Mod Pathol 2000;13:202A.
45. Kumar S, Perlman E, Harris CA, et al: Myogenin is a specific marker for rhabdomyosarcoma: An immunohistochemical study in paraffin-embedded tissues. Mod Pathol 2000;13:988.
46. Pinto A, Tallini G, Novak RW, et al: Undifferentiated rhabdomyosarcoma with lymphoid phenotype expression. Med Pediatr Oncol 1997;28:165.
47. Kilpatrick SE, Teot LA, Geisinger KR, et al: Relationship of DNA ploidy to histology and prognosis in rhabdomyosarcoma. Cancer 1994;74:3227.
48. Parham DM, Shapiro DN, Downing JR, et al: Solid alveolar rhabdomyosarcomas with the t(2;13): Report of two cases with diagnostic implications. Am J Surg Pathol 1994;18:474.
49. Lawrence W Jr, Anderson JR, Gehan EA, et al: Pretreatment TNM staging of childhood rhabdomyosarcoma: A report of the Intergroup Rhabdomyosarcoma Study Group. Cancer 1997;80:1165.
50. Coffin CM, Rulon J, Smith L, et al: Pathologic features of rhabdomyosarcoma before and after treatment: A clinicopathologic and immunohistochemical analysis. Mod Pathol 1997;10:1175.

Extracardiac Rhabdomyoma

51. Kapadia SB, Meis JM, Frisman DM, et al: Adult rhabdomyoma of the head and neck: A clinicopathologic and immunophenotypic study. Hum Pathol 1993;24:608.
52. Willis J, Abdul-Karim FW, Di Sant'Agnese PA: Extracardiac rhabdomyomas. Semin Diagn Pathol 1994;11:15.
53. Blaauwgeers JL, Troost D, Dingemans KP, et al: Multifocal rhabdomyoma of the neck: Report of a case studied by fine needle aspiration, light and electron microscopy, histochemistry and immunohistochemistry. Am J Surg Pathol 1989;13:791.
54. Dehner LP, Enzinger FM, Frisman DM, et al: Fetal rhabdomyoma: An analysis of nine cases. Cancer 1972;30:160.
55. Kapadia SB, Meis JM, Frisman DM, et al: Fetal rhabdomyoma of the head and neck: A clinicopathologic and immunophenotypic study of 24 cases. Hum Pathol 1993;24:754.
56. Kodet R, Fajstavr J, Kabelka Z, et al: Is fetal cellular rhabdomyoma an entity or a differentiated rhabdomyosarcoma? A study of patients with rhabdomyoma of the tongue and sarcoma of the tongue enrolled in the Intergroup Rhabdomyosarcoma Studies I, II and III. Cancer 1991;67:2907.
57. DiSanto S, Abt AB, Boal DK, et al: Fetal rhabdomyoma and nevoid basal cell carcinoma syndrome. Pediatr Pathol 1992;12:441.
58. Chabrel CM, Beilby JW: Vaginal rhabdomyoma. Histopathology 1980;4:645.
59. Sahn EE, Garen PD, Pai GS, et al: Multiple rhabdomyomatous mesenchymal hamartomas of the skin. Am J Dermatopathol 1990;12:485.

Mesenchymal Chondrosarcoma

60. Nakashima Y, Unni KK, Shives TC, et al: Mesenchymal chondrosarcoma of bone and soft tissue: A review of 111 cases. Cancer 1986;57:2444.
61. Huvos AG, Rosen G, Dabska M, Marcove RC: Mesenchymal chondrosarcoma: A clinicopathologic analysis of 35 patients with emphasis on treatment. Cancer 1983;51:1230.
62. Vencio EF, Reeve CM, Unni KK, et al: Mesenchymal chondrosarcoma of the jaw bones: Clinicopathologic study of 19 cases. Cancer 1998;82:2350.
63. Walaas L, Kindblom L-G, Gunterberg B, et al: Light and electron microscopic examination of fine needle aspirates in the preoperative diagnosis of cartilaginous tumors. Diagn Cytopathol 1990;6:396.
64. Martinez-Tello FJ, Navas-Palacios JJ: Ultrastructural study of conventional chondrosarcomas and myxoid and mesenchymal chondrosarcomas. Virchows Arch [A] 1982;396:197.
65. Granter SR, Renshaw AA, Fletcher CD, et al: CD99 reactivity in mesenchymal chondrosarcoma. Hum Pathol 1996;27:1273.
66. Hoang MP, Ayala AG, Suarez PA, et al: Mesenchymal chondrosarcoma: A small cell neoplasm with polyphenotypic differentiation (abstract). Mod Pathol 2000;13:11A.
67. Rushing EJ, Armonda RA, Ansari Q, et al: Mesenchymal chondrosarcoma: A clinicopathologic and flow cytometric study of 13 cases presenting in the central nervous system. Cancer 1996;77:1884.
68. Naumann S, Krallman PA, Unni KK, et al: Translocation der(13;21)(q10;q10) in skeletal and extraskeletal mesenchymal chondrosarcoma. Mod Pathol 2002;15:572.
69. Sainati L, Scapinello A, Montaldi A, et al: A mesenchymal chondrosarcoma of a child with the reciprocal translocation (11;22)(q24;q12). Cancer Genet Cytogenet 1993;71:144.

Desmoplastic Small Round Cell Tumor

70. Ordonez NG: Desmoplastic small round cell tumor: A histopathologic study of 39 cases with emphasis on unusual histological patterns. Am J Surg Pathol 1998;22:1303.
71. Parkash V, Gerald WL, Parma A, et al: Desmoplastic small round cell tumor of the pleura. Am J Surg Pathol 1995;19:659.
72. Zaloudek, C, Miller TR, Stern JL: Desmoplastic small cell tumor of the ovary: A unique polyphenotypic tumro with an unfavorable prognosis. Int J Gynecol Pathol 1995;14:260.
73. Cummings OW, Ulbright TM, Young RH, et al: Desmoplastic small round cell tumors of the paratesticular region: A report of six cases. Am J Surg Pathol 1997;21:219.
74. Tison V, Cerasoli S, Morigi F, et al: Intracranial desmoplastic small cell tumor: Report of a case. Am J Surg Pathol 1996;20:112.
75. Adsay V, Cheng J, Athanasian E, et al: Primary desmoplastic small cell tumor of soft tissues and bone of the hand. Am J Surg Pathol 1999;23:1408.
76. Parham DM, Weeks DA, Beckwith JB: The clinicopathologic spectrum of putative extrarenal rhabdoid tumors: An analysis of 42 cases studied with immunohistochemistry or electron microscopy. Am J Surg Pathol 1994;18:1010.
77. Ali SZ, Nicol TL, Port J, et al: Intraabdominal desmoplastic small round cell tumor: Cytologic findings in two cases. Diagn Cytopathol 1998;18:449.
78. Ordonez NG: Desmoplastic small round cell tumor: An ultrastructural and immunohistochemical study with emphasis on new immunohistochemical markers. Am J Surg Pathol 1998;22:1314.
79. Miettinen M, Chatten J, Paetau A, et al: Monoclonal antibody NB84 in the differential diagnosis of neuroblastoma and other small round cell tumors. Am J Surg Pathol 1998;22:327.
80. Hill DA, Pfeifer JD, Marley EF, et al: WT1 staining reliably differentiates desmoplastic small round cell tumor from Ewing sarcoma/primitive neuroectodermal tumor: An immunohistochemical and molecular diagnostic study. Am J Clin Pathol 2000;114:345.
81. Barnoud R, Sabourin J-C, Pasquier D, et al: Immunohistochemical expression of WT1 by desmoplastic small round cell tumor: A comparative study with other small round cell tumors. Am J Surg Pathol 2000;24:830.
82. Lae ME, Roche PC, Jin L, et al: Desmoplastic small round cell tumor: A clinicopathologic, immunohistochemical, and molecular study of 32 tumors. Am J Surg Pathol 2002;26:823.
83. Leuschner I, Radig K, Harms D: Desmoplastic small round cell tumor. Semin Diagn Pathol 1996;13:204.
84. Kilpatrick SE, Teot LA, Geisinger KR, et al: Relationship of DNA ploidy to histology and prognosis in rhabdomyosarcoma. Cancer 1994;74:3227.
85. Sawyer JR, Tryka AF, Lewis JM: A novel reciprocal chromosomal translocation t(11;22)(p13;q12) in an intra-abdominal desmoplastic small round cell tumor. Am J Surg Pathol 1992;16:411.
86. Kawano N, Inayama Y, Nagashima Y, et al: Desmoplastic small round cell tumor of the paratesticular region: Report of an adult case with demonstration of EWS and WT1 gene fusion using paraffin-embedded tissue. Mod Pathol 1999;12:729.

87. Katz Rl, Quezado M, Senderowicz AM, et al: An intra-abdominal small round cell neoplasm with features of primitive neuroectodermal and desmoplastic round cell tumor and an EWS/FLI-1 fusion transcript. Hum Pathol 1997;28:502.
88. Ordi J, de Alava E, Torne A, et al: Intraabdominal desmoplastic small round cell tumor with EWS/ERG fusion transcript. Am J Surg Pathol 1998;22:1026.
89. Amato RJ, Ellershorst JA, Ayala AG: Intraabdominal desmoplastic small cell tumor: Report and discussion of five cases. Cancer 1996;78:845.

Olfactory Neuroblastoma

90. Elkon D, Hightower SI, Lim ML, et al: Esthesioneuroblastoma. Cancer 1979;44:1087.
91. Mills SE, Frierson HF Jr: Olfactory neuroblastoma: A clinicopathologic study of 21 cases. Am J Surg Pathol 1985;9:317.
92. Oberman HA, Rice DH: Olfactory neuroblastomas: A clinicopathologic study. Cancer 1976;38:2494.
93. Miller DC, Goodman ML, Pilch BZ, et al: Mixed ofactory neuroblastoma and carcinoma: Report of two cases. Cancer 1984;54:2019.
94. Fagan MF, Rone R: Esthesioneuroblastoma: Cytologic features with differential diagnostic considerations. Diagn Cytopathol 1985;1:322.
95. Ferris CA, Schnadig VJ, Quinn FB, et al: Olfactory neuroblastoma: Cytodiagnostic features in a case with ultrastructural and immunohistochemical correlation. Acta Cytol 1988;32:381.
96. Osamara RY, Fine G: Ultrastructure of the esthesioneuroblastoma. Cancer 1976;38:173.
97. Argani P, Perez-Ordonez B, Xiao H, et al: Olfactory neuroblastoma is not related to the Ewing family of tumors: Absence of EWS/FLI1 gene fusion and MIC2 expression. Am J Surg Pathol 1998;22:391.
98. Hirose T, Scheithauer BW, Lopes MB, et al: Olfactory neuroblastoma: An immunohistochemical, ultrastructural, and flow cytometric study. Cancer 1996;77:1957.
99. Whang-Peng J, Freter CE, Knutsen T, et al: Translocation t(11;22) in esthesioneuroblastoma. Cancer Genet Cytogenet 1987;29:155.
100. Kadish S, Goodman M, Wang CC: Olfactory neuroblastoma: A clinicopathologic analysis of 17 cases. Cancer 1976;37:1571.
101. Zappia JJ, Carroll WR, Wolf GT, et al: Olfactory neuroblastoma: The results of modern treatment approaches at the University of Michigan. Head Neck 1993;15:190.
102. Polin RS, Sheehan JP, Chenelle AG, et al: The role of preoperative adjuvant treatment in the management of esthesioneuroblastoma: The University of Virginia experience. Neurosurgery 1998;42:1029.

Melanotic Neuroectodermal Tumor of Infancy

103. Pettinato G, Manivel JC, d'Amore ES, et al: Melanotic neuroectodermal tumor of infancy: A reexamination of a histogenetic problem based on immunohistochemical, flow cytometric, and ultrastructural study of 10 cases. Am J Surg Pathol 1991;15:233.
104. Kapadia SB, Frisman DM, Hitchcock CL, et al: Melanotic neuroectodermal tumor of infancy: Clinicopathological, immunohistochemical, and flow cytometric study. Am J Surg Pathol 1993;17:566.
105. Calabrese F, Danieli D, Valente M: Melanotic neuroectodermal tumor of the epididymis of infancy: Case report and review of the literature. Urology 1995;46:415.
106. Rao CR, Visweshwaraiah LD, Veerapaiah KS, et al: Melanotic neuroectodermal tumor of infancy initially diagnosed by fine needle aspiration cytology. Acta Cytol 1990;34:681.
107. Rege JD, Shet T, Sawant HV, et al: Cytologic diagnosis of melanotic neuroectodermal tumor of infancy occurring in the cranial bones. Diagn Cytopathol 1999;21:280.
108. Khoddami M, Squire J, Zielenska M, et al: Melanotic neuroectodermal tumor of infancy: A molecular genetic study. Pediatr Dev Pathol 1998;1:295.
109. Mast BA, Kapadia SB, Yunis E, et al: Subtotal maxillectomy for melanotic neuroectodermal tumor of infancy. Plast Reconstr Surg 1999;103:1961.

Malignant Lymphoma and Hodgkin's Disease

110. Petit CK, Zuckerberg LR, Gray MH, et al: Primary lymphoma of bone: A B-cell neoplasm with a high frequency of multilobated cells. Cancer 1990;14:329.
111. Ostrowski ML, Inwards CY, Strickler JG, et al: Osseous Hodgkin disease. Cancer 1999;85:1166.
112. Jones D, Kraus MD, Dorfman DM: Lymphoma presenting as a solitary bone lesion. Am J Clin Pathol 1999;111:171.
113. Ostrowski ML, Unni KK, Banks PM, et al: Malignant lymphoma of bone. Cancer 1986;58:2646.
114. Lanham GR, Weiss SW, Enzinger FM: Malignant lymphoma: A study of 75 cases presenting in soft tissue. Am J Surg Pathol 1989;13:1.
115. Htwe HM, Lucas DR, Bedrossian CW, et al: Fine needle aspirate of primary lymphoma of bone. Diagn Cytopathol 1996;15:421.
116. Fulciniti F, Vetrani A, Aeppa P, et al: Hodgkin's disease: Diagnostic accuracy of fine needle aspiration, a report of 62 consecutive cases. Cytopathology 1994;5:226.

Plasmacytoma

117. Brown LM, Linet MS, Greenberg RS, et al: Multiple myeloma and family history of cancer among blacks and whites in the U.S. Cancer 1999;85:2385.
118. Osserman EF, Merlini G, Butler VP Jr: Multiple myeloma and related plasma cell dyscrasias. JAMA 1987;258:2930.
119. Kyle RA: Multiple myeloma: A review of 869 cases. Mayo Clin Proc 1975;50:29.
120. Pambuccian SE, Horyd ID, Cawte T, et al: Amyloidoma of bone, a plasma cell/plasmacytoid neoplasm: Report of three cases and review of the literature. Am J Surg Pathol 1997;21:179.
121. Tani E, Santos GC, Svedmyr E, et al: Fine-needle aspiration cytology and immunohistochemistry of soft-tissue extramedullary plasma-cell neoplasms. Diagn Cytopathol 1999;20:120.
122. Meis JM, Butler JJ, Osborne BM, et al: Solitary plasmacytomas of bone and extramedullary plasmacytomas: A clinicopathologic and immunohistochemical study. Cancer 1987;59:1475.

CHAPTER 4

Epithelioid/Polygonal Cell Tumors of Bone and Soft Tissue

The category of epithelioid/polygonal cell tumors encompasses a group of diverse entities, all of which share the presence of an epithelioid-to-polygonal–shaped cell usually with abundant cytoplasm and a mostly round to slightly ovoid nucleus. The spectrum of epithelioid/polygonal cell tumors is presented in Table 4.1. Entities that, by definition, have an epithelioid component in most cases, such as epithelioid sarcoma or clear cell sarcoma, are discussed in this chapter. Despite having a predominant epithelioid phenotype, epithelioid hemangioendothelioma is discussed in Chapter 10 on vascular tumors. Other tumors, included in the differential diagnosis but less commonly exhibiting epithelioid morphology, such as angiosarcoma and malignant peripheral nerve sheath tumor, are discussed in other chapters. Because rhabdomyoma, especially the fetal type, is more likely to cause diagnostic confusion with rhabdomyosarcoma, it is discussed along with the differential diagnosis of rhabdomyosarcoma. Some neoplasms included in this chapter, especially synovial sarcoma, may be included within the differential diagnosis of spindle cell tumors. Metastatic carcinoma and malignant melanoma occasionally exhibit spindle cell features but are included in this categorization because of their more common histologic presentation of epithelioid morphology.

Although the reader may assume that these tumors share little in their biologic characteristics, common features exist among many of these neoplasms, especially the primary sarcomas, which deserve special consideration. The origin (bone versus soft tissue) of epithelioid/polygonal cell tumors is summarized in Table 4.2. With the exception of adamantinoma and Langerhans' cell histiocytosis, most of these primary lesions arise predominantly within extraskeletal soft tissues.

Despite distinct morphologic and immunohistochemical properties, epithelioid, synovial, alveolar soft part, and clear

TABLE 4.1 Epithelioid/Polygonal Cell Tumors with Typical Age Ranges

Histologic Type	Usual Age Range (yr)
Epithelioid sarcoma	10-40
Extrarenal rhabdoid tumor	Birth-1
Epithelioid hemangioendothelioma	20-60
Epithelioid angiosarcoma	>50
Epithelioid malignant peripheral nerve sheath tumor	20-40
Clear cell sarcoma	15-40
Alveolar soft part sarcoma	15-40
Synovial sarcoma	20-40
Granular cell tumor	15-50
Rhabdomyoma, adult type	>40
Adamantinoma	10-30
Langerhans' cell histiocytosis	Birth-20
Metastatic carcinoma	>50
Malignant melanoma	>50

TABLE 4.2 Origin of Primary Musculoskeletal Epithelioid/Polygonal Cell Tumors (Bone versus Soft Tissue)

Bone Origin	Soft Tissue Origin
Adamantinoma	Epithelioid sarcoma
Epithelioid hemangioendothelioma	Epithelioid hemangioendothelioma
Langerhans' cell histiocytosis*	Synovial sarcoma
	Clear cell sarcoma
	Alveolar soft part sarcoma
	Granular cell tumor
	Rhabdomyoma, adult type
	Extrarenal rhabdoid tumor

*Although Langerhans' cell histiocytosis may manifest as a cutaneous lesion, it does not typically present as a solitary soft tissue mass.

cell sarcomas exhibit similar epidemiologic and biologic characteristics. All tend to affect adolescents and young adults, arising mostly within the extremities. Although 5-year survival rates may range from 60% to 75%, continued declines in 10- and 15-year survival rates classically are observed. It is not unusual for an affected patient to die of metastatic disease 20 years after initial presentation. Another feature shared by these tumors is their relatively high frequency of regional lymph node involvement, a finding uncommonly observed among most soft tissue sarcomas. Consequently, these sarcomas are considered high-grade lesions and, at most institutions, are treated with adjuvant radiation therapy or chemotherapy or both.

Synovial Sarcoma

Synovial sarcoma is a soft tissue malignancy of uncertain histogenesis. Based on its morphologic and immunohistochemical properties, it may be characterized more accurately as a *carcinosarcoma* of soft tissues. The original designation of *synovial sarcoma* was partly due to the fact that these tumors frequently arose in soft tissues near, but rarely within, large joints and, histologically, had an epithelial component that was likened to synovium. Normal synovium lacks immunoreactivity to keratins, however.

Clinical Features

Synovial sarcoma typically arises in adolescents and young adults, with a peak incidence between 20 and 40 years of age. The most frequent anatomic location is the extremities, especially near joints, and the lower extremity is affected more commonly than the upper extremity and proximal more often than distal. Synovial sarcoma may arise in areas largely devoid of synovium, such as the head and neck, abdomen, and retroperitoneum. Presenting symptoms usually are related to the presence of an asymptomatic soft tissue mass; complaints of pain are observed less commonly.[1,2]

Radiologically, synovial sarcomas almost always are deeply seated, presenting as deceptively well-circumscribed but nonspecific soft tissue masses. Stippled calcifications, a well-known feature of synovial sarcoma, are present in one third of cases (Fig. 4.1).[3] Less commonly, tumors may display extensive calcifications and metaplastic bone formation, mimicking myositis ossificans.[4]

Pathologic Findings

Histology

On the basis of morphologic features, synovial sarcoma may be subtyped into four distinct categories: monophasic fibrous,

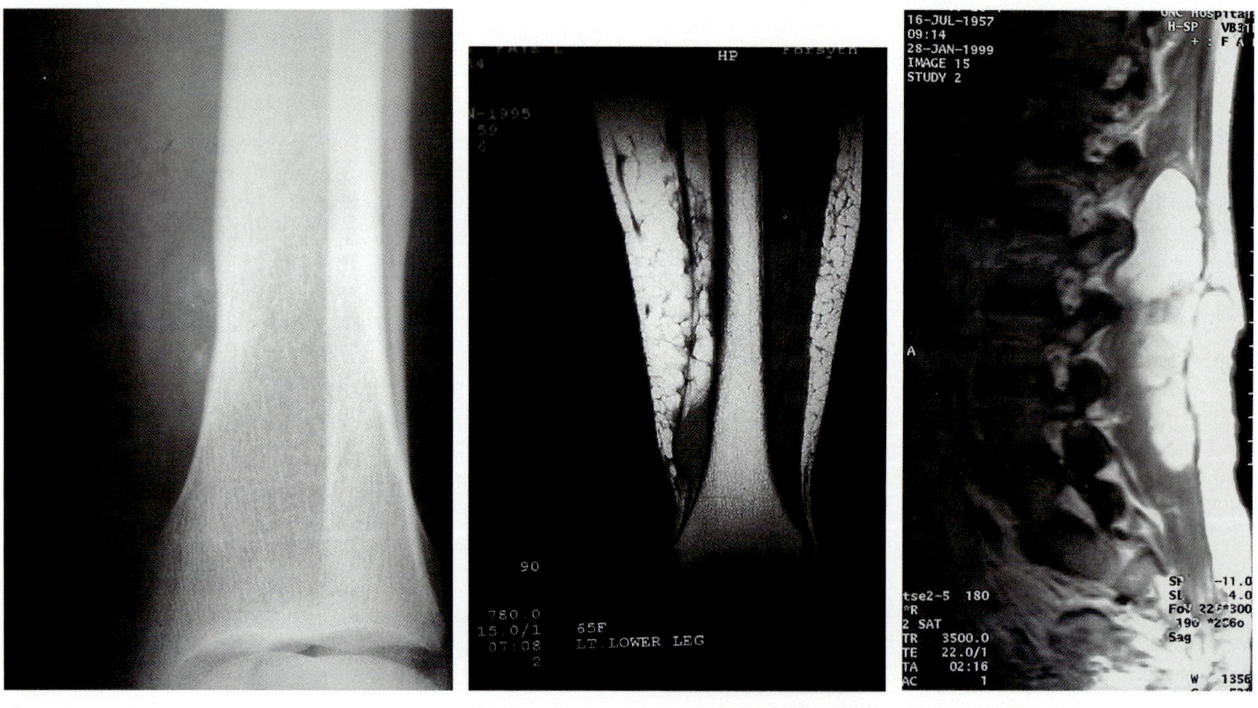

A B C

FIGURE 4.1 Synovial sarcoma. A lateral view of the distal tibia shows irregular calcifications anterior to the distal tibia and an adjacent, smooth pressure erosion of the underlying cortex **(A)**. A T1-weighted coronal magnetic resonance image of the same tumor shows a soft tissue mass adjacent to and abutting the tibial cortex **(B)**. A T2-weighted sagittal magnetic resonance image in another patient shows a multilobulated mass in the paraspinous muculature posterior to the spine **(C)**.

monophasic epithelial, biphasic, and poorly differentiated. The last-mentioned category likely represents a poorly differentiated form of monophasic fibrous subtype. The monophasic fibrous subtype, according to more recent series, is the most common variant, followed in decreasing order of frequency by biphasic, poorly differentiated, and monophasic epithelial subtypes.[1] Many, if not most, examples of monophasic epithelial subtype are biphasic tumors with an overwhelmingly predominant epithelial component.[5] Regardless of subtype, synovial sarcomas often exhibit intratumoral calcifications and may undergo cystic degeneration.

Monophasic fibrous synovial sarcoma is characterized by a relatively uniform population of monotonous, slightly spindled tumor cells arranged in short fascicular patterns, sometimes resembling fibrosarcoma, and associated with variable amounts of stromal collagen deposition. Alternating hypercellular and hypocellular, loose-appearing areas are observed frequently (Fig. 4.2). Less commonly, synovial sarcoma may be abundantly mucinous, so extensive in some cases as to confound the diagnosis (Fig. 4.3).[6] A hemangiopericytoma-like vascular pattern and focal intratumoral calcifications are observed frequently in the more cellular regions (Fig. 4.4). Metaplastic bone is rarely so extensive as to cause confusion with a bone-forming neoplasm (Fig. 4.5). Cytologically, individual tumor cells appear slightly spindled with a round-to-ovoid, hyperchromatic nucleus and inconspicuous nucleoli (Fig. 4.6). Nuclear-to-cytoplasmic ratios are generally high with scant amounts of slightly tapering cytoplasm. Mitotic activity may be low, ranging from less than 1 mitosis to greater than 10 mitoses per 10 high-power fields.

Poorly differentiated synovial sarcomas also generally are composed of a mostly uniform population of rounded-to-polygonal or slightly spindled cells with round-to-ovoid

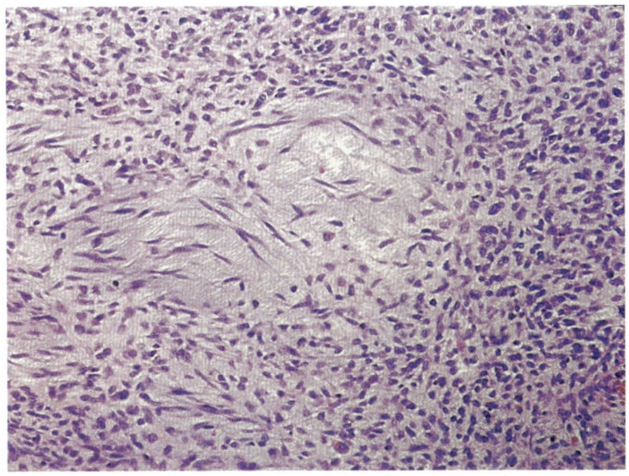

FIGURE 4.3 Synovial sarcoma, monophasic fibrous subtype, with myxoid stroma. (H&E.)

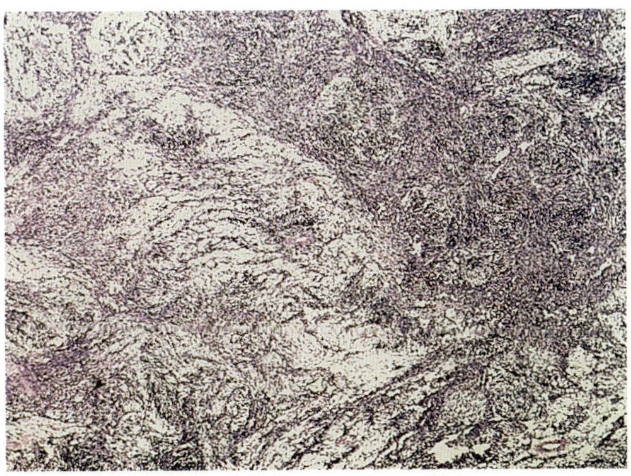

A

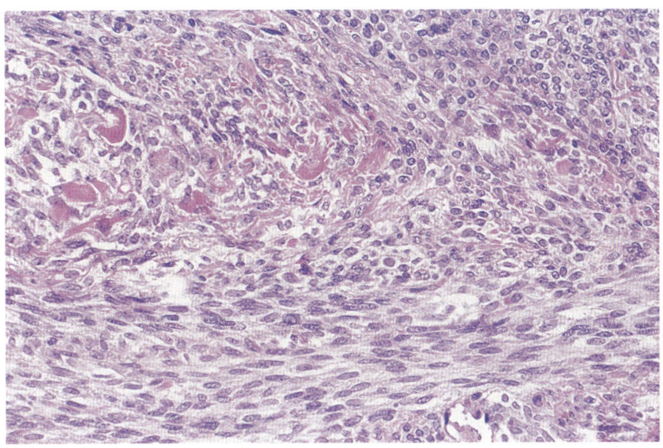

B

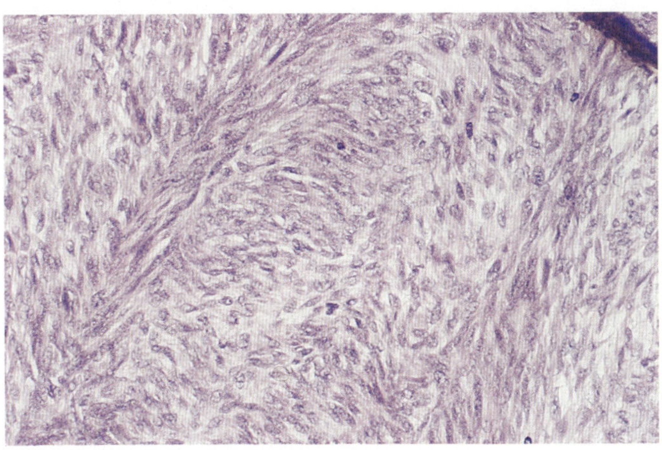

C

FIGURE 4.2 Synovial sarcoma. Monophasic fibrous subtype with characteristic alternating hypercellular and hypocellular areas **(A)** and fascicles of mostly uniform, ovoid to slightly spindled tumor cells with variable collagen stromal deposition **(B)**. Fibrosarcoma-like appearance with intersecting fascicles creating a "herringbone" pattern **(C)**. (**A**, low power; **B**, **C**, high power, H&E.)

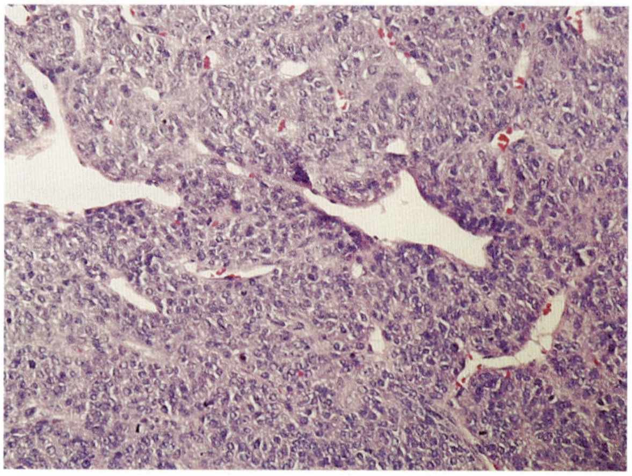

FIGURE 4.4 Synovial sarcoma, monophasic fibrous subtype, with background hemaniopericytoma-like vascular pattern. This pattern is observed frequently in the poorly differentiated form. (H&E.)

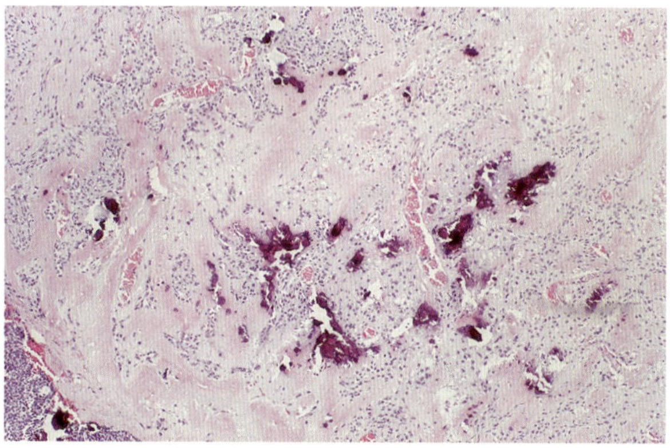

FIGURE 4.5 Synovial sarcomas frequently contain calcifications and metaplastic bone. (H&E.)

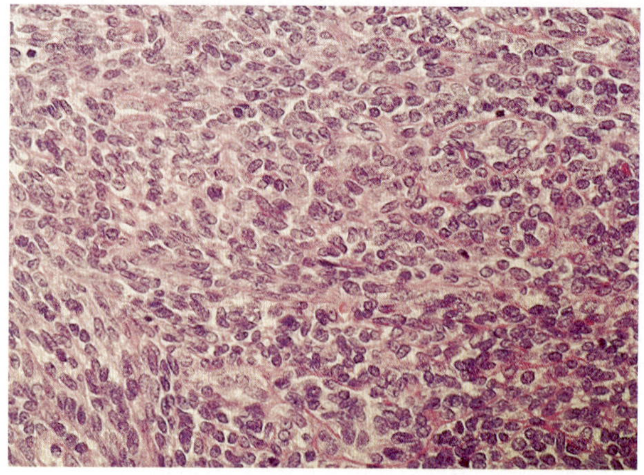

FIGURE 4.6 Synovial sarcoma, monophasic fibrous subtype, with characteristic cytomorphology. Note the remarkably uniform population of round-to-ovoid tumor cells with scant cytoplasm, inconspicuous nucleoli, and a paucity of mitotic activity. (H&E.)

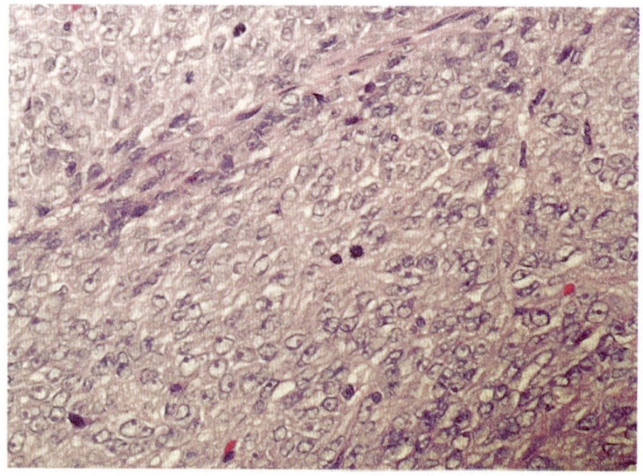

FIGURE 4.7 Synovial sarcoma, poorly differentiated subtype, characterized by a population of larger tumor cells with vesicular nuclei, prominent nucleoli, and abundant mitotic figures. (H&E.)

nuclei. A vesicular or coarsely granular chromatin pattern and prominent nucleoli are characteristic, however. A high mitotic rate (>20 mitoses per 10 high-power fields) frequently is observed (Fig. 4.7).[7] These tumors usually lack obvious epithelial or glandular differentiation. Infrequently, poorly differentiated synovial sarcoma may be composed of small round cells with more uniformly hyperchromatic nuclei, resembling Ewing's sarcoma.

The epithelial component of monophasic epithelial and biphasic subtypes is most commonly glandular, resembling a moderately differentiated to well-differentiated adenocarcinoma (Figs. 4.8 and 4.9). Less common patterns include papillary fronds, solid nests of poorly differentiated glandular cells, and squamous differentiation (see Fig. 4.9).

Fine Needle Aspiration Biopsy

Cytologic preparations from synovial sarcomas are generally highly cellular and composed of a mostly discohesive tumor cell population accompanied by occasional tumor cell aggregates.[8] In most cases, individual tumor cells are remarkably uniform with high nuclear-to-cytoplasmic ratios; round-to-ovoid hyperchromatic nuclei; inconspicuous nucleoli; and absent-to-scant, slightly tapering cytoplasm (Fig. 4.10). As expected, the epithelial tumor cells typically exhibit a mostly round, vesicular nucleus and occasional prominent nucleoli (Fig. 4.11). In our experience, most synovial sarcomas, including the biphasic variant, lack such cells on cytologic smears.[8] This situation is usually not problematic because the diagnosis is easily rendered when material is available for ancillary studies.

Ancillary Studies

Ultrastructurally the more fibroblast-like spindled cells exhibit nuclei with marginated chromatin, irregular membranes, and often small nucleoli. The cytoplasm usually contains mitochondria, Golgi apparatus, and rough endoplasmic reticulum. Separating the epithelial cells from the more spindle-shaped cells is a continuous basal lamina. The latter

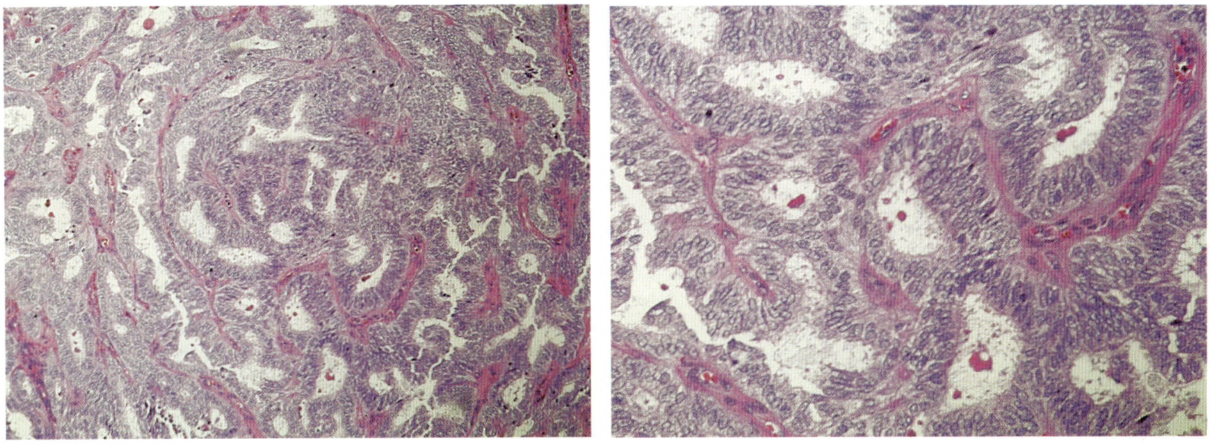

A B

FIGURE 4.8 Synovial sarcoma, monophasic epithelial subtype, composed entirely of glandular epithelium resembling colonic or endometrial adenocarcinoma **(A** and **B). (A,** Low power; **B,** high power, H&E.)

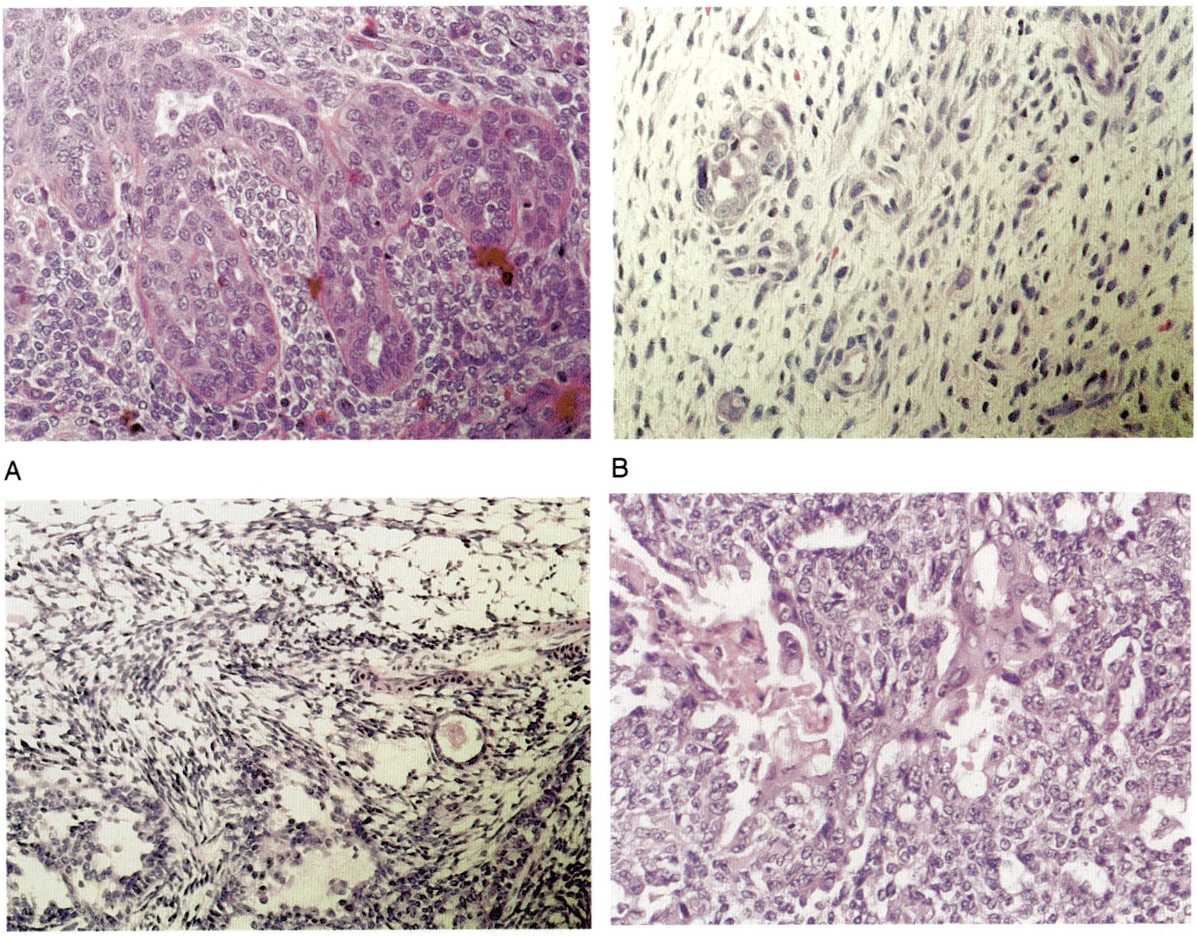

A B C D

FIGURE 4.9 Synovial sarcoma, biphasic type, may display a variety of epithelial forms, including obvious glandular epithelium **(A)**, endothelial-like epithelium **(B)**, serrated-to-cystic epithelium **(C)**, and rarely squamous differentiation **(D)**. (H&E.)

is not observed in normal synovium, adding further evidence that the term *synovial sarcoma* is likely a misnomer. The epithelial cells display mostly ovoid-to-round nuclei with well-defined regular membranes and occasional prominent nucleoli. Intermediate filaments, usually paranuclear in distribution, are within the cytoplasm.

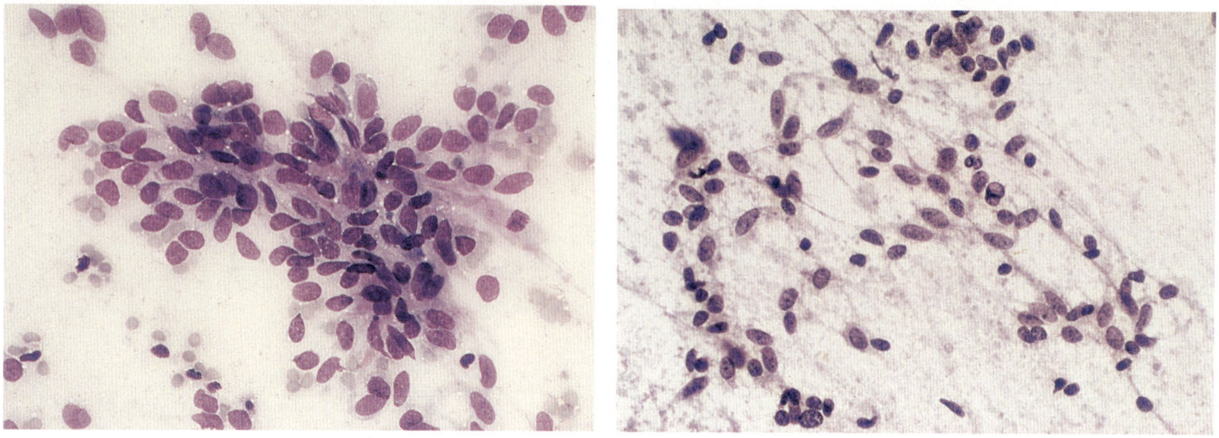

A B

FIGURE 4.10 In monophasic fibrous and biphasic subtypes, fine needle aspiration biopsy of synovial sarcoma generally yields hypercellular smears composed of a uniform population of ovoid cells with high nuclear-to-cytoplasmic ratios, scanty tapering cytoplasm, and inconspicuous nucleoli **(A and B). (A,** Diff-Quik; **B,** Papanicolaou.)

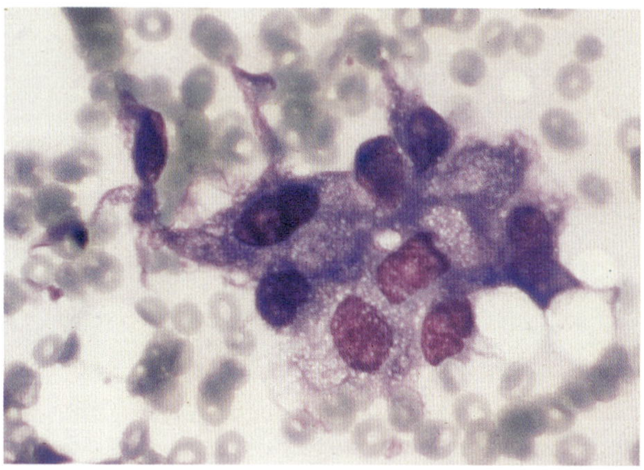

FIGURE 4.11 Epithelial cell component composed of a cohesive aggregate of large tumor cells with abundant cytoplasm, resembling adenocarcinoma. Even in biphasic synovial sarcomas, the presence of an obvious epithelial component is rarely observed. (Diff-Quik.)

The immunohistochemical profile of synovial sarcoma is summarized in Table 4.3. Monophasic and epithelial components usually express keratins and epithelial membrane antigen, at least focally. Epithelial membrane antigen seems to represent a more sensitive marker than cytokeratin, especially for the poorly differentiated subtype of synovial sarcoma.[6,7] Cytoplasmic CD99 reactivity has been reported in greater than 50% of tumors.[9] A potential source of confusion with the differential diagnosis of malignant peripheral nerve sheath tumor is the fact that approximately one third of synovial sarcomas show at least focal positivity for S-100 protein.[10]

Because malignant peripheral nerve sheath tumor occasionally may exhibit cytokeratin positivity or epithelial membrane antigen positivity or both, some have advocated the use of cytokeratin subsets for distinguishing monophasic fibrous synovial sarcoma from malignant peripheral nerve sheath tumor. Using cytokeratins 7 and 19, Smith and colleagues[10] evaluated 29 cases of monophasic fibrous synovial sarcoma. Of these cases, 23 expressed both cytokeratin subsets, whereas only 2 appeared negative for both cytokeratins. Conversely, among 22 malignant peripheral nerve sheath tumors, 2 cases expressed cytokeratin 7, 1 case stained with cytokeratin 19, but no examples expressed both cytokeratins.[10]

In most cases, conventional cytogenetic analysis reveals a balanced, arguably specific translocation t(X;18)(p11.2;11.2) with the fusion product SYT-SSX. This finding is observed in biphasic and monophasic subtypes. We now know that two related but distinct X-chromosomal genes may be rearranged in this translocation, producing distinct fusion products, SYT-SSX1 and SYT-SSX2.[11,12] Kawai and associates[13] documented an association between synovial sarcoma subtype and the SYT-SSX subtype. In their series, biphasic tumors exclusively harbored the SYT-SSX1 rearrangement, whereas monophasic fibrous types were predominantly (but not exclusively) found to have the SYT-SSX2 rearrangement. Other investigators have not shown such a relationship, however.[14] Fine needle aspirates have proved successful in detecting the t(X;18) and its fusion product, SYT-SSX.[15]

O'Sullivan and colleagues[16] at Washington University Medical Center evaluated RNA extracted from 34 synovial sarcoma specimens and 20 malignant peripheral nerve sheath tumor specimens for the presence of the t(X;18) by reverse-transcriptase polymerase chain reaction. Approximately 85% of synovial sarcomas and 75% of malignant peripheral nerve sheath tumors showed the translocations. Of the 15 cases of malignant peripheral nerve sheath tumors bearing the translocation, 3 were malignant triton tumors and 6 arose in patients with neurofibromatosis. The authors pointed out that the results could not be attributed to diagnostic inaccuracies or errors because "diagnoses were based on well-established morphologic, immunohistochemical, and electron-microscopic criteria, and were carefully scrutinized because synovial sarcoma, especially the monophasic variant, and malignant peripheral nerve sheath tumors have substantial morphologic and immunophenotypic overlap."[16]

TABLE 4.3 Immunohistochemical Profile of Synovial Sarcoma

	Monophasic Fibrous	Biphasic	Poorly Differentiated
Antibody	PERCENT REACTIVITY	PERCENT REACTIVITY	PERCENT REACTIVITY
Vimentin	100	100	100
EMA	60-95	100	>90
Cytokeratin	50-85	100	30-50
CD99	40-70	60-70	>90
S-100 protein	10-35	10-35	NA

EMA, epithelial membrane antigen; NA, not available.

Prognosis and Therapy

Estimated 5-, 10-, and 15-year survival rates for synovial sarcoma range from 50% to 65%, 20% to 50%, and 10% to 45%.[1,2] Risk factors for disease progression have included older age of patient (>25 years), large tumor size (≥5 cm), poorly differentiated subtype (high nuclear grade), extensive tumor necrosis (>50%), the presence of rhabdoid morphology, and high tumor stage.[1,2] Bergh and colleagues[1] retrospectively reviewed their experience with 121 patients with synovial sarcoma, dividing them into two prognostic categories: low and high risk. The low-risk group included patients aged younger than 25 years, tumor size less than 5 cm, and the absence of poorly differentiated histology. Overall disease-free survival among patients in the latter group was estimated at 88%. Conversely, the high-risk category, defined as patient age 25 years and older, tumor size 5 cm and larger, and presence of poorly differentiated histology, had an overall disease-free survival of approximately 18%.[1]

Synovial sarcomas containing the SYT-SSX1–type fusion seem to be associated with worse prognosis than sarcomas harboring the SYT-SSX2 subtype.[13,14] Inagaki and coworkers[14] documented a statistically significant relationship between the SYT-SSX1 fusion and high Ki-67 expression and a high mitotic rate, suggesting that the SYT-SSX fusion subtype is associated with the tumor cell proliferative activity.

At most institutions, synovial sarcoma is considered an intermediate-grade to high-grade sarcoma requiring not only surgical resection, but also adjuvant therapy, including chemotherapy or radiation therapy or both. Adequate primary surgery seems to represent the most significant factor in local control and the prevention of recurrence.[1]

Epithelioid Sarcoma

Similar to synovial sarcoma, the histogenesis of epithelioid sarcoma is uncertain. The morphologic and immunohistochemical profile of epithelioid sarcoma suggests that it may represent a "carcinoma" of soft parts.

Clinical Features

Epithelioid sarcoma typically arises in adolescents and young adults, with a usual age range of 10 to 40 years. It predominantly occurs in the distal extremities and has a propensity, in contrast to most sarcomas, to involve the upper extremity, especially the hands and forearms (Fig. 4.12).[17] Consequently, epithelioid sarcoma often presents as a painless, soft tissue mass, superficially located within the dermis and subcutis, especially along the fascial planes and tendon sheaths. Radiologically, epithelial sarcomas are generally solitary but often multinodular masses that, similar to synovial sarcoma, frequently harbor calcifications, in approximately 20% to 30% of cases.[17]

Pathologic Findings

Histology

Epithelioid sarcomas typically grow as multinodular proliferations composed of epithelioid-to-polygonal–appearing tumor cells with round-to-ovoid vesicular nuclei, inconspicuous-to-prominent nucleoli, and abundant eosinophilic cytoplasm. When abundant necrosis is present, the multinodular growth pattern exhibits a "granulomatous" appearance, reminiscent of rheumatoid nodule or granuloma annulare. These necrotic zones are composed of acellular debris or abundant hyalinized collagen or both (Figs. 4.13 and 4.14).[17,18] Nuclear pleomorphism generally ranges from slight to moderate with occasional binucleated forms and rhabdoid features (Fig. 4.15). Less commonly, focal areas of myxoid change may be observed. Rarely, multinucleated giant cells may be scattered haphazardly among the cellular regions.[17] Such cells may result in an erroneous interpretation of giant cell tumor of tender sheath. Although virtually all cases exhibit predominant epithelioid morphology, focal areas displaying spindle cell patterns and even storiform growth may occur (Fig. 4.16). Dystrophic calcifications with or without osseous metaplasia are seen in one fifth of cases.[17] Mitotic activity is variable, ranging from less than 1 mitotic figure to greater than 20 mitotic figures per 10 high-power fields.[18] Guillou

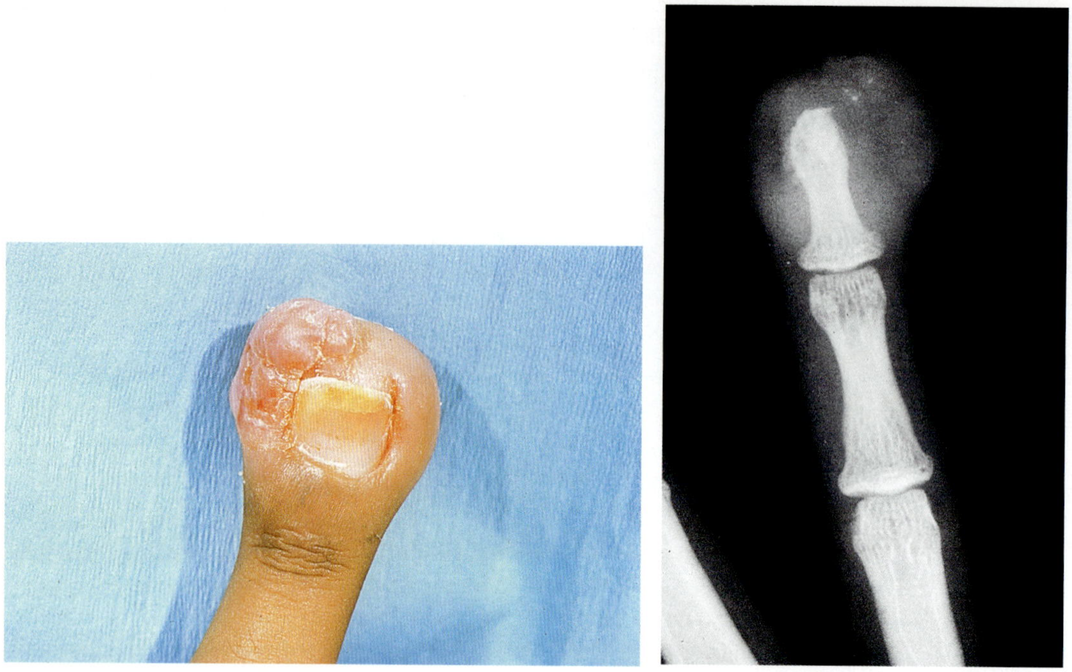

A B

FIGURE 4.12 Epithelioid sarcoma. A verrucous, fungating mass arises on the palmar surface and nail bed of the middle finger **(A).** An anteroposterior radiograph of the finger shows an extraosseous soft tissue mass medial to the distal phalanx containing multiple, small, and irregular dystrophic calcifications **(B).**

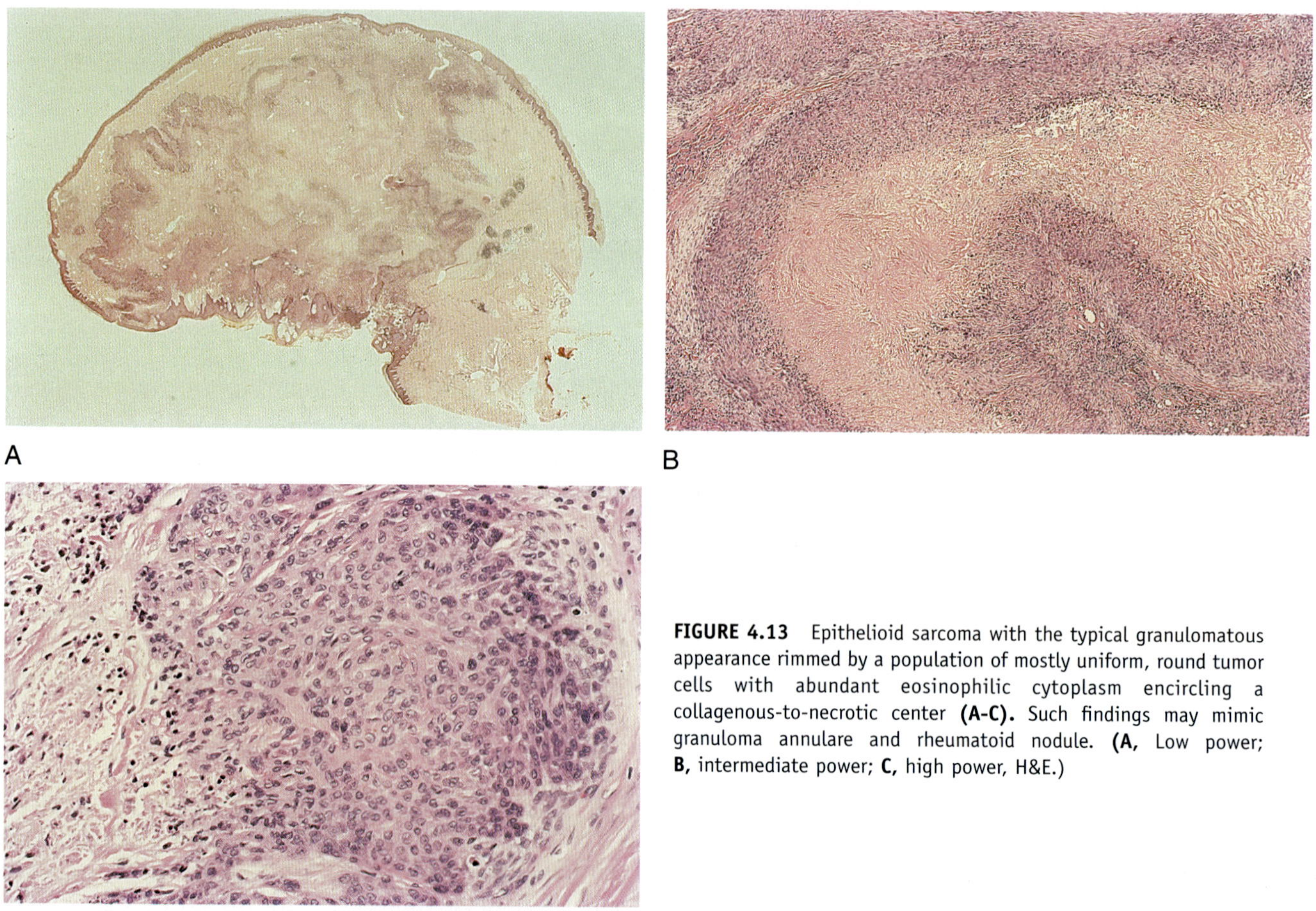

A B C

FIGURE 4.13 Epithelioid sarcoma with the typical granulomatous appearance rimmed by a population of mostly uniform, round tumor cells with abundant eosinophilic cytoplasm encircling a collagenous-to-necrotic center **(A-C).** Such findings may mimic granuloma annulare and rheumatoid nodule. **(A,** Low power; **B,** intermediate power; **C,** high power, H&E.)

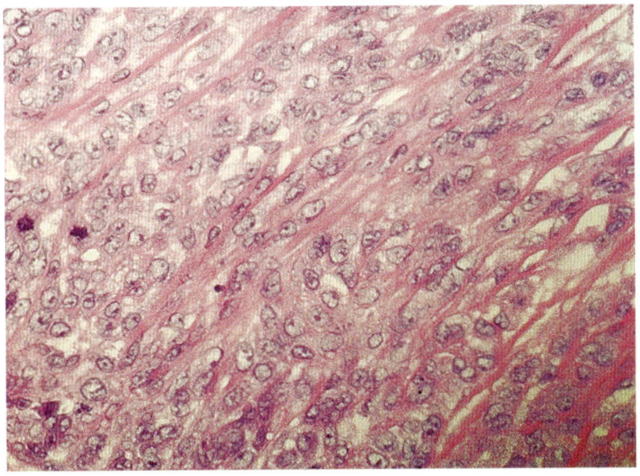

FIGURE 4.14 Epithelioid sarcoma with uniform epithelioid cells with vesicular nuclei, minimal nuclear pleomorphism, a single nucleolus, and abundant eosinophilic cytoplasm. Note the presence of occasional mitotic figures. (H&E.)

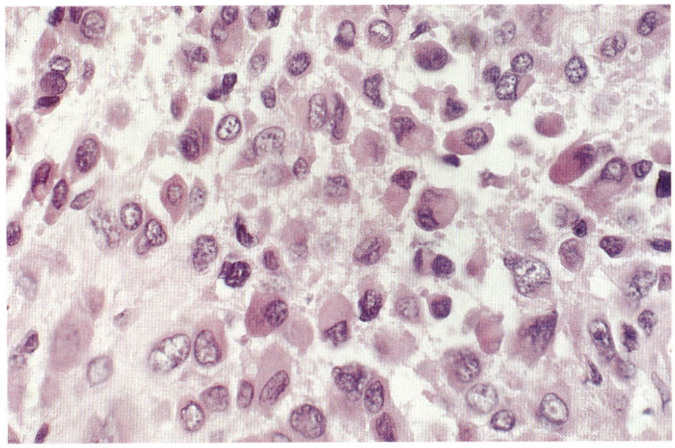

FIGURE 4.15 Occasional examples, especially those arising in the proximal extremities, may show whorls of eosinophilic cytoplasm pushing aside the adjacent nucleus, creating a so-called rhabdoid appearance. (H&E.)

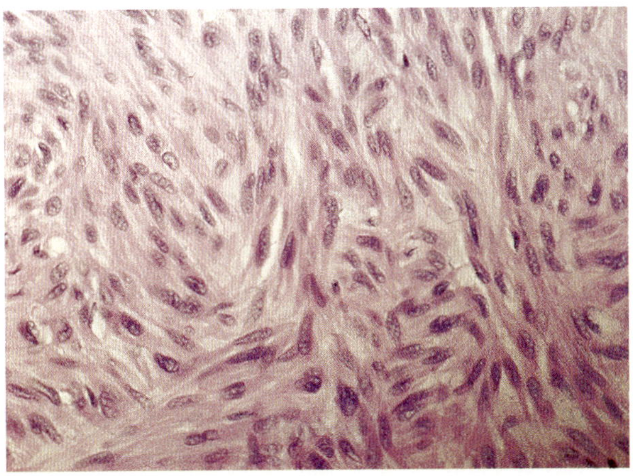

FIGURE 4.16 Epithelioid sarcoma may exhibit more spindled areas sometimes displaying storiform patterns. (H&E.)

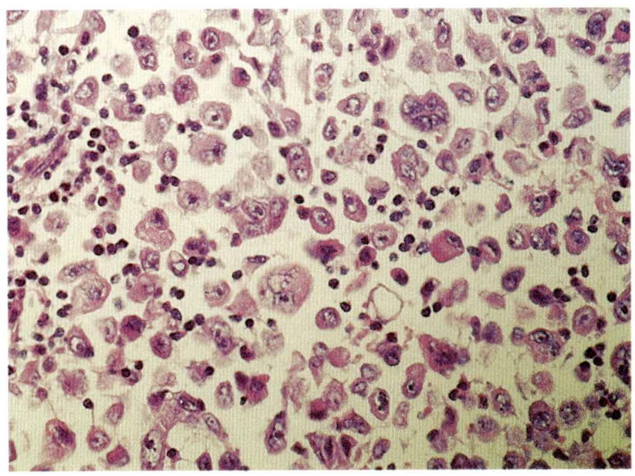

FIGURE 4.17 "Proximal-type" epithelioid sarcoma exhibiting significant nuclear atypia, pleomorphism, and prominent nucleoli. (H&E.)

and colleagues[19] described a "proximal type" of epithelioid sarcoma displaying marked cytologic atypia and rhabdoid features and arising within more proximal anatomic sites, including the pelvis and perineal regions, buttocks, and hips (Fig. 4.17). Limited follow-up data suggest that this unusual variant of epithelioid sarcoma may behave more aggressively.

Fine Needle Aspiration Biopsy

Cytologic smears generally range from moderately to highly cellular with mostly individually dispersed tumor cells ranging from epithelioid and polygonal to slightly spindled. Nuclei are generally large, round to ovoid, with a slightly granular-to-vesicular chromatin pattern, and occasional prominent nucleoli. The cytoplasm is dense and often abundant and may be slightly tapering (Fig. 4.18).[20] Intracytoplasmic vacuoles, presumably degenerative, appear at least focally present in most cases, mimicking epithelioid hemangioendothelioma (Fig. 4.19).

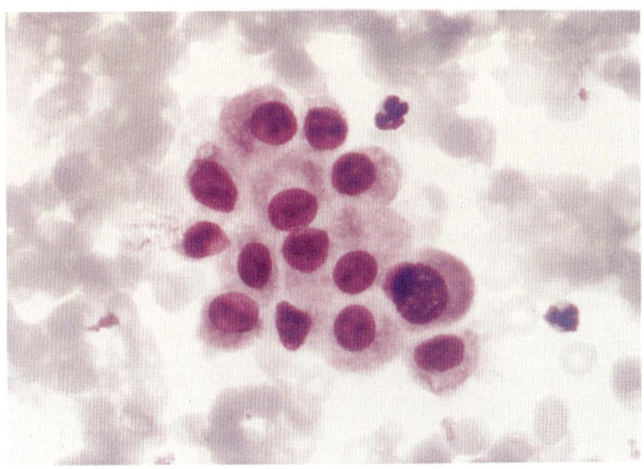

FIGURE 4.18 Cytologic features of epithelioid sarcoma characterized by clusters and solitary tumor cells with a mostly round nucleus and abundant, eccentrically placed cytoplasm, resembling a carcinoma. (Diff-Quik.)

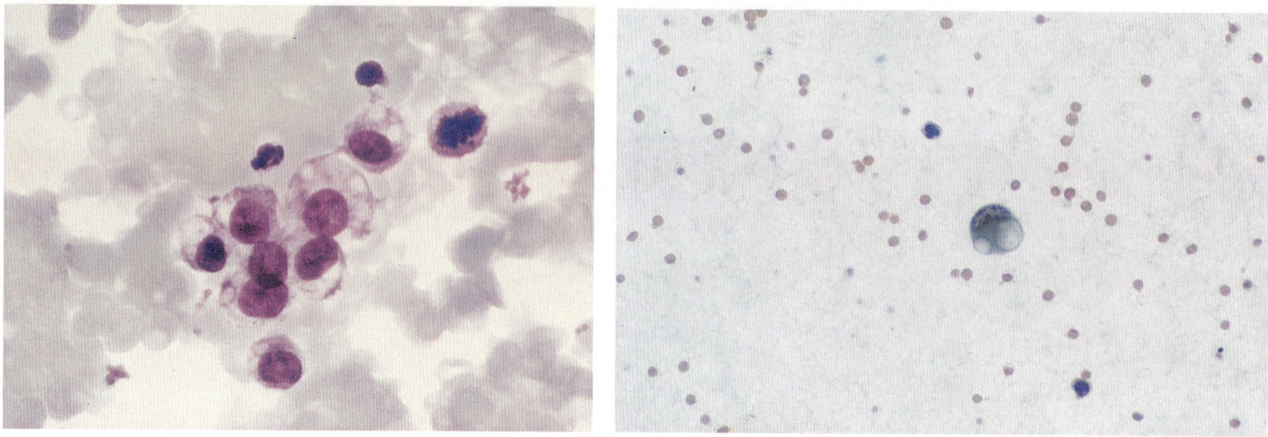

A B

FIGURE 4.19 Cytoplasmic vacuolation, presumably degenerative, is common and may cause diagnostic confusion with epithelioid hemangioendothelioma (**A** and **B**). (**A,** Diff-Quik; **B,** Papanicolaou.)

Ancillary Studies

Ultrastructurally the round to slightly spindle-shaped cells contain round-to-ovoid nuclei surrounded by abundant cytoplasm. Within the cytoplasm are a prominent Golgi apparatus, rough endoplasmic reticulum, and bundles of intermediate filaments. Basal laminae are not observed. Intercellular junctions may be present.

The immunohistochemical profile of epithelioid sarcoma is summarized in Table 4.4. Immunohistochemically, most epithelioid sarcomas express cytokeratin and epithelial membrane antigen. Likewise, vimentin is positive in greater than 95% of cases. Up to 50% of cases express CD34 at least focally.[19,21] Because metastatic carcinomas are almost always negative for this marker, the use of CD34 may help distinguish these two entities in difficult cases.[21] In contrast to epithelioid hemangioendothelioma, CD31 is uniformly negative in epithelioid sarcoma. Although S-100 protein also typically has produced negative results, HMB45 rarely has been reported as positive.[19]

Cytogenetic analysis has revealed no reproducible chromosomal abnormalities characteristic of epithelioid sarcoma. Cordoba and colleagues[22] reported a single case of epithelioid sarcoma with a t(8;22)(q22;11).

TABLE 4.4 Immunohistochemical Profile of Epithelioid Sarcoma

Antibody	Percent Reactivity
Vimentin	>95
Cytokeratin	70-95
EMA	70-95
CD34	50
CEA	10-40
HMB 45	0-10
S-100 protein	0-10
CD31	Negative

CEA, carcinoembryonic antigen; EMA, epithelial membrane antigen.

Prognosis and Therapy

Local recurrence and metastatic rates in epithelioid sarcoma are high, ranging from 38% to 77% and 40% to 50%.[17,18,23] As with synovial sarcoma, prolonged follow-up is mandatory in these patients. Tumor-related death may be observed 20 years after initial presentation. A more aggressive clinical course has been associated with tumor size ($\geq$5 cm), proximal location, and histologic features such as necrosis, mitotic activity, and the presence of vascular invasion.[17,23] Evans and Baer[18] emphasized that the initial treatment has a strong relationship with local recurrence but does not affect ultimate clinical outcome. Regional lymph node metastasis seems to be strongly correlated with tumor size.

Alveolar Soft Part Sarcoma

Alveolar soft part sarcoma is a rare but histologically distinct neoplasm, the histogenesis of which is unknown, despite extensive investigation during the last several decades.

Clinical Features

Most cases arise in young adult and adolescent patients; however, the reported ages of patients range from 16 months to 71 years.[24] Overall, the most common location is the lower extremity, especially the buttock and thigh. Nevertheless, in children, alveolar soft part sarcoma most often arises in the head and neck regions, especially the orbit and less commonly in the tongue. Regardless of anatomic origin, alveolar

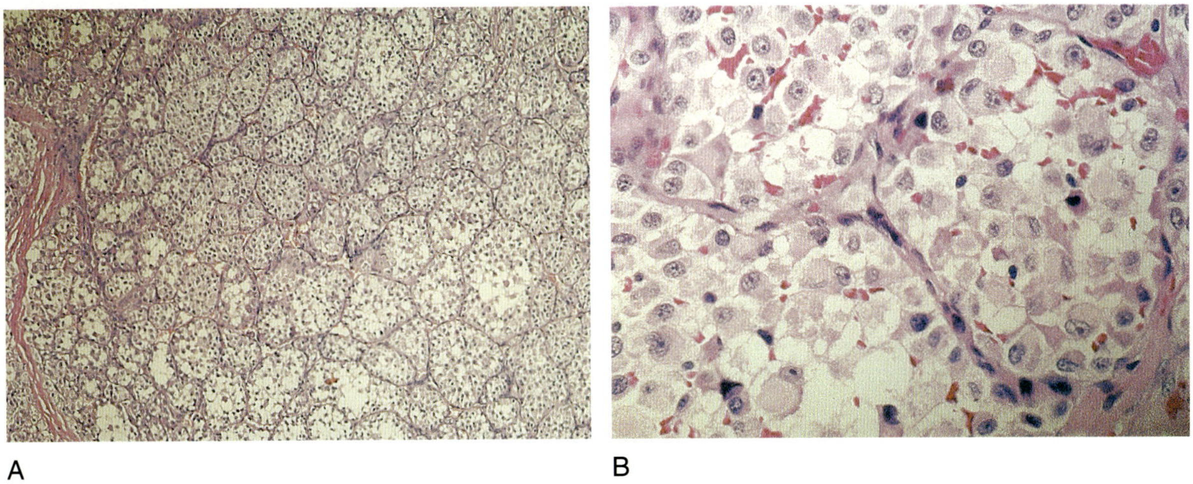

FIGURE 4.20 Alveolar soft part sarcoma with neoplastic cells arranged in well-defined nests separated by thin-walled fibrovascular septa **(A).** At high power, the individual cells are quite large but generally uniform with a round-to-ovoid vesicular nucleus, prominent nucleoli, and abundant, lightly granular-to-eosinophilic cytoplasm **(B).** (H&E.)

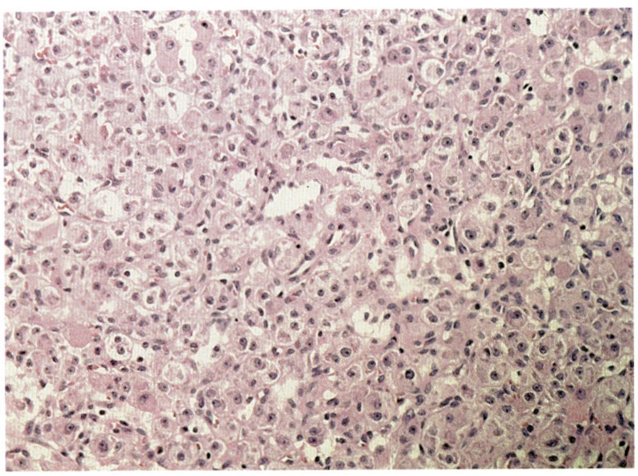

FIGURE 4.21 Alveolar soft part sarcoma may contain more solid-appearing areas. (H&E.)

soft part sarcoma usually presents as a relatively slow-growing, painless soft tissue mass.

Pathologic Findings

Histology

Alveolar soft part sarcoma usually appears well circumscribed but distinctly lacks a true capsule. Most commonly, the neoplastic cells are arranged in well-defined nests separated by thin-walled fibrovascular septa (Fig. 4.20). These nests of tumor cells often appear uniform but may range from solid to so-called pseudoalveolar patterns (Fig. 4.21). Presumably the latter is due to a loss of cohesiveness among the tumor cells and is likely the result of the type of fixation employed, being usually observed in routinely formalin-fixed histologic preparations.[25] Less common histologic patterns include diffuse sheets of cells and a hemangiopericytoma-like vascular pattern. Equally distinctive are the high-power properties. Individual tumor cells are generally relatively uniform in size, round to polygonal, and contain one to two round nuclei. The chromatin pattern is generally vesicular and associated with prominent nucleoli. In most cases, the cytoplasm is abundant, clearly defined, and eosinophilic (see Fig. 4.20). Rarely, cytoplasmic vacuolation, nuclear hyperchromasia with atypia, and clear cell features, mimicking renal cell carcinoma, may be observed (Fig. 4.22).[25] Despite a high-grade biologic behavior, mitotic figures are uncommon. Intracytoplasmic eosinophilic rod-shaped structures are observed faintly in some cells on routine hematoxylin and eosin staining; however, they are shown more easily using periodic acid–Schiff (PAS) stain with diastase digestion. The number of intracytoplasmic crystals is highly variable; crystals may be seen in virtually all or almost none of the individual tumor cells (Fig. 4.23).[25]

Fine Needle Aspiration Biopsy

Fine needle aspiration biopsy of alveolar soft part sarcoma generally yields slightly to moderately cellular smears containing mostly discohesive, large, round-to-polygonal–shaped tumor cells.[26] Despite their relatively large size, the neoplastic cells tend to be mostly uniform, exhibiting only slight variations in size and configuration (Fig. 4.24). Nuclear pleomorphism is generally not a feature of this neoplasm. The nuclei tend to be eccentrically placed, round to ovoid, with a vesicular chromatin pattern and a single prominent nucleolus. The cytoplasm is abundant and dense to granular. Although the histologic features may be distinctive, in our limited experience, the cytologic features tend to show significant overlap with other epithelioid/polygonal cell tumors, necessitating ancillary studies for definitive diagnosis.

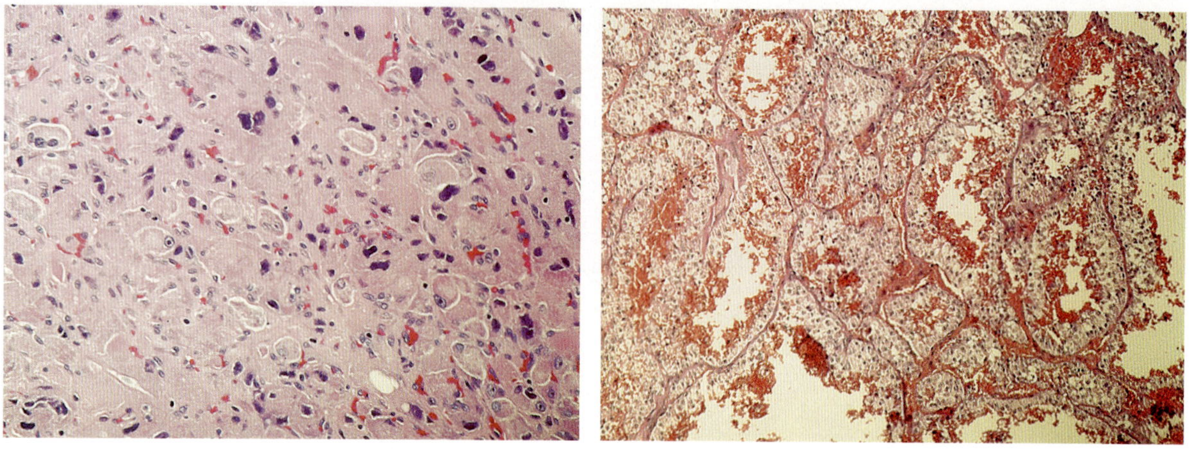

A B

FIGURE 4.22 Less commonly, alveolar soft part sarcoma may display nuclear atypia, probably degenerative, with a "smudgy" hyperchromasia **(A).** Hypervascular forms may closely mimic clear cell, renal cell carcinoma **(B).** (H&E.)

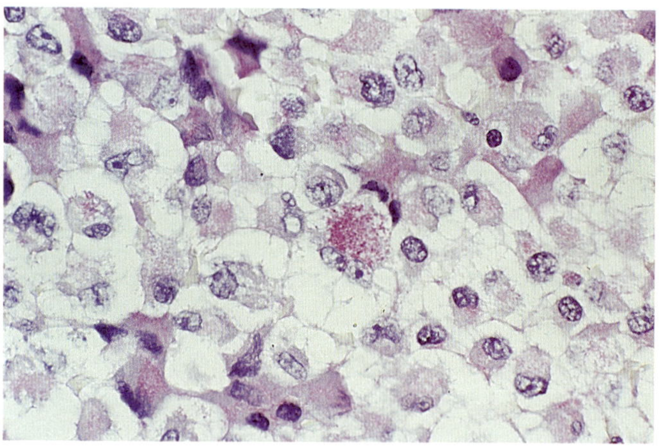

FIGURE 4.23 Intracytoplasmic, PAS-positive crystals in alveolar soft part sarcoma are a helpful diagnostic clue. (PAS.)

Ancillary Studies

Ultrastructural studies have shown that distinctive tumor cell nests usually are surrounded by a continuous-to-discontinuous basal lamina. Helpful diagnostic features include the presence of prominent Golgi complexes often accompanied by dense-core granules. Mitochondria are frequently numerous. Nevertheless, the most distinctive feature of alveolar soft part sarcoma are the rhomboid-shaped crystals (Fig. 4.25).[27]

The immunohistochemical profile of alveolar soft part sarcoma is summarized in Table 4.5. Despite its distinctive histologic appearance, no single immunohistochemical marker has proved reliable for confirming the diagnosis of alveolar soft part sarcoma. In the literature, approximately 78% of cases express, at least focally, desmin immunoreactivity.[24,25,28] Actin positivity has been observed less commonly. Because of

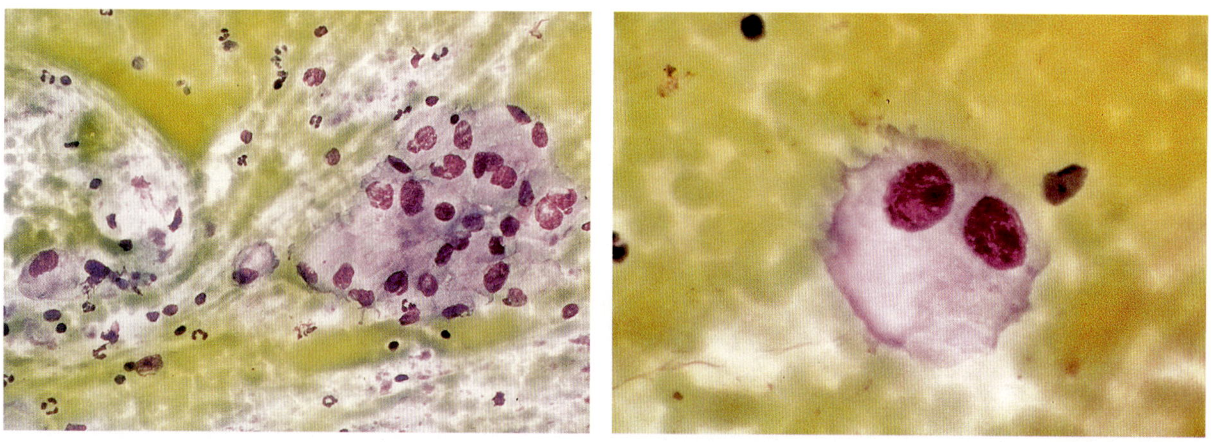

A B

FIGURE 4.24 Fine needle aspiration biopsy of alveolar soft part sarcoma yields moderately cellular smears with clusters and solitary, large but uniform tumor cells with abundant cytoplasm, one or more round nuclei, and prominent nucleoli **(A** and **B).** (Diff-Quik.)

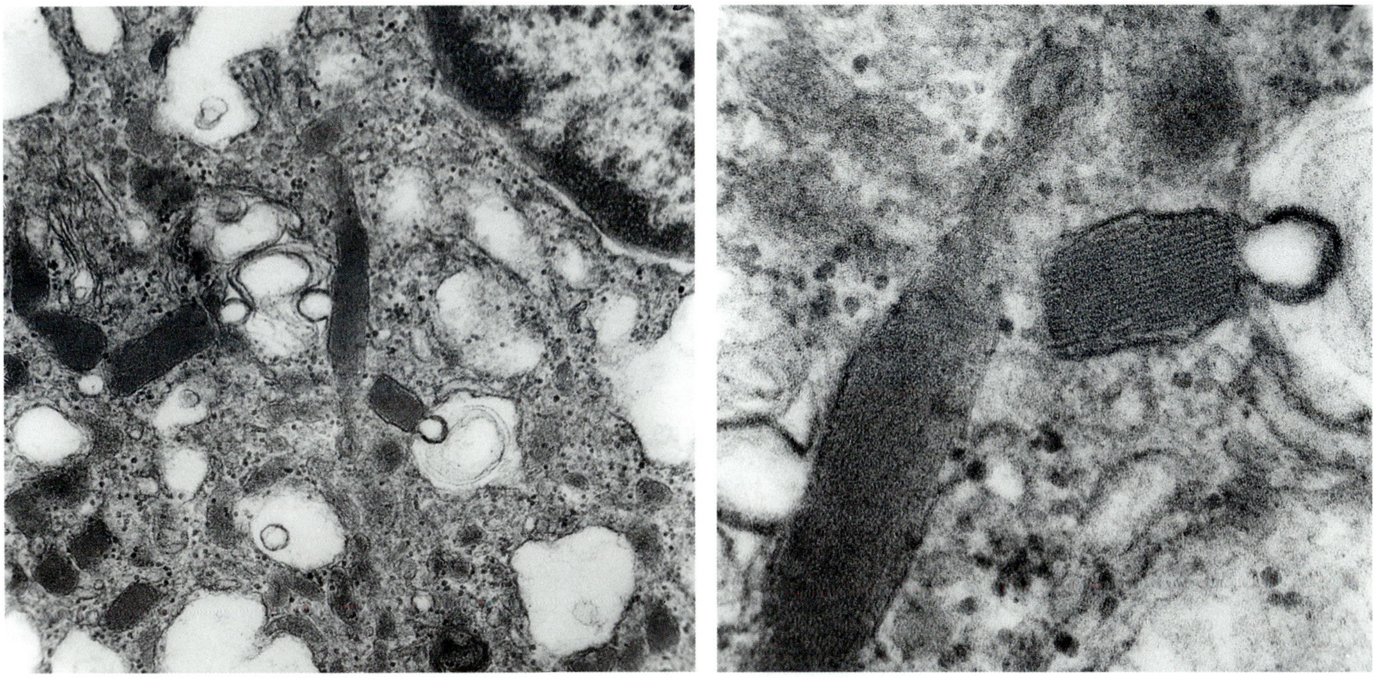

A B

FIGURE 4.25 Ultrastructurally, the most distinctive feature of alveolar soft part sarcoma is the intracytoplasmic, rhomboid-shaped crystals **(A** and **B)**.

these findings, earlier studies suggested skeletal muscle origin or differentiation for alveolar soft part sarcoma. More recent studies have not confirmed immunoreactivity, however, for specific myogenic regulatory proteins, such as MyoD1 and myogenin.[29,30]

Cytogenetic analysis of alveolar soft part sarcoma has been reported only more recently in the literature. The most frequently described chromosomal abnormality seems to represent a t(X;17)(p11;q25) with the *ASPL-TFE3* gene fusion.[31]

Prognosis and Therapy

According to larger series, 5-year survival rates range from 60% to 70%, 10-year survival rates range from 30% to 40%, and 20-year survival rates approach 15%.[24,32] Favorable prognostic indicators have included younger age at presentation, tumor size less than 5 cm, and the absence of metastases at the initial diagnosis.[24,33] Among patients with localized disease at presentation, 5-year survival rates have been reported approaching 87%.[34] There seem to be no histologic indicators predictive of survival. Because local recurrence may occur in 20% of cases, complete surgical excision is the primary recommended treatment. The role of chemotherapy and radiation therapy for alveolar soft part sarcoma is unclear. Lieberman and coworkers,[24] in a review of more than 50 years' experience, showed no evidence, however, that either chemotherapy or radiation therapy improved survival in patients with alveolar soft part sarcoma.[24]

TABLE 4.5 Immunohistochemical Profile of Alveolar Soft Part Sarcoma

Antibody	Percent Reactivity
Desmin	78
Vimentin	38
NSE	35
S-100 protein	23
Muscle-specific actin	13
Smooth muscle actin	7
Cytokeratin	<5
EMA	Negative
Myogenin	Negative

EMA, epithelial membrane antigen; NSE, neuron-specific enolase.
Based on a review of the literature by Ordonez NG: Alveolar soft part sarcoma: A review and update. Adv Anat Pathol 1999;6:125.

Clear Cell Sarcoma of Soft Tissues

Clear cell sarcoma, also known as malignant melanoma of soft parts, is a rare soft tissue malignancy most commonly involving the extremities of young adults.[35,36] Despite morphologic and immunohistochemical similarities to malignant melanoma, clear cell sarcoma should not be thought of merely as a deeply seated malignant melanoma. Its behavior tends to parallel that of other members of the epithelial polygonal cell sarcoma group. A specific cytogenetic abnormality present in most cases adds further support to the concept that clear cell sarcoma should be regarded as an entity distinct from malignant melanoma.

Clinical Features

Clear cell sarcoma predominantly afflicts young adults between the ages of 20 and 40 years. Men and women are affected approximately equally. The extremities, especially the lower limb and foot, account for most cases (Fig. 4.26).[35,36] Rarely, clear cell sarcoma may involve the head and neck or trunk regions. Most patients present with a palpable but painless soft tissue mass.

Pathologic Findings

Histology

At low power, clear cell sarcoma appears predominantly in clusters and nests of tumor cells of variable size separated by fibrous tissue septa. The number and thickness of the fibrous tissue bands tend to vary (Fig. 4.27). Individual tumor cells range from round to ovoid with abundant, clear to slightly basophilic cytoplasm containing a round-to-ovoid nucleus with a vesicular chromatin pattern and usually a prominent nucleolus (Fig. 4.28). Although the overall architecture tends toward an organoid pattern, clear cell sarcoma may be composed partly or virtually entirely of spindle-shaped cells arranged in short fascicles without intervening stroma (Fig. 4.29). Nuclear pleomorphism is generally mild. For most

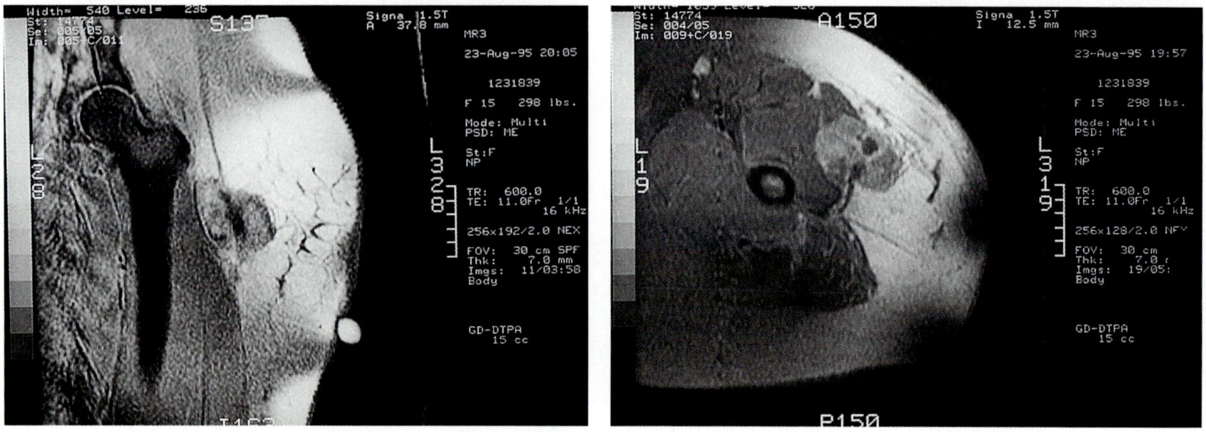

A B

FIGURE 4.26 Clear cell sarcoma. A T1-weighted coronal magnetic resonance image obtained after administration of intravenous gadolinium-DTPA shows a heterogeneous, enhancing mass in the lateral aspect of the proximal thigh abutting the quadriceps musculature **(A).** An axial T1-weighted, gadolinium-enhanced magnetic resonance image shows the heterogeneous mass invading the posterior aspect of the vastus lateralis muscle. No involvement of the overlying skin is observed **(B).**

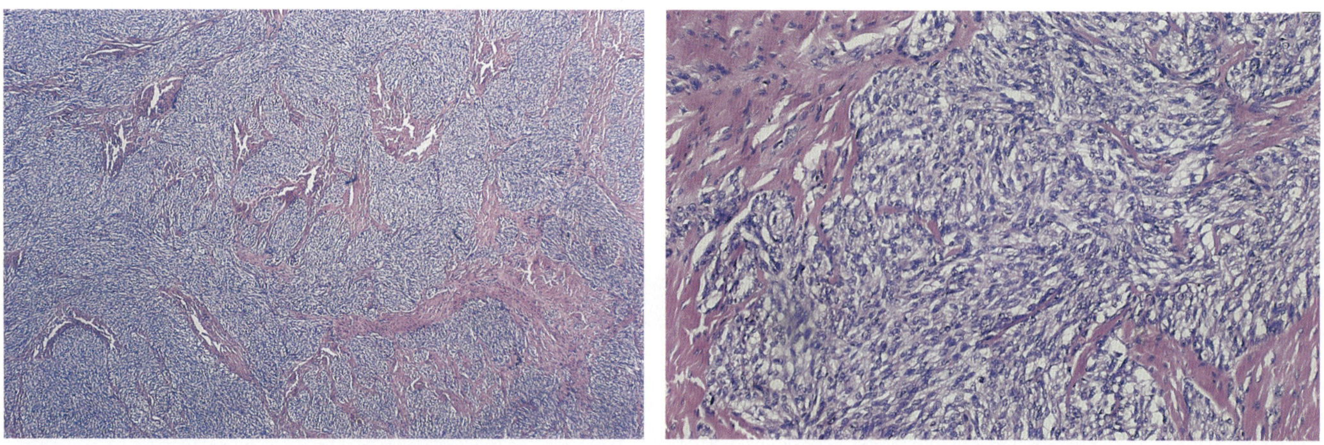

A B

FIGURE 4.27 Clear cell sarcoma with variably sized clusters of tumor cells separated by fibrous tissue septa, creating a vague organoid pattern **(A** and **B).** The number and thickness of the fibrous tissue bands also tend to vary. **(A,** Low power; **B,** intermediate power, H&E.)

cases, the mitotic rate is less than 5 mitoses per 10 high-power fields.[36] Multinucleated giant cells, resembling Touton giant cells with nuclei arranged in a "garland-like" pattern, may be present in 50% of cases and are a helpful diagnostic clue (Fig. 4.30). Despite its resemblance to melanoma, in our experience, intracytoplasmic melanin pigment is observed in only a few tumors (Fig. 4.31).[36]

Fine Needle Aspiration Biopsy

Fine needle aspiration biopsy yields moderately cellular aspirates composed mostly of a dispersed population of uniform, ovoid, slightly round-appearing tumor cells with vesicular nuclei and a single prominent nucleolus.[37] The cytoplasm ranges from scant to abundant but generally stains clear to pale (Fig. 4.32). Multinucleated giant cells of the Touton type are a rare but helpful finding. Intranuclear cytoplasmic pseudoinclusions and intracytoplasmic melanin, in our experience, are extraordinarily rare features in cytologic smears. Ancillary studies, principally immunohistochemistry, are generally required to establish a diagnosis.

Ancillary Studies

Ultrastructural analysis generally reveals nuclei with slightly regular-to-irregular nuclear membranes and one or more prominent nucleoli. Cytoplasm is usually abundant but contains sparse organelles and varying amounts of glycogen. Rare intracytoplasmic premelanosomes are usually observed, but their numbers often vary from cell to cell and even case to case.

The immunohistochemical profile of clear cell sarcoma is summarized in Table 4.6. HMB 45 and S-100 protein are usually positive in more than 70% of cases. Likewise, most examples also express vimentin. Although most tumors appear negative for cytokeratins, a study showed at least focal positivity for keratins in one third of cases.[38] Cytogenetic

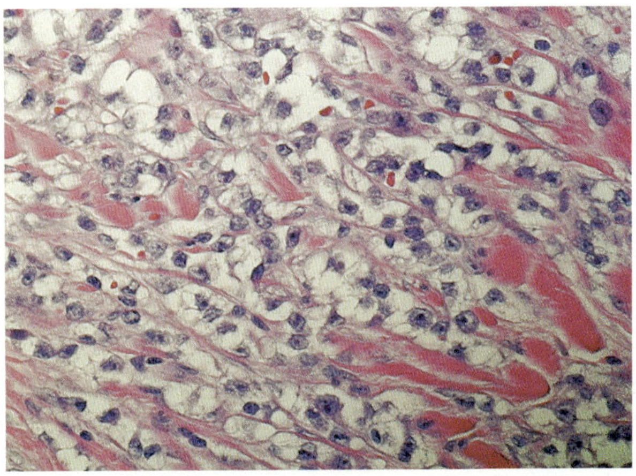

FIGURE 4.28 Individual tumor cells in clear cell sarcoma range from round to ovoid with abundant, clear to slightly basophilic cytoplasm, a round-to-ovoid nucleus with a vesicular chromatin pattern, and a prominent nucleolus. Nuclear pleomorphism is minimal. (H&E.)

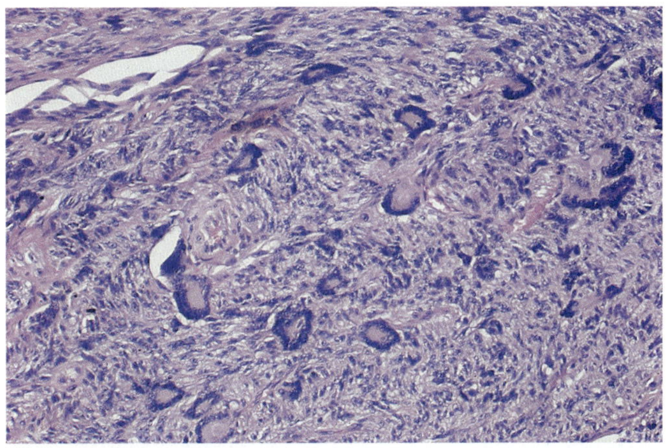

FIGURE 4.30 Multinucleated giant cells, resembling Touton giant cells with nuclei arranged in a "garland-like" pattern, are a helpful diagnostic clue in clear cell sarcoma. (H&E.)

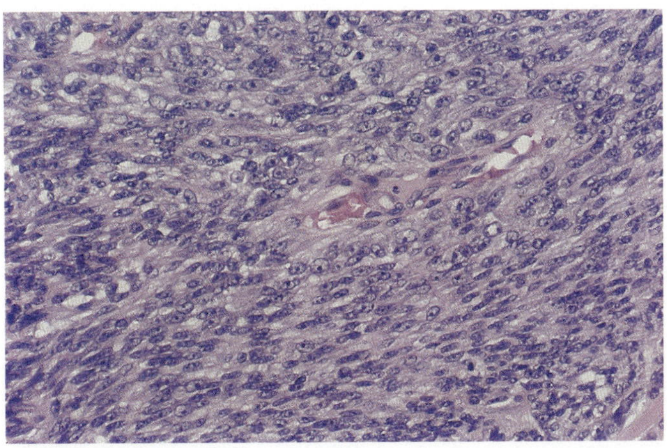

FIGURE 4.29 Clear cell sarcoma may be composed partly or virtually entirely of spindle-shaped cells arranged in short fascicles without intervening stroma. (H&E.)

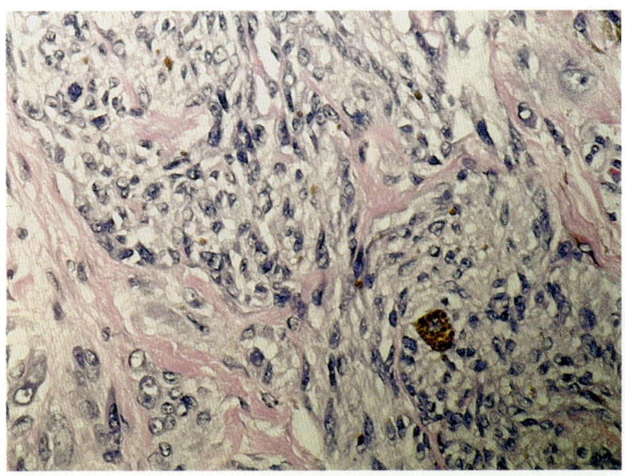

FIGURE 4.31 Intracytoplasmic melanin pigment is observed in only occasional cases of clear cell sarcoma. (H&E.)

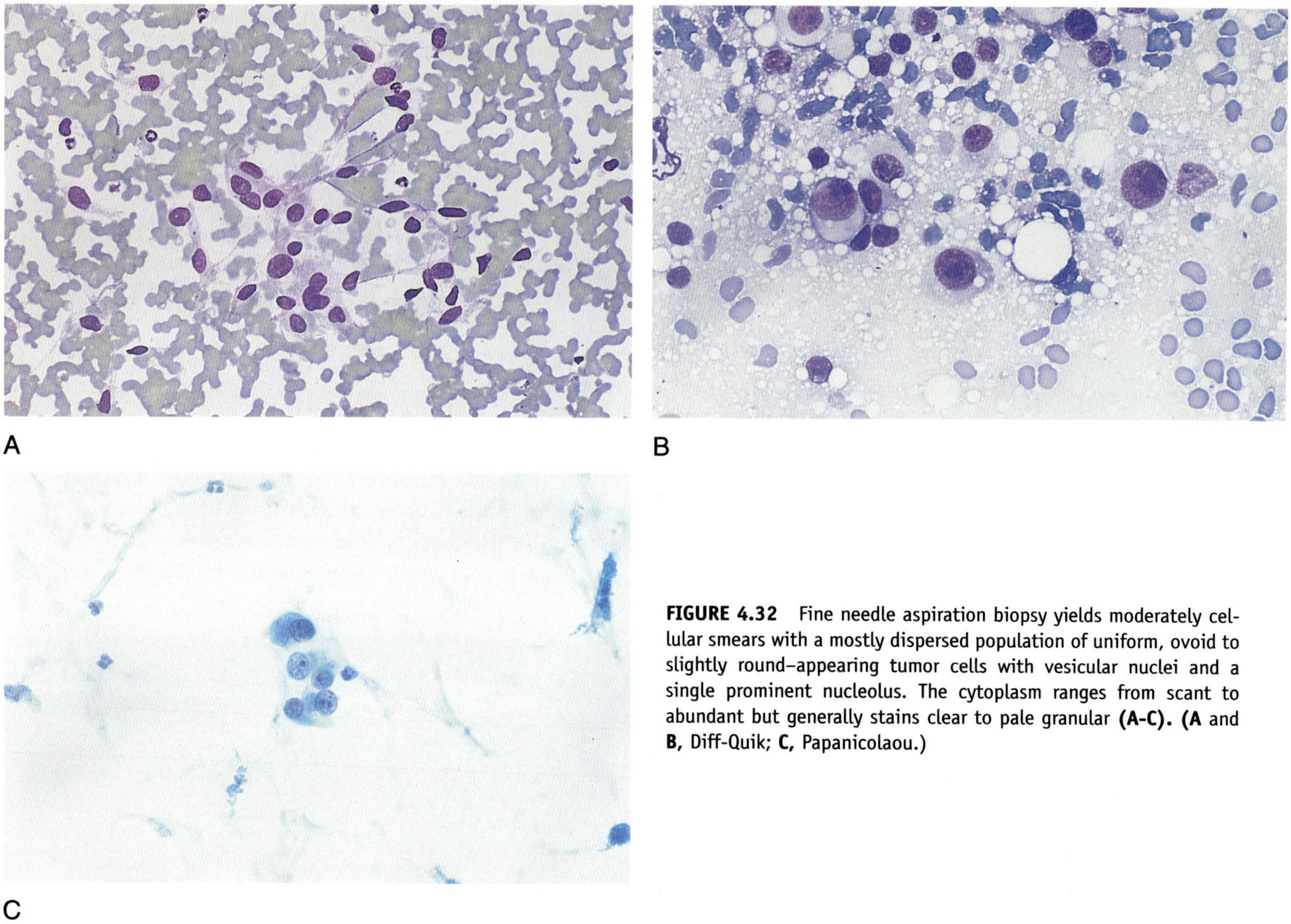

FIGURE 4.32 Fine needle aspiration biopsy yields moderately cellular smears with a mostly dispersed population of uniform, ovoid to slightly round-appearing tumor cells with vesicular nuclei and a single prominent nucleolus. The cytoplasm ranges from scant to abundant but generally stains clear to pale granular **(A-C)**. **(A** and **B,** Diff-Quik; **C,** Papanicolaou.)

TABLE 4.6 Immunohistochemical Profile of Clear Cell Sarcoma

Antibody	Percent Reactivity
Vimentin	75-100
HMB 45	70-95
S-100 protein	65-80
Cytokeratin	0-30
CD34	Negative
CD31	Negative

analysis has revealed a consistent translocation involving chromosomes 12 and 22, t(12;22)(q13;q12) with the ATF1-EWS fusion product, in more than 75% of cases analyzed.[39]

Prognosis and Therapy

The 5-year survival rate of clear cell sarcoma ranges from 54% to 70%.[36,38] Survival declines with 10- and 20-year survival rates approaching 33% and 10%.[36] In contrast to many soft tissue sarcomas, clear cell sarcoma frequently metastases to regional lymph nodes. Reported rates of lymph node metastases have ranged from 33% to 53%, raising the question of whether prophylactic regional lymph node dissection should be part of the therapeutic management of clear cell sarcoma.[35,40] Tumor size greater than 5 cm, the presence of tumor necrosis, and metastases (including regional lymph nodes) at initial presentation seem to be adverse prognostic factors.[35,36,38] At present, there are no histologic variables that seem to be prognostically significant. Complete resection of the primary tumor is the optimal form of treatment. Some investigators have reported adjuvant radiation therapy to the primary tumor site as having a "beneficial effect on survival."[38] The role of chemotherapy in the management of clear cell sarcoma is unclear.

Granular Cell Tumor

The histogenesis of granular cell tumor has resulted in speculation and controversy. Originally, granular cell tumor was proposed as having a myoblastic origin and initially was designated as granular cell myoblastoma. At present, most investigators favor a nerve sheath or schwannian derivation, predominantly based on immunohistochemical and ultrastructural features.

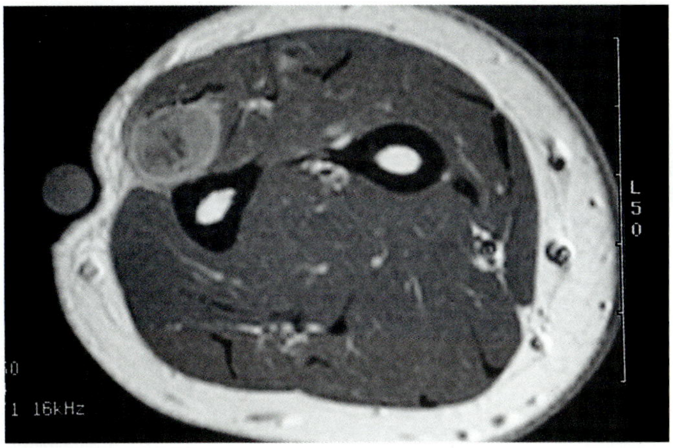

FIGURE 4.33 Granular cell tumor. A T1-weighted axial magnetic resonance image of the right forearm reveals a heterogeneous mass dorsal to the shaft of the ulna in the extensor carpi ulnaris muscle.

Clinical Features

Similar to most of the epithelioid/polygonal cell tumors, granular cell tumor may arise at any age but most commonly occurs in patients between the ages of 20 and 40 years.[41,42] Granular cell tumor may occur in virtually any anatomic location, but almost 50% of reported cases involve the head and neck (Fig. 4.33). In the latter, localization within the tongue is the most common site of origin. Of patients with granular cell tumor, 10% to 15% have multiple lesions within the same organ or at multiple sites.[43] Symptoms usually are related to the tumefaction and are most often painless.

Pathologic Findings

Histology

Granular cell tumors are usually small lesions (<2 cm) and often infiltrative. Malignant tumors tend to be larger, often exceeding 5 cm in greatest dimension.[44] At low power, the neoplastic cells are arranged in ill-defined groups that may be partially separated by slender fibrous tissue septa. Generally, there is little to no architectural or "pattern" arrangement of the tumor cells within granular cell tumors.[42] Subepithelial or submucosal forms of the tumor may be associated with pseudoepitheliomatous changes in the overlying epithelium (Fig. 4.34). Consequently, such examples may be mistaken for squamous cell carcinoma. At high power, the neoplastic cells appear ovoid to polygonal with abundant, slightly eosinophilic but coarsely granular cytoplasm surrounding mostly hyperchromatic but uniform nuclei (Fig. 4.35). Occasional binucleation may be observed. The cytoplasmic granules are characteristically PAS positive and diastase resistant. Significant mitotic activity and nuclear pleomorphism usually are not features of benign granular cell tumor. Although histology is an imperfect predictor of prognosis in granular cell tumors, certain features suggest potential for more aggressive behavior. Granular cell tumors exhibiting increased cellularity and prominent spindling of the tumor cells; tumor necrosis; and individual cells with high nuclear-to-cytoplasmic ratios, nuclear pleomorphism, vesicular nuclei with prominent nucleoli, and numerous mitotic figures (>2 mitoses per 10 high-power fields) are more likely to behave in a malignant fashion.[44] Fanburg-Smith and colleagues[44] proposed that any tumor exhibiting three or more of the aforementioned criteria be classified as malignant, whereas tumors with only one or two of the criteria be designated as "atypical." Despite limited data, this histologic classification seems to be prognostically significant. Benign and malignant granular cell tumors may display invasion of surrounding tissues.

The granular nature of the individual tumor cells is not specific for granular cell tumors; granular cells have been observed in other benign and malignant lesions, including carcinomas, leiomyomas, leiomyosarcomas, malignant peripheral nerve sheath tumors, and melanomas.[42,45,46] Meticulous examination for nongranular cell tumor areas and judicious use of ancillary studies when necessary generally avoid this pitfall. For this reason, some investigators consider the diagnosis of granular cell tumor to be one of exclusion.

Fine Needle Aspiration Biopsy

Fine needle aspiration biopsy of granular cell tumor yields cellular smears composed of mostly discohesive, uniform-appearing, polygonal-shaped tumor cells with round-to-ovoid regular nuclei, inconspicuous-to-prominent nuclei, and abundant granular cytoplasm (Fig. 4.36).[47] Bare nuclei, stripped of their cytoplasm, and occasional intranuclear cytoplasmic invaginations may be observed. Although the diagnosis of granular cell tumor may be rendered in cytologic material, a frank diagnosis of malignancy probably should be avoided because assessment of certain features, such as mitotic activity and necrosis, usually cannot be determined.

Ancillary Studies

Ultrastructural examination reveals groups of neoplastic cells surrounded by a basal lamina that may appear disrupted. As expected, the cytoplasm is abundant and filled with numerous lysosomes, causing the intense granularity observed by light microscopy. Overall, the ultrastructural appearance of malignant lesions does not differ significantly from benign tumors, although irregular nuclear membranes are more commonly observed in the former.[42]

The immunohistochemical profile of granular cell tumors is summarized in Table 4.7. They are virtually always positive for vimentin, S-100 protein, and NK1-C3 but are uniformly negative for HMB-45 and GFAP.[44,48]

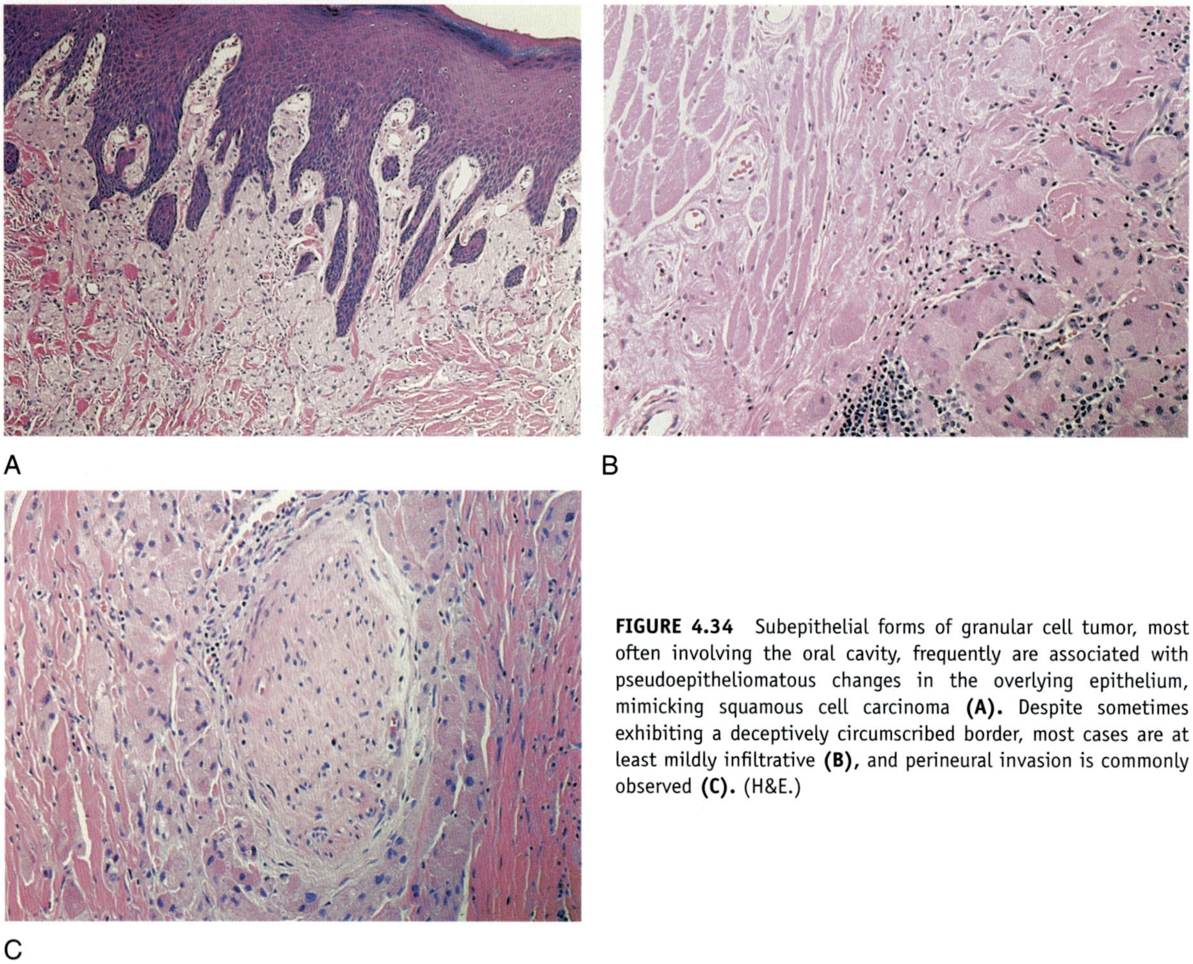

FIGURE 4.34 Subepithelial forms of granular cell tumor, most often involving the oral cavity, frequently are associated with pseudoepitheliomatous changes in the overlying epithelium, mimicking squamous cell carcinoma **(A).** Despite sometimes exhibiting a deceptively circumscribed border, most cases are at least mildly infiltrative **(B),** and perineural invasion is commonly observed **(C).** (H&E.)

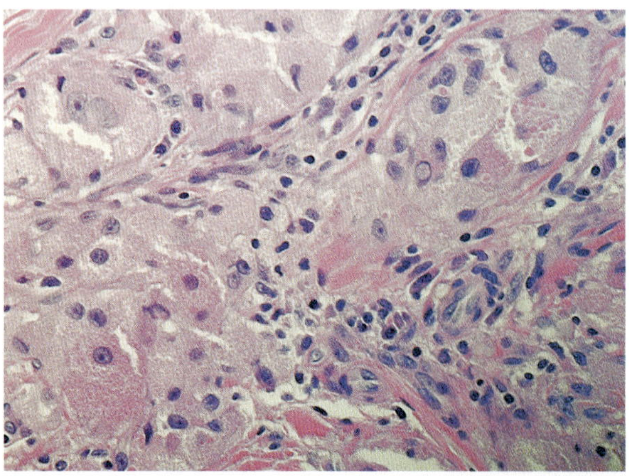

FIGURE 4.35 Cytologically, granular cell tumor cells usually appear ovoid to polygonal with abundant, slightly eosinophilic and coarsely granular cytoplasm; hyperchromatic to vesicular but uniform nuclei; and occasional prominent nucleoli. (H&E.)

Prognosis and Therapy

Because only 1% to 2% of granular cell tumors are malignant, most may be treated by local excision, and recurrence tends to be rare. Among malignant granular cell tumors, metastases most commonly are observed to regional lymph nodes, lung, and bone. Fanburg-Smith and colleagues[44] reported 28 malignant granular cell tumors of soft tissue with follow-up information. Of these patients, 11 (39%) died of their disease, 8 remained alive with disease, and the remaining 9 were alive without evidence of disease at a median interval of 7 years after diagnosis. Important prognostic features included local recurrence, size of the primary tumor, histologic classification as malignant, and the presence of metastases at diagnosis. High Ki67 values and immunostaining with p53 also correlated with malignant classification and clinical course.[44] Wide surgical excision seems to represent the therapy of choice for malignant granular cell tumors. At present, the role of radiation therapy or chemotherapy in the management of malignant lesions is unclear.

Malignant Extrarenal Rhabdoid Tumor

Malignant rhabdoid tumor originally was described as a highly malignant, childhood renal tumor composed of large, round-to-polygonal cells with vesicular nuclei, prominent

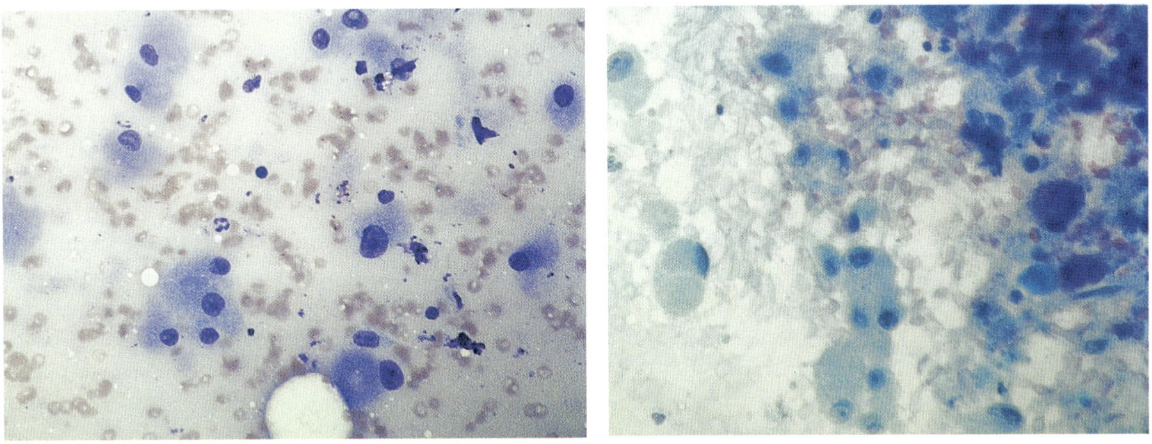

A B

FIGURE 4.36 Fine needle aspirates of granular cell tumor yield cellular smears of mostly discohesive but uniform-appearing, polygonal-shaped cells with round-to-ovoid nuclei, inconspicuous-to-prominent nucleoli, and abundant granular cytoplasm **(A** and **B). (A,** Diff-Quik; **B,** Papanicolaou.)

TABLE 4.7 Immunohistochemical Profile of Granular Cell Tumor

Antibody	Percent Reactivity
Vimentin	>95
S-100 protein	>95
NK1-C3	>95
NSE	90-95
CD68	60-95
CD57	60-70
MAC387	Negative
HMB 45	Negative
GFAP	Negative
α smooth muscle actin	Negative

GFAP, glial fibrillary acidic protein; NSE, neuron-specific enolase.

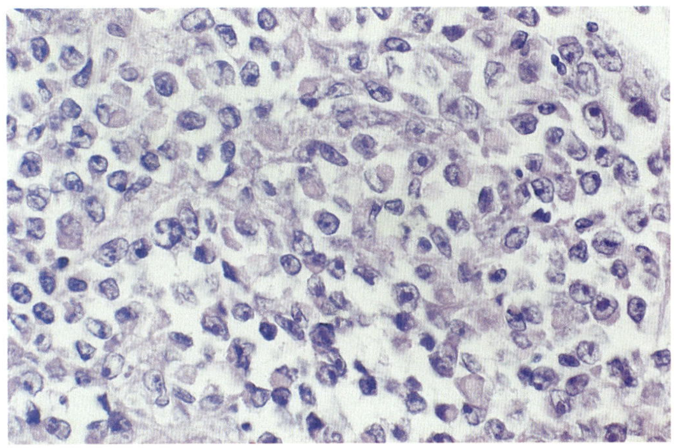

FIGURE 4.37 Malignant rhabdoid tumor with epithelioid-to-polygonal-shaped tumor cells containing round-to-ovoid, vesicular nuclei, prominent nucleoli, and abundant eosinophilic cytoplasm, sometimes exhibiting inclusion-like, intracytoplasmic "whorls." Such "rhabdoid" morphologic features are not specific for rhabdoid tumor and may be observed in other sarcomas, melanoma, and some poorly differentiated carcinomas. (H&E.)

nucleoli, and abundant eosinophilic cytoplasm, closely resembling rhabdomyosarcoma (rhabdoid) but lacking cross striations.[49] Some cells exhibited whorled to globoid intracytoplasmic inclusions that by ultrastructural examination appear to represent intracytoplasmic intermediate filaments. After the discovery of the well-characterized renal form of malignant rhabdoid tumor, reports of an extrarenal counterpart emerged. In contrast to renal malignant rhabdoid tumors, the extrarenal tumors appeared to represent a less cohesive group with wide age ranges and clinical features coupled with variable clinical behavior. It became clear that the so-called rhabdoid features were not specific to malignant rhabdoid tumors and subsequently were reported in a wider variety of tumor types, including melanoma, carcinoma, synovial sarcoma, epithelioid sarcoma, angiosarcoma, malignant peripheral nerve sheath tumor, and rhabdomyosarcoma.[50-52] Consequently, many investigators questioned the existence of extrarenal malignant rhabdoid tumors. In 1999, White and colleagues[53] reported a congenital form of disseminated malignant rhabdoid tumor associated with an aggressive biologic behavior and abnormalities of chromosome 22q11-12. Pathologically, all cases showed slightly spindled-to-polygonal cells arranged in nests or organoid patterns (Fig. 4.37). The rhabdoid pattern was observed in all tumors. Mitotic figures were numerous and often atypical. Immunohistochemically, all nine cases were vimentin positive, and of tumors examined, all but one expressed cytokeratin and epithelial membrane antigen. Actin positivity was observed in six cases, desmin in three, and membranous reactivity for CD99 in five. All patients died of their disease (average survival time, <6 weeks after diagnosis).[53] A renal and an extrarenal form of malignant rhabdoid tumor clearly exist. Outside of the setting of a widely disseminated tumor of infancy, however, we believe the diagnosis of extrarenal malignant rhabdoid tumor is one of exclusion, given the wide variety of biologically distinct neoplasms that may exhibit the so-called rhabdoid phenotype.

Langerhans' Cell Histiocytosis

Langerhans' cell histiocytosis, also known as Langerhans' cell granulomatosis, encompasses a group of histologically similar but biologically distinct clinical syndromes, including eosinophilic granuloma, Hand-Schüller-Christian disease, and Letterer-Siwe syndrome.[54] All share the histologic finding of the Langerhans' cell histiocyte. In the past, whether Langerhans' cell histiocytosis represented a true neoplasm or reflected an inflammatory or immune response has been disputed. Evidence suggests that Langerhans' cell histiocytosis is a clonal proliferation, supporting a neoplastic origin.[55,56]

Clinical Features

Langerhans' cell histiocytosis may be found at any age, but most occur in children, usually before 5 years, and males are affected more commonly than females. The skeleton is the most frequent site of involvement, specifically the craniofacial region followed by the femur, pelvis, ribs, and spine (Fig. 4.38).[54] In adult patients, the most common skeletal site is the ribs.[57] Extraosseous manifestations include diabetes insipidus (usually irreversible), a seborrhea-like skin rash, interstitial pulmonary abnormalities, lymphadenopathy, hepatosplenomegaly, and pancytopenia. Presenting symptoms vary depending on the site affected. Langerhans' cell histiocytosis of the skeleton usually is associated with pain and less commonly a soft tissue mass. Involvement of the mandible may manifest as loose teeth, whereas otitis media and diminished hearing often occur with disease of the mastoid region. The classic Hand-Schüller-Christian disease triad (diabetes insipidus, osteolytic bone lesions, and exophthalmos) is uncommon, generally occurring in less than 5% of patients.

Radiologically, regardless of anatomic site, Langerhans' cell histiocytosis tends to form osteolytic intramedullary lesions that are sharply marginated but typically lack a zone of reactive sclerosis. Concomitant cortical destruction is common and may be associated with a periosteal reaction. Less frequently, a permeative ill-defined pattern of bone destruction may mimic a malignancy. When Langerhans' cell histiocytosis occurs in the long bones of the extremities, the lesions are usually diaphyseal-centered, and these cases rarely may suggest Ewing's sarcoma (Fig. 4.39).[58]

Pathologic Findings

Histology

Morphologically, Langerhans' cell histiocytes usually are arranged in loose nests or clusters and occasionally as individual cells. At high power, these cells are characterized by ovoid, indented-to-folded or grooved nuclei and inconspicuous-to-prominent nucleoli surrounded by clear-to-eosinophilic cytoplasm (Figs. 4.40 and 4.41). Binucleated and multinucleated forms frequently are observed (Fig. 4. 42). Mitotic figures are generally sparse but may range up to 10 mitoses per 10 high-power fields. Atypical mitotic figures are never observed, however. Destruction of bony trabeculae may be seen in one third of cases.[54] Variable numbers of inflammatory cells, principally eosinophils but also neutrophils and lymphocytes, are often present within the background. Coagulative necrosis, when extensive, may make interpretation difficult. Although

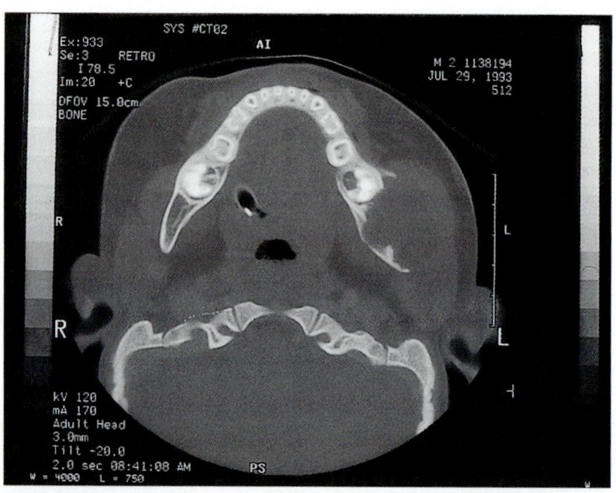

FIGURE 4.38 Langerhans' cell histiocytosis. An axial computed tomographic scan shows an area of bone lysis in the left angle of the mandible with endosteal scalloping and extension to the adjacent molar and adjoining soft tissues.

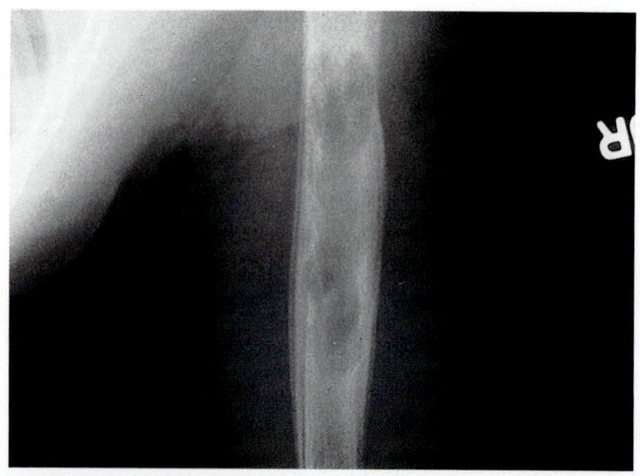

FIGURE 4.39 Langerhans' cell histiocytosis. An anteroposterior view of the humerus shows an extensive area of medullary osteolysis with multiple foci of endosteal erosion. An immature, lamellated pattern of periosteal new bone production encircles the humerus, reminiscent of the periosteal response evoked by Ewing's sarcoma.

ancillary studies, such as electron microscopy or immunohistochemistry, are helpful, we believe that in most cases the diagnosis of Langerhans' cell histiocytosis of bone can be established easily with light microscopy alone, especially when correlated with clinical and radiologic data.

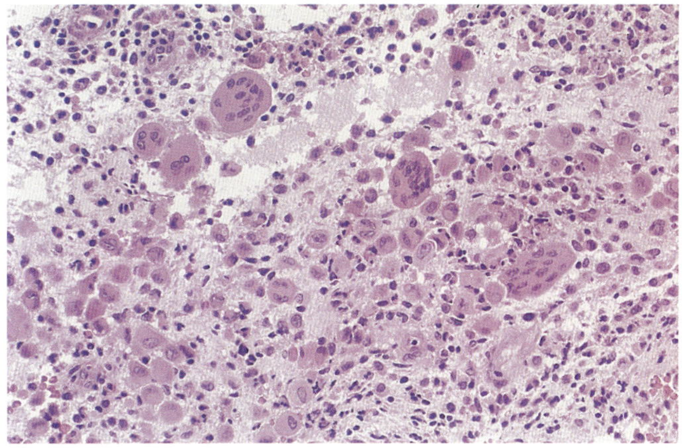

FIGURE 4.42 Langerhans' cell histiocytosis often displays binucleated and multinucleated histiocytes. (H&E.)

Fine Needle Aspiration Biopsy

Cytologic smears are usually hypercellular and composed of individually dispersed Langerhans' cell histiocytes with characteristic ovoid-to-reniform or convoluted nuclei, often exhibiting distinct longitudinal grooves (Fig. 4.43). Nucleoli are typically small and inconspicuous but rarely may be prominent. Binucleated and multinucleated forms are virtually always present. Accompanying the diagnostic histiocytes are variable numbers of eosinophils, lymphocytes, and neutrophils

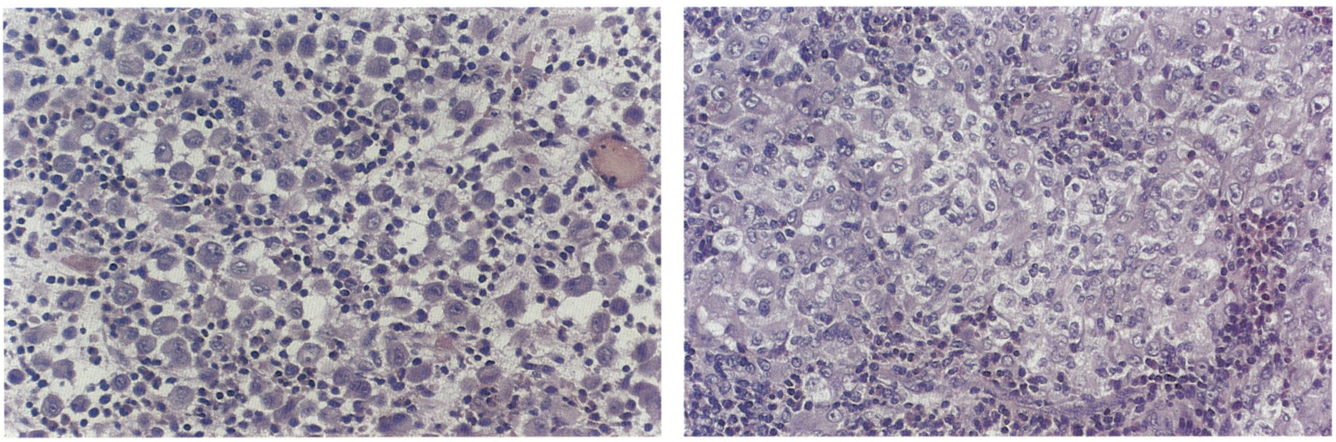

A B

FIGURE 4.40 Langerhans' cell histiocytosis composed of the characteristic histiocytes arranged in loose sheets, nests, or clusters and occasionally as individual cells and accompanied by a mixed inflammatory infiltrate, primarily lymphocytes and eosinophils **(A** and **B).** (H&E.)

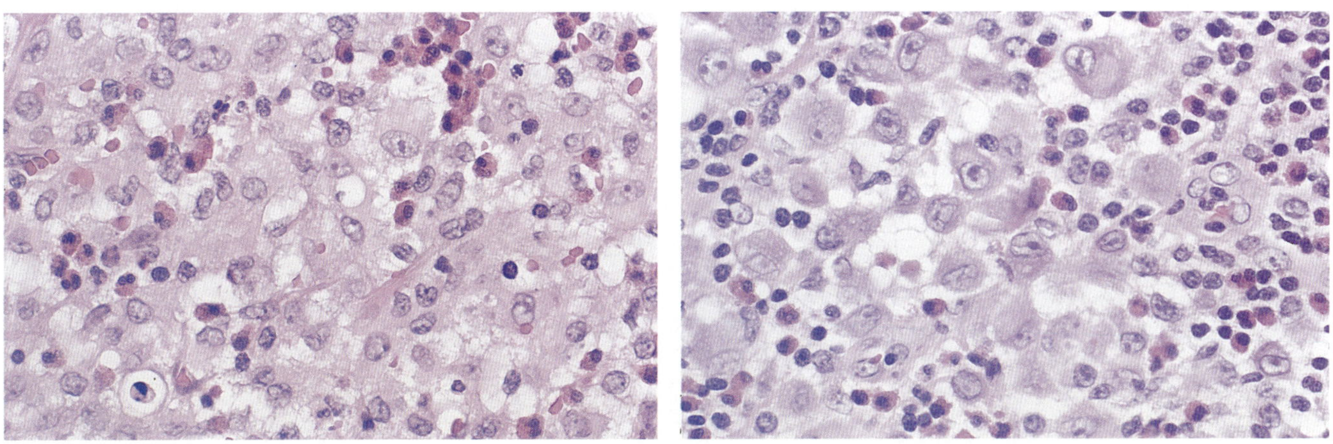

A B

FIGURE 4.41 At high power, Langerhans' cell histiocytes are characterized by ovoid, indented-to-folded or grooved nuclei and inconspicuous-to-prominent nucleoli and are surrounded by clear-to-eosinophilic cytoplasm. Note the variable numbers of eosinophils and lymphocytes **(A** and **B).** (H&E.)

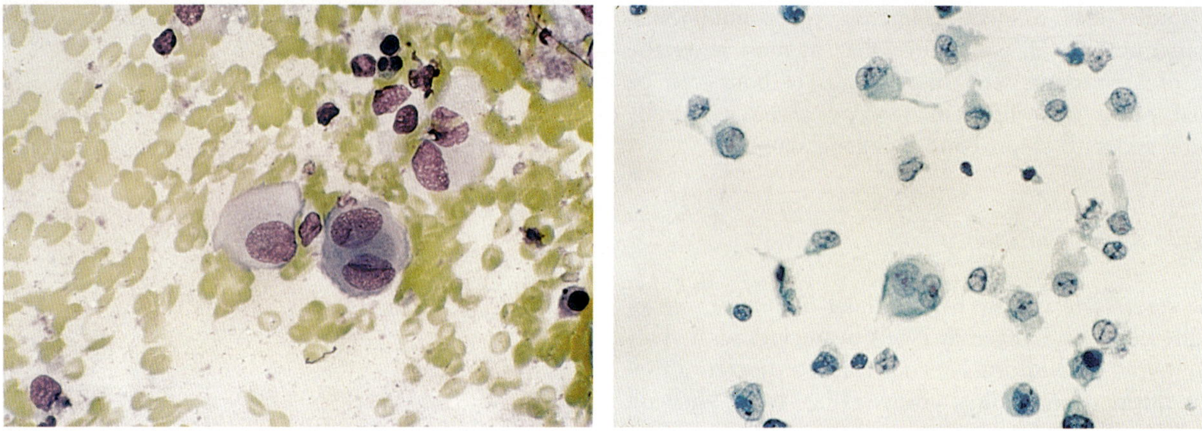

A B

FIGURE 4.43 Fine needle aspiration biopsy of Langerhans' cell histiocytosis yields hypercellular smears composed of individually dispersed Langerhans' cell histiocytes with the characteristic ovoid-to-reniform or convoluted nuclei, often exhibiting distinct longitudinal grooves. Nucleoli are usually small and inconspicuous but rarely may be prominent. Note the binucleated cells **(A** and **B). (A,** Diff-Quik; **B,** Papanicolaou.)

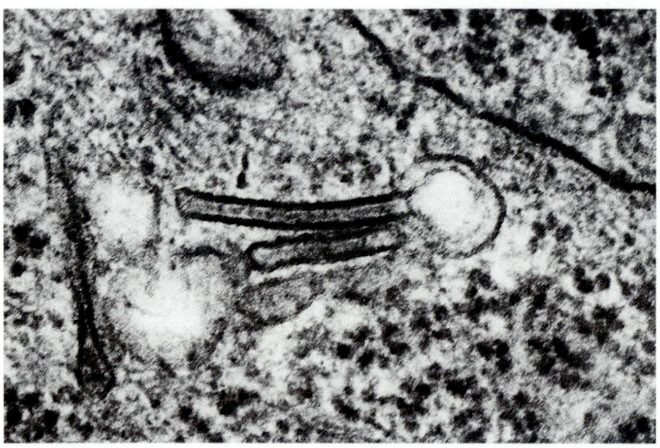

FIGURE 4.44 Ultrastructurally, the most distinctive feature of Langerhans' cell histiocytosis is the presence of intracytoplasmic tennis racket–shaped structures referred to as *Birbeck granules*.

that may predominate.[59] Erythrophagocytosis and leukophagocytosis are never present. The absence of matrix material and the clinicopathologic features generally allow distinction from chondroblastoma. In most cases, the diagnosis of Langerhans' cell histiocytosis can be established easily in cytologic material.

Ancillary Studies

Ultrastructural examination reveals the classic histiocytic/dendritic cells with an ovoid-to-folded nucleus, abundant cytoplasm, and the presence of intracytoplasmic tennis racket–shaped structures, so-called Birbeck granules (Fig. 4.44). Additional features include free ribosomes, rough endoplasmic reticulum, mitochondria, filopodia at the cell surface, and primary lysosomes.

Immunohistochemically, virtually all cases of Langerhans' cell histiocytosis express S-100 protein, and most express CD1a, its more specific marker. Additional immunohistochemical stains that also are frequently positive include vimentin and CD68. Langerhans' cell histiocytosis is generally negative, at least in paraffin, for CD45, α_1-antitrypsin, CD15, and epithelial membrane antigen.

Prognosis and Therapy

Overall the biologic behavior of Langerhans' cell histiocytosis is variable and sometimes unpredictable. Generally, patients with solitary bone lesions have an excellent prognosis, however, and usually can be treated successfully by surgical curettage or excision alone. Patients with polyostotic disease (more than three bones involved) are more likely to develop disseminated disease. Additional poor prognostic indicators include younger age at diagnosis (<3 years), hepatosplenomegaly, and thrombocytopenia.[54,60-62] The role of chemotherapy is unclear, but chemotherapy generally is used only in patients with disseminated disease. In our experience, the disease course of Langerhans' cell histiocytosis seems largely independent of treatment, and some cases show spontaneous resolution.

Adamantinoma

Clinical Features

Adamantinoma is an extraordinarily rare low-grade malignancy of bone. Although it may occur at virtually any age, most patients are between 10 and 30 years old at diagnosis. Adamantinoma almost always arises from the diaphysis (midshaft) of the tibia.[63,64] Concomitant involvement of the tibia and fibula is observed in 15% of cases.[63] Rarely, other long

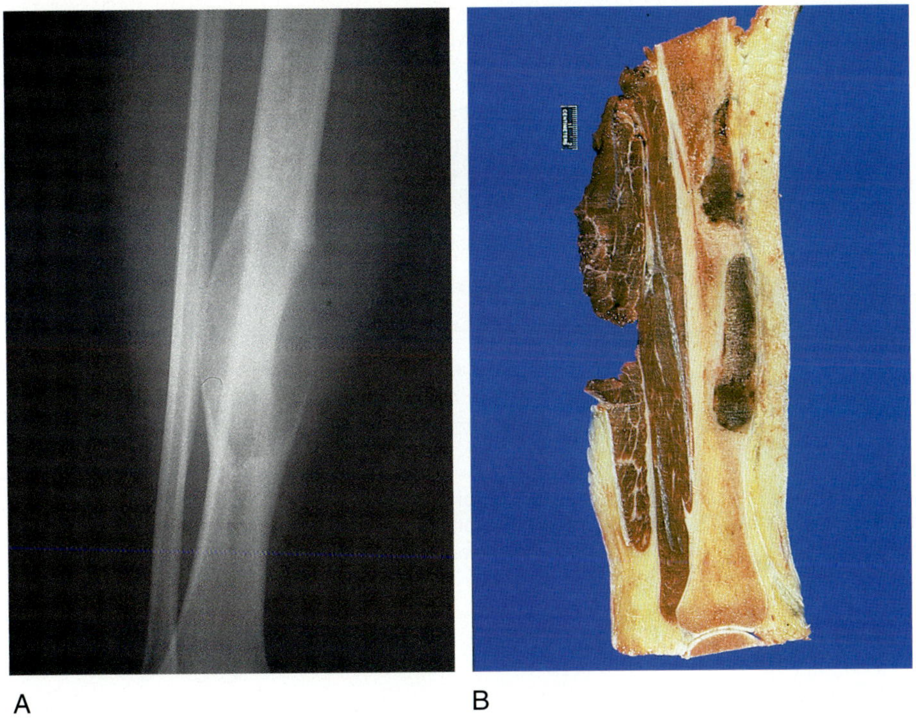

FIGURE 4.45 Adamantinoma. An anteroposterior radiograph of the tibia shows an extensive lesion of the midshaft of the tibia. The cortex is centrifugally ballooned and partially eroded medially **(A).** The corresponding amputation specimen reveals the eccentric tibial shaft lesion arising in and extending through the cortex of the tibia **(B).**

bones may be involved, including the fibula, femur, ulna, and humerus. Although generally considered a primary bone tumor, there are a few reports of adamantinomas arising in pretibial soft tissues.[63,65] Presenting symptoms typically consist of pain and soft tissue swelling. The duration of the complaints is often prolonged, exceeding several years. Keeney and associates[63] reported a patient with symptoms of 50 years' duration before diagnosis.

Radiologically, adamantinomas are usually eccentric, cortical-based lesions within the diaphysis or metadiaphysis of the tibia or fibula or both (Fig. 4.45). They share many radiologic features with osteofibrous dysplasia, including a multiloculated, lytic appearance with sharply defined, sclerotic margins. Less commonly, multicentric lesions may span the entire shaft of the tibia.[63] Differing from osteofibrous dysplasia, however, adamantinoma may erode the overlying cortical bone, extending into adjacent soft tissues. Additionally, most cases extend into the medullary canal at least focally, a feature not seen in osteofibrous dysplasia.

Pathologic Findings

Histology

Morphologically, most adamantinomas show variably sized clusters and nests of epithelial cells within a fibrous-to-fibro-osseous stroma, the latter of which may resemble osteofibrous dysplasia (Fig. 4.46). Because of the extensive clinicoradiologic and pathologic overlap between adamantinoma and osteofibrous dysplasia, it is essential that all suspected cases of osteofibrous dysplasia be sampled extensively to exclude adamantinoma. Most commonly, the epithelial component of adamantinoma resembles basal cell carcinoma of the skin with characteristic peripheral palisading of the epithelial nests (see Fig. 4.46). In some examples, the epithelium forms glandular or cystic spaces, and squamous differentiation may be observed. Kuruvilla and Steiner[66] reported five cases of osteofibrous dysplasia–like adamantinoma in which no obvious epithelial cells by routine light microscopy were observed, but instead scattered keratin-positive cells were identified in all cases. Three of the tumors recurred locally. These findings and reports of cases of adamantinoma preceded by biopsy-proven osteofibrous dysplasia prompted some investigators to suggest a possible relationship between the two.[66,67] Among 80 patients with osteofibrous dysplasia retrospectively reviewed at the Mayo Clinic, Park and coworkers[68] documented no cases of osteofibrous dysplasia progressing to adamantinoma.

Perhaps the most unusual and rarest histologic pattern is the spindle cell "fibrosarcomatous" appearance, virtually devoid of morphologically characteristic epithelial cells (Fig. 4.47).[63] Nevertheless, in all cases, the cytologic features are unusually bland and monomorphic. Likewise, mitotic figures tend to be rare. Significant nuclear pleomorphism is not a feature of adamantinoma and, if present, should suggest the possibility of metastatic carcinoma, or if the spindle cells predominate, a primary bone sarcoma should be considered.

Fine Needle Aspiration Biopsy

Cytologic smears most often contain varying proportions of benign-appearing, spindle-shaped cells, which may predomi-

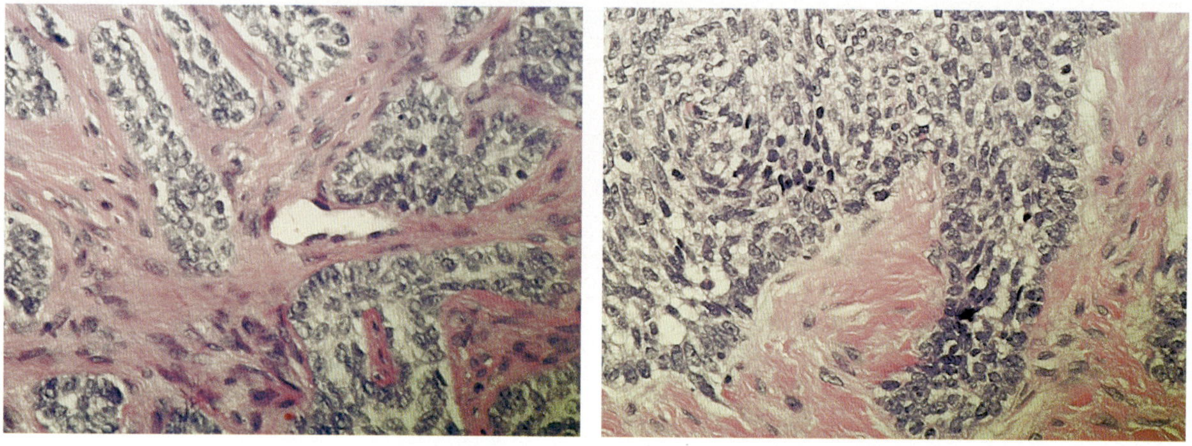

A B

FIGURE 4.46 Adamantinomas generally show variably sized clusters and nests of epithelial cells within a fibrous-to-fibro-osseous stroma. The epithelial component shows only minimal atypia and often resembles cutaneous basal carcinoma with peripheral nuclear palisading **(A** and **B)**. **(A,** Low power; **B,** high power, H&E.)

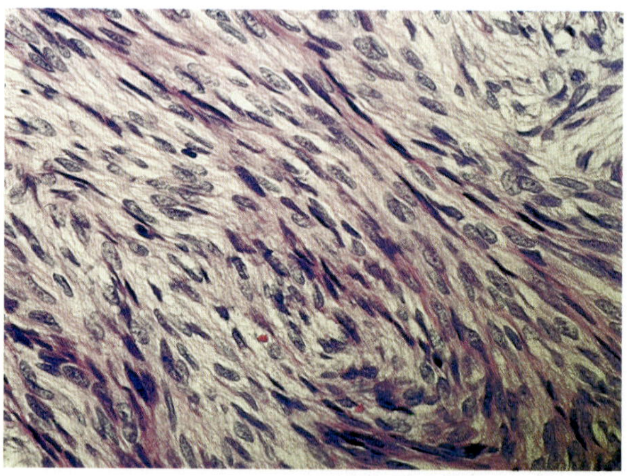

FIGURE 4.47 Adamantinoma rarely displays a spindle cell "fibrosarcomatous" appearance, devoid of epithelial cells. Note the bland and monomorphic cytologic features. (H&E.)

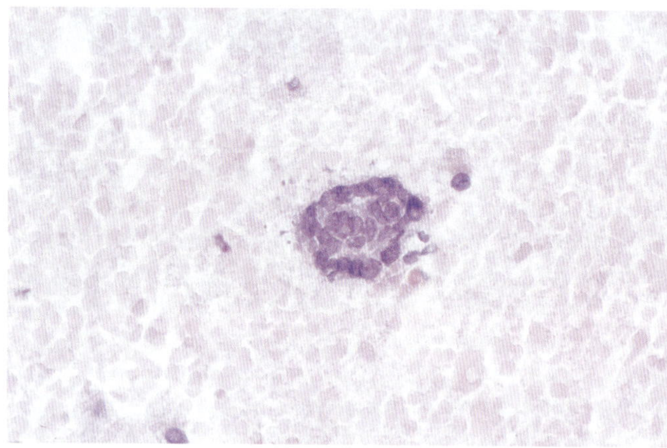

FIGURE 4.48 Fine needle aspiration biopsy of adamantinoma with a nest of mostly bland-appearing epithelial cells. (H&E.)

nate, admixed with cohesive clusters of uniform and monotonous epithelial cells.[69,70] The latter typically exhibit round, mostly uniform nuclei with a finely granular chromatin pattern and inconspicuous-to-small nucleoli (Fig. 4.48). Significant nuclear atypia is never seen and should suggest metastatic carcinoma. If correlated with clinicoradiologic features, the diagnosis can be established easily by fine needle aspiration biopsy.

Ancillary Studies

Ultrastructural examination reveals a constellation of features, including intracellular bundles of type I microfilaments, moderate numbers of mitochondria, rough endoplasmic reticulum, occasional Golgi bodies and lysosomes, and scattered glycogen. Microvilli and desmosomes are found in virtually all tumors. Basement membranes tend to be well formed, and intercellular basement membrane–like material may be deposited focally in pools.[71]

Immunohistochemically the epithelial component always expresses keratins and generally vimentin. Occasionally, keratin immunopositivity is observed in the spindle cell component.

Prognosis and Therapy

Adamantinomas should be regarded as low-grade malignancies. Because of the potential for local recurrence, the preferred therapy is surgical excision, usually wide en bloc resection and limb salvage therapy. In most cases, amputation can be reserved for recurrent disease. Metastases occur in 15% to 25% of patients but may not become apparent for several years after primary therapy.[63] Prognosis seems to be related primarily to the adequacy of surgical therapy.[63,64]

Oureshi and colleagues[72] reported preservation and 10-year survival rates of 84% and 87% among 70 patients treated with limb salvage therapy.

REFERENCES

Synovial Sarcoma

1. Bergh P, Meis-Kindblom JM, Gherlinzoni F, et al: Synovial sarcoma: Identification of low and high risk groups. Cancer 1999;85:2596.
2. Oda Y, Hashimoto H, Tsuneyoshi M, et al: Survival in synovial sarcoma: A multivariate study of prognostic factors with special emphasis on the comparison between early death and long-term survival. Am J Surg Pathol 1993;17:35.
3. Varela-Duran J, Enzinger FM: Calcifying synovial sarcoma. Cancer 1982;50:345.
4. Milchgrub S, Ghandur-Mnaymneh L, Dorfman HD, et al: Synovial sarcoma with extensive osteoid and bone formation. Am J Surg Pathol 1993;17:357.
5. Majeste RM, Beckman EN: Synovial sarcoma with an overwhelming epithelial component. Cancer 1988;61:2527.
6. Krane JF, Bertoni F, Fletcher CDM: Myxoid synovial sarcoma: An underappreciated morphologic subset. Mod Pathol 1999;12:456.
7. Folpe AL, Schmidt RA, Chapman D, Gown AM: Poorly differentiated synovial sarcoma: Immunohistochemical distinction from primitive neuroectodermal tumors and high-grade malignant peripheral nerve sheath tumors. Am J Surg Pathol 1998;22:673.
8. Kilpatrick SE, Teot LA, Stanley MW, et al: Fine-needle aspiration biopsy of synovial sarcoma: A cytomorphologic analysis of primary, recurrent, and metastatic tumors. Am J Clin Pathol 1996;106:769.
9. Dei Tos AP, Wadden C, Calonje E, et al: Immunohistochemical demonstration of glycoprotein p30/32mic2 (CD99) in synovial sarcoma: A potential cause of diagnostic confusion. Appl Immunohistochem 1995;3:168.
10. Smith TA, Machen SK, Fisher C, et al: Usefulness of cytokeratin subsets for distinguishing monophasic synovial sarcoma from malignant peripheral nerve sheath tumor. Am J Clin Pathol 1999;112:641.
11. De Leeuw B, Balemans M, Olde Weghuis D, et al: Identification of two alternative fusion genes, SYT-SSX1 and SYT-SSX2, in t(X;18)(p11.2;q11.2)-positive synovial sarcoma. Hum Mol Genet 1995;4:1097.
12. Crew AJ, Clark J, Fisher C, et al: Fusion of SYT to two genes, SSX1 and SSX2, encoding proteins with homology to the Kruppel-associated box in human synovial sarcoma. EMBO J 1995;14:2333.
13. Kawai A, Woodruff J, Healey JH, et al: SYT-SSX gene fusion as a determinant of morphology and prognosis in synovial sarcoma. N Engl J Med 1998;338:153.
14. Inagaki H, Nagasaka T, Otsuka T, et al: Association of SYT-SSX fusion types with proliferative activity and prognosis in synovial sarcoma. Mod Pathol 2000;13:482.
15. Nilsson G, Wang M, Wejde J, et al: Reverse transcriptase polymerase chain reaction on fine needle aspirates for rapid detection of translocations in synovial sarcoma. Acta Cytol 1998;42:1317.
16. O'Sullivan MJ, Kyriakos M, Zhu X, et al: Malignant peripheral nerve sheath tumors with t(X;18): A pathologic and molecular genetic study. Mod Pathol 2000;13:1336.

Epithelioid Sarcoma

17. Chase DR, Enzinger FM: Epithelioid sarcoma: Diagnosis, prognostic indicators, and treatment. Am J Surg Pathol 1985;9:241.
18. Evans HL, Baer SC: Epithelioid sarcoma: A clinicopathologic and prognostic study of 26 cases. Semin Diagn Pathol 1993;10:286.
19. Guillou L, Wadden C, Coindre JM, et al: "Proximal-type" epithelioid sarcoma, a distinctive aggressive neoplasm showing rhabdoid features. Am J Surg Pathol 1997;21:130.
20. Pohar-Marinsek Z, Zidar A: Epithelioid sarcoma in FNAB smears. Diagn Cytopathol 1994;11:367.
21. Arber DA, Kandalaft PL, Mehta P, et al: Vimentin-negative epithelioid sarcoma: The value of an immunohistochemical panel that includes CD34. Am J Surg Pathol 1993;17:302.
22. Cordoba JC, Parham DM, Meyer WH, et al: A new cytogenetic finding in an epithelioid sarcoma, t(8;22)(q22;q11). Cancer Genet Cytogenet 1994;72:151.
23. Halling AC, Wollan PC, Pritchard DJ, et al: Epithelioid sarcoma: A clinicopathologic review of 55 cases. Mayo Clin Proc 1996;71:636.

Alveolar Soft Part Sarcoma

24. Lieberman PH, Brennan MF, Kimmel M, et al: Alveolar soft part sarcoma: A clinicopathologic study of half a century. Cancer 1989;63:1.
25. Ordonez NG: Alveolar soft part sarcoma: A review and update. Adv Anat Pathol 1999;6:125.
26. Shabb N, Sneige N, Fanning CV, et al: Fine needle aspiration cytology of alveolar soft part sarcoma. Diagn Cytopathol 1991;63:1.
27. Unni KK, Soule EH: Alveolar soft part sarcoma: An electron microscopic study. Mayo Clin Proc 1975;50:591.
28. Ordonez NG, Hickey RC, Brooks TE: Alveolar soft part sarcoma: A cytologic and immunohistochemical study. Cancer 1988;61:525.
29. Wang NP, Bacchi CE, Jiang JJ, et al: Does alveolar soft-part sarcoma exhibit skeletal muscle differentiation? An immunocytochemical and biochemical study of myogenic regulatory protein expression. Mod Pathol 1996;9:496.
30. Ordonez NG, Mackay B: Alveolar soft part sarcoma: A review of the pathology and histogenesis. Ultrastruct Pathol 1998;22:275.
31. Ladanyi M, Lui MY, Antonescu CR, et al: Cloning of the der(17)t(X;17)(p11;q25) of alveolar soft part sarcoma identifies the ASPL-TFE3 gene fusion, a new molecular marker (abstract). Mod Pathol 2001;14:14A.
32. Auerbach HE, Brooks JJ: Alveolar soft-part sarcoma: A clinicopathologic and immunohistochemical study. Cancer 1987;60:66.
33. Evans HL: Alveolar soft-part sarcoma: A study of 13 typical examples and one with a histologically atypical component. Cancer 1985;55:912.
34. Portera CA Jr, Ho CA, Patel SR, et al: Alveolar soft part sarcoma: Clinical course and patterns of metastasis in 70 patients treated at a single institution. Cancer 2001;91:585.

Clear Cell Sarcoma

35. Chung EB, Enzinger FM: Malignant melanoma of soft parts. A reassessment of clear cell sarcoma. Am J Surg Pathol 1983;7:405.
36. Lucas DR, Nascimento AG, Sim FH: Clear cell sarcoma of soft tissues: Mayo Clinic experience with 35 cases. Am J Surg Pathol 1992;16:1197.
37. Caraway NP, Fanning CV, Wojcik EM, et al: Cytology of malignant melanoma of soft parts: Fine-needle aspirates and exfoliative specimens. Diagn Cytopathol 1993;9:632.
38. Deenik W, Mooi WJ, Rutgers EJ, et al: Clear cell sarcoma (malignant melanoma) of soft parts: A clinicopathologic study of 30 cases. Cancer 1999;86:969.
39. Zucman J, Delattre O, Desmaze C, et al: EWS and ATF-1 gene fusion induced by t(12;22) translocation in malignant melanoma of soft parts. Nat Genet 1993;4:341.
40. Eckardt JJ, Pritchard DJ, Soule EH: Clear cell sarcoma: A clinicopathologic study of 27 cases. Cancer 1983;52:1482.

Granular Cell Tumor

41. Strong EW, McDivitt RW, Brasfield RD: Granular cell myoblastoma. Cancer 1970;25:415.
42. Ordonez NG: Granular cell tumor: A review and update. Adv Anat Pathol 1999;6:186.
43. Boraf CS, Bender B: Multiple cutaneous granular cell myoblastoma. Arch Dermatol 1964;89:243.

44. Fanburg-Smith JC, Meis-Kindblom JM, Fante R, et al: Malignant granular cell tumor of soft tissue: Diagnostic criteria and clinicopathologic correlation. Am J Surg Pathol 1998;22:779.
45. McWilliam LJ, Harris M: Granular cell angiosarcoma of the skin: Histology, electron microscopy, and immunohistochemistry of a newly recognized tumor. Histopathology 1985;9:1205.
46. Shimokama T, Watanabe T: Leiomyoma exhibiting a marked granular cell change: Granular cell leiomyoma vs. granular cell schwannoma. Hum Pathol 1992;23:327.
47. Liu K, Madden JF, Olatidoye BA, et al: Features of benign granular cell tumor on fine needle aspiration. Acta Cytol 1999;43:552.
48. Mazur MT, Shultz JJ, Myers JL: Granular cell tumor: Immunohistochemical analysis of 21 benign tumors and one malignant tumor. Arch Pathol Lab Med 1990;114:692.

Malignant Extrarenal Rhabdoid Tumor

49. Haas JE, Palmer NF, Weinberg AG, et al: Ultrastructure of malignant rhabdoid tumor of the kidney. Hum Pathol 1981;12:646.
50. Kumar S, Kumar D, Cowan DF: Transitional cell carcinoma with rhabdoid features. Am J Surg Pathol 1992;16:515.
51. Kodet R, Newton WA Jr, Hamoudi AB, et al: Rhabdomyosarcomas with intermediate-filament inclusions and features of rhabdoid tumors: Light microscopic and immunohistochemical study. Am J Surg Pathol 1991;15:257.
52. Parham DM, Weeks DA, Beckwith JB: The clinicopathologic spectrum of putative extrarenal rhabdoid tumors: An analysis of 42 cases studied with immunhistochemistry or electron microscopy. Am J Surg Pathol 1994;18:1010.
53. White FV, Dehner LP, Belchis DA, et al: Congenital disseminated malignant rhabdoid tumor: A distinct clinicopathologic entity demonstrating abnormalities of chromosome 22q11. Am J Surg Pathol 1999;23:249.

Langerhans' Cell Histiocytosis

54. Kilpatrick SE, Wenger DE, Gilchrist GS, et al: Langerhans' cell histiocytosis (histiocytosis X) of bone: A clinicopathologic analysis of 263 pediatric and adult cases. Cancer 1995;76:2471.
55. Yu RC, Chu C, Buluwela L, et al: Clonal proliferation of Langerhans cells in Langerhans' cell histiocytosis. Lancet 1994;343:767.
56. Wilman CL, Busque L, Griffith BB, et al: Langerhans' cell histiocytosis (histiocytosis X): A clonal proliferative disease. N Engl J Med 1994;331:154.
57. Wester SM, Unni KK, Beabout JW, et al: Langerhans' cell granulomatosis (histiocytosis X) of bone in adults. Am J Surg Pathol 1982;1:413.
58. Biswal BM, Lai P, Uppal R, et al: Unifocal Langerhans' cell histiocytosis (eosinophilic granuloma) resembling Ewing's sarcoma. Australas Radiol 1994;38:313.
59. Kilpatrick SE: Fine-needle aspiration biopsy of Langerhans' cell histiocytosis of bone: Are ancillary studies necessary for "definitive" diagnosis? Acta Cytol 1998;42:820.
60. Raney RB Jr, D'Angio GT: Langerhans' cell histiocytosis (histiocytosis X): Experience at the Children's Hospital of Philadelphia, 1970-1984. Med Pediatr Oncol 1989;17:20.
61. Nezelof C, Frileux-Herbert F, Cronier-Sachot J: Disseminated histiocytosis X: Analysis of prognostic factors based on a retrospective study of 50 cases. Cancer 1979;44:1824.
62. Komp DM, Herson J, Starling KA, et al: A staging system for histiocytosis X: A Southwest Oncology Group study. Cancer 1981;47:798.

Adamantinoma

63. Keeney GL, Unni KK, Beabout JW, et al: Adamantinoma of long bones: A clinicopathologic study of 85 cases. Cancer 1989;64:730.
64. Campanacci M, Giunti A, Bertoni F, et al: Adamantinoma of the long bones: The experience at the Instituto Orthopedico Rizzoli. Am J Surg Pathol 1981;5:533.
65. Mills SE, Rosai J: Adamantinoma of the pretibial soft tissue: Clinicopathologic features, differential diagnosis, and possible relationship to intraosseous disease. Am J Clin Pathol 1985;83:108.
66. Kuruvilla G, Steiner GC: Osteofibrous dysplasia-like adamantinoma of bone: A report of five cases with immunohistochemical and ultrastructural studies. Hum Pathol 1998;29:809.
67. Springfield DS, Rosenberg AE, Mankin HJ, et al: Relationship between osteofibrous dysplasia and adamantinoma. Clin Orthop 1994;309:234.
68. Park YK, Unni KK, McLeod RA, et al: Osteofibrous dysplasia: Clinicopathologic study of 80 cases. Hum Pathol 1993;24:1339.
69. Laucirica R, Mody D, MacLeay L, et al: Adamantinoma: A case report with aspiration cytology and differential diagnostic and immunohistochemical considerations. Acta Cytol 1992;36:951.
70. Galera-Davidson H, Fernandez-Rodriquez A, Torres-Olivera FJ, et al: Cytologic diagnosis of a case of recurrent adamantinoma. Acta Cytol 1989;33:635.
71. Knapp RH, Wick MR, Scheithauer BW, et al: Adamantinoma of bone: An electron microscopic and immunohistochemical study. Virchows Arch A Pathol Anat Histopathol 1982;398:75.
72. Oureshi AA, Shot S, Mallin BA, et al: Current trends in the management of adamantinoma of long bones: An international study. J Bone Joint Surg Am 2000;82:1122.

CHAPTER 5

Spindle Cell Tumors of Bone and Soft Tissue in Infants and Children

A variety of spindle cell tumors may arise during infancy and childhood. Some of these lesions are virtually never observed in adults—fibrous hamartoma of infancy, fibromatosis colli, infantile digital fibromatosis, and giant cell fibroblastoma. The other spindle cell lesions discussed in this chapter occur predominantly in children, although they may be seen rarely in adults. All of these lesions are summarized in Table 5.1. From a histogenetic perspective, virtually all of these spindle cell tumors are of fibroblastic/myofibroblastic origin. Consequently, immunohistochemical stains generally are not useful for establishing their diagnosis. Likewise, the role of fine needle aspiration biopsy (FNAB) is limited because diagnostic architectural features cannot be seen. With the exception of fibromatosis colli, rendering a specific histogenetic diagnosis by FNAB generally is not possible. Osteosarcoma is discussed in Chapter 12; embryonal rhabdomyosarcoma is discussed in Chapter 3.

TABLE 5.1 Spindle Cell Tumors of Bone and Soft Tissue Occurring Predominantly in Infancy and Childhood

Bone Origin	Soft Tissue Origin
Avulsive cortical irregularity	Fibrous hamartoma of infancy
Myofibroma/myofibromatosis	Myofibroma/myofibromatosis
Metaphyseal fibrous defect	Fibromatosis colli
Desmoplastic fibroma	Infantile digital fibromatosis
Osteosarcoma	Infantile fibromatosis
	Infantile fibrosarcoma
	Calcifying aponeurotic fibroma
	Giant cell fibroblastoma
	Inflammatory myofibroblastic tumor
	Angiomatoid fibrous histiocytoma
	Embryonal rhabdomyosarcoma

Metaphyseal Fibrous Defect (Nonossifying Fibroma)

Metaphyseal fibrous defects typically involve the metaphysis of a long bone and most likely do not represent true neoplastic change. The terms *nonossifying fibroma*, *fibroma*, and *fibrous cortical defect* generally are considered synonymous.

Clinical Features

In general, metaphyseal fibrous defects are incidental findings, usually presenting between 10 and 20 years of age. Males and females are affected roughly equally. Physical examination rarely reveals any significant soft tissue swelling or overlying skin changes. Occasionally, patients present with pathologic fracture. The most common anatomic locations in decreasing order of frequency are the distal femur, distal tibia, proximal tibia, and proximal fibula. Rare examples involve the clavicle or the ribs. Although usually solitary, multiple lesions are seen rarely and may be associated with extraosseous features (Jaffe-Campanacci syndrome). These extraosseous stigmata may include café-au-lait–like skin patches (in the absence of neurofibromas), cryptorchidism, and mental retardation.[1,2]

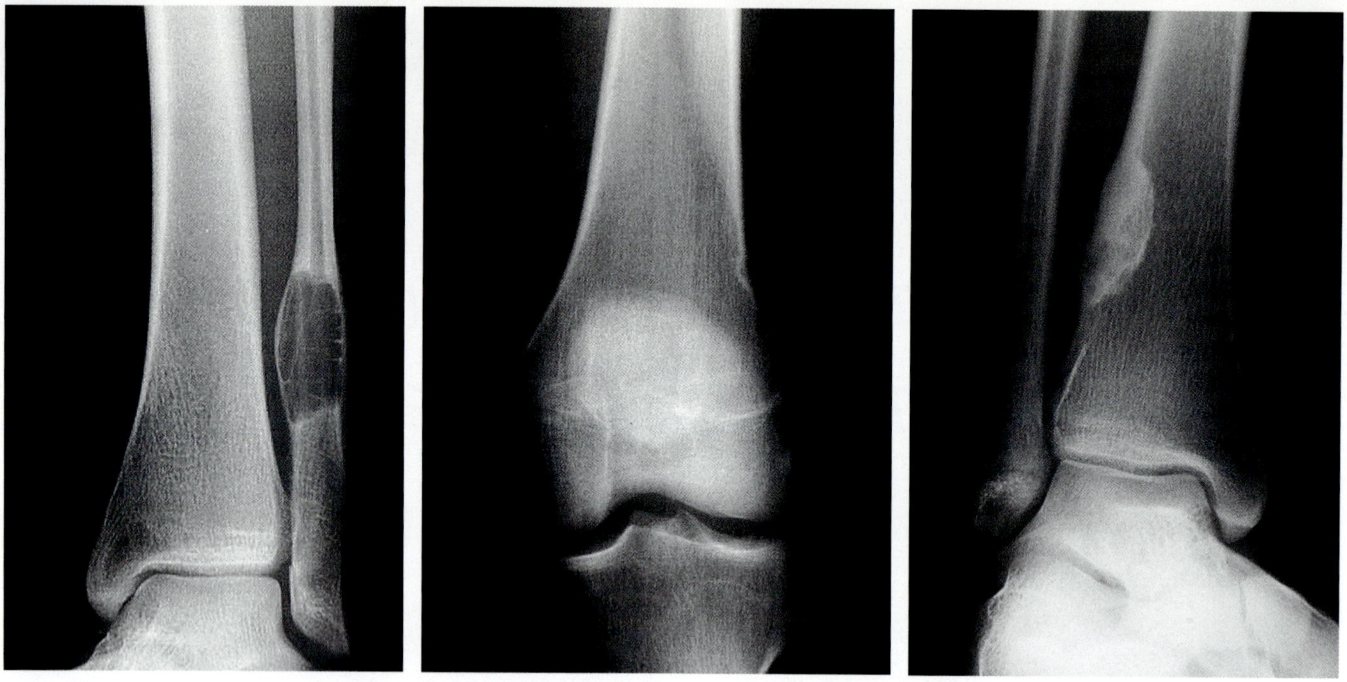

A B C

FIGURE 5.1 Metaphyseal fibrous defect. An oblique radiograph of the distal fibula shows a well-defined lytic lesion in the distal fibula **(A)**. The lesion occupies the entire medullary canal and results in enlargement of the bone with smooth cortical thinning. An anteroposterior radiograph of the knee in another patient reveals a tiny cortical lesion in the lateral cortex of the distal femur **(B)**. An oblique radiograph of the ankle in a third patient shows a sharply defined area of cortical thickening in the lateral aspect of the distal tibia **(C)**. Residual areas of radiolucency are seen within the sclerotic bone.

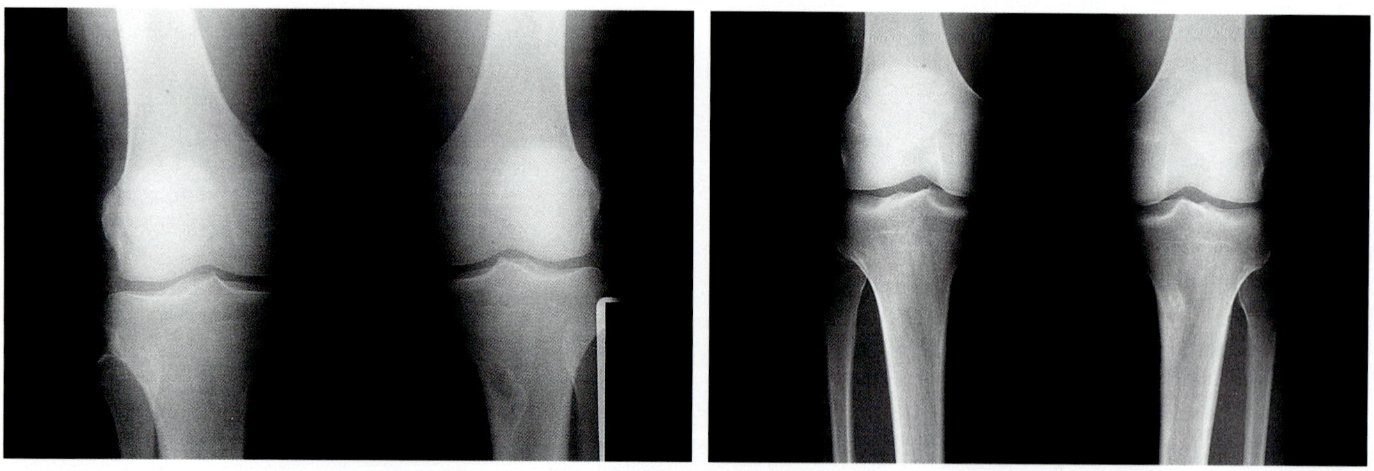

A B

FIGURE 5.2 Healing metaphyseal fibrous defect. An anteroposterior radiograph of the knees shows a well-defined, sharply demarcated lucent lesion in the medial metaphysis of the proximal left tibia **(A)**. Six years later, the lesion in the proximal left tibia has largely healed, leaving behind an area of medullary sclerosis **(B)**. No bone destruction or periosteal new bone production is seen to suggest an aggressive lesion.

Radiographically, metaphyseal fibrous defects are eccentrically positioned, generally along the long axis of the metaphysis of a long bone (Fig. 5.1). Size is variable, ranging from small intracortical lesions to lesions involving virtually the entire diameter of the bone. When metaphyseal fibrous defects are observed in adults, the lesions may be diaphyseal centered and show mineralization (healing) (Fig. 5.2). Metaphyseal fibrous defects may be expansile but almost always are sharply marginated with a sclerotic rim.

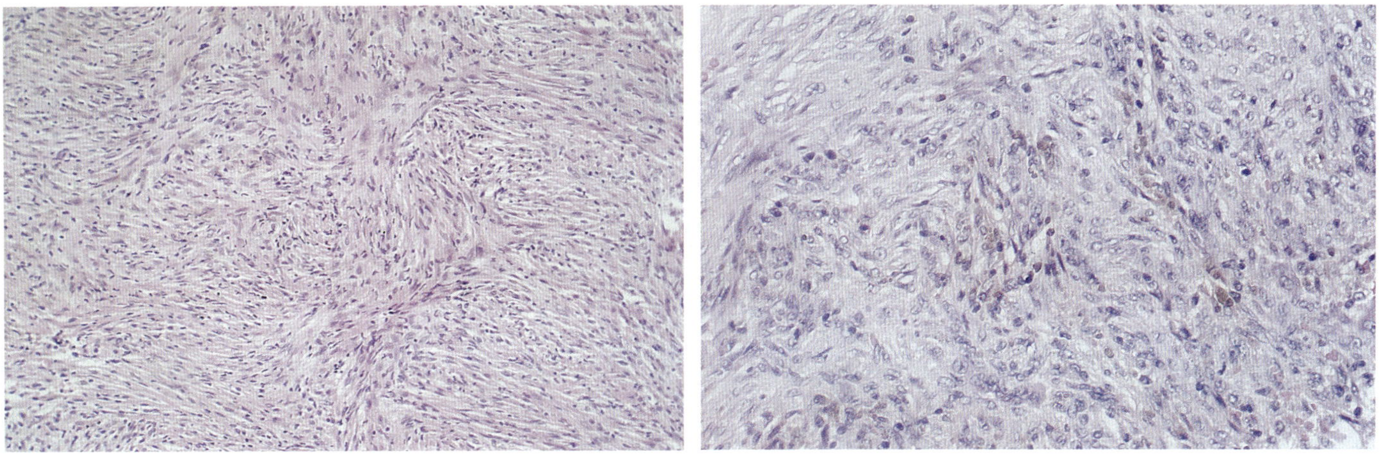

A B

FIGURE 5.3 Metaphyseal fibrous defect appears hypercellular and composed of monotonous cells arranged in short fascicles and storiform patterns **(A** and **B)**. Note the hemosiderin pigment deposition. **(A** and **B,** H&E.)

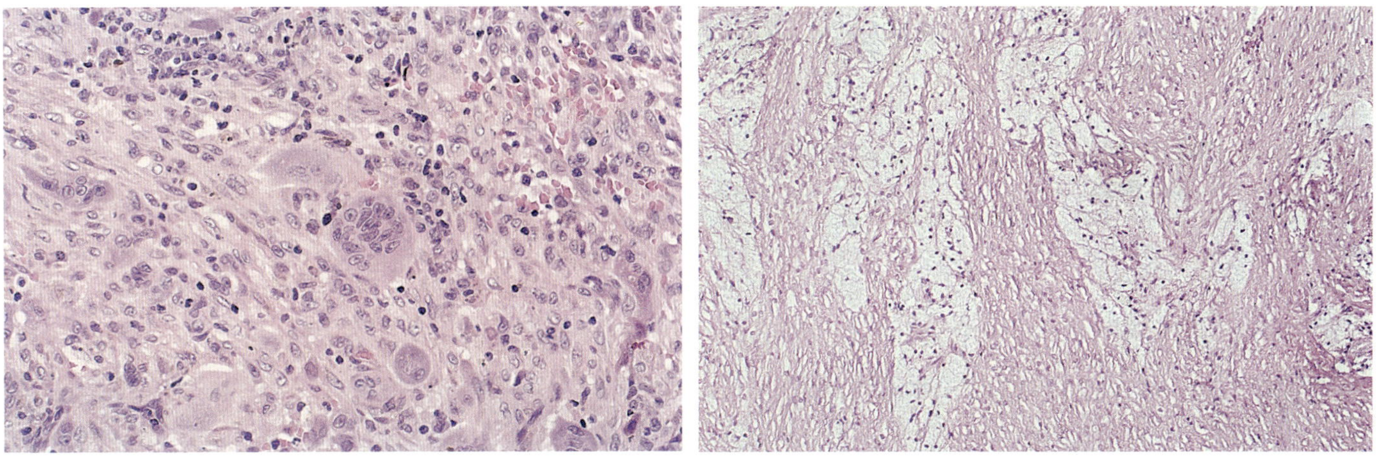

A B

FIGURE 5.4 Metaphyseal fibrous defect often exhibits scattered osteoclast-type giant cells **(A)** and more fibrotic areas with aggregates of foamy histiocytes **(B)**. **(A** and **B,** H&E.)

Pathologic Findings

Histology

Microscopically, metaphyseal fibrous defects are hypercellular lesions comprising a uniform population of spindle cells characteristically arranged in fascicles and storiform patterns. The nuclei of the spindle cells often contain prominent nucleoli but remain regular and monotonous (Fig. 5.3). Numerous mitotic figures may be present, but atypical forms are never seen. Randomly distributed throughout the lesion are numerous osteoclast-type giant cells, foamy histiocytes, and occasional hemosiderin-laden macrophages (Fig. 5.4). Reactive new bone formation rimmed by a thin layer of osteoblasts may be present, especially in the presence of pathologic fracture (Fig. 5.5). Older lesions often show increased mature trabecular bone. For these reasons, the term *nonossifying fibroma* probably should be avoided.

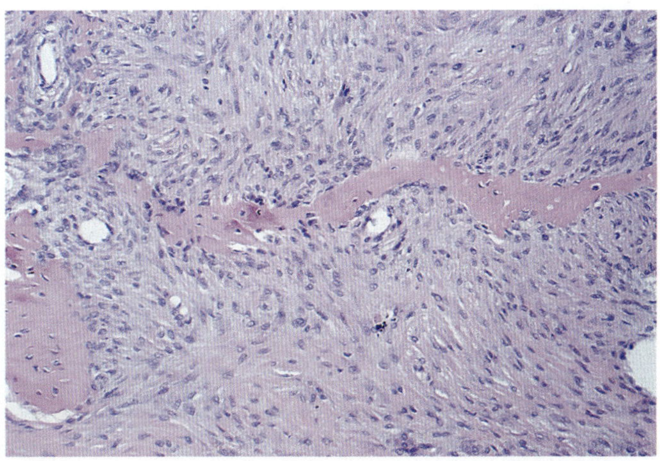

FIGURE 5.5 Metaphyseal fibrous defect often contains focal reactive bone formation. For this reason, we tend to avoid the term *nonossifying fibroma*. (H&E.)

Ancillary Studies

Immunohistochemistry is not necessary for the diagnosis of metaphyseal fibrous defect. Most cases show positivity for vimentin and variable expression for actin. Cytokeratin is uniformly negative.

Prognosis and Therapy

In cases in which the integrity of the bone is not compromised, simple observation is adequate treatment. Most metaphyseal fibrous defects ultimately heal, probably by cortical remodeling and reparative ossification. Lesions occupying more than 50% of the bone diameter pose a significant risk for fracture.[3] In these examples, bone curettage with grafting is generally curative.

Avulsive Cortical Irregularity (Periosteal Desmoid)

Synonyms of avulsive cortical irregularity include periosteal desmoid, cortical desmoid, distal metaphyseal femoral defect, distal femoral cortical defect, and cortical irregularity syndrome. Avulsive cortical irregularity is found almost exclusively on the posterior medial distal femur at or near the insertion of the adductor magnus muscle. Similar lesions also have been described involving the humerus at the insertion of the pectoralis major muscle.[4] Most patients are younger than 20 years old at diagnosis; boys are affected more often than girls. Some of the lesions are bilateral.[5] Most cases present as incidental findings after minor trauma. Radiologically, avulsive cortical irregularity usually presents as a radiolucent, eccentric area located along the medial posterior subcondylar ridges, superior to the epiphyseal plate (Fig. 5.6). Pathologically the lesion is composed of abundant stromal collagen reminiscent of tendon-like fibrous tissue. It generally is only moderately cellular. Individual spindle cells are uniform and lack significant nuclear atypia. A few benign-appearing, osteoclast-like giant cells may be scattered throughout the lesion. Rarely, reactive bone or cartilage resembling callus may be observed. In most cases with classic radiographic features, no therapy is recommended. Biopsy or curettage is indicated in patients in whom the radiographic features are atypical. Treated or untreated, the overall prognosis is excellent, and recurrence does not occur after biopsy.[6]

Desmoplastic Fibroma

Clinical Features

Desmoplastic fibroma is an extraordinarily rare primary bone tumor and represents the intraosseous equivalent of soft

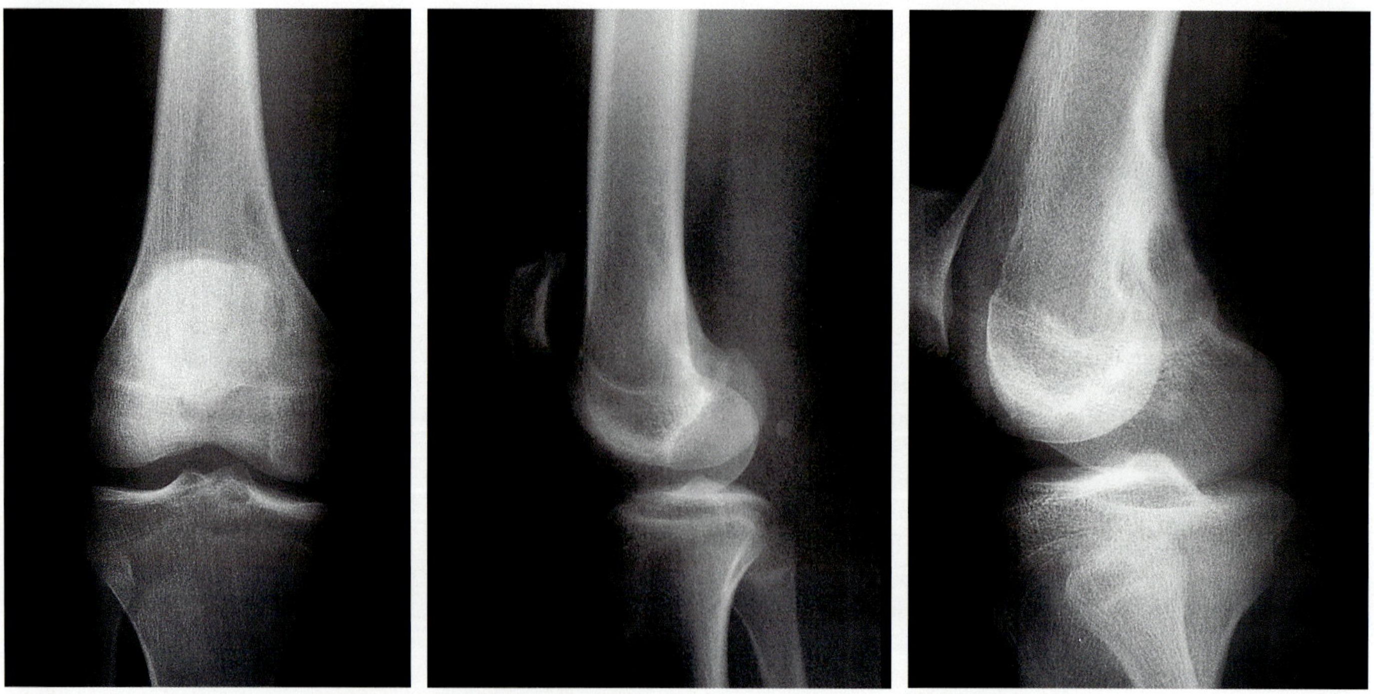

A B C

FIGURE 5.6 Avulsive cortical irregularity. Anteroposterior **(A)** and lateral **(B)** radiographs of the knee show a subtle area of mixed sclerosis and lucency in the posteromedial aspect of the distal femur. An external oblique radiograph of the knee **(C)** shows the obvious lesion in the posteromedial cortex of the femur with irregular periosteal new bone production overlying the lesion.

tissue desmoid tumor. The age at diagnosis ranges from 1 to 70 years; however, most patients are diagnosed before age 30. There seems to be a slight male predominance. The most common anatomic site is the mandible. When involving the long bones, desmoplastic fibroma usually arises from the metaphysis or metadiaphysis of the femur, tibia, or humerus.[7] The most common presenting complaint is localized pain. Rare examples have been reported associated with Paget's disease and fibrous dysplasia.[8,9]

Radiographically, desmoplastic fibroma most commonly presents as an expansile, lytic, and lobulated lesion, sometimes described as having a "soap bubble" appearance, devoid of matrix production (Fig. 5.7). Periosteal reaction usually is not seen, and the margin is sharply defined with occasional sclerosis. Less commonly, more obvious bone destruction associated with soft tissue extension may simulate a malignancy.[10]

Pathologic Findings

Histology

The morphology of desmoplastic fibroma is identical to that of fibromatosis (desmoid) of deep soft tissue. Characteristic microscopic features include sweeping fascicles of uniform-appearing spindle cells within a variably collagenized stroma. Although the tumor usually is relatively hypocellular, occasional foci of hypercellularity may be present. The stromal collagen ranges from thin, wavy fibers to thickened, keloid-like bundles (Fig. 5.8). In areas of absent or sparse collagen production, myxoid changes also may be apparent.[7] Individual spindle cells exhibit slender-to-elongated, monotonous nuclei and inconspicuous nucleoli. Significant nuclear pleomorphism is not observed. Mitotic activity tends to be rare. Sections from

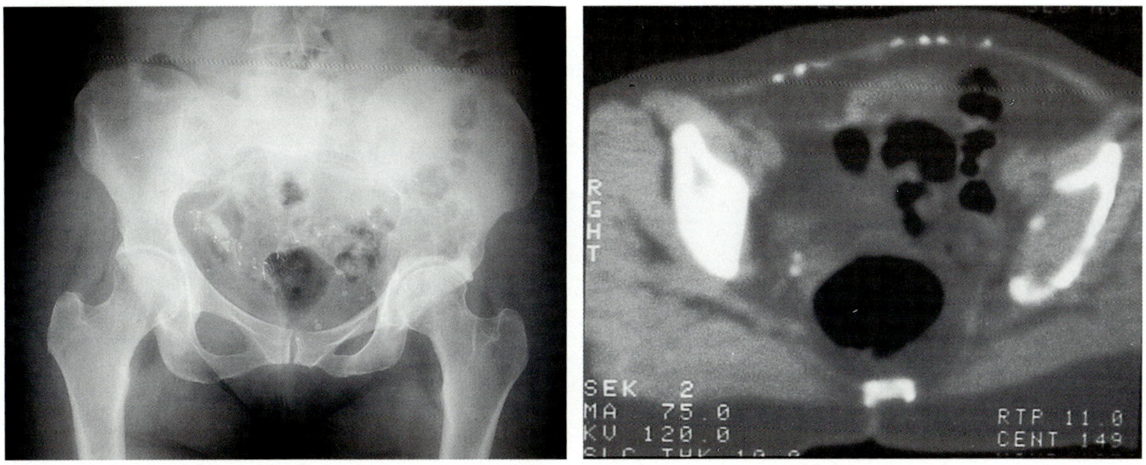

A B

FIGURE 5.7 Desmoplastic fibroma. An anteroposterior radiograph of the pelvis shows an extensive, destructive lesion in the left ilium. The supra-acetabulum portion of the ilium and the medial ilium extending to the sacroiliac joint are destroyed **(A)**. An axial computed tomography scan shows the destructive lesion in the left ilium with dissolution of the medial margin of the pelvis **(B)**.

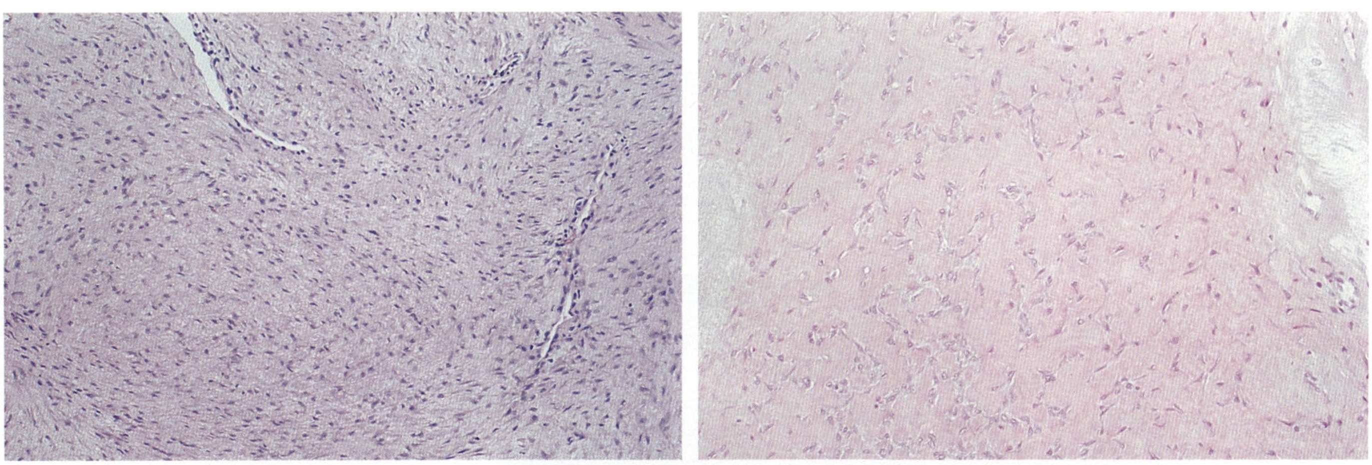

A B

FIGURE 5.8 Most cases of desmoplastic fibroma are indistinguishable from soft tissue desmoid, being moderately cellular and composed of sweeping fascicles of mostly uniform-appearing tumor cells within a variably collagenous stroma **(A)**. Less frequently, the stroma may appear more hyalinized or exhibit focal myxoid changes **(B)**. (**A** and **B**, H&E.)

the periphery of the tumor may reveal permeation of existing bone trabeculae with extension into surrounding soft tissue.

Ancillary Studies

Immunohistochemically, desmoplastic fibromas are diffusely positive for vimentin and show variable, weak immunoreactivity for actin and smooth muscle actin. Desmin and S-100 protein are usually negative.[10]

Prognosis and Therapy

Desmoplastic fibroma of bone should be regarded as a low-grade or borderline malignancy because of its tendency toward locally aggressive behavior but absence of metastatic potential. Recurrence rates after surgery approach 47%. For this reason, en bloc resection with a wide margin is generally recommended.[7,10] At present, there appears to be no role for radiation therapy or chemotherapy in the treatment of desmoplastic fibroma.

Myofibroma/Myofibromatosis

Myofibroma and *myofibromatosis* are terms referring to a similar entity that may be solitary (myofibroma) or multicentric (myofibromatosis). In bone, myofibroma/myofibromatosis also is called *congenital fibromatosis*.

Clinical Features

Myofibroma/myofibromatosis is a rare disease, most commonly observed in infancy and childhood. Age at diagnosis ranges from newborn to the elderly; however, most patients are less than 2 years old at presentation. Males are affected more commonly than females. It may present as a solitary subcutaneous nodule or multiple masses involving the skeleton and soft tissues with multiple visceral organ involvement.[11] Multicentric lesions are observed more often in children than in adults. Within soft tissues, myofibroma/myofibromatosis most commonly arises in the cutaneous and subcutaneous tissues of the head and neck region, followed by the trunk and proximal extremities.[11] Distal extremity involvement (e.g., hands or feet) does not usually occur. The craniofacial skeleton, specifically the skull followed by the mandible, is the most frequent site of osseous involvement (Fig. 5.9).[12] The multicentric form (myofibromatosis) may involve soft tissue, bone, and a variety of viscera, including the lungs, heart, and gastrointestinal tract. Patients generally present with cutaneous or subcutaneous lesions, usually described as mobile and painless.

Regardless of whether the lesion is solitary or multicentric, osseous forms typically present radiologically as a lucent lesion with or without a sclerotic rim.[12] Within the mandible, these lesions are lucent and sharply marginated but generally lack sclerosis. In the multicentric form (myofibromatosis), multiple, bilateral, and symmetric lesions are seen frequently in the metaphyses of the long bones. Often, as patients mature, the lesions spontaneously heal. Whether some of these lesions in the long bones represent concomitant metaphyseal fibrous defects is unclear. Extraskeletal soft tissue lesions may present on radiographs as focally calcified soft tissue masses.[11]

Pathologic Findings

Histology

Myofibroma/myofibromatosis characteristically shows pale-staining bundles, whorls, and nodules of smooth muscle–appearing cells alternating with fascicles of spindled fibroblast-like cells. Within the fascicular areas between the nodules and more centrally within the lesion are slit-like

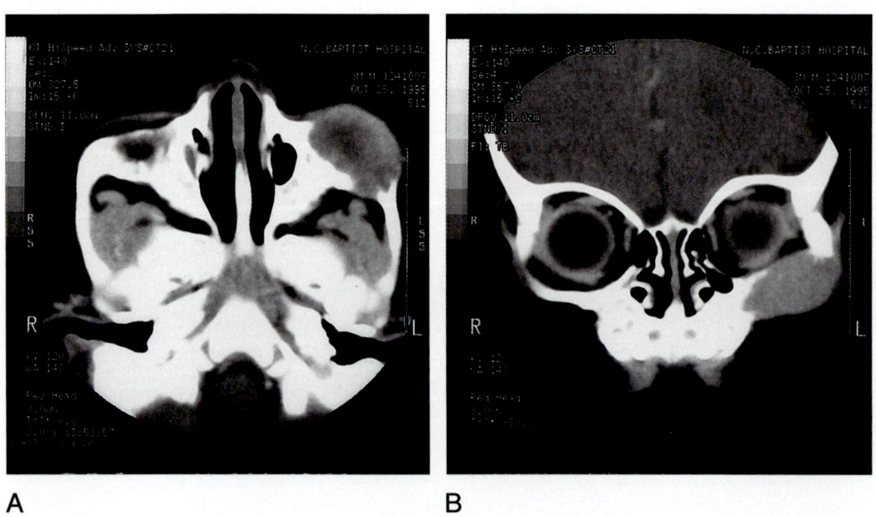

FIGURE 5.9 Infantile myofibroma/myofibromatosis. Axial **(A)** and coronal **(B)** computed tomography scans show a destructive, expansile lesion involving the inferior orbital rim and floor of the orbit on the left. No matrix calcification is present.

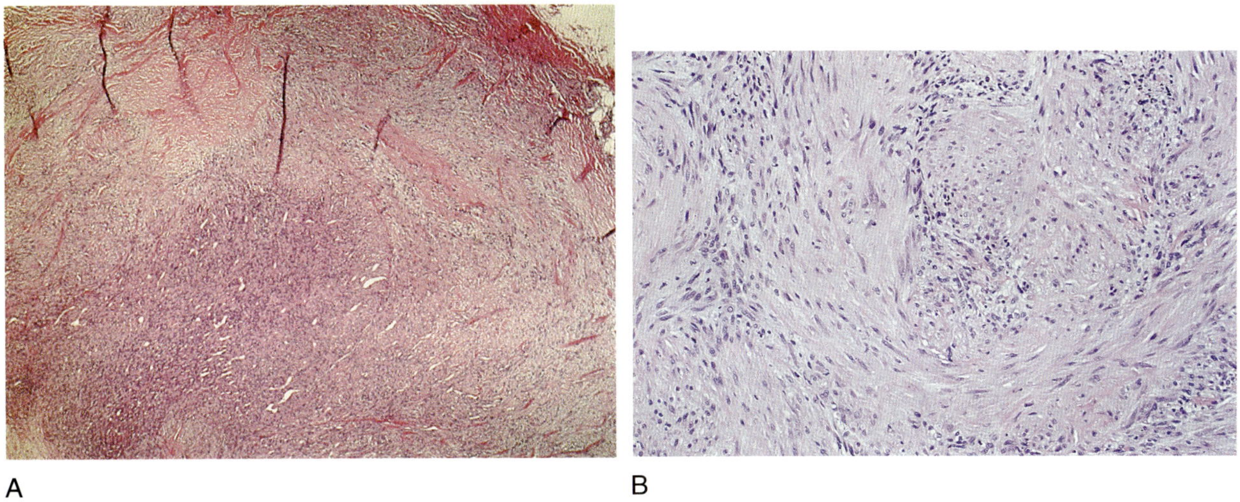

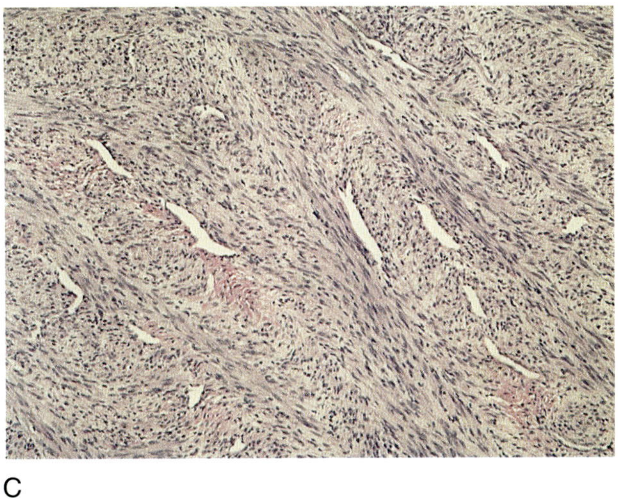

FIGURE 5.10 Infantile myofibroma/myofibromatosis characterized by pale-staining nodules and fascicles of bland-appearing tumor cells surrounding a more cellular central zone with a hemangiopericytoma-like vascular pattern **(A-C)**. **(A,** Low power, H&E; **B,** intermediate power, H&E; **C,** intermediate power, H&E.)

to staghorn-shaped vascular spaces, simulating hemangiopericytoma (Fig. 5.10). Infantile hemangiopericytoma and some adult forms are believed to represent a spectrum of myofibroma/myofibromatosis.[13,14] The background stroma usually appears loose and focally may show myxoid or chondroid changes. Occasionally, foci of necrosis or dystrophic calcifications also are apparent. Individual myofibroblasts appear mostly spindled with elongated, tapering, and uniform nuclei; one or more small nucleoli; and abundant tapering pink cytoplasm. Significant nuclear atypia is not present. Mitotic figures are usually not numerous, and atypical forms are never seen. Within the center of the lesion, where the hemangiopericytoma-like areas predominate, the cells often appear more primitive and round to polygonal but remain uniform. Intravascular growths may be observed but have no prognostic significance (Fig. 5.11).

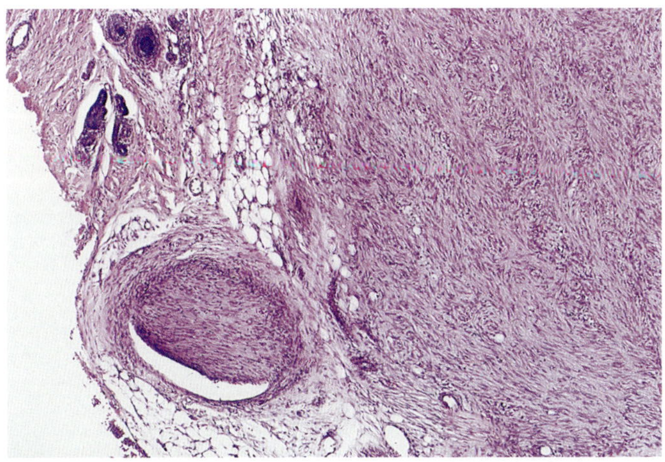

FIGURE 5.11 Infantile myofibroma/myofibromatosis rarely shows intravascular invasion. (H&E.)

Ancillary Studies

The ultrastructural features are generally nonspecific and include dilated rough endoplasmic reticulum, prominent Golgi apparatus, bundles of microfilaments with dense bodies, and focal basal lamina, suggesting myofibroblastic differentiation.[15]

Immunohistochemically, myofibroma/myofibromatosis usually expresses vimentin and smooth muscle actin but tends to be negative for S-100 protein, CD31, and epithelial membrane antigen. Rare positivity for keratin has been reported.[13]

Little is known about the cytogenetic features of myofibroma/myofibromatosis. Rare examples of familial occurrence with a possible autosomal dominant inheritance pattern have been observed.[16,17]

Prognosis and Therapy

In the solitary form of the disease, conservative surgical treatment with simple excision is recommended. Local recurrence is uncommon but almost always is cured by re-excision. When the diagnosis of myofibroma has been established, further studies should be performed to exclude multicentric (myofibromatosis) disease. Most patients do well, even in the presence of multiple bone and soft tissue lesions. Chung and Enzinger[11] reported 15 patients with multicentric involvement; 12 of these patients were alive and without active disease at last contact, and 5 of the 12 showed spontaneous regression. Patients with extensive visceral involvement have a significantly higher risk of disease progression and death; of the four patients in this study with extensive visceral involvement, three died shortly after birth.[11]

Fibrous Hamartoma of Infancy

Clinical Features

Fibrous hamartoma of infancy is rare but is seen more commonly than most of the other fibrous lesions of childhood. Table 5.2 lists the various fibrous lesions of infancy and childhood with their respective clinical features. Most patients with fibrous hamartomas are diagnosed before age 2 years. Boys are affected more commonly than girls. Most patients present with solitary lesions usually involving the anterior or posterior axillary folds. Other common locations include the upper arm, trunk, inguinal region, and external genitalia.[18,19] Involvement of the distal extremities (e.g., hands and feet) is extraordinarily rare. The most likely presentation is a rapidly growing, mobile cutaneous/subcutaneous mass. No familial tendency has been described.

Pathologic Findings

Histology

Fibrous hamartoma of infancy is a poorly circumscribed, superficial soft tissue lesion consisting of variable amounts of three distinct components—intersecting fibroblastic/myofibroblastic fascicles; loose, more primitive-appearing mesenchymal cells within a myxoid matrix; and adipose tissue. The fibroblastic fascicles resemble fibromatosis and often contain abundant collagen. Conversely the more primitive-appearing areas are arranged in nests and islands consisting of a more rounded but uniform cell population. Adipose tissue is interspersed between both components (Fig. 5.12).[19] In older lesions, significant amounts of sclerosis may be present, replacing large portions of the lesion. Rarely, fibrous hamartoma may show infiltration of skeletal muscle. Significant nuclear atypia is absent; mitotic figures are scant.

Ancillary Studies

Ultrastructural features of fibrous hamartoma of infancy are those of fibroblastic/myofibroblastic differentiation. The cells within the dense, fascicular areas exhibit dilated rough

TABLE 5.2 Clinical Features of Fibroblastic/Myofibroblastic Soft Tissue Tumors of Infancy and Childhood

	Peak Age	Congenital*	Gender	Location†	Regression‡
Myofibroma/myofibromatosis	<2	+	M>F	Head and neck, trunk, proximal extremities	+
Fibrous hamartoma of infancy	<2	+	M>F	Axilla, upper arm, trunk	–
Fibromatosis colli	<1	+	M=F	Sternocleidomastoid	+
Infantile digital fibromatosis	<1	+	M=F	Dorsal digits, spares first digits of hands and feet	+
Infantile fibromatosis	<8	+	M=F	Head and neck, proximal extremities	–
Infantile fibrosarcoma	<2	+	M>F	Extremities, trunk, head, neck	+
Calcifying aponeurotic fibroma	8-15	–	M>F	Palms, soles, wrists, ankles	–
Giant cell fibroblastoma	<5	–	M>F	Trunk, extremities	–
Inflammatory myofibroblastic tumor	<15	–	F>M	Intra-abdominal/retroperitoneum, head and neck	–
Angiomatoid MFH	<20	–	F>M	Extremities, trunk, head, neck	–

*May be present at birth.
†Common anatomic locations in decreasing order of frequency.
‡Refers to whether spontaneous regression of the lesion occurs.
MFH, malignant fibrous histiocytoma.

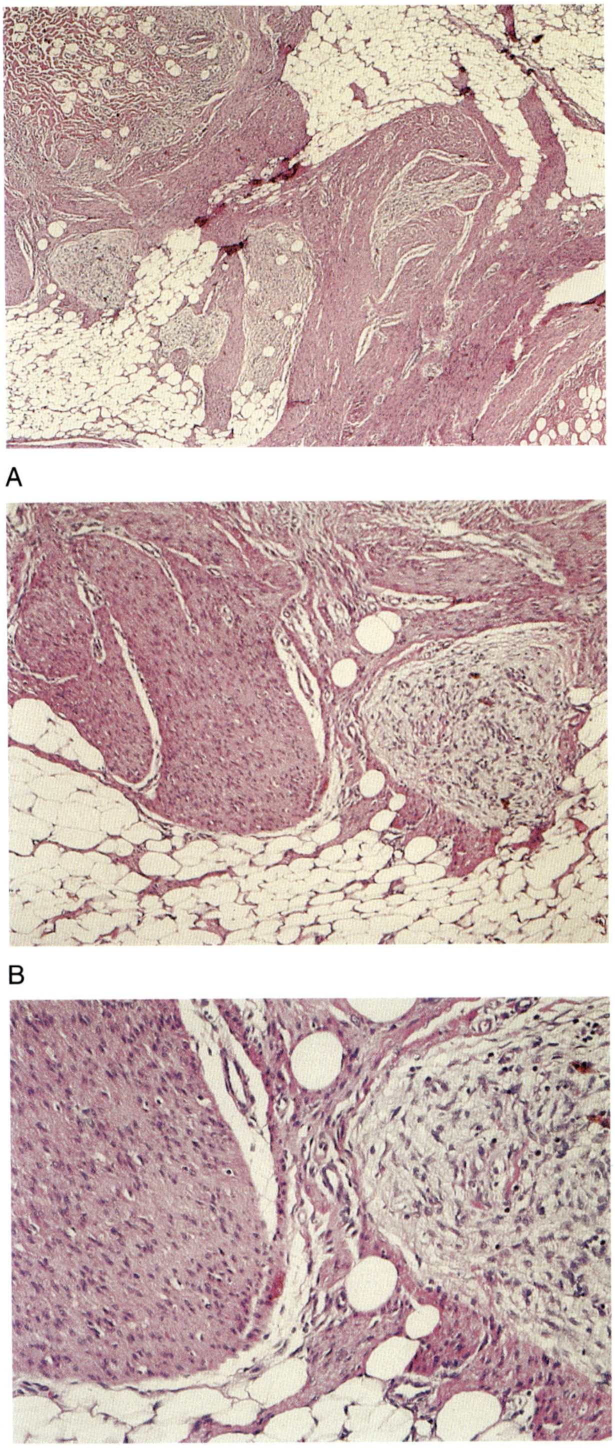

A

B

C

FIGURE 5.12 Fibrous hamartoma is defined as having varying amounts of three components—dense fibrous trabeculae resembling fibromatosis, more primitive-appearing myxoid nodules, and interspersed mature adipose tissue. Cytologic atypia is not a feature of any of the components **(A-C)**. (**A,** Low power, H&E; **B,** intermediate power, H&E; **C,** high power, H&E.)

endoplasmic reticulum, prominent Golgi apparatus, filaments with dense bodies, and close association with collagen.[20,21] The more primitive-appearing cells are largely undifferentiated, characterized by slender cytoplasmic processes and few intracytoplasmic organelles.

Immunohistochemically, fibrous hamartoma shows positivity for vimentin and variable reactivity for actin and desmin, mostly in the trabecular, fibromatosis-like areas.[22] The myxoid islands of primitive-appearing cells generally express only vimentin. S-100 protein is positive in the adipose tissue component.

Prognosis and Therapy

Fibrous hamartoma of infancy is a benign lesion that almost always is cured by local excision. Rarely, local recurrence occurs but is curable by re-excision. Spontaneous regression has not been reported.

Fibromatosis Colli

Clinical Features

Fibromatosis colli, also called *congenital muscular torticollis* and *sternocleidomastoid tumor of infancy,* is a rare but benign lesion arising in the distal sternocleidomastoid muscle of infants. Males and females are affected equally. Additionally, there seems to be an association with the development of fibromatosis colli and abnormal intrauterine positioning and difficulties in obstetric delivery.[23] Fibromatosis colli exclusively affects the distal third of the sternocleidomastoid muscle, resulting in asymmetric soft tissue swelling, shortening of the muscle, and torticollis.

Pathologic Findings

Histology

Fibromatosis colli is characterized by a diffuse, hypocellular, scar-like fibroblastic proliferation that appears to expand and to separate individual skeletal muscle fibers, many of which show degenerative changes. The background stroma is variably collagenous (Fig. 5.13). Individual cells appear uniform with ovoid-to-spindled, bland-appearing nuclei and abundant tapering cytoplasm. Significant nuclear atypia is not observed; mitotic activity is rarely present.

Fine Needle Aspiration Biopsy

Because of its classic clinical presentation, the diagnosis of fibromatosis colli may be rendered easily by FNAB, obviating the need for surgical biopsy. Cytologic smears generally are moderately cellular with aggregates and solitary, uniform-appearing fibroblasts/myofibroblasts with ovoid-to-spindled nuclei, inconspicuous-to-small nucleoli, and tapering cytoplasm.[24] Multinucleated skeletal myocytes are typically present throughout the smear.

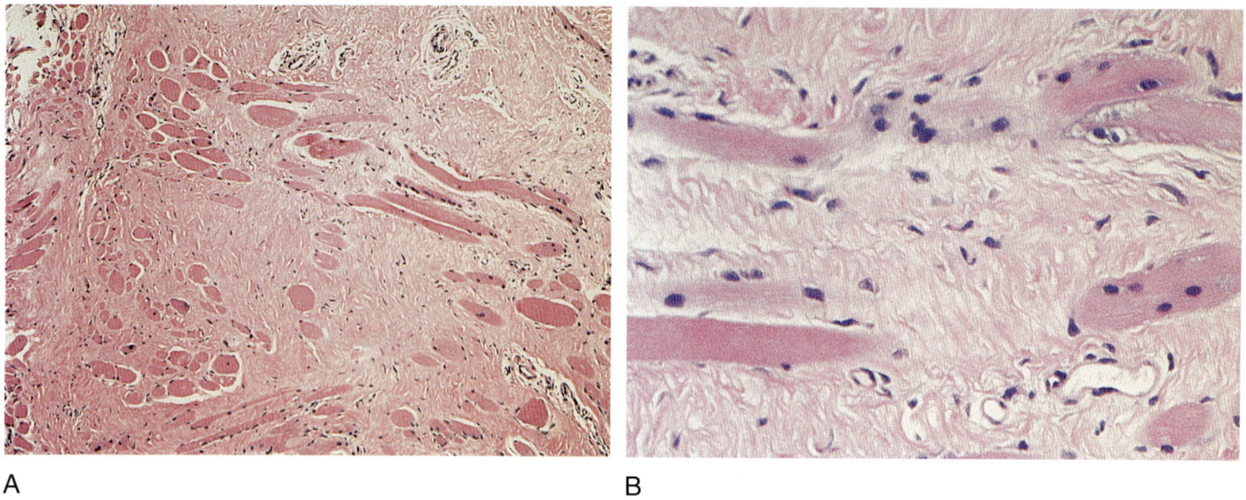

FIGURE 5.13 Fibromatosis colli with a hypocellular, scar-like fibrous proliferation infiltrating and separating muscle fibers, some of which show degenerative changes **(A** and **B)**. **(A,** Low power, H&E; **B,** high power, H&E.)

Ancillary Studies

Immunohistochemistry is usually not needed for the diagnosis of fibromatosis colli. Individual cells appear uniformly positive for vimentin and show variable actin expression.

Prognosis and Therapy

The early therapy for fibromatosis colli is principally not surgical and involves physical therapy and stretching. Complete resolution of the mass is the rule rather than the exception. Less commonly, surgical intervention may be required. Even among the latter group of patients, however, resolution and restoration of normal function generally is observed.[23] Favorable therapeutic results are achieved best in infants younger than age 1 year.

Infantile Digital Fibromatosis (Inclusion Body Fibromatosis)

Clinical Features

As the nomenclature implies, infantile digital fibromatosis almost always is observed in infants younger than 1 year old and arises on the dorsal aspect of the digits of the hands and feet.[25,26] Boys and girls are affected equally. Infantile digital fibromatosis also has been reported in older patients and involving extradigital sites.[27,28] Most are solitary, producing dome-shaped soft tissue swellings overlying the distal or middle phalanges or both. For reasons that are unclear, the thumb and great toe almost always are spared. Infrequently the lesions may be multiple, affecting one or more digits of the same hand or foot. Presenting complaints include functional impairment, soft tissue swelling, and pain.

Pathologic Findings

Histology

Infantile digital fibromatosis is a cutaneous lesion, composed of intradermal fascicles of uniform-appearing fibroblasts with a densely collagenized stroma, closely resembling adult desmoid tumor. The overlying epidermis is intact, with generally only slight hyperkeratosis. Overall the lesion is poorly circumscribed and frequently extends into and around dermal appendages and may involve subcutaneous adipose tissue. Individual tumor cells have ovoid-to-elongated nuclei, inconspicuous-to-small nucleoli, and tapering cytoplasm. The most characteristic feature of infantile digital fibromatosis is the presence of intracytoplasmic spherical and eosinophilic perinuclear inclusions (Fig. 5.14).[25,28,29] These inclusions may be difficult to demonstrate because they are not distributed uniformly and only present in a few cells. Special stains, especially the Masson trichrome stain, frequently highlight these inclusions, however.

Ancillary Studies

The ultrastructural features of infantile fibromatosis are those of fibroblasts/myofibroblasts with dilated rough endoplasmic reticulum and intracytoplasmic intermediate filaments.[25,29] The characteristic inclusions are adjacent to the nucleus but lie free within the cytoplasm. These inclusion bodies consist of granular and fibrillary material that is continuous with actin filaments.[25]

Immunohistochemically, infantile fibromatosis usually shows positivity for vimentin and less frequently reactivity for actin.[29] The eosinophilic inclusions appear variably actin positive, possibly depending on prior tissue preparation.

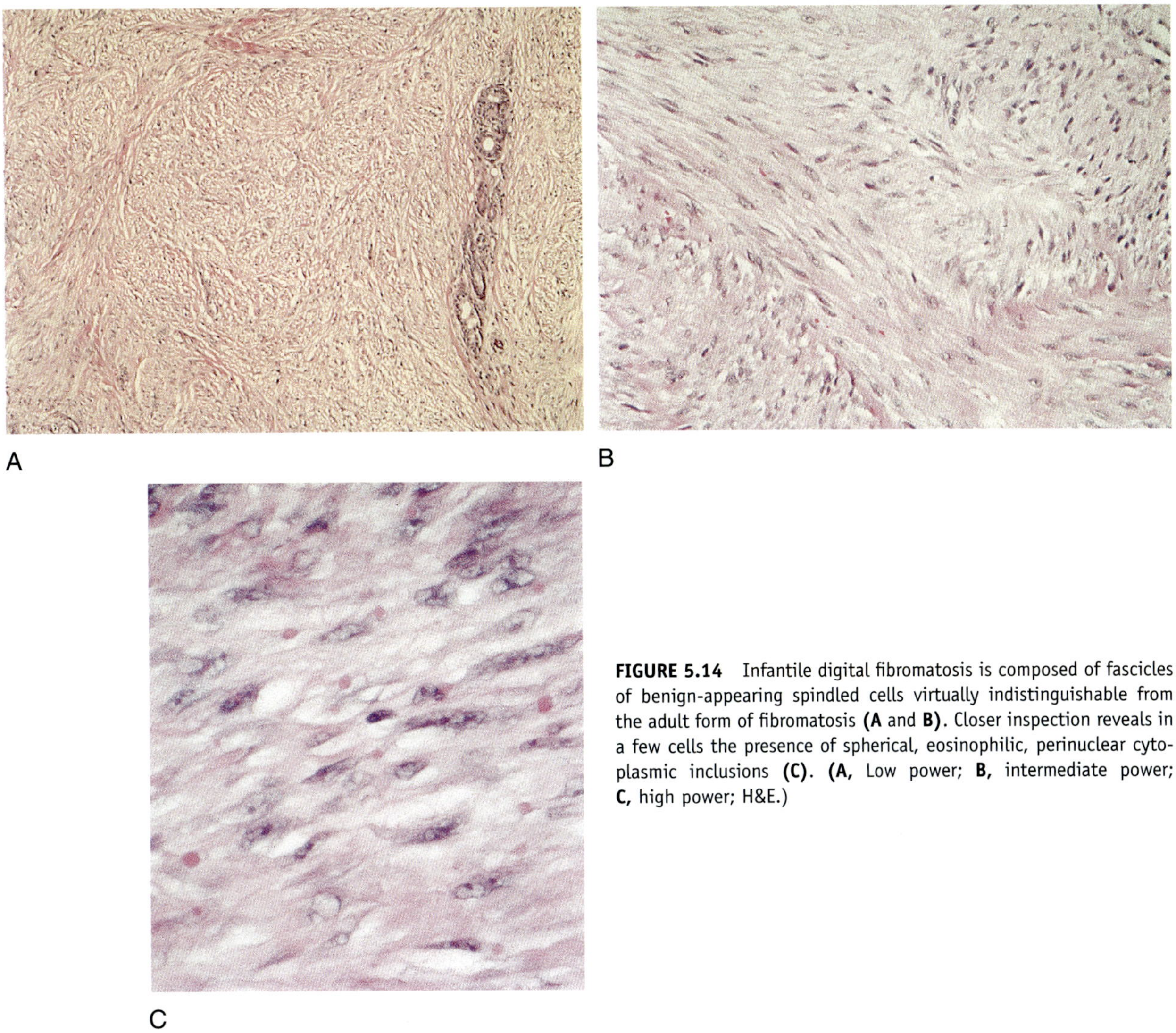

FIGURE 5.14 Infantile digital fibromatosis is composed of fascicles of benign-appearing spindled cells virtually indistinguishable from the adult form of fibromatosis **(A** and **B)**. Closer inspection reveals in a few cells the presence of spherical, eosinophilic, perinuclear cytoplasmic inclusions **(C)**. **(A,** Low power; **B,** intermediate power; **C,** high power; H&E.)

Prognosis and Therapy

Conservative surgical resection generally is recommended. Local recurrences are observed in 50% of cases, but more aggressive behavior or evidence of malignancy is lacking.[26] Spontaneous regression frequently occurs. The risk of local recurrence is related most strongly to the adequacy of the primary excision.

Infantile Fibromatosis

Clinical Features

Infantile fibromatosis usually is seen between birth and 10 years of age, with most patients younger than age 2 years. Boys and girls are affected roughly equally. Most patients present within painless, deeply seated, soft tissue masses of the head and neck region or proximal extremities.[30,31] Involvement of the hands or feet is extraordinarily rare, helping to distinguish it from infantile digital fibromatosis. A few patients report previous trauma to the affected area.[30] Similar to fibrous hamartoma of infancy, there seems to be no familial association.

Pathologic Findings

Histology

Infantile fibromatosis is an infiltrative, ill-defined lesion (Fig. 5.15). Compared with adult desmoid tumors, infantile fibromatosis exhibits a wide morphologic spectrum, reflecting varying degrees of differentiation. The diffuse mesenchymal form (cellular fibromatosis), occurring almost exclusively in infants, comprises uniformly round-to-ovoid, primitive-appearing cells markedly infiltrating individual skeletal muscle fibers and fat. The background stroma appears myxoid (Fig. 5.16). The desmoid or adult type is seen more often in children older than age 5 years and is indistinguishable from aggressive fibromatosis in adults (Fig. 5.17).[32] Sweeping fascicles of mostly uniform-appearing spindled cells are within a heavily collagenized stroma.

Ancillary Studies

The ultrastructural features of infantile fibromatosis show evidence of fibroblastic/myofibroblastic differentiation, including dilated rough endoplasmic reticulum, prominent Golgi apparatus, and abundant intermediate filaments. Immunohistochemistry is not usually helpful for the diagnosis of infantile fibromatosis. Vimentin is always positive, and variable immunoreactivity is observed with smooth muscle actin, actin, and desmin.[32] Although much of the data concern adult patients, cytogenetic analysis in childhood fibromatosis reveals a variety of chromosomal aberrations, the most common being gains of chromosomes 8 and 20.

Prognosis and Therapy

Local recurrence may occur in up to 65% of cases and seems correlated most strongly with the adequacy of the initial surgical resection.[30] Wide surgical resection with negative margins is the recommended therapy. Adjuvant radiation therapy or chemotherapy may be beneficial in some cases, but data are limited. Infantile fibromatosis does not metastasize.

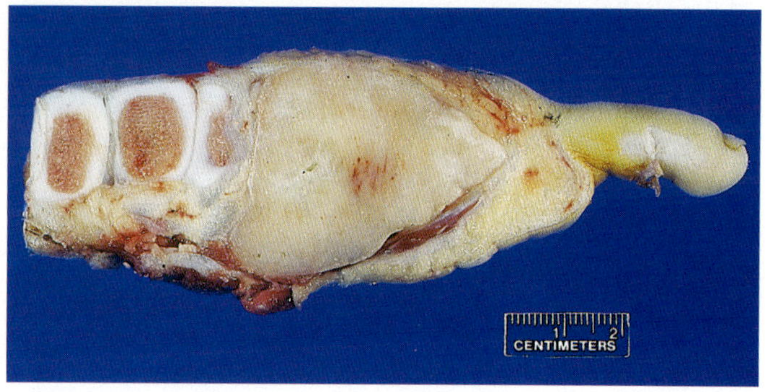

FIGURE 5.15 Infantile fibromatosis shows infiltration of the adjacent soft tissues surrounding the tarsal bones, ultimately leading to amputation.

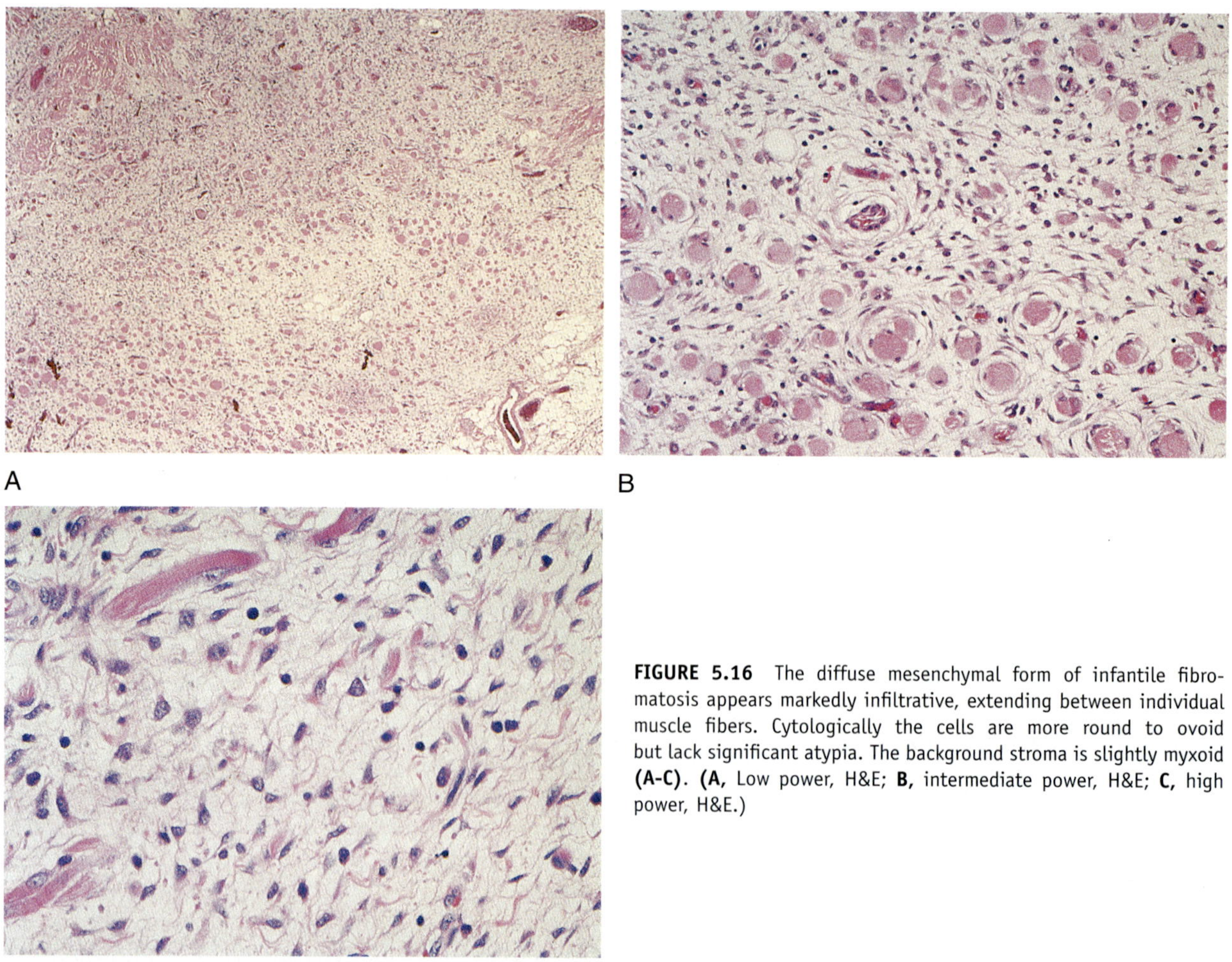

FIGURE 5.16 The diffuse mesenchymal form of infantile fibromatosis appears markedly infiltrative, extending between individual muscle fibers. Cytologically the cells are more round to ovoid but lack significant atypia. The background stroma is slightly myxoid **(A-C)**. (**A,** Low power, H&E; **B,** intermediate power, H&E; **C,** high power, H&E.)

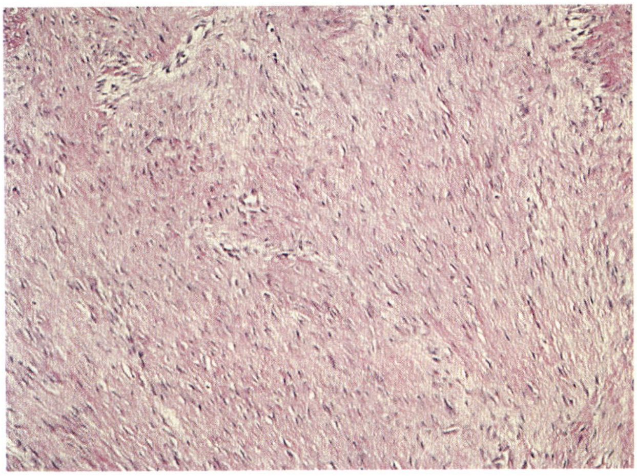

FIGURE 5.17 The adult form of infantile fibromatosis is composed of the typical features of desmoid tumor with sweeping fascicles of bland-appearing, spindle-shaped cells within a collagenized stroma. (H&E.)

Infantile Fibrosarcoma

Clinical Features

Infantile fibrosarcoma, also called *congenital fibrosarcoma* and *juvenile fibrosarcoma*, usually is diagnosed in infants and children younger than 2 years old. There seems to be a slight male predominance. The most common anatomic sites in decreasing order of frequency are the extremities, trunk, and head and neck regions.[33,34] Intra-abdominal and retroperitoneal forms are extraordinarily rare. Most patients present with rapidly growing but solitary soft tissue swelling. Congenital and infantile cases may be extraordinarily large, encompassing virtually an entire extremity.

Pathologic Findings

Histology

Infantile fibrosarcoma is a poorly circumscribed, infiltrative lesion that may resemble closely the adult form of fibrosarcoma. Characteristic histologic features include a cellular spindle cell proliferation composed of intersecting fascicles and bundles with the characteristic "herringbone" pattern and variable amounts of collagen deposition (Fig. 5.18). Dystrophic calcifications, necrosis, and hemorrhage may be observed.[33,34] Less commonly, infantile fibrosarcoma shows hemangiopericytoma-like areas and myxoid regions. Individual tumor cells usually are spindled with ovoid to spindle-shaped, hyperchromatic nuclei and variable amounts of tapering cytoplasm. Significant nuclear pleomorphism is not present. Mitotic figures may be numerous. Rarely, infantile fibrosarcoma may be composed of a predominantly round cell proliferation.

Ancillary Studies

Similar to most of the fibrous tumors of infancy, infantile fibrosarcoma shows ultrastructural features of fibroblastic and myofibroblastic differentiation with dilated rough endoplasmic reticulum, intracytoplasmic intermediate filaments, lysosomes, and focal basement membrane–like material.[35] Immunohistochemical features are relatively nonspecific and generally not helpful in establishing the diagnosis of infantile fibrosarcoma. Immunohistochemically, most cases show diffuse and strong positivity for vimentin and variable positivity for actin and smooth muscle actin. A few cases focally express desmin, S-100 protein, cytokeratin, and CD-34.[36,37]

Cytogenetic analysis reveals that most infantile fibrosarcomas show a t(12;15)(p13;q26) with the ETV6/NTRK3 fusion product.[36,38] Trisomies 8, 11, 17, and 20 are additional chromosomal aberrations often observed in infantile fibrosarcoma.

Prognosis and Therapy

Compared with adult fibrosarcoma, the prognosis in infantile fibrosarcoma is significantly better. Local recurrence rates after excision range up to 50%; however, distant metastasis is rare.[33,34] No morphologic or genetic factors predict the clinical outcome. Spontaneous regression has been reported.[39] Surgical resection with a wide margin generally is recommended, but more recent studies have shown some benefit from chemotherapy.[40]

Calcifying Aponeurotic Fibroma

Calcifying aponeurotic fibroma is an extraordinarily rare lesion. Although the age range is variable, most cases present in childhood and adolescence. Males are affected slightly more often than females. The most common anatomic locations are the soft tissues of the palms of the hands, wrists, soles of the feet, and ankles. Calcifying aponeurotic fibroma generally does not involve the digits. Less commonly, calcifying aponeurotic fibroma may involve the trunk and proximal extremities.[41,42] Most cases arise adjacent to tendons and fascia.

Patients typically present with slowly growing soft tissue masses that, by imaging studies, show calcifications. Morphologically, calcifying aponeurotic fibroma is a biphasic lesion, composed of a moderately cellular collagenous component resembling fibromatosis and nodules of dystrophic calcification surrounded by more rounded, histiocyte-like cells. The fibroblastic, desmoid-like component is infiltrative, accounting for the increased incidence of local recurrence. The stroma in the region of the calcified nodules ranges from hyalinized to focally chondroid. Individual cells of both components are typically uniform and lack significant nuclear atypia. Mitotic figures tend to be uncommon. With immunohistochemical

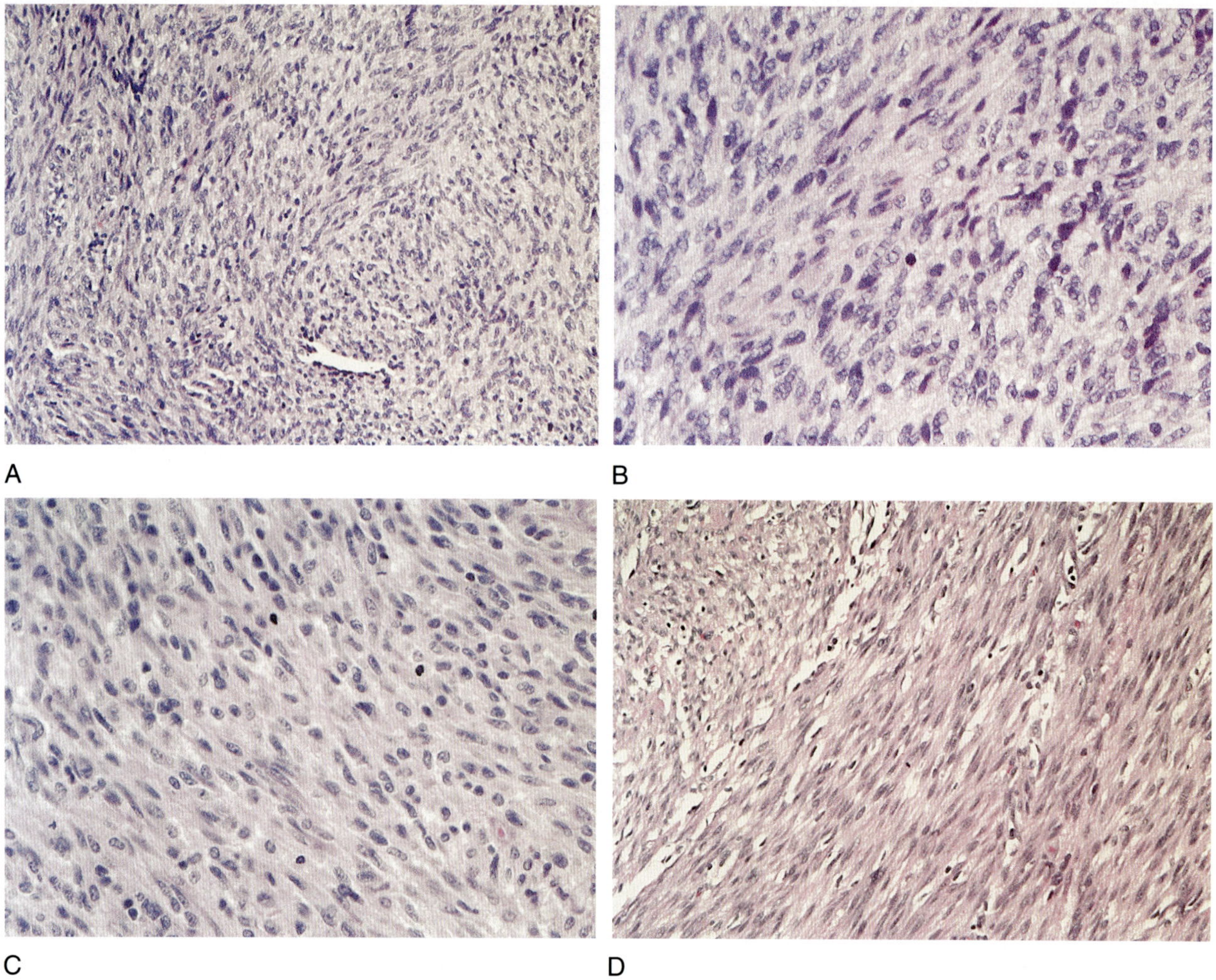

FIGURE 5.18 Infantile fibrosarcoma comprises sweeping and intersecting, cellular fascicles of mostly uniform-appearing, ovoid-to-spindled tumor cells. Significant nuclear pleomorphism is not a feature of infantile fibrosarcoma (A-C). Occasional examples may show more stromal collagen, but the degree of cellularity exceeds that typically observed in infantile fibromatosis (D). (A, Low power, H&E; B, high power, H&E; C, high power, H&E; D, low power, H&E.)

staining, most cases show positive expression for vimentin, actin, and smooth muscle actin. CD-99 and S-100 protein also may be expressed by the lesional cells.[41]

Conservative surgical resection with preservation of function is generally recommended. Local recurrence occurs in 50% of patients but is not generally destructive. The risk of local recurrence seems higher in young children (<5 years old) but does not appear related to anatomic location, pathologic features, or adequacy of surgical resection. Distant metastasis does not occur.

Giant Cell Fibroblastoma

Giant cell fibroblastoma, also called *juvenile dermatofibrosarcoma protuberans*, most likely is a rare histologic variant of the adult form of dermatofibrosarcoma protuberans. Morphologic, immunohistochemical, and cytogenetic studies have confirmed this association.[43–46]

Clinical Features

Although rarely occurring in adults, giant cell fibroblastoma most commonly arises in children younger than age 5 years.[43] Boys are affected more often than girls. Common anatomic locations include the trunk and inguinal region, followed by the extremities. Most patients present with painless, dermal or subcutaneous soft tissue swelling. The overlying skin is usually normal.

Pathologic Findings

Histology

Giant cell fibroblastoma forms an infiltrative lesion, extending into the dermis or subcutaneous tissues, entrapping adnexal structures. Cellularity ranges from hypocellular and myxoid/hyalinized to more cellular regions resembling dermatofibrosarcoma protuberans (Figs. 5.19 and 5.20).

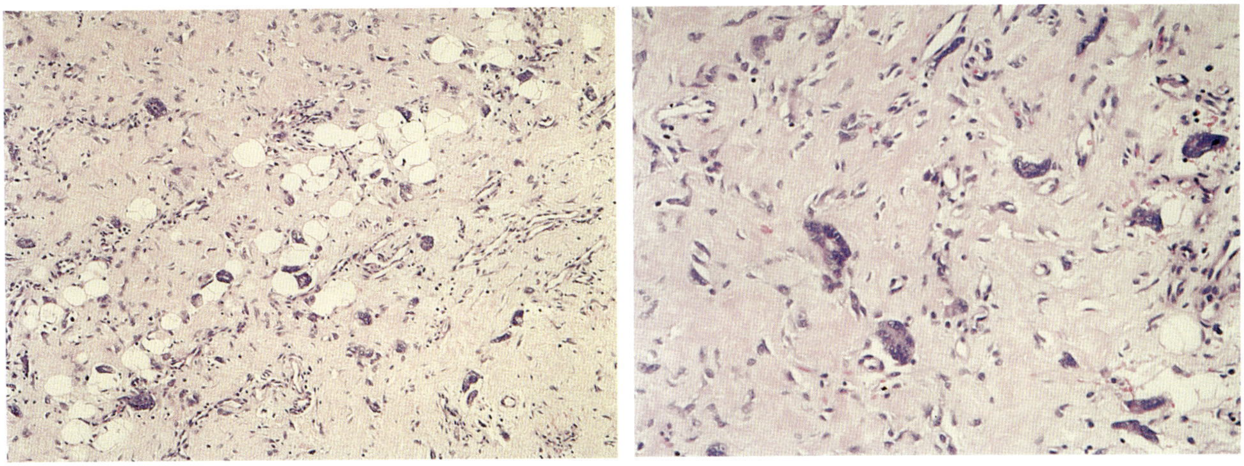

A B

FIGURE 5.19 Giant cell fibroblastoma arising from the ear of a 1-year-old boy (**A** and **B**). The histologic features are typical with scattered ovoid-to-spindle-shaped cells and giant cells within a myxohyalinized stroma. (**A** and **B**, H&E.)

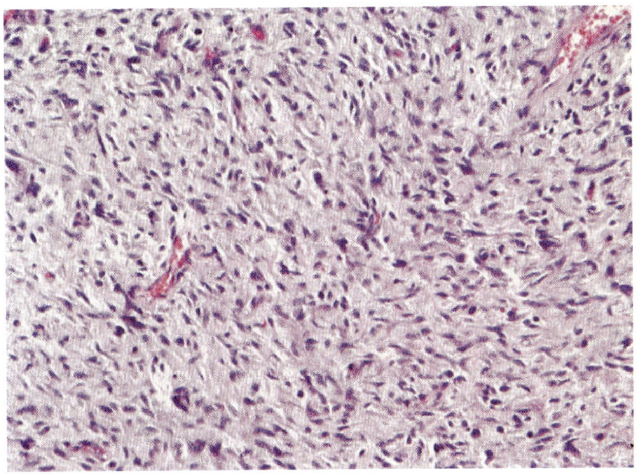

FIGURE 5.20 Occasional examples of giant cell fibroblastoma may appear more cellular, and the giant cells are less conspicuous. (H&E.)

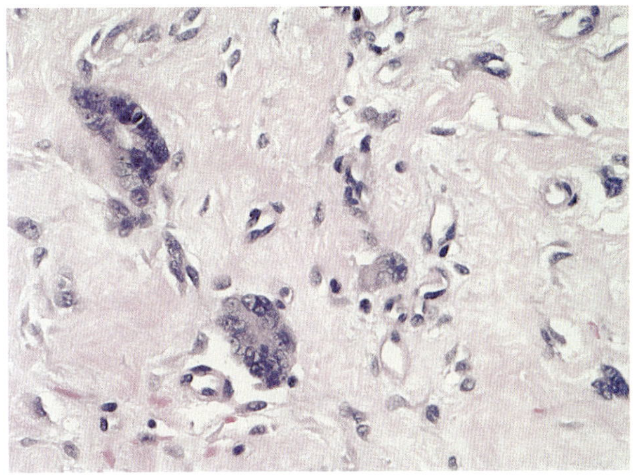

FIGURE 5.21 Closer inspection of the giant cells in giant cell fibroblastoma shows multilobated, overlapping nuclei often arranged in a floret-like pattern. (H&E.)

Most of the tumor cells appear uniform and spindled to stellate. The characteristic giant cells exhibit multilobated, hyperchromatic nuclei often arranged in a floret-like pattern (Fig. 5.21). These cells may be present anywhere within the lesion but have a predilection for angiectatic spaces, where they often form a discontinuous line along the surface (Fig. 5.22). Mitotic activity generally does not exceed one mitosis per 10 high-power fields. Transition forms between giant cell fibroblastoma and dermatofibrosarcoma protuberans are well documented; giant cell fibroblastoma may recur locally as a dermatofibrosarcoma protuberans (Fig. 5.23).[44]

Fine Needle Aspiration Biopsy

FNAB of giant cell fibroblastoma has been described only rarely.[47] Cytologic smears consist of mostly mononuclear, ovoid-to-stellate, bland-appearing cells arranged singly and in small clusters, occasionally associated with metachromatic stroma. Rare giant cells are seen.[47] Because of the distinctness of the latter, it may be possible, in contrast to the other fibrous lesions of childhood, to render a diagnosis of giant cell fibroblastoma by FNAB. Current data are too limited, however, to draw any specific conclusions.

Ancillary Studies

The ultrastructural features are essentially those of fibroblasts. The giant cells show nuclear segmentations and multilobations with multiple centrioles, suggesting that abnormalities of cellular division may lead to their development.[48]

Immunohistochemically the neoplastic cells are positive for vimentin and frequently express CD34.[44] Desmin, myoglobin, smooth muscle actin, S-100 protein, epithelial membrane antigen, and factor 8 are negative.[49,50] With cytogenetic

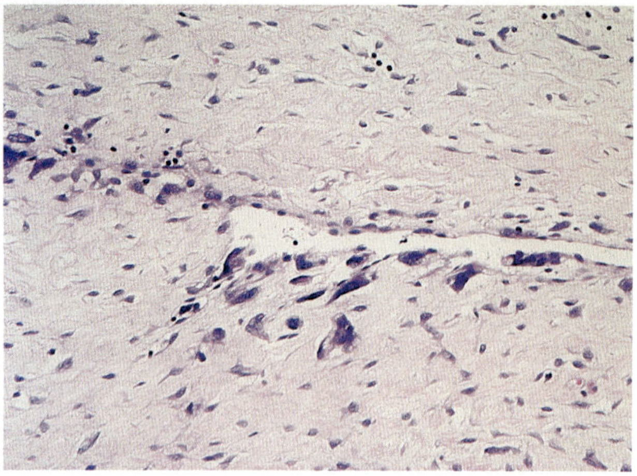

FIGURE 5.22 The giant cells in giant cell fibroblastoma frequently form a discontinuous layer along the surface of angiectatic spaces. (H&E.)

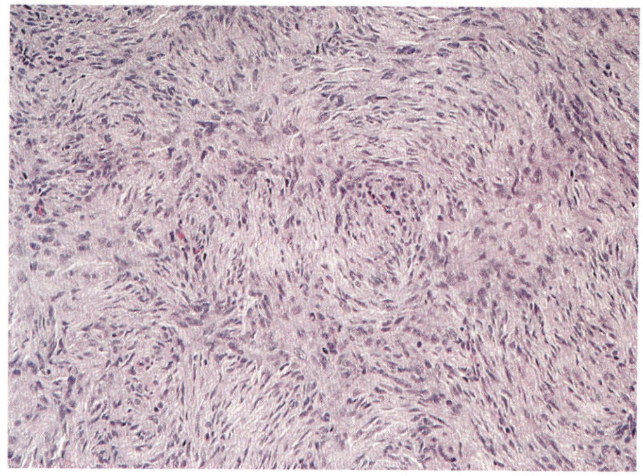

FIGURE 5.23 Same patient as in Figure 5.19. Approximately 6 years after excision of the giant cell fibroblastoma of the ear, the lesion locally recurred as a dermatofibrosarcoma protuberans, appearing highly cellular with spindled cells arranged in prominent storiform patterns. No evidence of residual giant cell fibroblastoma was observed. (H&E.)

analysis, dermatofibrosarcoma protuberans and giant cell fibroblastoma frequently show translocations of chromosomes 17 and 22 with the COL1A1/PDGFB fusion product.[45,46,50]

Prognosis and Therapy

Giant cell fibroblastoma should be considered a low-grade malignancy. Local recurrence occurs in 50% of cases, especially after marginal excision.[43,49] Wide excision almost always results in cure, however.[50] It is well known that giant cell fibroblastoma may recur locally as dermatofibrosarcoma protuberans and vice versa.[44] There are no histologic features predictive of prognosis. Wide surgical resection with negative margins is recommended. Metastasis has not been reported.

Inflammatory Myofibroblastic Tumor

In the past, inflammatory myofibroblastic tumor was known by a variety of designations, many of which have caused considerable confusion—*plasma cell granuloma, inflammatory pseudotumor, plasma cell pseudotumor,* and *inflammatory fibrosarcoma*.[51,52] Although it remains controversial, we believe that inflammatory myofibroblastic tumor and inflammatory fibrosarcoma represent a spectrum of a similar disease. Most of this discussion pertains to the extrapulmonary form.

Clinical Features

Although sometimes seen in adulthood, extrapulmonary inflammatory myofibroblastic tumor generally occurs in children and young adults (mean age, 10 years); this is in contrast to the pulmonary form, which is observed more commonly in midadulthood. Females are affected more commonly than males.[52] Overall, the most common anatomic site is the lung; frequent extrapulmonary sites include the mesentery, omentum, and intra-abdominal viscera and soft tissues. Less commonly, the head and neck region may be involved. As expected, the clinical symptoms vary depending on the anatomic site in which inflammatory myofibroblastic tumor arises. Primary lung inflammatory myofibroblastic tumor may be asymptomatic but often is associated with dyspnea and chest pain. Intra-abdominal tumors may present as soft tissue swelling, gastrointestinal obstruction, fever, or weight loss. Additional sequelae may include hematopoietic manifestations, including anemia and thrombocytosis.[52]

Pathologic Findings

Histology

Inflammatory myofibroblastic tumors typically are multinodular and circumscribed but rarely may be multicentric within the same anatomic region. Populations of mostly uniform-appearing, plump to spindle-shaped cells are arranged loosely within sheets and vague fascicles. The background stroma ranges from myxoid to collagenous and contains a variable mixture of lymphocytes, plasma cells, and eosinophils. Individual spindle cells show ovoid to slightly spindled vesicular nuclei, one or more small nucleoli, and variable amounts of cytoplasm (Fig. 5.24).[52] Occasional cells may resemble closely ganglion cells with large ovoid, vesicular nuclei; prominent nucleoli; and abundant basophilic cytoplasm (Fig. 5.25). Significant nuclear pleomorphism is generally not present. Mitotic activity may exceed 10 mitoses per 10 high-power fields, but atypical forms are never observed.

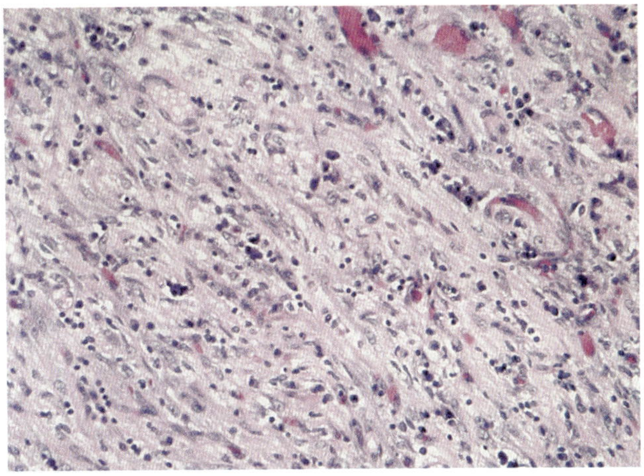

A

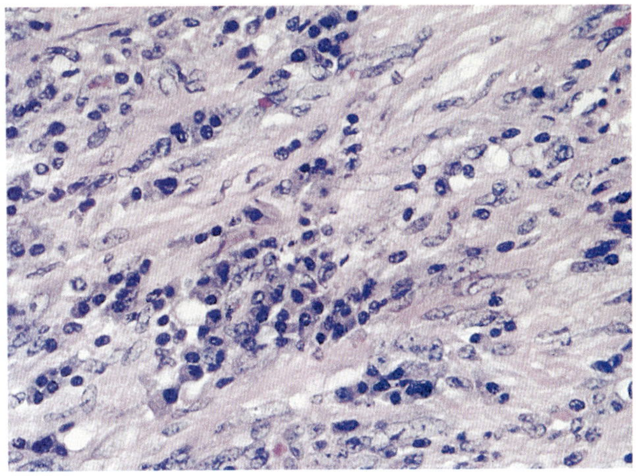

B

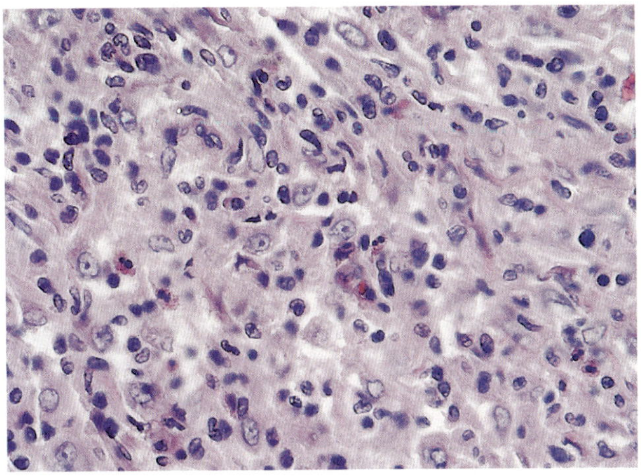

C

FIGURE 5.24 Inflammatory myofibroblastic tumor is characterized by a population of reactive-appearing fibroblasts with vesicular nuclei and prominent nucleoli, within a variably collagenous stroma and accompanied by randomly distributed but inconstant mixtures of lymphocytes, plasma cells, and eosinophils **(A-C)**. (**A,** Low power, H&E; **B,** high power, H&E; **C,** high power, H&E.)

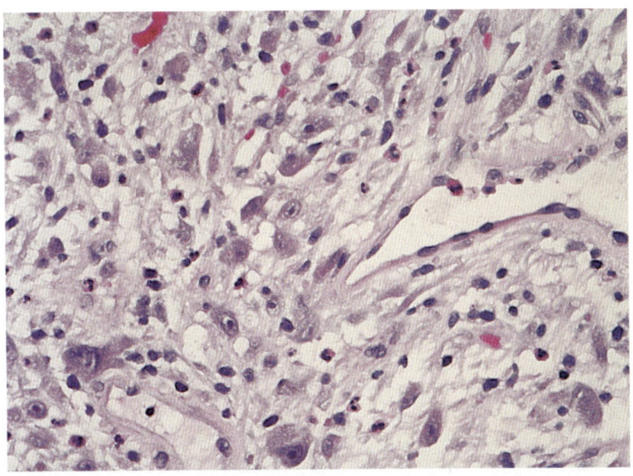

FIGURE 5.25 Less frequently, inflammatory myofibroblastic tumor reveals ganglion-like fibroblasts/myofibroblasts, sometimes mimicking Hodgkin's disease. (H&E.)

Ancillary Studies

Inflammatory myofibroblastic tumor shows ultrastructural features of fibroblastic/myofibroblastic differentiation with prominent rough endoplasmic reticulum, well-developed Golgi apparatus, intracytoplasmic filaments, and extracellular collagen deposition.[52] Immunohistochemically, inflammatory myofibroblastic tumors typically show positivity for vimentin, muscle-specific actin, and smooth muscle actin.[52] Desmin reactivity is observed less commonly. In one third of cases, focal cytokeratin positivity may be seen, potentially confounding the diagnosis.[52] CD117, S-100 protein, and myogenin are uniformly negative. ALK1 (anaplastic lymphoma kinase) cytoplasmic positivity is observed in one third of patients and is most common in tumors arising in children and young adults.[53,54]

Cytogenetic analysis of inflammatory myofibroblastic tumor has yielded variable results. Cases arising in children and adolescence, usually intra-abdominal or of pulmonary origin, often reveal chromosomal rearrangements involving band 2p23, specifically the *ALK* receptor tyrosine kinase gene.[54]

Prognosis and Therapy

The prognosis of patients with extrapulmonary inflammatory myofibroblastic tumor is generally worse than that observed with the pulmonary form. Local recurrence rates are 25% and seem related to anatomic location and resectability. No histologic features predict clinical outcome.[55] Surgical resection is the primary recommended form of therapy. Distant metastasis is seen rarely, likely occurring in less than 5% of cases.

Angiomatoid Malignant Fibrous Histiocytoma

Angiomatoid malignant fibrous histiocytoma has been renamed *angiomatoid fibrous histiocytoma* by the World Health Organization to reflect the rarity of distant metastases and death.

Clinical Features

Angiomatoid fibrous histiocytoma arises in children and young adults (mean age, 17 years).[56] Females are affected more often than males. The most common anatomic location is the subcutaneous tissues of the extremities, followed by the trunk and head and neck region.[56,57] Most patients present with superficial, slowly growing, painless soft tissue masses. Often the initial clinical impression is a cyst. Constitutional symptoms, including anemia and fever, are rarely observed.[56]

Pathologic Findings

Histology

Most angiomatoid fibrous histiocytomas appear circumscribed with a densely fibrous pseudocapsule associated with a variable lymphoplasmacytic infiltrate. In some cases, the latter contain prominent lymphoid follicles, simulating the appearance of a lymph node. Individual tumor cells are arranged in sheets, whorls, and ill-defined fascicles and appear spindled to round. In a few cases, significant nuclear pleomorphism with multinucleated tumor giant cells is observed (Fig. 5.26). Mitotic activity rarely exceeds five mitoses per 10 high-power fields.[56] Cystic areas with hemorrhage, occasionally accompanied by hemosiderin-laden macrophages, frequently occupy the central portion of the tumor (Fig. 5.27). These cysts are not lined by endothelial cells.

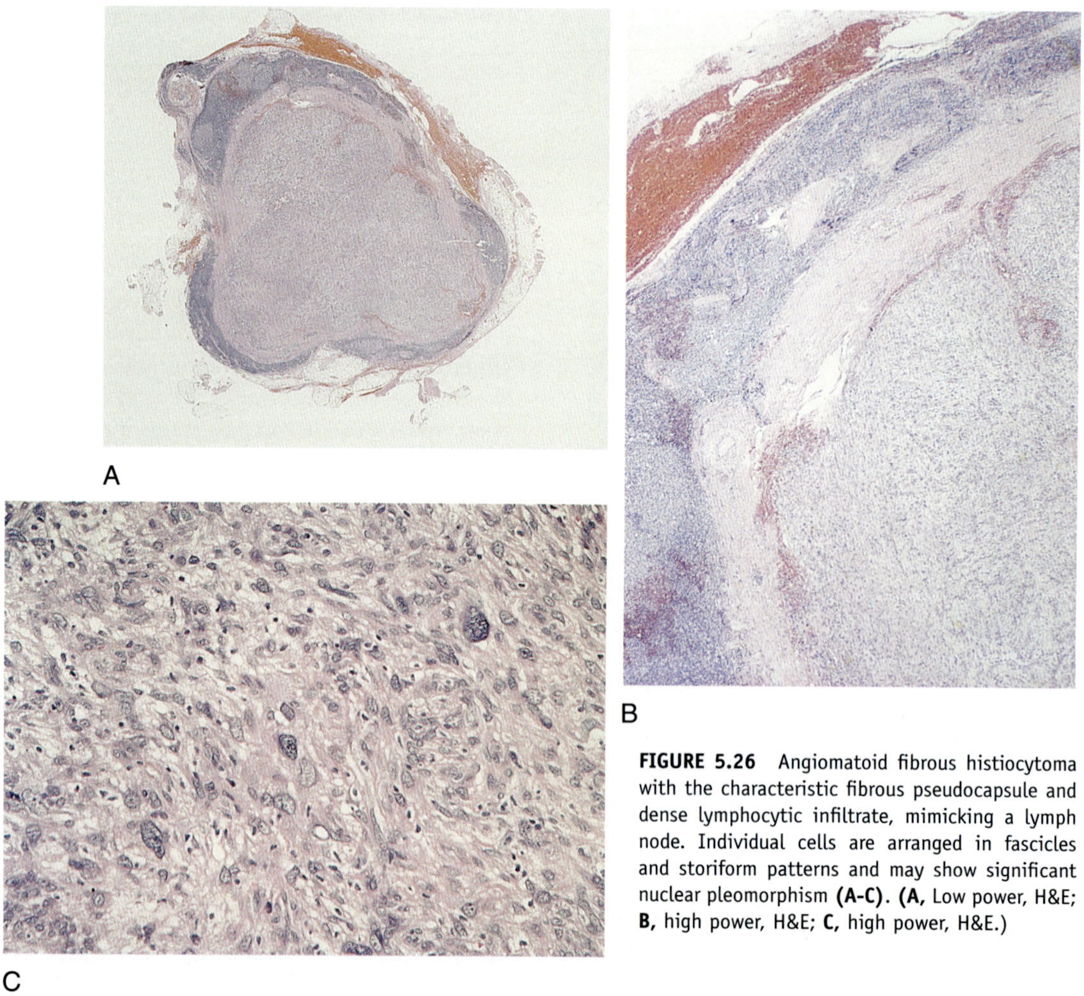

FIGURE 5.26 Angiomatoid fibrous histiocytoma with the characteristic fibrous pseudocapsule and dense lymphocytic infiltrate, mimicking a lymph node. Individual cells are arranged in fascicles and storiform patterns and may show significant nuclear pleomorphism **(A-C)**. **(A,** Low power, H&E; **B,** high power, H&E; **C,** high power, H&E.)

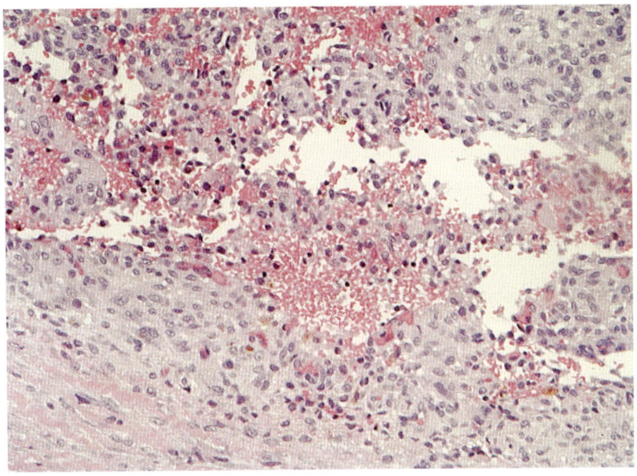

FIGURE 5.27 A characteristic feature of angiomatoid fibrous histiocytoma is the presence of hemorrhagic cystic areas often accompanied by hemosiderin pigment deposition. (H&E.)

Ancillary Studies

The ultrastructural features of angiomatoid fibrous histiocytoma show evidence of fibroblastic, histiocytic, and myofibroblastic differentiation, including cytoplasmic processes, intermediate filaments, and dense-core granules.[58] Angiomatoid fibrous histiocytoma is virtually always positive for vimentin and desmin, and CD99 positivity is seen in 50% of cases.[58,59] Smooth muscle actin and muscle-specific actin positivity are observed less frequently. Positivity for epithelial membrane antigen and synaptophysin has been reported.[58] MyoD1, myogenin, myoglobin, CD34, keratin, CD21, and CD35 are negative.

Cytogenetic analysis in a single case revealed a chromosomal translocation involving bands 12q13 and 16p11 with the FUS/ATF-1 fusion product.[60] We also have seen a consultation case (unpublished personal observations) with this same anomaly.

Prognosis and Therapy

Angiomatoid fibrous histiocytoma should be considered a low-grade or borderline malignancy. Long-term follow-up including more recent data indicates a local recurrence rate of 20% after excision and a metastatic rate of 1%. Increased risk of local recurrence is associated with deep subfascial/skeletal muscle origin, infiltrative margins, and localization to the head and neck.[56] Complete surgical resection with negative margins is recommended.

REFERENCES

Metaphyseal Fibrous Defect

1. Campanacci M, Laus M, Boriani S: Multiple non-ossifying fibromata with extraskeletal anomalies: A new syndrome? J Bone Joint Surg Br 1983;65:627.
2. Mirra JM, Gold RH, Rand F: Disseminated non-ossifying fibromas in association with cafe-au-lait spots (Jaffe-Campanacci syndrome). Clin Orthop 1982;168:192.
3. Arata MA, Peterson HA, Dahlin DC: Pathological fracture through non-ossifying fibromas: Review of the Mayo Clinic experience. J Bone Joint Surg Am 1981;63:980.

Avulsive Cortical Irregularity

4. Chadwick CJ: Tendinitis of the pectoralis major insertion with humeral lesions: A report of two cases. J Bone Joint Surg Br 1989;71:816.
5. Dunham WK, Marcus NW, Enneking WF, et al: Developmental defects of the distal femoral metaphysis. J Bone Joint Surg Am 1980;62:801.
6. Resnick D, Greenway G: Distal femoral cortical defects, irregularities, and excavations: A critical review of the literature with the addition of histologic and paleopathologic data. Radiology 1982;143:345.

Desmoplastic Fibroma

7. Inwards CY, Unni KK, Beabout JW, et al: Desmoplastic fibroma of bone. Cancer 1991;68:1978.
8. West R, Huvos AG, Lane JM: Desmoplastic fibroma of bone arising in fibrous dysplasia. Am J Clin Pathol 1983;79:630.
9. Hillman JS, Mesgarzadeh M, Tang CK, et al: Case report 481: Benign intraosseous fibroma (desmoplastic fibroma) associated with Paget's disease of the iliac bone. Skeletal Radiol 1988;17:356.
10. Bohm P, Krober S, Greschniok A, et al: Desmoplastic fibroma of the bone: A report of two patients, review of the literature, and therapeutic implications. Cancer 1996;78:1011.

Myofibroma/Myofibromatosis

11. Chung EB, Enzinger FM: Infantile myofibromatosis. Cancer 1981;48:1807.
12. Inwards CY, Unni KK, Beabout JW, et al: Solitary congenital fibromatosis (infantile myofibromatosis) of bone. Am J Surg Pathol 1991;15:935.
13. Mentzel T, Calonje E, Nascimento AG, et al: Infantile hemangiopericytoma versus infantile myofibromatosis: Study of a series suggesting a continuous spectrum of infantile myofibroblastic lesions. Am J Surg Pathol 1994;18:922.
14. Granter SR, Badizadegan K, Fletcher CDM: Myofibromatosis in adults, glomangiopericytoma, and myopericytoma: A spectrum of tumors showing perivascular myoid differentiation. Am J Surg Pathol 1998;22:513.
15. Hasegawa T, Hirose T, Seki K, et al: Solitary infantile myofibromatosis of bone: An immunohistochemical and ultrastructural study. Am J Surg Pathol 1993;17:308.
16. Venencie PY, Bigel P, Desgruelles C, et al: Infantile myofibromatosis: Report of two cases in one family. Br J Dermatol 1987;117:255.
17. Jennings TA, Duray PH, Collins FS, et al: Infantile myofibromatosis: Evidence for an autosomal dominant disorder. Am J Surg Pathol 1984;8:529.

Fibrous Hamartoma of Infancy

18. Dickey GE, Sotello-Avila C: Fibrous hamartoma of infancy: Current review. Pediatr Dev Pathol 1999;2:236.
19. Enzinger FM: Fibrous hamartoma of infancy. Cancer 1965;18:241.
20. Fletcher CDM, Powell G, Van Noorden S, et al: Fibrous hamartoma of infancy: A histochemical and immunohistochemical study. Histopathology 1988;12:65.
21. Greco MA, Schinella RA, Vuletin JC: Fibrous hamartoma of infancy: An ultrastructural study. Hum Pathol 1984;15:717.
22. Groisman G, Lichtig C: Fibrous hamartoma of infancy: An immunohistochemical and ultrastructural study. Hum Pathol 1991;22:914.

Fibromatosis Colli

23. Binder H, Eng GD, Gaiser JF, et al: Congenital muscular torticollis: Results of conservative management with long-term follow-up in 85 cases. Arch Phys Med Rehabil 1987;68:222.
24. Kurtycz DF, Logrono R, Hoerl HD, et al: Diagnosis of fibromatosis colli by fine needle aspiration. Diagn Cytopathol 2000;23:338.

Infantile Digital Fibromatosis

25. Hayashi T, Tsuda N, Chowbhury PR, et al: Infantile digital fibromatosis: A study of the development and regression of cytoplasmic inclusion bodies. Mod Pathol 1995;8:548.
26. Bekett JH, Jacobs AH: Recurring digital fibrous tumors of childhood: A review. Pediatrics 1977;59:401.
27. Pettinato G, Manivel JC, Gould EW, et al: Inclusion body fibromatosis of the breast: Two cases with immunohistochemical and ultrastructural findings. Am J Clin Pathol 1994;101:714.
28. Purdy LJ, Colby TV: Infantile digital fibromatosis occurring outside the digit. Am J Surg Pathol 1984;8:787.
29. Choi KC, Hashimoto K, Setoyama M, et al: Infantile digital fibromatosis: Immunohistochemical and electron microscopic studies. J Cutan Pathol 1990;17:225.

Infantile Fibromatosis

30. Faulkner LD, Hajdu SI, Kher U, et al: Pediatric desmoid tumor: Retrospective analysis of 63 cases. J Clin Oncol 1995;13:2813.
31. Ayala AG, Ro JY, Goepfert H, et al: Desmoid fibromatosis: A clinicopathologic study of 25 children. Semin Diagn Pathol 1986;3:138.
32. Weiss SW, Goldblum JR: Infantile fibromatosis. In: Weiss SW, Goldbloom JR (eds): Enzinger and Weiss's Soft Tissue Tumors, 4th ed. Philadelphia: Mosby, 2001, pp 371–376.

Infantile Fibrosarcoma

33. Chung EB, Enzinger FM: Infantile fibrosarcoma. Cancer 1976;38:729.
34. Coffin CM, Jaszcz W, O'Shea PA, et al: So-called congenital-infantile fibrosarcoma: Does it exist and what is it? Pediatr Pathol 1994;14:133.
35. Argyle JC, Tomlinson GE, Stewart D, et al: Ultrastructural, immunocytochemical, and cytogenetic characterization of a large congenital fibrosarcoma. Arch Pathol Lab Med 1992;116:972.
36. Sheng WQ, Hisaoka M, Okamoto S, et al: Congenital-infantile fibrosarcoma: A clinicopathologic study of 10 cases and molecular detection of the ETV6-NTRK3 fusion transcripts using paraffin-embedded tissues. Am J Clin Pathol 2001;115:348.
37. Variend S, Bax NM, van Gorp J: Are infantile myofibromatosis, congenital fibrosarcoma and congenital haemangiopericytoma histogenetically related? Histopathology 1995;26:57.
38. Bourgeois JM, Knezevich SR, Mathers JA, et al: Molecular detection of the ETV6-NTRK3 gene fusion differentiates congenital fibrosarcoma from other childhood spindle cell tumors. Am J Surg Pathol 2000;24:937.
39. Madden NP, Spicer RD, Allibone EB, et al: Spontaneous regression of neonatal fibrosarcoma. Br J Cancer 1992;18(suppl):S72.
40. Shetty AK, Yu LC, Gardner RV, et al: Role of chemotherapy in the treatment of infantile fibrosarcoma. Med Pediatr Oncol 1999;33:425.

Calcifying Aponeurotic Fibroma

41. Fetsch JF, Miettinen M: Calcifying aponeurotic fibroma: A clinicopathologic study of 22 cases arising in uncommon sites. Hum Pathol 1998;29:1504.
42. Murphy BA, Kilpatrick SE, Panella MJ, et al: Extra-acral calcifying aponeurotic fibroma: A distinctive case with 23-year follow-up. J Cutan Pathol 1996;23:369.

Giant Cell Fibroblastoma

43. Shmookler BM, Enzinger FM, Weiss SW: Giant cell fibroblastoma: A juvenile form of dermatofibrosarcoma protuberans. Cancer 1989;64:2154.
44. Harvell JD, Kilpatrick SE, White WL: Histogenetic relations between giant cell fibroblastoma and dermatofibrosarcoma protuberans: CD34 staining showing the spectrum and a simulator. Am J Dermatopathol 1998;20:339.
45. Dal Cin P, Polito P, Van Eyken P, et al: Anomalies of chromosomes 17 and 22 in giant cell fibroblastoma. Cancer Genet Cytogenet 1997;97:165.
46. Cin PD, Sciot R, de Wever I, et al: Cytogenetic and immunohistochemical evidence that giant cell fibroblastoma is related to dermatofibrosarcoma protuberans. Genes Chromosomes Cancer 1996;15:73.
47. Layfield LJ, Gopez EV: Fine-needle aspiration cytology of giant cell fibroblastoma: Case report and review of the literature. Diagn Cytopathol 2002;26:398.
48. Pinto A, Hwang WS, Wong AL, et al: Giant cell fibroblastoma in childhood: Immunohistochemical and ultrastructural study. Mod Pathol 1992;5:639.
49. Fletcher CD: Giant cell fibroblastoma of soft tissue: A clinicopathological and immunohistochemical study. Histopathology 1988;13:499.
50. Terrier-Lacombe MJ, Guillou L, Maire G, et al: Dermatofibrosarcoma protuberans, giant cell fibroblastoma, and hybrid lesions in children: Clinicopathologic analysis of 28 cases with molecular data: A study from the French Federation of Cancer Centers Sarcoma Group. Am J Surg Pathol 2003;27:27.

Inflammatory Myofibroblastic Tumor

51. Meis JM, Enzinger FM: Inflammatory fibrosarcoma of the mesentery and retroperitoneum. Am J Surg Pathol 1991;15:1146.
52. Coffin CM, Watterson J, Priest JR, et al: Extrapulmonary inflammatory myofibroblastic tumor (inflammatory pseudotumor): A clinicopathologic and immunohistochemical study of 84 cases. Am J Surg Pathol 1995;19:859.
53. Chan JKC, Cheuk W, Shimizu M: Anaplastic lymphoma kinase expression in inflammatory pseudotumors. Am J Surg Pathol 2001;25:761.
54. Coffin CM, Patel A, Perkins S, et al: ALK1 and p80 expression and chromosomal rearrangements involving 2p23 in inflammatory myofibroblastic tumor. Mod Pathol 2001;14:569.
55. Hussong JW, Brown M, Perkins S, et al: Comparison of DNA ploidy, histologic, and immunohistochemical findings with clinical outcome in inflammatory myofibroblastic tumors. Mod Pathol 1999;12:279.

Angiomatoid Malignant Fibrous Histiocytoma

56. Costa MJ, Weiss SW: Angiomatoid fibrous histiocytoma: A follow-up study of 108 cases with evaluation of possible histologic predictors of outcome. Am J Surg Pathol 1990;14:1126.
57. Fletcher CDM: Angiomatoid "malignant fibrous histiocytoma": An immunohistochemical study indicative of myoid differentiation. Hum Pathol 1991;22:563.
58. Hasegawa T, Seki K, Ono K, et al: Angiomatoid (malignant) fibrous histiocytoma: A peculiar low grade tumor showing immunophenotypic heterogeneity and ultrastructural variations. Pathol Int 2000;50:731.
59. Fanburg-Smith JC, Miettinen M: Angiomatoid "malignant" fibrous histiocytoma: A clinicopathologic study of 158 cases and further exploration of the myoid phenotype. Hum Pathol 1999;30:1336.
60. Waters BL, Panagopoulos I, Allen EF: Genetic characterization of angiomatoid fibrous histiocytoma identifies fusion of the FUS and ATF-1 genes induced by a chromosomal translocation involving bands 12q13 and 16p11. Cancer Genet Cytogenet 2000;121:109.

CHAPTER 6

Spindle Cell Tumors of Bone and Soft Tissue Occurring Predominantly in Adults

Spindle cell tumors that occur predominantly in adult patients encompass a large, broad group of tumors (Table 6.1). Synovial sarcoma may be included with this category of tumors, but we discuss it with the epithelioid/polygonal cell tumors in Chapter 4. Most adult spindle cell tumors show evidence of fibroblastic or myofibroblastic differentiation. This category of lesions also includes nerve sheath and smooth muscle tumors, however. Despite advances in immunohistochemistry and molecular genetics, the diagnosis of most of these tumors still depends largely on recognition of their specific clinical features and routine light microscopic findings. Immunohistochemistry can be misleading in these tumors. We have encountered several cases of nodular fasciitis initially misdiagnosed as leiomyosarcoma solely because of immunopositivity for smooth muscle actin. Immunohistochemistry should never be used as the sole criterion for separating fibroblastic and myofibroblastic lesions from smooth muscle tumors. In contrast to the small round cell tumors, reproducible diagnostic chromosomal aberrations and translocations have yet to be described for most adult spindle cell tumors.

TABLE 6.1 Spindle Cell Tumors of Bone and Soft Tissue Occurring Predominantly in Adults

Bone Origin	Soft Tissue Origin
Benign fibrous histiocytoma	Nodular fasciitis
Malignant fibrous histiocytoma	Proliferative fasciitis/myositis
Adult fibrosarcoma	Fibroma of tendon sheath
Schwannoma	Superficial and deep fibromatoses
Leiomyoma	Solitary fibrous tumor/hemangiopericytoma
Leiomyosarcoma	Elastofibroma
	Nuchal fibroma
	Benign fibrous histiocytoma
	Malignant fibrous histiocytoma
	Dermatofibrosarcoma protuberans
	Low-grade fibromyxoid sarcoma
	Adult fibrosarcoma
	Neurofibroma
	Schwannoma
	Malignant peripheral nerve sheath tumor
	Angioleiomyoma
	Leiomyoma
	Leiomyosarcoma
	Extraskeletal osteosarcoma

Fine needle aspiration biopsy (FNAB) is only marginally accurate for the histologic subtyping of spindle cell lesions. Our greatest successes have involved the cytologic diagnoses of nodular fasciitis and schwannoma. Because the diagnosis of many of these spindle cell tumors depends on a combination of architectural features and ancillary studies, it is doubtful that most can be diagnosed reliably and consistently by FNAB.

Nodular Fasciitis

Clinical Features

Nodular fasciitis is a relatively common soft tissue mass that occurs over a wide age range but predominantly affects adults 20 to 40 years old. There is no gender bias.[1,2] Most cases arise within deep dermis and subcutaneous adipose tissue and are less than 2 cm in greatest dimension. Less frequently, nodular fasciitis may arise within skeletal muscle; these lesions are often quite large, measuring up to 5 cm in greatest dimension. The most common anatomic location is the extremities, especially the forearm and arm, followed by the trunk and head and neck region. In children, nodular fasciitis is seen most commonly in the superficial soft tissues of the head and neck. Involvement of the hand or foot is rare.[1] Patients typically complain of a rapidly growing, painless superficial mass. Radiographic features of nodular fasciitis are nondistinct.

Intravascular fasciitis is a rare form of nodular fasciitis arising within small-to-medium, muscular-walled blood vessels. Cranial fasciitis is an extraordinarily rare form of nodular fasciitis predominantly occurring in infants, causing erosion of the outer table of the skull.[3] Radiographically, cranial fasciitis is seen as a soft tissue mass with a lytic cranial defect and an associated sclerotic rim. It is possible that some cases of cranial fasciitis may be the result of birth trauma.

Pathologic Findings

Histology

Nodular fasciitis characteristically forms a well-circumscribed but unencapsulated lesion (<2 cm) with minimally infiltrative margins, sometimes streaming into adjacent fat or skeletal muscle, simulating a sarcoma (Figs. 6.1 and 6.2). Histologically the lesion comprises proliferating but uniform-appearing, plump fibroblasts arranged loosely (e.g., tissue culture appearance) in short fascicles, bundles, and vague storiform patterns.[1] In places, the lesional tissue frequently appears to "tear apart," creating pseudocystic spaces (Fig. 6.3). The background stroma is variably collagenous (Fig. 6.4) but may be significantly myxoid, especially among cases arising in children (Fig. 6.5). Mitotic figures may be abundant but are never atypical. Lymphocytes, plasma cells, and histiocytes are variably scattered among the lesional cells, but the presence of neutrophils tends to be an unusual finding. Extravasated red blood cells and osteoclast-type giant cells also are identified frequently within nodular fasciitis (Fig. 6.6). Osseous metaplasia rarely is observed in nodular fasciitis and cranial fasciitis.[4]

Fine Needle Aspiration Biopsy

FNAB of nodular fasciitis typically yields hypercellular smears composed of mostly discohesive fibroblasts and myofibroblasts with occasional cellular clusters (Fig. 6.7). Individual cells range from spindled-to-stellate forms with mostly round-to-ovoid, uniform nuclei, surrounded by delicate-to-dense, tapering cytoplasm. Generally the nuclei are vesicular with an evenly distributed chromatin pattern and small-to-prominent nucleoli. A myxoid granular background film or clusters of cells intimately associated with metachromatic stroma often are observed in smears procured from relatively "young," actively growing lesions (Fig. 6.8). Background inflammatory cells, especially histiocytes and

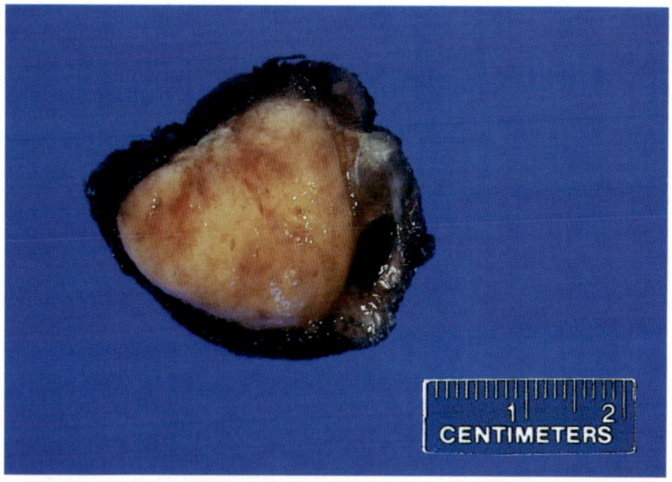

FIGURE 6.1 Intramuscular nodular fasciitis appears well circumscribed grossly.

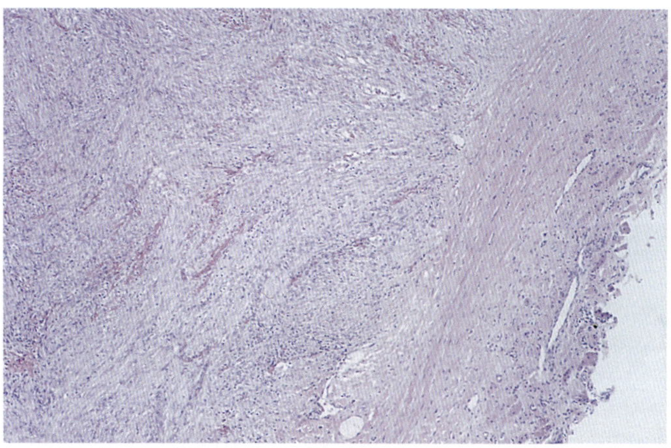

A

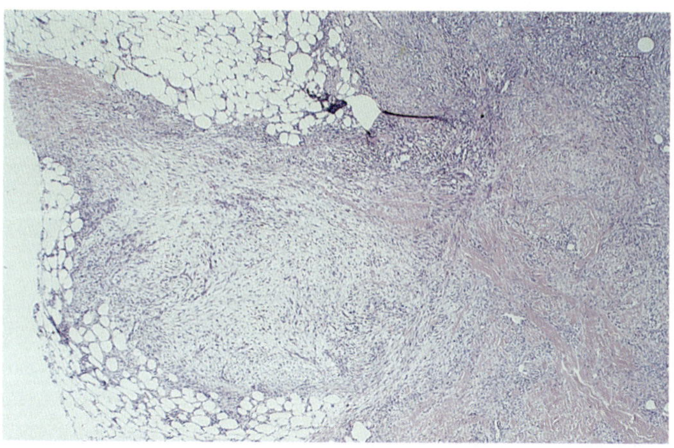

B

FIGURE 6.2 Nodular fasciitis usually appears well circumscribed but unencapsulated **(A)**. Occasional examples may show strands of infiltration peripherally **(B)**. **(A** and **B,** H&E.)

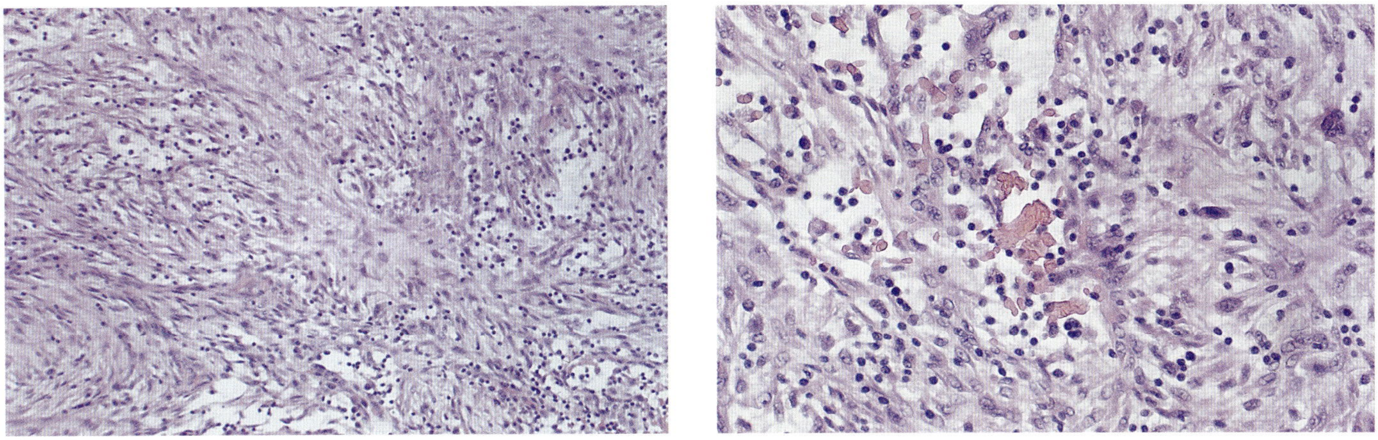

A B

FIGURE 6.3 Classic nodular fasciitis characterized by a loose proliferation of plump, reactive-appearing fibroblasts arranged in short fascicles and storiform patterns. Focally the tissue appears to tear apart. Extravasated erythrocytes and lymphocytes frequently are observed **(A** and **B)**. **(A,** Low power, H&E; **B,** high power, H&E.)

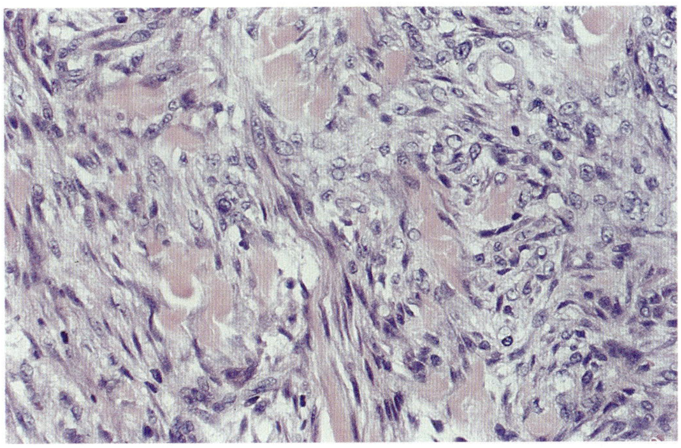

FIGURE 6.4 The background stroma of nodular fasciitis is variably collagenous, ranging from bundles of collagen to focally hyalinized areas. (H&E.)

lymphocytes, are seen frequently (Fig. 6.9). In the appropriate clinical setting, FNAB is diagnostic of nodular fasciitis.[5] Nevertheless, after an FNAB diagnosis of nodular fasciitis, we generally recommend close clinical follow-up and rebiopsy if the lesion continues to grow or fails to resolve in at least 2 months.

Ancillary Studies

Ultrastructurally, nodular fasciitis shows evidence of fibroblastic and myofibroblastic differentiation. Individual cells may contain intracytoplasmic intermediate filaments, dilated rough endoplasmic reticulum, and cellular junctions.

Similar to most myofibroblastic lesions, the cells of nodular fasciitis may show positivity for actin, smooth muscle actin, or

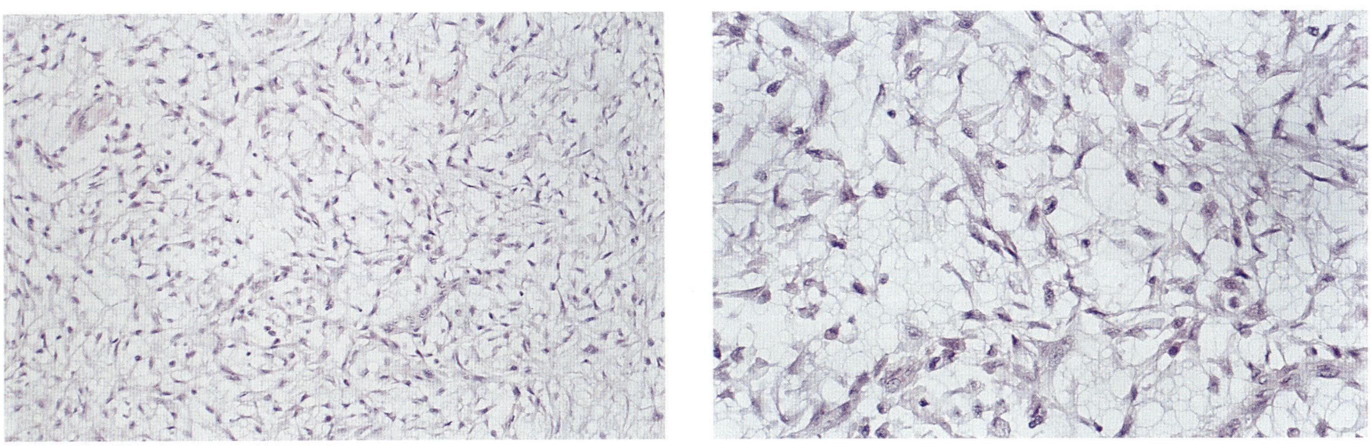

A B

FIGURE 6.5 Although the overall cytologic and histologic features remain the same, nodular fasciitis may be focally to diffusely myxoid, causing confusion with myxofibrosarcoma **(A** and **B)**. **(A,** Low power, H&E; **B,** high power, H&E.)

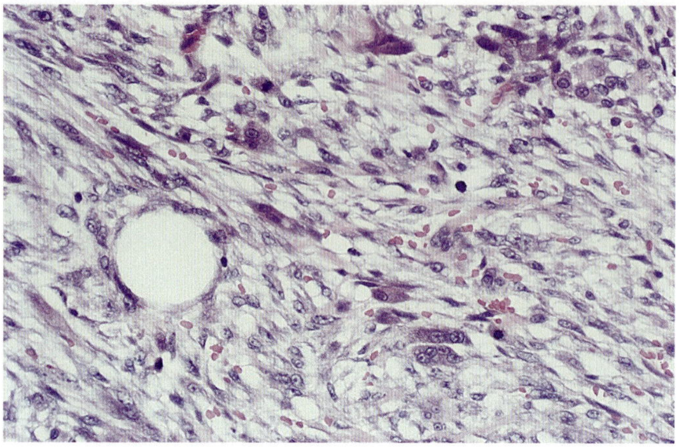

FIGURE 6.6 Nodular fasciitis frequently contains scattered osteoclast-type giant cells. Although mitotic figures are often present, they are never atypical. (H&E.)

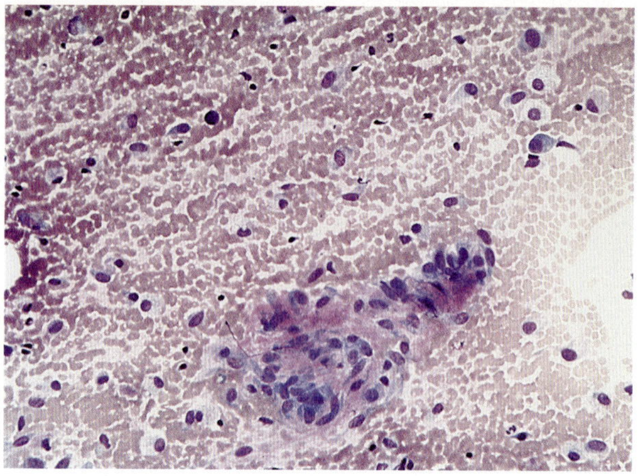

FIGURE 6.8 Cellular clusters of spindled cells surrounding metachromatic stromal material frequently are seen in the cytologic preparations of early nodular fasciitis. (Diff-Quik.)

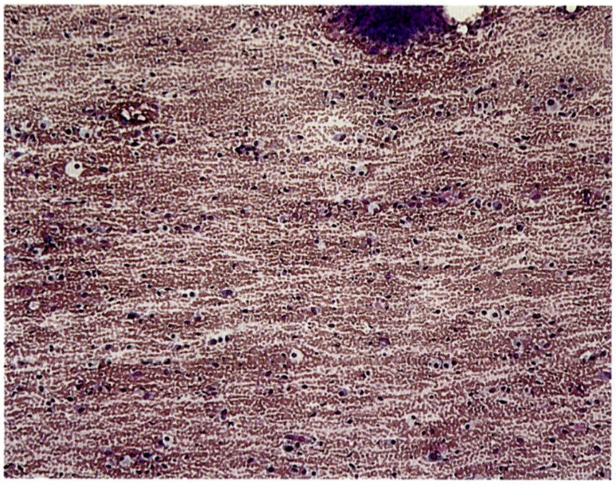

A

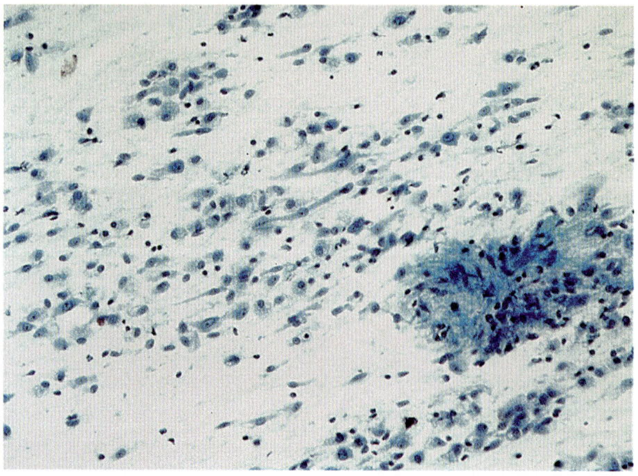

B

FIGURE 6.7 Fine needle aspiration biopsy of nodular fasciitis yields highly cellular smears of mostly discohesive, spindled cells with scattered cellular clusters **(A** and **B)**. **(A,** Diff-Quik; **B,** Papanicolaou.)

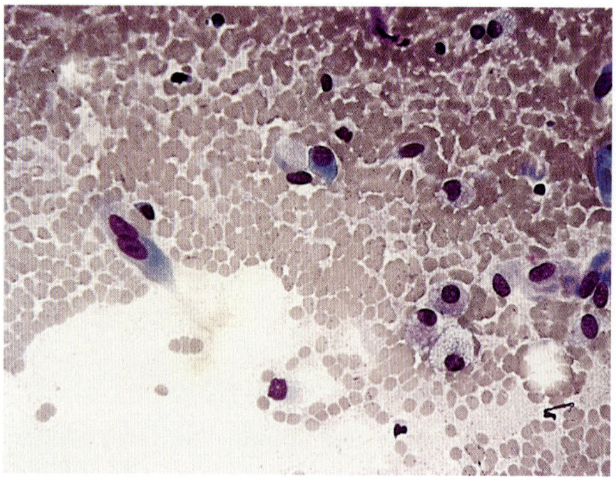

A

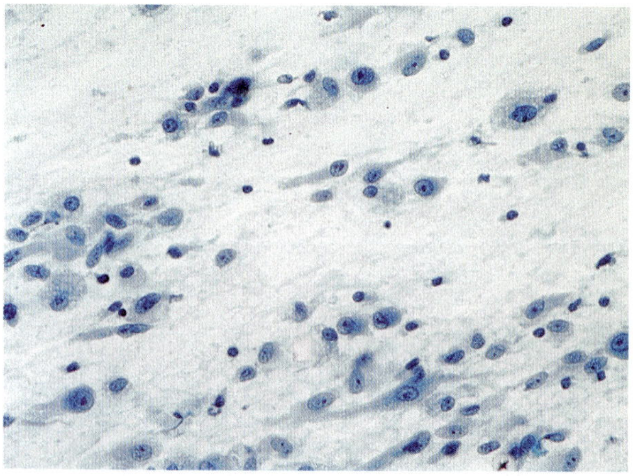

B

FIGURE 6.9 Fine needle aspiration biopsy specimen of nodular fasciitis typically contains numerous, discohesive spindled fibroblasts, some of which are binucleated, admixed with variable numbers of lymphocytes and histiocytes. The fibroblastic cells have round-to-ovoid, vesicular nuclei and often exhibit prominent nucleoli, surrounded by abundant cytoplasm **(A** and **B)**. **(A,** Diff-Quik; **B,** Papanicolaou.)

desmin, in virtually any combination. Actin is expressed more commonly than desmin.[6] Nevertheless, immunohistochemical studies generally are not helpful (and may be misleading) in distinguishing nodular fasciitis from leiomyoma/leiomyosarcoma. The background histiocytes and osteoclast-type giant cells express CD68. Cytokeratin, epithelial membrane antigen (EMA), and S-100 protein are negative.

Cytogenetic analysis has revealed clonal abnormalities in rare cases of nodular fasciitis. No reproducible and diagnostic translocations or aberrations have been found, however.[7] Nodular fasciitis is a diploid lesion.

Prognosis and Therapy

Nodular fasciitis is a self-limited process, and spontaneous resolution even after incomplete excision or FNAB is the rule rather than the exception.[5] Local recurrence is seen rarely, occurring in less than 1% of cases, usually after incomplete excision. Nevertheless, when a lesion originally diagnosed as nodular fasciitis locally recurs, review of the original material is necessary to exclude a misdiagnosis.[1]

Proliferative Fasciitis and Myositis

Clinical Features

Proliferative fasciitis and myositis are uncommon lesions, typically affecting adults 40 to 60 years old.[8,9] Rarely, proliferative fasciitis has been documented in children.[10] There is no gender predilection. By definition, proliferative fasciitis involves subcutaneous adipose tissue, whereas proliferative myositis is an intramuscular lesion. Similar to nodular fasciitis, most examples of proliferative fasciitis arise in the extremities, especially the upper extremities. Proliferative myositis more commonly arises in the skeletal muscles of the trunk or shoulder girdle. Involvement of the head and neck rarely is observed in either proliferative fasciitis or myositis. Patients typically report rapidly growing but painless soft tissue swelling. Some patients report a history of prior trauma to the affected area.[8]

Pathologic Findings

Histology

In contrast to the circumscription of nodular fasciitis, proliferative fasciitis and myositis form infiltrative, frequently stellate-appearing lesions, involving the deep subcutaneous fat and skeletal muscle, respectively.[8,9] In addition to loosely packed, plump spindled cells and a myxoid/collagenous stroma, the proliferative lesions display variable numbers of large ganglion-like cells with large, round-to-ovoid, vesicular nuclei; one or more prominent nucleoli; and abundant basophilic cytoplasm. Binucleated and multinucleated forms frequently are present. In proliferative fasciitis, these ganglion-like cells often are less evenly distributed, whereas in proliferative myositis, they tend to be more prominent and diffusely spread throughout the lesion (Figs. 6.10 and 6.11). Mitoses may be abundant but, as in nodular fasciitis, are not atypical. Scattered lymphocytes often are observed. Osseous metaplasia is seen rarely.

Fine Needle Aspiration Biopsy

FNAB of proliferative fasciitis and myositis produces similar cytologic smears to that observed in nodular fasciitis. Variable numbers of relatively large, polygonal-shaped cells with round-to-ovoid nuclei, prominent nucleoli, and abundant dense cytoplasm are scattered among the benign-appearing fibroblastic cells.[11] Correlation with clinical features generally yields the correct diagnosis.

Ancillary Studies

Ultrastructurally the lesional cells of proliferative fasciitis and myositis show evidence of fibroblastic and myofibroblastic differentiation. These features are virtually identical to those observed in nodular fasciitis. Likewise, the spindle cells of proliferative fasciitis and myositis show variable expression of actin, smooth muscle actin, and, less frequently, desmin, reflecting myofibroblastic differentiation.[11,12] Immunopositivity for actin also is observed in the ganglion cells but may be weak and focal in distribution. Cytokeratin, S-100 protein, and myoglobin are uniformly negative. Using routine cytogenetic analysis, trisomy 2 has been detected in one case each of proliferative fasciitis and proliferative myositis.[13,14]

Prognosis and Therapy

Proliferative fasciitis and myositis are benign, self-limited lesions that rarely recur locally. Local excision is considered adequate therapy. Distant metastasis has not been reported.

Fibroma of Tendon Sheath

Clinical Features

Fibroma of tendon sheath usually is observed in patients 20 to 40 years old; men are affected more commonly than women.[15] The most common anatomic site is the distal upper extremity, especially the fingers and hand. Patients frequently present with complaints of a small (<2 cm) soft tissue mass

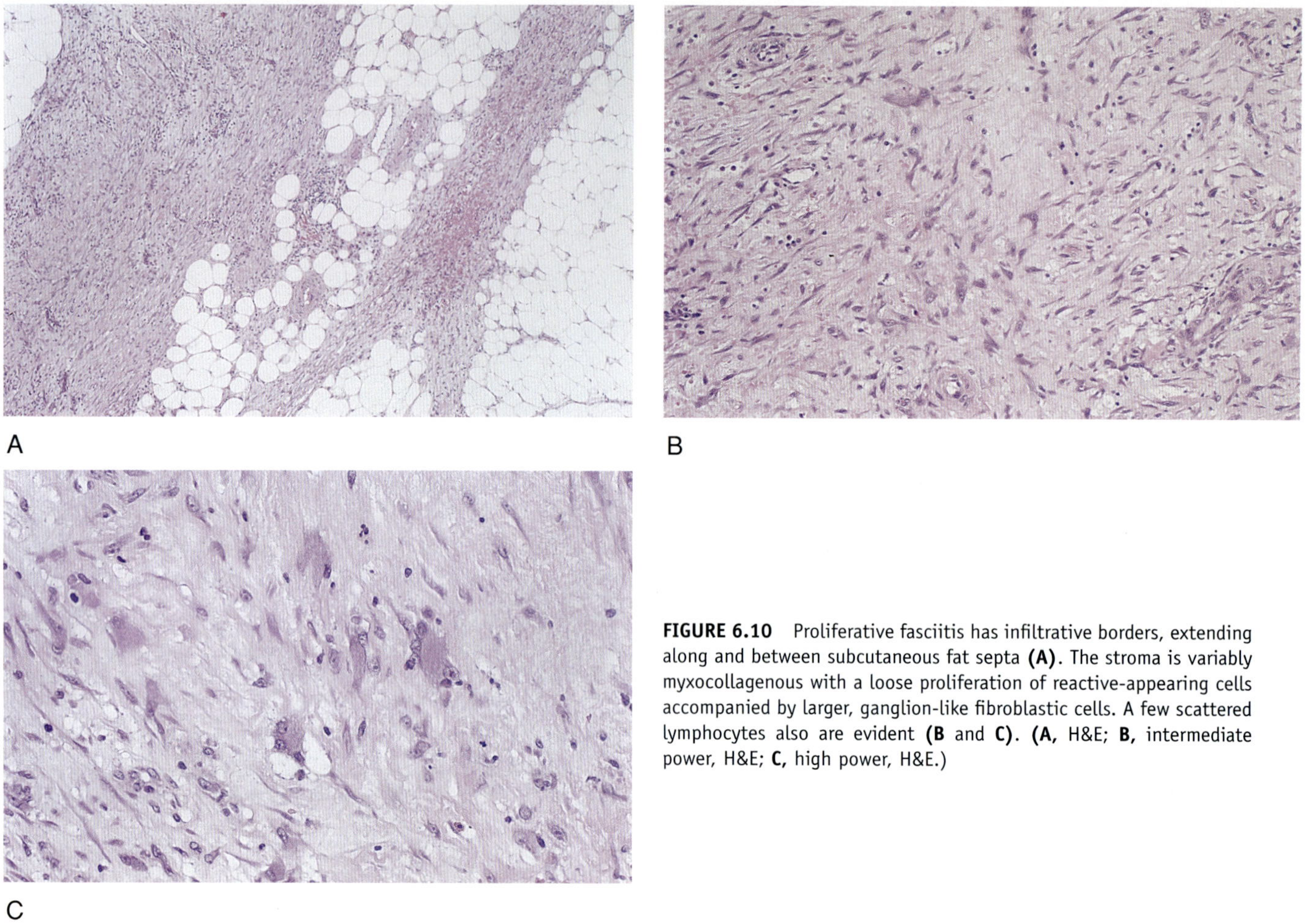

FIGURE 6.10 Proliferative fasciitis has infiltrative borders, extending along and between subcutaneous fat septa **(A)**. The stroma is variably myxocollagenous with a loose proliferation of reactive-appearing cells accompanied by larger, ganglion-like fibroblastic cells. A few scattered lymphocytes also are evident **(B** and **C)**. **(A,** H&E; **B,** intermediate power, H&E; **C,** high power, H&E.)

that may have been present for some time and is increasing slowly in size. Less frequently, patients report associated localized pain. A history of trauma or prior injury is observed in approximately 10% of cases.[15,16]

Pathologic Findings

Histology

Fibroma of tendon sheath is characterized by sharp circumscription and a multinodular appearance with individual nodules partially separated by clefts (Fig. 6.12). Most cases are hypocellular and composed of a bland-appearing population of spindled to stellate-appearing fibroblasts in a heavily collagenized-to-hyalinized stroma. Slit-like vascular channels and clefts are seen frequently. Areas of hypercellularity, resembling nodular fasciitis, always blend with the more typical hypocellular zones (Fig. 6.13). Myxoid change is seen less frequently in the hypocellular areas.

Ancillary Studies

Ultrastructurally, fibroma of tendon sheath shows evidence of fibroblastic and myofibroblastic differentiation, including dilated rough endoplasmic reticulum and intracytoplasmic intermediate filaments with dense bodies. Immunohistochemically, the lesional cells appear positive for vimentin, actin, and smooth muscle actin; desmin generally is negative. Data regarding cytogenetic analysis is too limited to draw any definite conclusions. One case reportedly had a clonal chromosomal abnormality, t(2;11) (q31-32;q12).[17]

Prognosis and Therapy

Fibroma of tendon sheath is an entirely benign process that may recur locally but does not metastasize. Given its frequent localization within the hands, surgical resection should be undertaken with the aim to preserve function. Local recurrence has been documented in up to one fourth of cases.[15] Re-excision of recurrent lesions is usually curative.

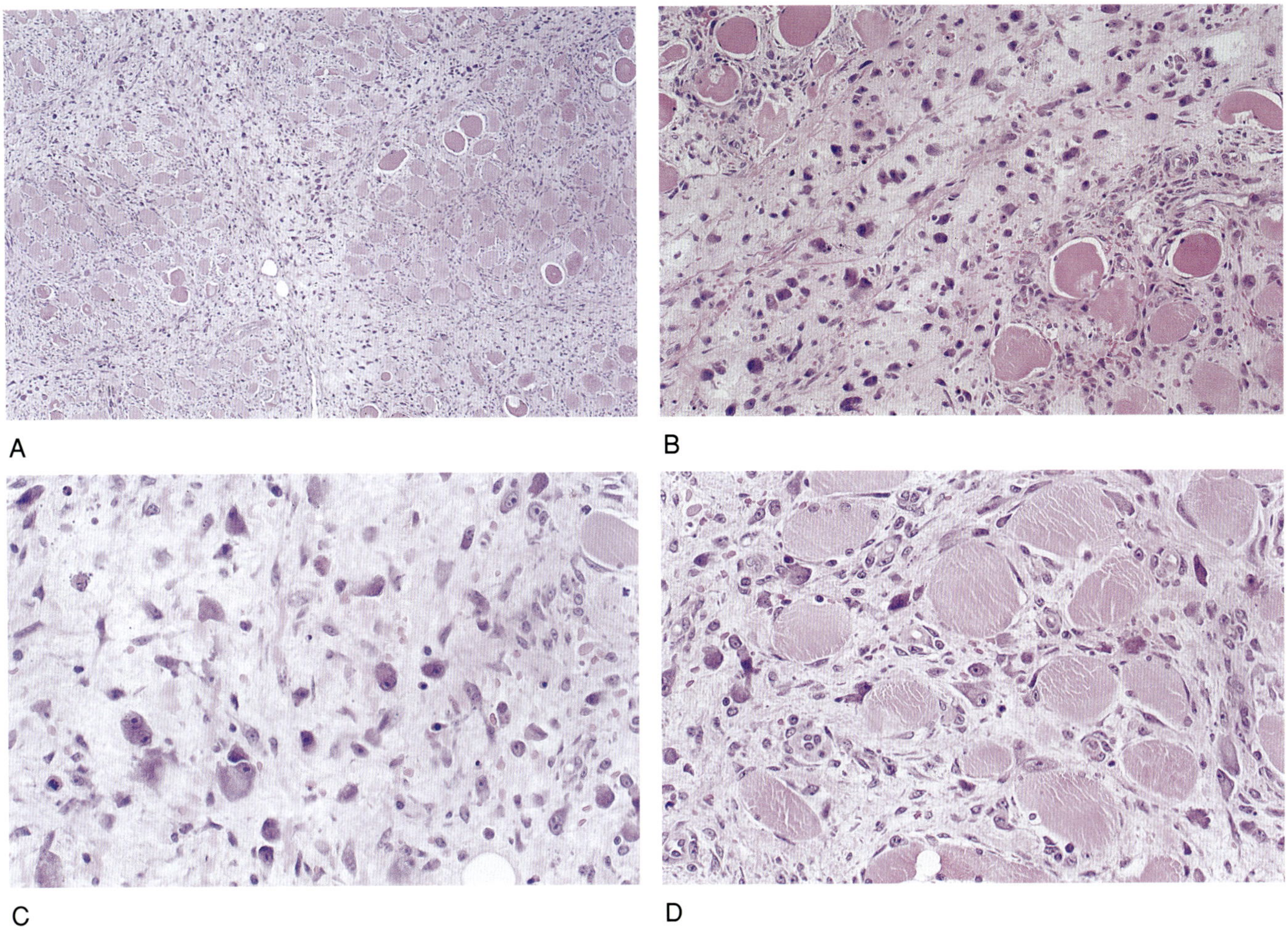

FIGURE 6.11 Proliferative myositis characterized by a slightly myxoid stroma and an abundant population of ganglion-like fibroblasts infiltrating (but preserving) skeletal muscle fascicles and in between individual skeletal muscle cells **(A-D)**. (**A**, Low power, H&E; **B**, intermediate power, H&E; **C** and **D**, high power, H&E.)

Nuchal Fibroma

Nuchal fibroma is a rare benign fibrosing lesion generally encountered in adults and involving the superficial tissues of the posterior neck region. There is a male predominance, and most patients are 20 to 40 years old.[18,19] "Extranuchal" fibromas have been described involving the face, buttock, and extremities.[20] For this reason, the designation *nuchal-type fibroma* may be more appropriate for this group of lesions. Patients typically present with painless soft tissue swelling in the cervicodorsal region. There seems to be a strong association with diabetes and possibly Gardner's syndrome.[18]

Histologically, nuchal fibroma is a poorly circumscribed and infiltrative lesion composed virtually entirely of dense hypocellular-to-acellular collagenous bundles. Scattered mature fibroblasts may be distributed within the dense collagen fibers. Entrapment of peripheral nerve and lobules of subcutaneous adipose tissue by the hypocellular collagenous bundles is typical (Fig. 6.14). Immunohistochemically, nuchal fibromas are usually positive for vimentin, CD34, and CD99 but generally negative for EMA, smooth muscle actin, and desmin.[18,21] Although nuchal fibroma may recur locally after excision, distant metastasis has not been documented.

Elastofibroma

Clinical Features

Elastofibroma usually is seen in patients older than age 50. There is a definite female predominance.[22,23] Many patients report a history of intensive manual labor. Elastofibromas typically arise within the connective tissues between the lower scapula and the chest wall. Bilateral cases rarely have been reported but may be more common than most data suggest; autopsy findings have revealed elastofibroma and pre-elastofibroma–like changes in up to 17% of patients.[24] Clinical symptoms are generally those of a slow-growing, soft tissue mass rarely associated with pain or tenderness. Radiographic studies reveal a poorly circumscribed but heterogeneous soft

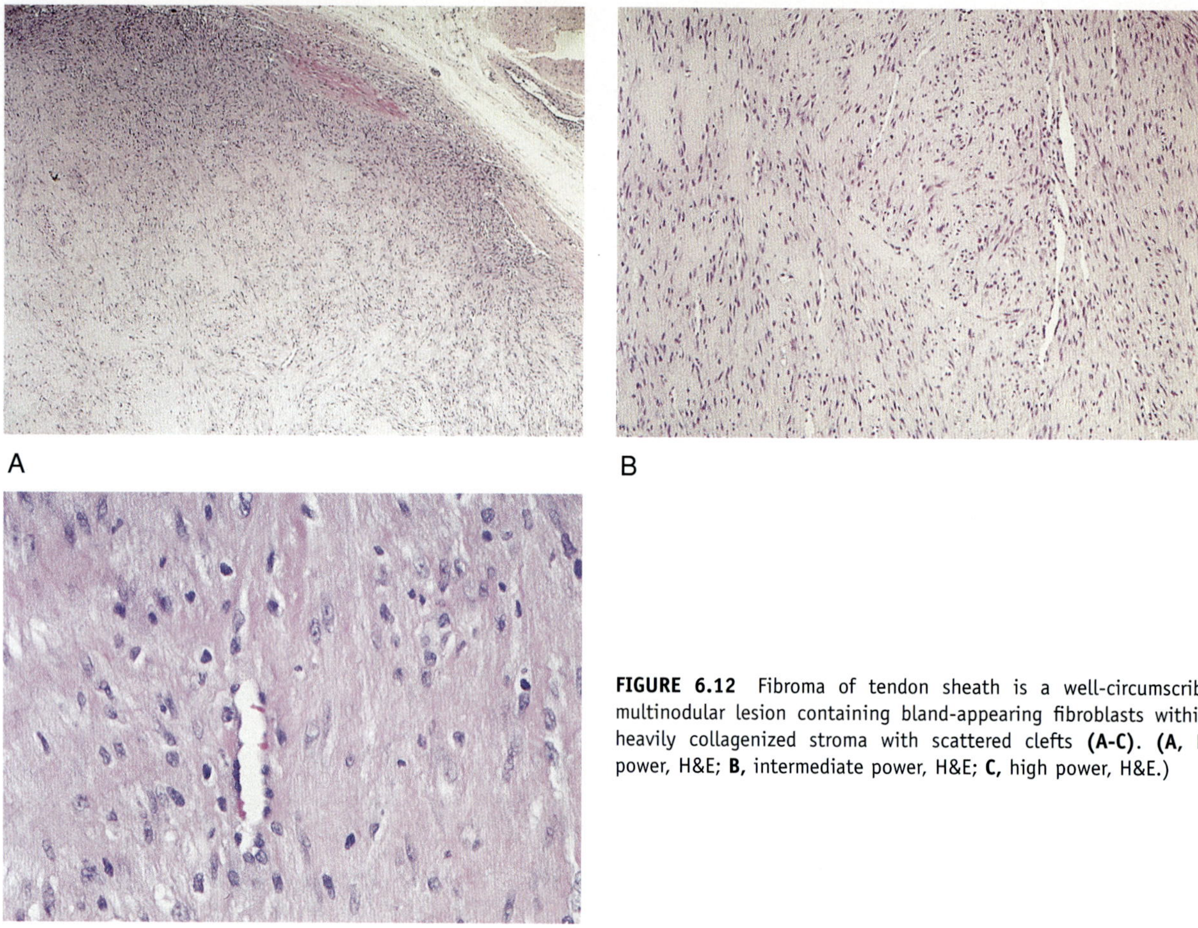

A B C

FIGURE 6.12 Fibroma of tendon sheath is a well-circumscribed, multinodular lesion containing bland-appearing fibroblasts within a heavily collagenized stroma with scattered clefts **(A-C)**. **(A,** Low power, H&E; **B,** intermediate power, H&E; **C,** high power, H&E.)

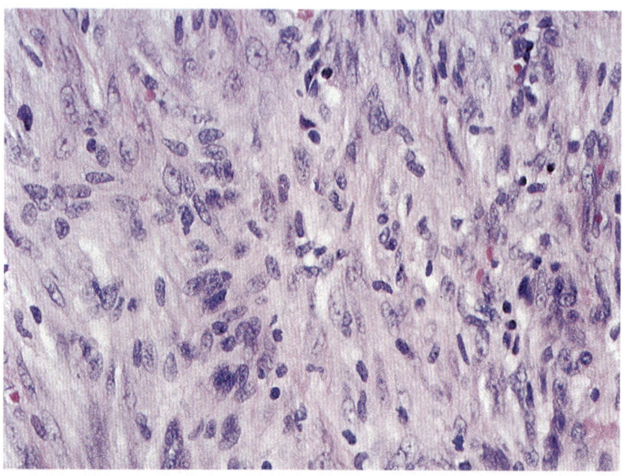

FIGURE 6.13 Fibroma of tendon sheath may contain focal, hypercellular areas resembling nodular fasciitis. (H&E.)

tissue mass with a signal intensity on magnetic resonance imaging similar to that of skeletal muscle. These findings coupled with the presence of interspersed adipose tissue and its classic location allow a presumptive clinical diagnosis of elastofibroma.[25,26]

Pathologic Findings

Histology

Microscopically, elastofibroma comprises a mixture of adipose tissue and strands of hypocellular collagen, often exhibiting myxoid changes. The margins of elastofibroma are irregular, and infiltration of adjacent skeletal muscle often occurs. Within the myocollagenous areas, variably fragmented elastic fibers, seen as beads of serrated disks or globules in linear arrangements, are distributed randomly among occasional fibroblasts and next to lobules of adipocytes (Fig. 6.15). These fibers are identified more easily with elastic stains.

Fine Needle Aspiration Biopsy

Despite the fact that only a few reports exist regarding the FNAB findings of elastofibroma, in the appropriate clinical setting, FNAB may be diagnostic.[27,28] Cytologic smears are typically hypocellular, but the characteristic elastic fibers are identified easily when present and meticulously sought.

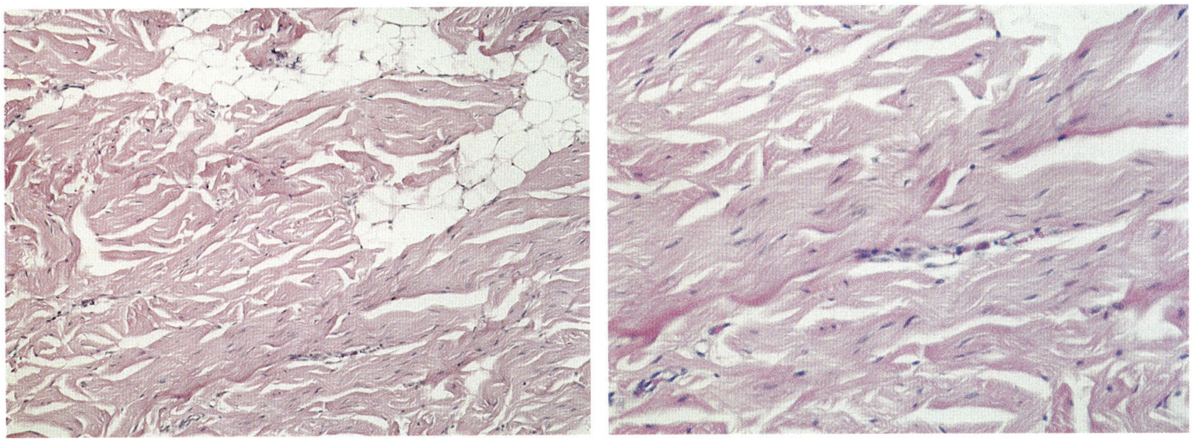

A B

FIGURE 6.14 Nuchal fibroma is an infiltrative lesion, frequently entrapping adipose tissue and peripheral nerve. It is composed of acellular-to-hypocellular collagenous bundles containing benign-appearing fibroblasts **(A** and **B)**. **(A,** Low power, H&E; **B,** high power, H&E.)

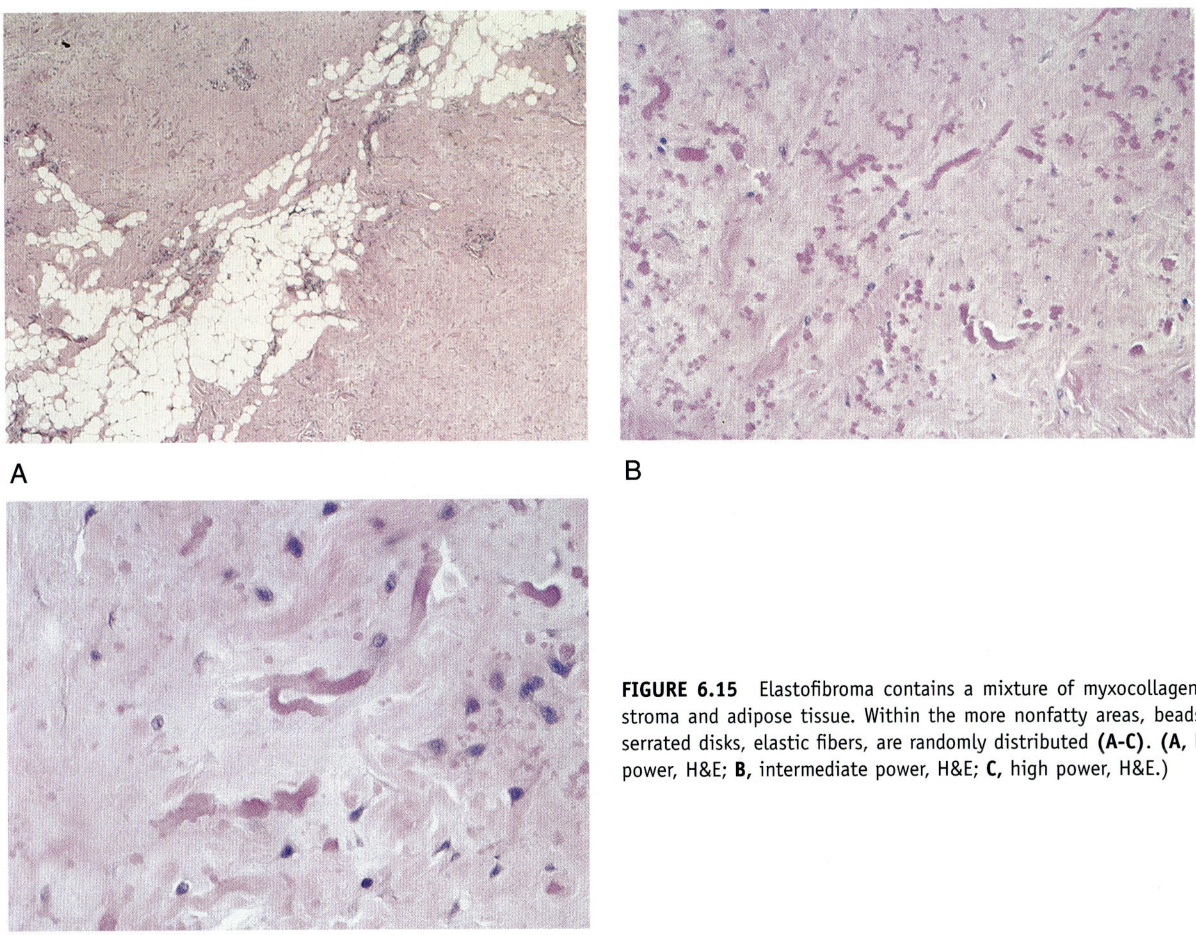

A B C

FIGURE 6.15 Elastofibroma contains a mixture of myxocollagenous stroma and adipose tissue. Within the more nonfatty areas, beads of serrated disks, elastic fibers, are randomly distributed **(A-C)**. **(A,** Low power, H&E; **B,** intermediate power, H&E; **C,** high power, H&E.)

Ancillary Studies

Electron microscopy of the linear elastic fibers reveals elongated masses composed of a central core of electron-lucent material resembling mature elastic tissue; the lucent material is surrounded by a less mature, fibrillary electron-dense substance resembling elastin. Individual cells within the fibrous areas show features of fibroblasts and myofibroblasts, and some contain granular bodies similar to extracellular elastin. These findings suggest that the fibroblasts are the origin of the extracellular elastic fibers.[29] Immunohistochemical stains are not necessary to establish a diagnosis of elastofibroma.

No reproducible chromosomal abnormality has been found in elastofibroma. Chromosomal aberrations involving chromosome 1p represent the most common abnormality.[30]

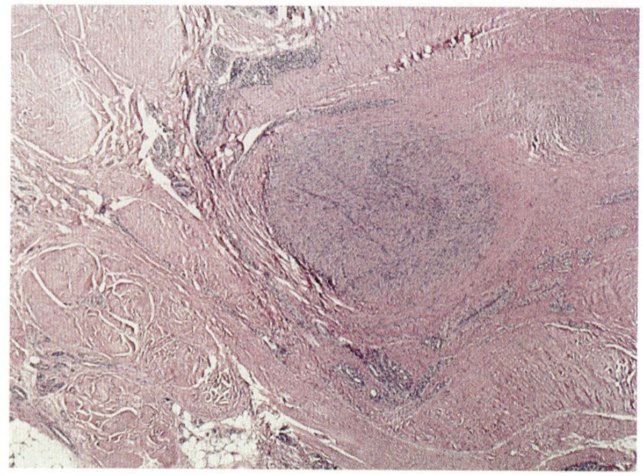

FIGURE 6.16 Superfical fibromatosis often begins as a multinodular growth within tendoaponeurotic fibrous tissue. (H&E.)

Prognosis and Therapy

Elastofibroma should be considered a totally benign lesion. Local excision rarely leads to recurrence. Distant metastasis has not been documented.

Superficial Fibromatoses

Superficial fibromatoses encompass palmar fibromatosis (Dupuytren's contracture), plantar fibromatosis (Ledderhose's syndrome), and penile fibromatosis (Peyronie's disease).[31-33] All are characterized by moderately cellular fibroblastic proliferations, arise in superficial soft tissues, and have an infiltrative growth pattern. These lesions may recur locally but do not metastasize.

Clinical Features

The most common form of fibromatosis is palmar fibromatosis. Palmar fibromatosis arises in adults, almost always older than 30 years. Men are affected more commonly than women. For unclear reasons, palmar fibromatosis has a predilection for Northern Europeans but is uncommon in individuals of African descent. Clinically, palmar fibromatosis manifests with a slow-growing, firm, nodular mass on the volvar aspect of the hand.[31] Up to 50% of cases may be bilateral. With progression, flexion contractures, predominantly affecting the fourth and fifth digits of the hand, develop. A few patients with palmar fibromatosis have concomitant plantar or penile lesions.[33]

Plantar fibromatosis, similar to its palmar counterpart, predominantly involves adults. Compared with palmar fibromatosis, it is has a higher incidence in children, however. There is a male predilection, and half of cases are bilateral. Patients generally present with a firm nodular thickening within the plantar fascia, involving the non–weight-bearing, medial aspect of the foot.[32] The anteromedial heel pad is the favored location in children. Although patients frequently complain of pain after prolonged standing or exercise, flexion contractures do not generally occur.

Penile fibromatosis is observed primarily in men older than age 40.[33] Most patients are white; the disease is uncommon in blacks and Asians. Patients complain of a plaque-like growth or thickening on the dorsal-lateral penile shaft, which with erection causes an abnormal curvature. Consequently, patients complain of difficulties achieving erection, painful erection, or painful sexual intercourse.

Pathologic Findings

Histology

Initially, all forms of superficial fibromatosis are characterized by a moderately cellular and nodular proliferation of mostly uniform-appearing fibroblasts (Fig. 6.16). Individual fibroblasts have bland, ovoid nuclei, small-to-inconspicuous nucleoli, and wavy-to-tapering eosinophilic cytoplasm. Mitotic figures are usually scarce (Fig. 6.17). With progression, the cellularity of the lesion often decreases accompanied by an increase in extracellular collagen. Infrequent histologic findings include osseous and chondroid metaplasia and aggregates of osteoclast-type giant cells.

Ancillary Studies

Ultrastructurally the cells of superficial fibromatosis show features of fibroblastic and myofibroblastic differentiation, including prominent rough endoplasmic reticulum and occasional intermediate filaments with dense bodies All forms of superficial fibromatosis show immunohistochemical expression of vimentin but variable positivity for smooth muscle actin and actin.

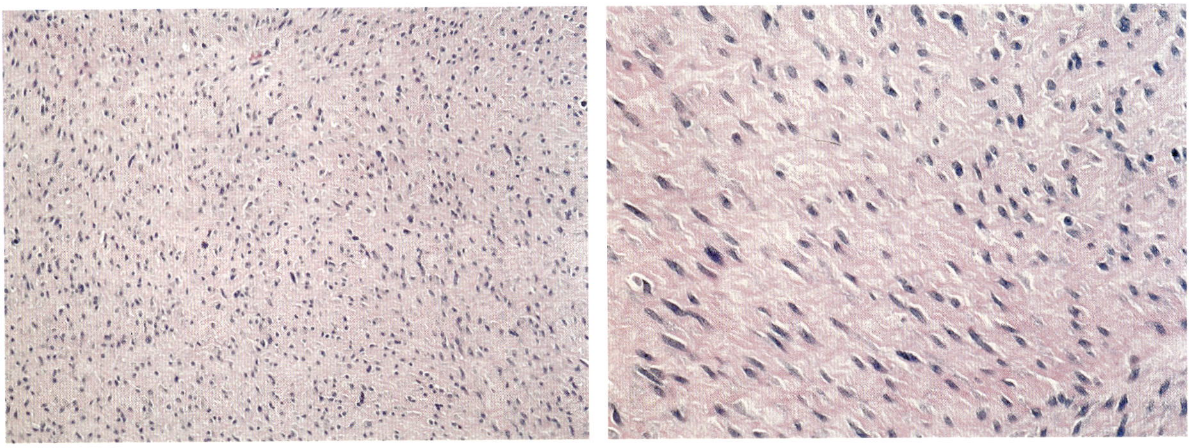

FIGURE 6.17 Superficial fibromatosis is characterized by moderately cellular fascicles of fibroblasts with bland, ovoid nuclei; small-to-inconspicuous nucleoli; and wavy-to-tapering eosinophilic cytoplasm **(A** and **B)**. **(A,** Low power, H&E; **B,** high power, H&E.)

Many patients have a significant family history of the disease.[34] Cytogenetic analysis reveals near-diploid karyotypes in virtually all cases of superficial fibromatosis. Although a specific translocation in superficial fibromatosis has not been identified, clonal chromosomal abnormalities, including gains of chromosomes 8 or 20, often are observed but tend to occur less frequently than with deep fibromatosis.[35]

Prognosis and Therapy

All forms of superficial fibromatosis have a risk of local recurrence; this risk is correlated most strongly with the adequacy of surgical excision.

Deep (Desmoid-Type) Fibromatosis

Clinical Features

Deep fibromatoses tend to be rarer than the superficial forms. Most patients are young to middle-aged adults. In contrast to superficial fibromatosis, there is a definite female predominance.[36] The most common anatomic location is the abdominal musculature, particularly in women during or after pregnancy. Among older adults, deep fibromatoses frequently involve extra-abdominal sites, especially the proximal extremities and limb girdles (Fig. 6.18). Regardless of anatomic site, most patients present with deeply seated, infiltrative masses unassociated with pain. Intra-abdominal and mesenteric forms are more likely to occur in patients with Gardner's syndrome. These patients are usually asymptomatic but may exhibit an abdominal mass on physical examination. Rare signs and symptoms include weight loss, acute abdomen, and fever.[37]

Pathologic Findings

Histology

Regardless of site of origin, deep fibromatoses are poorly circumscribed lesions composed of a mostly uniform population of spindled to stellate-shaped cells with ovoid nuclei and inconspicuous-to-small nucleoli. Individual cells are arranged in sweeping fascicles that infiltrate adjacent skeletal muscle and/or adipose tissue (Fig. 6.19). The stroma tends to be uniformly collagenous but may contain focal myxoid areas, extensive hyalinization, or keloid-like collagen deposition (Fig. 6.20). Aggregates of lymphocytes are often present, most frequently observed at the periphery of the lesion.

Fine Needle Aspiration Biopsy

FNAB of fibromatoses are usually nondiagnostic. Smears generally consist mostly of blood with scattered solitary and rare groups of fibroblasts, indistinguishable from normal connective tissue elements (Fig. 6.21). Open biopsy usually is required for definitive diagnosis.[38]

Ancillary Studies

Ultrastructurally, the lesional cells of fibromatoses show features of fibroblastic and myofibroblastic differentiation, including dilated rough endoplasmic reticulum, focal well-formed basal lamina, and aggregates of intracytoplasmic filaments. Immunohistochemically, deep fibromatosis shows strong and diffuse immunoexpression for vimentin and is usually positive for smooth muscle actin. Desmin positivity is observed in about 50% of cases. Cytokeratin, CD34, and S-100 protein are negative. Yantiss and colleagues[39] documented CD117 (c-kit)

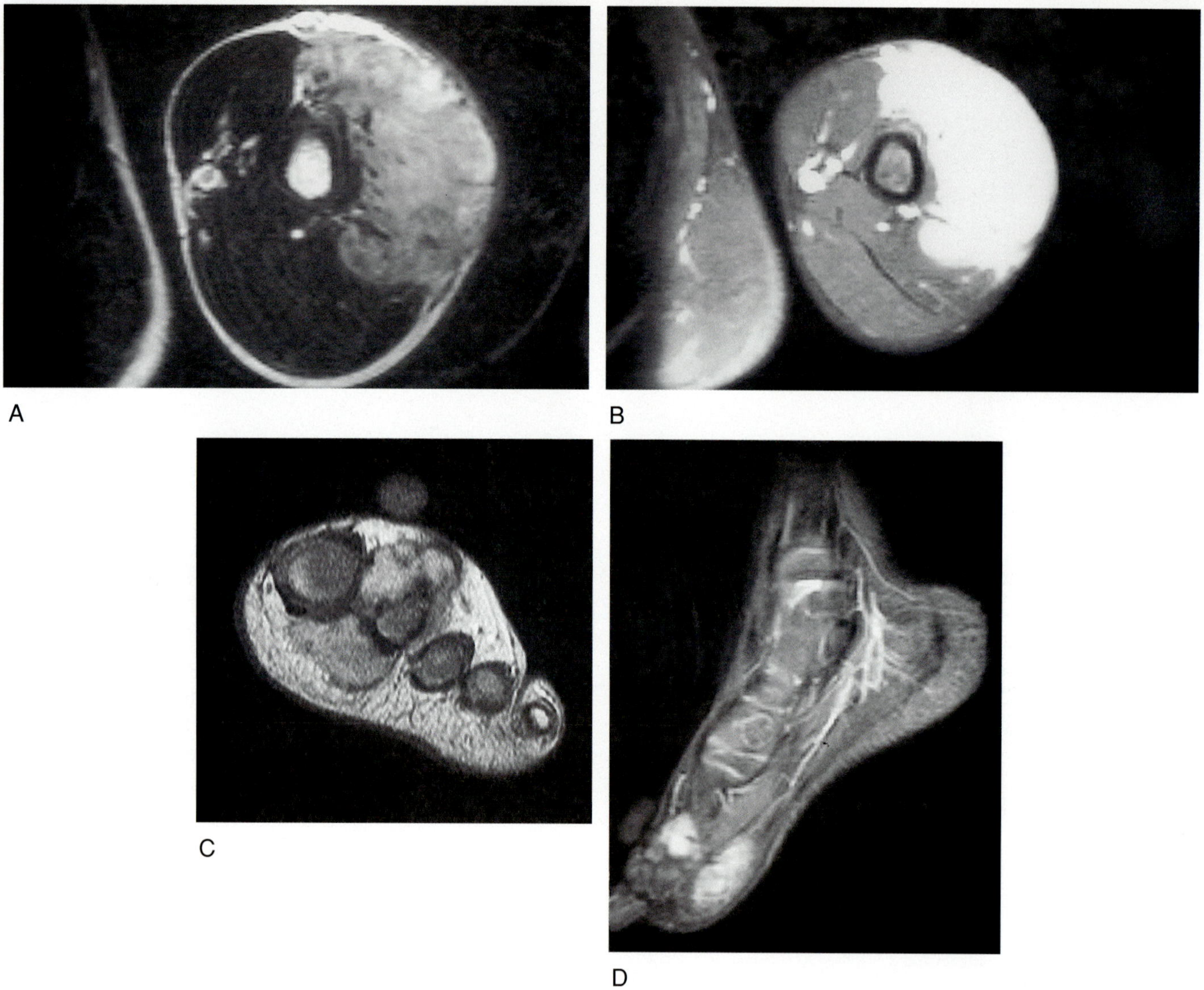

FIGURE 6.18 Deep fibromatosis. T2-weighted **(A)** and gadolinium-enhanced, fat-suppressed T1-weighted **(B)** magnetic resonance images of the upper arm show a large, heterogeneous, enhancing mass in the lateral musculature extending into the triceps and flexor compartments of the arm. In another patient, coronal proton density **(C)** and sagittal short tau inversion recovery (STIR) **(D)** magnetic resonance images of the foot reveal a mass extending between the first and second metatarsals. The rounded mass dorsal to the foot is a vitamin E capsule placed on the foot as a marker during the scan.

cytoplasmic positivity in 75% of cases of intra-abdominal fibromatosis. For this reason, CD117 positivity should not be used as the sole determinant of distinguishing gastrointestinal stromal tumor from fibromatosis. No reproducible chromosomal translocations have been identified in deep fibromatoses. Clonal aberrations are common, however, especially trisomies 8 and 20 and loss of 5q material.[35]

Prognosis and Therapy

Deep fibromatoses are nonmetastasizing but locally aggressive lesions, often requiring extensive surgical resection for local control. The most important prognostic factor is the adequacy of the surgical excision. The goal of achieving negative margins should be balanced with a desire to preserve function and to limit morbidity because the presence of residual disease does not seem to affect survival adversely.[36] The role of chemotherapy and radiation therapy in deep fibromatosis is controversial and unclear.

Extrapleural Solitary Fibrous Tumor

Clinical Features

Solitary fibrous tumors most often arise from the pleural surface. This section focuses on the less common extrapleural form. Most soft tissue examples occur in middle-aged to older adults (mean, 50 to 60 years old), and there is no gender

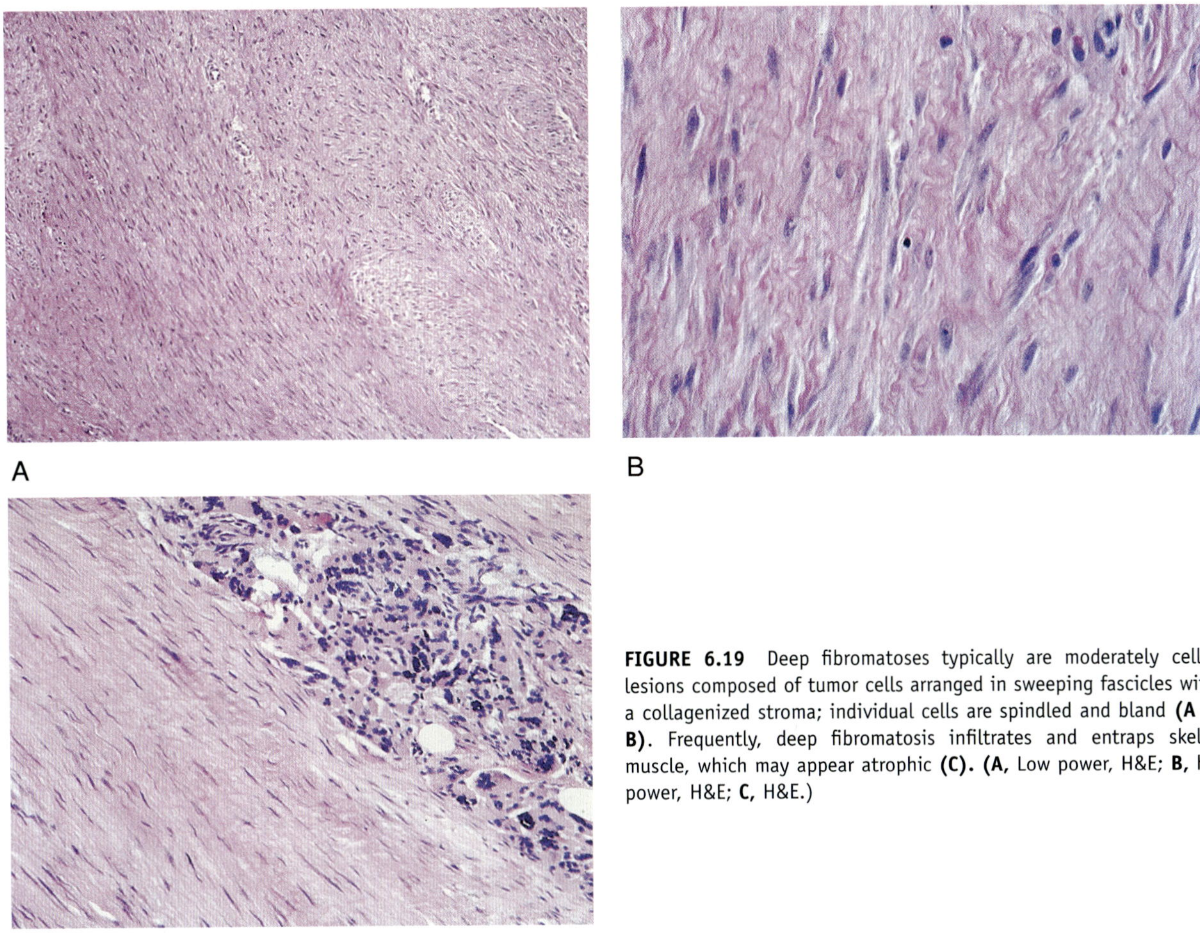

FIGURE 6.19 Deep fibromatoses typically are moderately cellular lesions composed of tumor cells arranged in sweeping fascicles within a collagenized stroma; individual cells are spindled and bland **(A** and **B)**. Frequently, deep fibromatosis infiltrates and entraps skeletal muscle, which may appear atrophic **(C)**. **(A,** Low power, H&E; **B,** high power, H&E; **C,** H&E.)

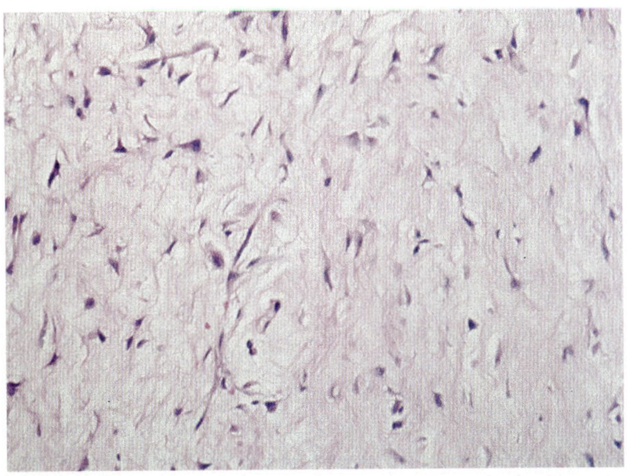

FIGURE 6.20 Myxoid areas occasionally are seen in deep fibromatoses. (H&E.)

preference. Solitary fibrous tumors have been described in virtually all locations, but most involve the subcutaneous and deep soft tissues of the head and neck region followed in frequency by the extremities and trunk.[40-42] Patients usually present with a slow-growing, painless soft tissue mass.

Pathologic Findings

Histology

Solitary fibrous tumors are typically well-circumscribed, partially encapsulated masses. The architecture has been described as patternless, consisting of a combination of alternating hypocellular and hypercellular regions with variable amounts of collagen deposition. A background of slit-like to staghorn-shaped blood vessels, creating a hemangiopericytoma-like pattern, frequently is observed and suggests a histologic spectrum between solitary fibrous tumor and so-called hemangiopericytoma.[40,42] The lesional cells are spindle-shaped with uniform-appearing, ovoid-to-spindled nuclei arranged in vague intersecting fascicles (Fig. 6.22). Myxoid stromal changes are common. Mitotic figures are seen rarely and should not exceed four mitoses per 10 high-power fields.

Approximately 10% of extrathoracic solitary fibrous tumors are characterized by increased cellularity, tumor necrosis, nuclear atypia, and a mitotic count exceeding four mitoses per 10 high-power fields. These findings are associated with more aggressive clinical behavior.[43]

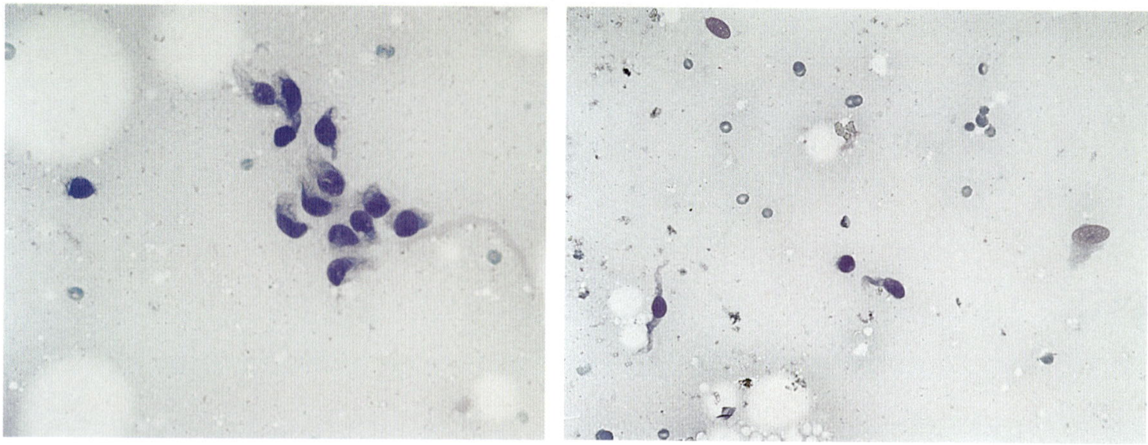

A B

FIGURE 6.21 Fine needle aspiration biopsy of deep fibromatoses is rarely diagnostic. Smears typically are hypocellular and composed of scattered, benign-appearing fibroblasts indistinguishable from inadvertently sampled normal connective tissue elements **(A** and **B)**. **(A,** and **B,** Diff-Quik.)

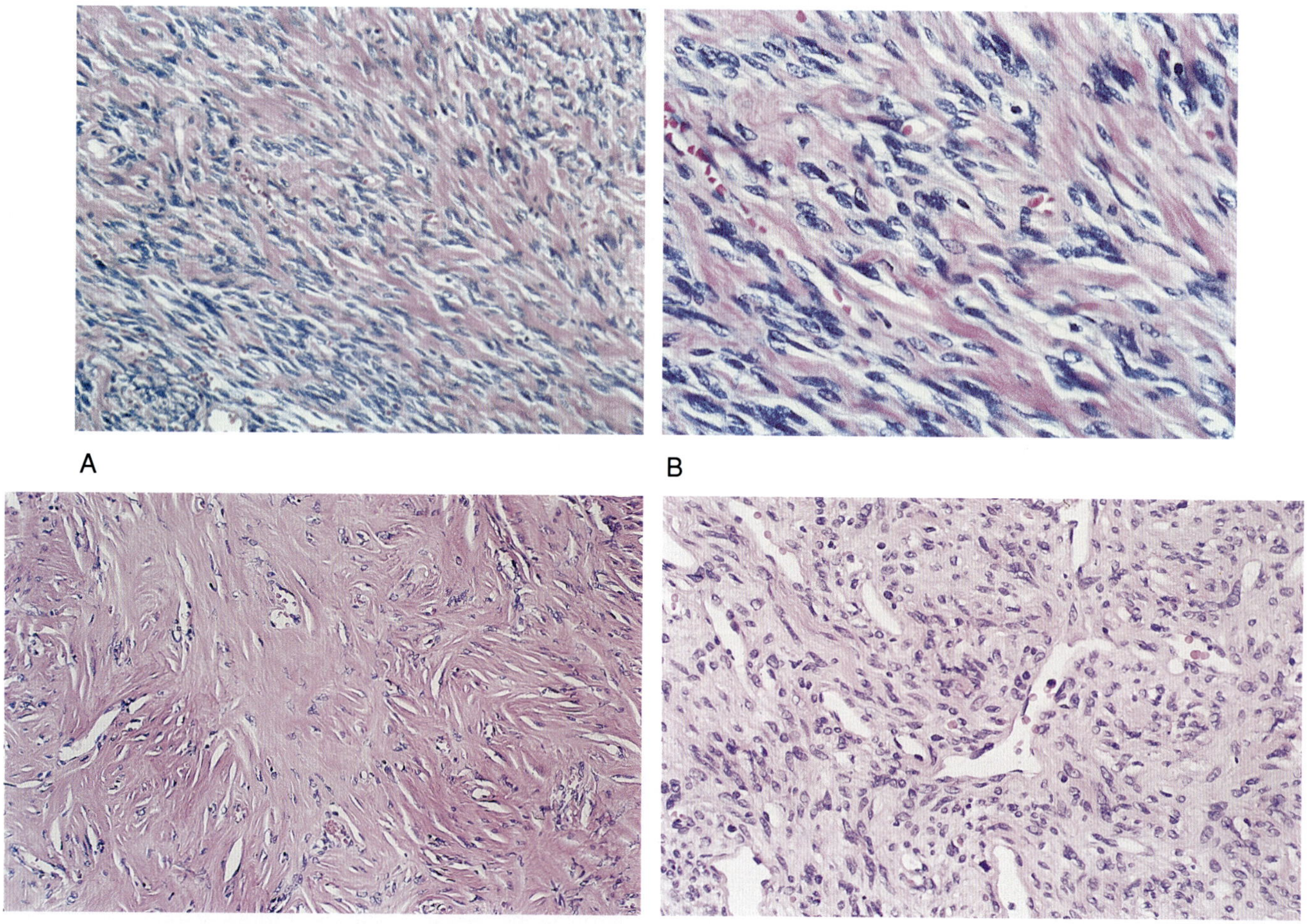

A B C D

FIGURE 6.22 Solitary fibrous tumor is characterized by a patternless to vague fascicular proliferation of uniform-appearing spindled cells accompanied by variable amounts of collagen **(A** and **B)**. Hypocellular, hyalinized regions are not unusual **(C)**. Overlapping histologic features, including the presence of at least a focal hemangiopericytoma-like vascular pattern, suggest a relationship between solitary fibrous tumor and classic hemangiopericytoma **(D)**. **(A,** Low power, H&E; **B,** high power, H&E; **C** and **D,** H&E.)

TABLE 6.2 Immunohistochemical Profile of Extrapleural Solitary Fibrous Tumor

Immunohistochemical Antibody	Estimated Incidence of Cases that Are Positive (%)
Vimentin	100
CD34	90-100
CD99	60-70
Smooth muscle actin	5-10
EMA	<5
Muscle-specific actin	<5
Cytokeratin	Negative
S-100 protein	Negative
Desmin	Negative

EMA, epithelial membrane antigen.

Fine Needle Aspiration Biopsy

FNAB smears range from scant to moderately cellular with mostly individually dispersed tumor cells and irregular, loose aggregates of cells embedded in a collagenous matrix.[44] The nuclei are uniform, ovoid, and bland appearing. "Ropy" irregular collagen fragments and occasional inflammatory cells are within the background.[44] Correlation with clinical features and the use of immunohistochemistry permit an accurate diagnosis.

Ancillary Studies

Ultrastructurally, the lesional cells of solitary fibrous tumor show features of fibroblastic and myofibroblastic differentiation, including dilated rough endoplasmic reticulum, prominent Golgi apparatuses, and, less frequently, intracytoplasmic filaments and dense bodies.[41] Table 6.2 summarizes the immunohistochemical profile of extrapleural solitary fibrous tumor. Strong and diffuse positivity for vimentin and CD34 is characteristic of solitary fibrous tumor (Fig. 6.23). Additionally, most also show positivity for CD99. Less frequently, solitary fibrous tumor displays immunoexpression for actin and smooth muscle actin. Desmin, cytokeratin, and S-100 protein are usually negative.[40,41,43,45] No reproducible cytogenetic abnormality has been found in solitary fibrous tumor.

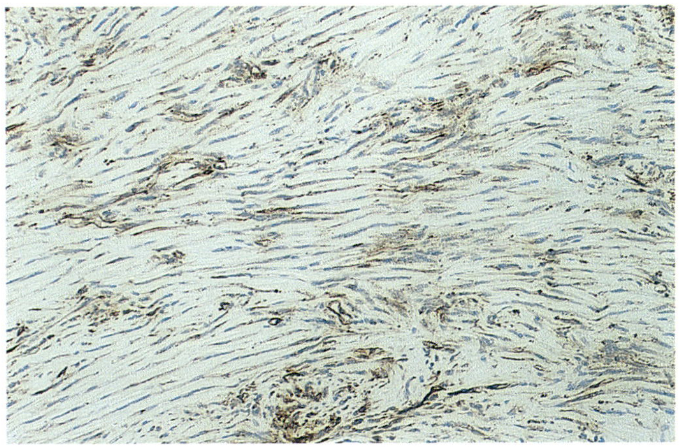

FIGURE 6.23 Diffuse CD34 positivity is a characteristic feature of solitary fibrous tumor. (Immunoperoxidase stain for CD34.)

TABLE 6.3 Bone and Soft Tissue Tumors Commonly Displaying a Hemangiopericytoma-Like Vascular Pattern

Benign fibrous histiocytoma
Myofibroma/myofibromatosis
Solitary fibrous tumor
Synovial sarcoma
Mesenchymal chondrosarcoma
Malignant peripheral nerve sheath tumor

Prognosis and Therapy

Most cases of solitary fibrous tumor behave in a benign fashion. Approximately 10% to 15% show aggressive (malignant) behavior; these tumors are more likely to display increased cellularity, nuclear atypia, necrosis, and a higher mitotic rate (>4 mitoses per 10 high-power fields). Histology is an imperfect predictor of clinical behavior, and all patients with solitary fibrous tumors require close clinical follow-up.

Hemangiopericytoma

Historically, hemangiopericytoma has been a relatively common tumor. In more recent years, it has become evident that the vascular pattern associated with hemangiopericytoma may be seen in a variety of tumors. Table 6.3 lists various bone and soft tissue tumors commonly exhibiting a hemangiopericytoma-like vascular pattern. Consequently, the diagnosis of hemangiopericytoma has become one of exclusion. At present, the World Health Organization considers

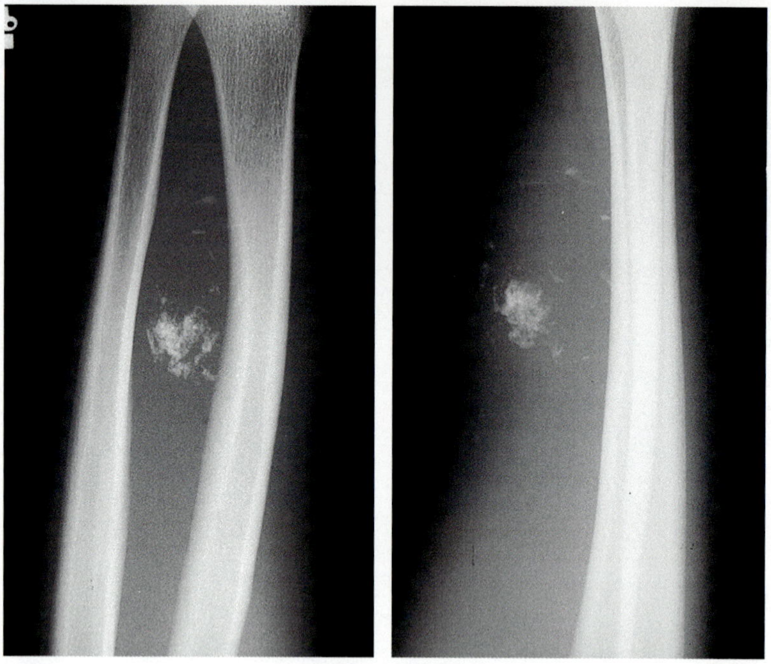

FIGURE 6.24 Hemangioperiocytoma. Anteroposterior **(A)** and lateral **(B)** radiographs of the forearm show a soft tissue mass in the flexor compartment of the arm with pleomorphic soft tissue calcifications.

many cases of hemangiopericytoma to represent a spectrum of solitary fibrous tumor.[46] Despite the name, hemangiopericytoma does not show the immunohistochemical or ultrastructural features of pericytes.

Clinical Features

Most cases arise in adults older than age 40, and there is a female predilection. The abdomen/retroperitoneum is the most common anatomic site, followed by the extremities (Fig. 6.24). Most cases occur in deep soft tissues and rarely may contain calcifications, especially if the lesion has been present for a long time. Patients usually present with painless soft tissue swelling. Retroperitoneal lesions may cause intestinal obstruction and/or urinary symptoms.[46,47]

Primary hemangiopericytoma of bone is extraordinarily rare. Similar to their soft tissue counterpart, most occur in adults, but there is no gender bias. Limited data suggest that the axial skeleton (spine and craniofacial region), followed in frequency by the pelvic girdle and ribs, is the most common anatomic site. Radiographically, skeletal hemangiopericytomas are typically lytic and may be well circumscribed or show some degree of cortical destruction. Overall, radiographic features are not specific for the diagnosis.[48]

Pathologic Findings

Histology

Hemangiopericytomas are typically well-circumscribed, unencapsulated lesions. Alternating hypocellular and hypercellular areas frequently are seen. The latter may resemble closely the more cellular areas of solitary fibrous tumor. Individual cells appear uniform and round to slightly spindled and may be closely packed. The background stroma is variably collagenous, ranging from strands of collagen to extensive hyalinization. The cardinal histologic feature of hemangiopericytoma is the presence of variably-sized, angulated to staghorn-shaped blood vessels, lined by a thin inconspicuous layer of flattened and bland endothelial cells (Fig. 6.25). Mitotic activity is not usually prominent and rarely exceeds four mitoses per 10 high-power fields. Tumors associated with greater mitotic activity should be designated as at least borderline or potentially malignant.[47] Rare examples of hemangiopericytoma are associated with a prominent adipocytic component, *lipomatous hemangiopericytoma.*[49]

Fine Needle Aspiration Biopsy

FNAB of hemangiopericytoma yields cellular smears composed of a uniform population of ovoid-to-spindled cells closely resembling those seen in synovial sarcoma; the cells appear singly and in small cohesive clusters (Fig. 6.26). Significant nuclear pleomorphism is not present. Some authors have described clusters of cells "aggregated around branched capillaries."[50] Without a concomitantly obtained cell block, the characteristic vascular pattern generally is not observed in cytologic preparations. We consider the diagnosis of hemangiopericytoma to be one of exclusion and do not believe that hemangiopericytoma can be diagnosed reliably by FNAB.

Ancillary Studies

Despite the name, the ultrastructural features of hemangiopericytoma show no evidence of true pericytic differentia-

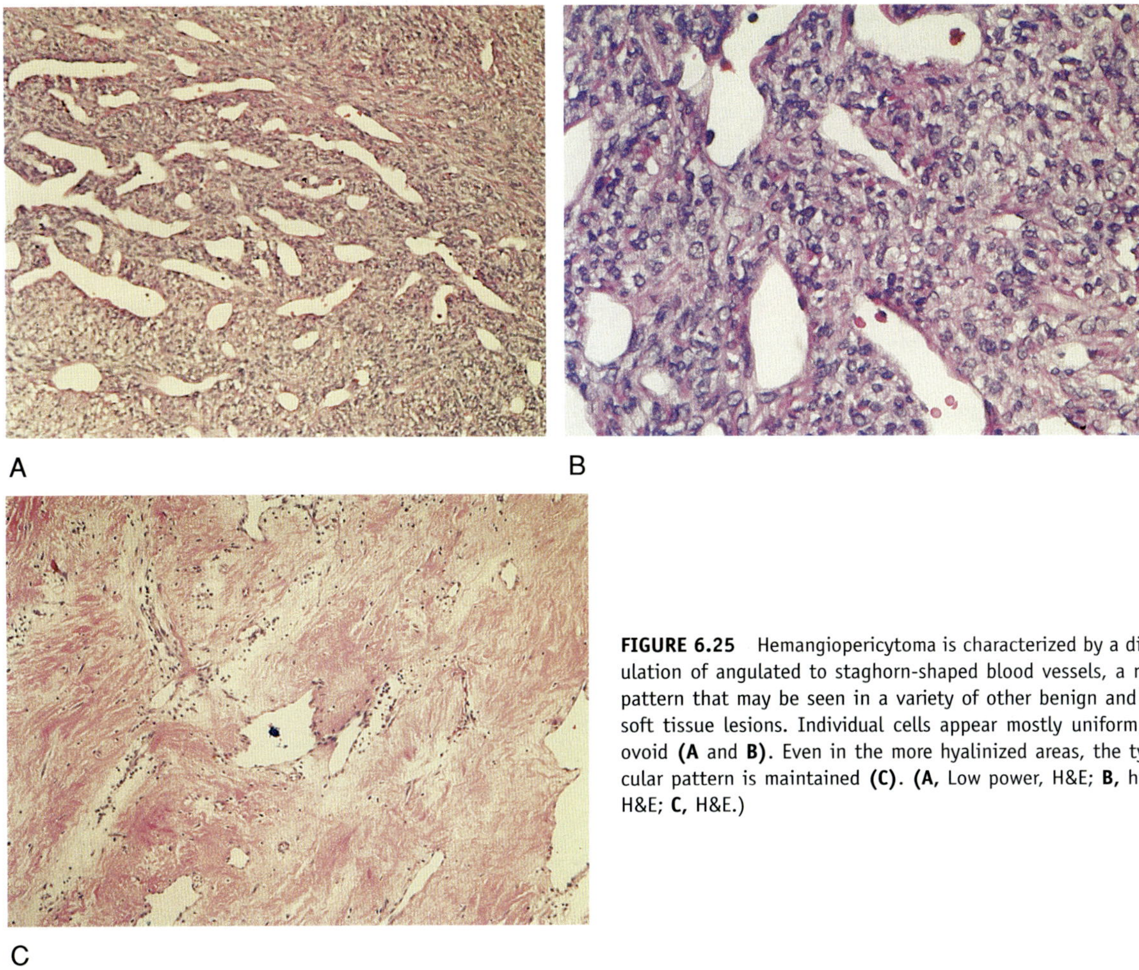

FIGURE 6.25 Hemangiopericytoma is characterized by a diffuse population of angulated to staghorn-shaped blood vessels, a nonspecific pattern that may be seen in a variety of other benign and malignant soft tissue lesions. Individual cells appear mostly uniform, round to ovoid **(A** and **B)**. Even in the more hyalinized areas, the typical vascular pattern is maintained **(C)**. **(A,** Low power, H&E; **B,** high power, H&E; **C,** H&E.)

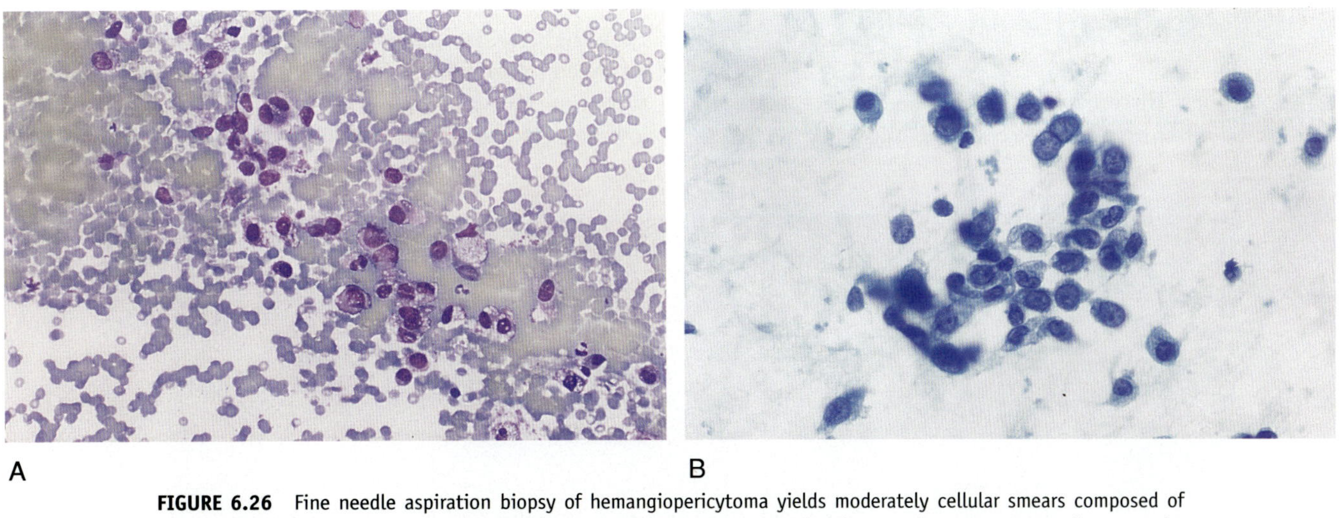

FIGURE 6.26 Fine needle aspiration biopsy of hemangiopericytoma yields moderately cellular smears composed of solitary and cohesive clusters of mostly uniform, round-to-ovoid tumor cells. The vascular pattern generally cannot be appreciated in cytologic smears **(A** and **B)**. **(A,** Diff-Quik; **B,** Papanicolaou.)

tion. Instead the electron microscopic findings reveal features of fibroblastic differentiation. After immunohistochemical exclusion of other entities, hemangiopericytomas typically show positivity for vimentin, CD99, and CD34.[46] Cytokeratin and CD31 are negative within the lesional cells.

At present, there is no reproducible chromosomal abnormality for hemangiopericytoma. Breakpoints involving 12q13-15 and 19q13 are present in approximately 50% and 25% of cases, respectively.[46]

Prognosis and Therapy

Histology is an imperfect predictor of prognosis in hemangiopericytoma, but most cases behave in a benign clinical fashion. Histologic features such as increased mitotic activity (>4 mitotic features per 10 high-power fields), necrosis, and nuclear pleomorphism suggest the potential for malignant behavior.[47] Wide surgical resection with negative margins is recommended. Lesions originating within bone may be treated with en bloc resection.

Collagenous Fibroma (Desmoplastic Fibroma)

Collagenous fibroma is a rare, more recently described lesion. It predominantly affects patients older than age 40, and there seems to be no gender bias.[51-53] The most common anatomic site is the subcutis and deep soft tissues of the extremities, followed by the neck and trunk. Patients present with a painless, slow-growing soft tissue mass. The tumor is typically well circumscribed and slightly lobulated. Histologically, it is characterized by a hypocellular and hypovascular collagenous stroma containing scattered bland, spindled to stellate-appearing fibroblasts. Myxoid stromal change may be focally evident. Immunohistochemically, the cells appear positive for vimentin and occasionally express smooth muscle actin and actin. Cytokeratin, EMA, S-100 protein, and CD34 are usually negative. Clonal chromosomal abnormalities, specifically involving band 11q12, have been reported in two cases of collagenous fibroma.[54] Simple excision is curative. There have been no reported recurrences or metastases.[51-53]

Benign Fibrous Histiocytoma

Benign fibrous histiocytomas most commonly arise in the dermis, where they are known to most clinicians as *dermatofibromas*. For this discussion, we focus primarily on cases that arise within subcutis, deep soft tissues, or bone.

Clinical Features

Compared with their cutaneous counterpart, deep benign fibrous histiocytomas are relatively rare lesions. Most occur in young to middle-aged adults, and there is a male predominance.[55] The most common anatomic sites are the lower extremities and head and neck region. Patients usually present with complaints of a slow-growing, soft tissue mass.

Benign (also called *atypical*) fibrous histiocytoma of bone is an extraordinarily rare (controversial) tumor. Women are affected slightly more commonly than men. The most common anatomic site is the ilium (Fig. 6.27), followed by the femur and tibia. In general, most patients are asymptomatic, and routine physical examination is unrevealing. Radiographically, benign fibrous histiocytoma is a lytic lesion with sharp margination and focal sclerosis. Matrix mineralization is absent.[56]

Pathologic Findings

Histology

Overall, deep soft tissue benign fibrous histiocytomas are generally larger, better circumscribed, and more monomorphic than their cutaneous counterparts. Individual tumor cells are arranged in short fascicles and prominent storiform patterns, often within a hemangiopericytoma-like background.[55] Cytologically the spindled cells have ovoid and vesicular

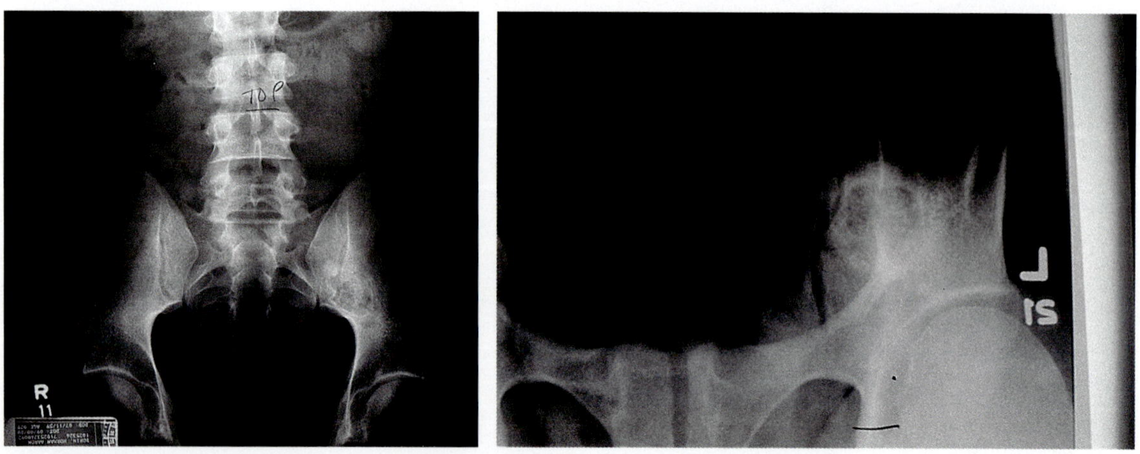

A B

FIGURE 6.27 Benign fibrous histiocytoma. An anteroposterior radiograph of the lower abdomen **(A)** and a coned radiograph of the ilium **(B)** reveal a lytic, slightly expansile lesion of the ilium. The margin of the lesion is sclerotic and well defined.

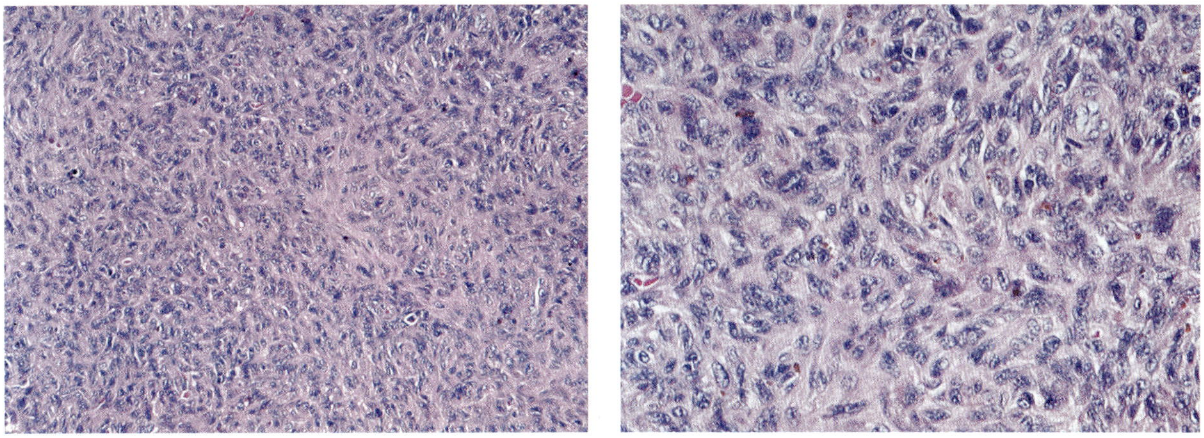

A B

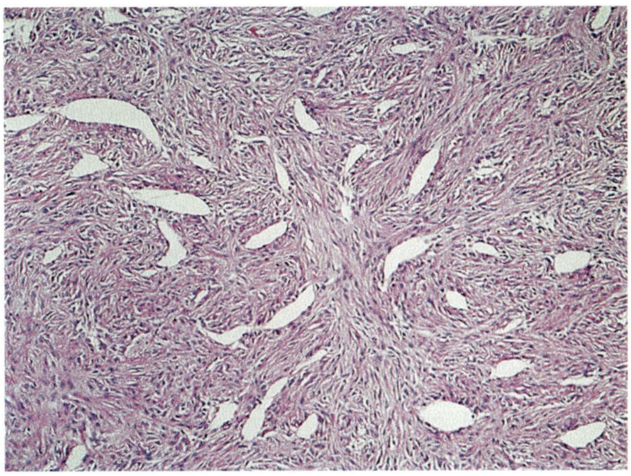

C

FIGURE 6.28 Deep fibrous histiocytoma is composed of a cellular, monomorphic population of cells arranged in fascicles and storiform patterns **(A** and **B)**. A hemangiopericytoma-like vascular pattern commonly is observed **(C)**. **(A,** Low power, H&E; **B,** high power, H&E; **C,** H&E.)

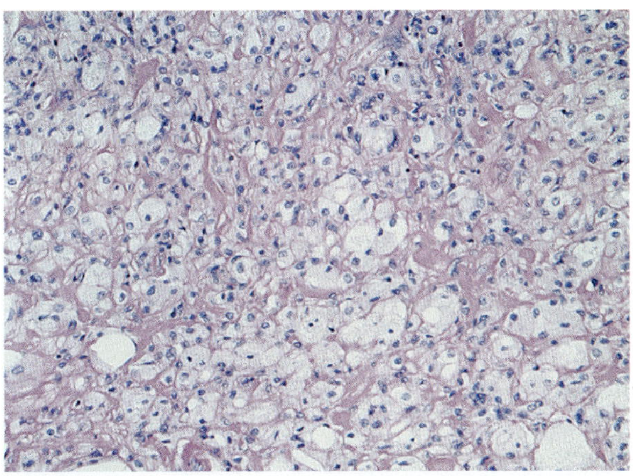

FIGURE 6.29 Less commonly observed in deep soft tissue forms, the finding of inflammatory elements, histiocytes and lymphocytes, is a helpful diagnostic feature in benign fibrous histiocytoma. (H&E.)

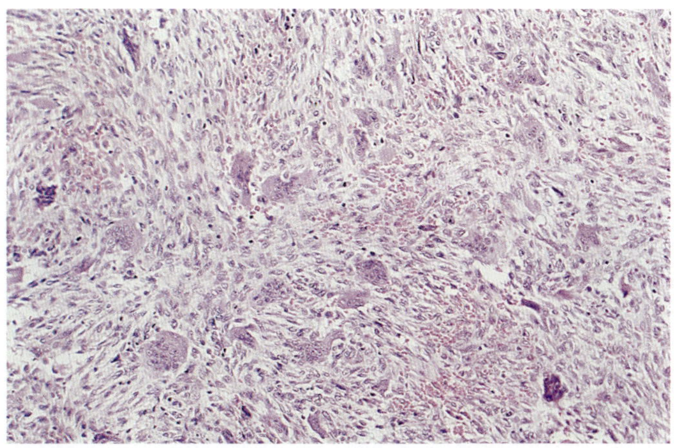

FIGURE 6.30 Benign fibrous histiocytoma of bone shows virtually identical features to those observed in metaphyseal fibrous defect. Correlation with clinical and radiographic findings avoids a misdiagnosis. (H&E.)

nuclei and inconspicuous-to-prominent nucleoli. Significant nuclear pleomorphism is not a feature (Fig. 6.28). Mitotic figures usually are identified easily but are never atypical. Inflammatory elements, such as foamy histiocytes and giant cells, are seen less commonly than in dermatofibroma, but lymphocytes often are scattered throughout the tumor proper (Fig. 6.29). When arising in bone, benign fibrous histiocytomas may mimic metaphyseal fibrous defect or giant cell tumor (Fig. 6.30). Meticulous attention to the clinical and radiographic features permits these distinctions.

Ancillary Studies

Immunohistochemically, benign fibrous histiocytoma of deep soft tissue shows no evidence of true histiocytic differentiation. Vimentin is always positive; variable reactivity is observed with smooth muscle actin. S-100 protein and desmin are negative.

Prognosis and Therapy

Deep benign fibrous histiocytoma is a benign lesion. Surgical resection is the recommended therapy. Local recurrence may occur in up to 33% of cases; however, distant metastasis has not been described.[55]

Benign fibrous histiocytoma of bone generally can be treated with simple curettage and bone grafting. En bloc resection may be necessary for lesions located in the ilium. Similar to its deep counterpart, local recurrence of benign fibrous histiocytoma of bone may occur.

Dermatofibrosarcoma Protuberans

Clinical Features

Dermatofibrosarcoma protuberans generally arises in adults 20 to 50 years old. Men and women are affected roughly equally.[57] Common anatomic locations include the trunk, groin, and lower extremities (Fig. 6.31). Less frequently, dermatofibrosarcoma protuberans may arise in the head and neck region. Origin in the palms of the hands, soles of the feet, or digits is extraordinarily rare. Patients typically present with exophytic, multinodular growths that are usually painless. When dermatofibrosarcoma protuberans occurs in children, a plaque-like growth pattern is typical.[58]

Pathologic Findings

Histology

Dermatofibrosarcoma protuberans is a poorly circumscribed lesion, usually originating in the dermis and often extending deep into the subcutis, entrapping adnexal structures and adipose tissue lobules. For unclear reasons, trails of adipocytes may extend into the upper dermis, unrelated solely to invasion of subcutaneous fat. Individual cells are remarkably uniform and appear ovoid with bland, round-to-ovoid nuclei and inconspicuous nucleoli. These cells often are arranged in prominent storiform patterns and short fascicles (Fig. 6.32). Background inflammatory cells, such as lymphocytes and histiocytes, are absent. Mitotic activity is usually not prominent (generally not exceeding 5 mitotic figures per 10 high-power fields). Bednar tumors are a variant of dermatofibrosarcoma protuberans containing scattered, heavily melanin-pigmented melanocytes.[59] The presence of these melanocytes has no clinical significance.

Transition forms between giant cell fibroblastoma, possibly a juvenile form of dermatofibrosarcoma protuberans, and classic dermatofibrosarcoma protuberans are well documented. Giant cell fibroblastoma may recur locally as a dermatofibrosarcoma protuberans and vice versa (Fig. 6.33).[60]

Fibrosarcomatous change in dermatofibrosarcoma protuberans is a relatively rare event and characterized by the presence of a cellular herringbone, fascicular growth pattern, associated with increased mitotic activity and cytologic atypia (Fig. 6.34).[61,62] Areas with pleomorphic tumor cells resembling malignant fibrous histiocytoma also may be evident. High-

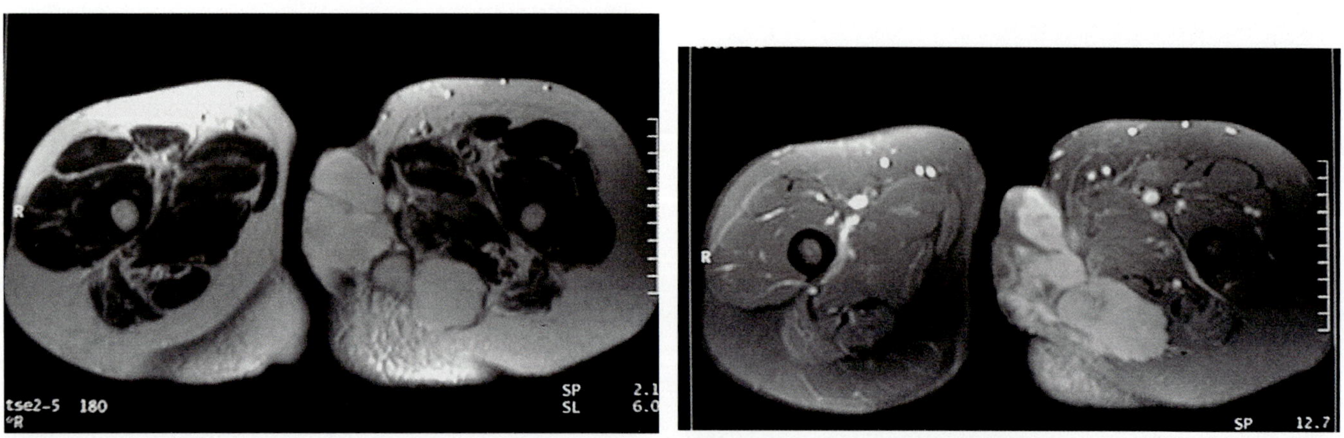

A B

FIGURE 6.31 Dermatofibrosarcoma protuberans. Axial T2-weighted **(A)** and fat-suppressed, gadolinium-enhanced T1-weighted **(B)** magnetic resonance images of the upper thighs show a large, heterogeneous, lobulated soft tissue mass extending from the posteromedial aspect of the hamstrings compartment of the thigh through the subcutaneous fat and projecting beyond the skin. The lesion enhances irregularly after gadolinium administration and is removed from the major neurovascular structures and the underlying femur.

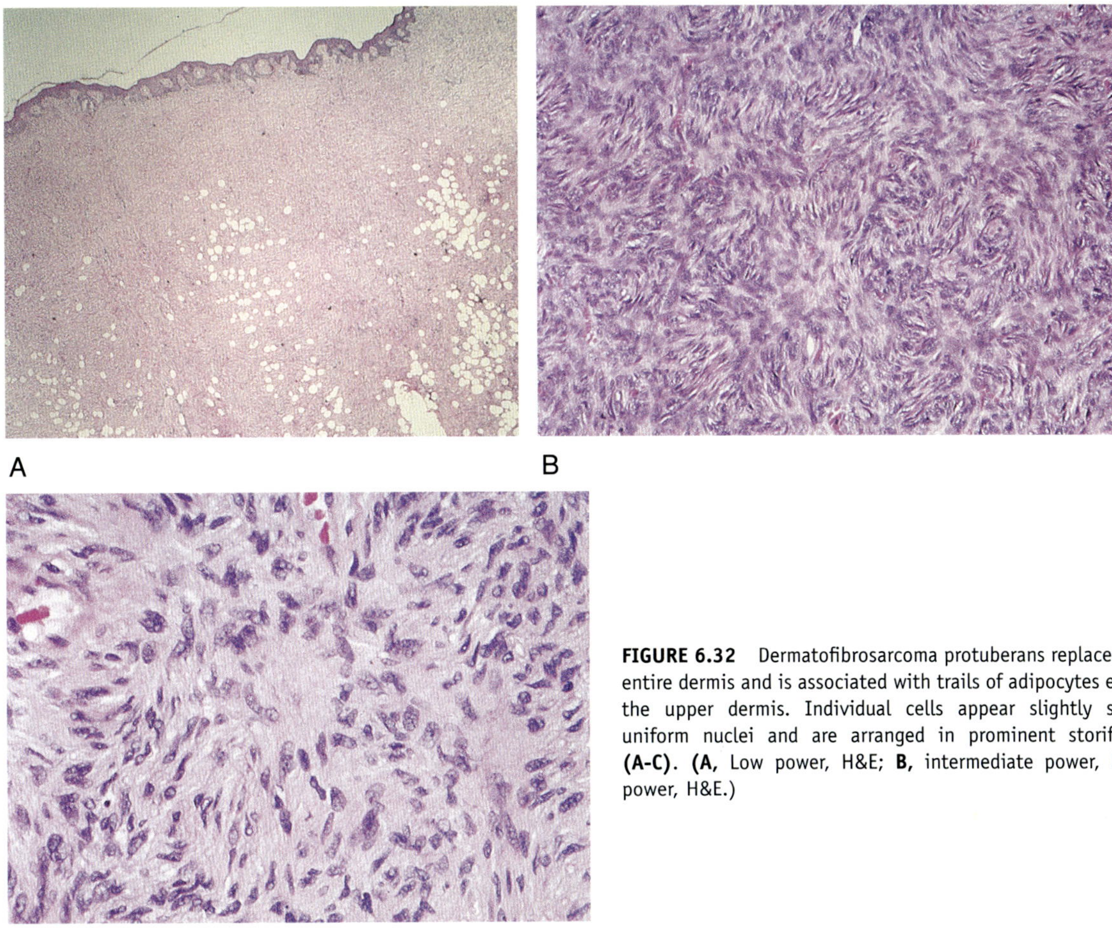

FIGURE 6.32 Dermatofibrosarcoma protuberans replaces virtually the entire dermis and is associated with trails of adipocytes extending into the upper dermis. Individual cells appear slightly spindled with uniform nuclei and are arranged in prominent storiform patterns **(A-C)**. **(A,** Low power, H&E; **B,** intermediate power, H&E; **C,** high power, H&E.)

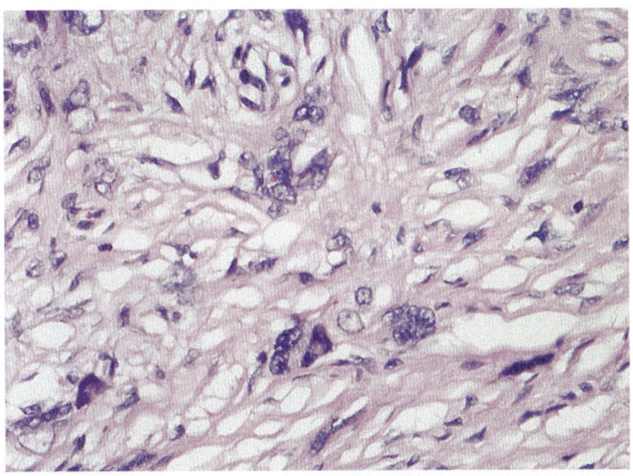

FIGURE 6.33 Giant cells, similar to cells observed with giant cell fibroblastoma, rarely are observed in dermatofibrosarcoma protuberans. (H&E.)

grade sarcomatous change is observed more often de novo among primary lesions and less frequently in recurrent ones.

Fine Needle Aspiration Biopsy

The diagnosis of dermatofibrosarcoma protuberans is difficult to render by FNAB analysis, but most cases are recognized as malignant. Cytologic features include tight cohesive clusters of uniform-appearing, spindled cells associated with a collagenous, metachromatic matrix. The classic storiform pattern is rarely recognizable, and ancillary studies are required for definitive diagnosis.[63]

Ancillary Studies

Ultrastructurally, individual tumor cells of dermatofibrosarcoma protuberans show features of fibroblasts, including dilated rough endoplasmic reticulum and extracellular collagen deposition. Most cases of dermatofibrosarcoma protuberans show diffuse and strong positivity for CD34 and vimentin. S-100 protein and smooth muscle actin expression are observed occasionally. Desmin, EMA, and cytokeratin are typically negative. When fibrosarcomatous change occurs, the high-grade sarcomatous portion is often negative for CD34.[61,62] Using cytogenetic analysis, dermatofibrosarcoma protuberans and giant cell fibroblastoma frequently show translocations of chromosomes 17 and 22 with the *COL1A1/PDGFB* fusion product, providing further evidence of a close kinship.[64,65]

Prognosis and Therapy

Wide surgical resection with negative margins is the therapy of choice. The most significant prognostic indicators in

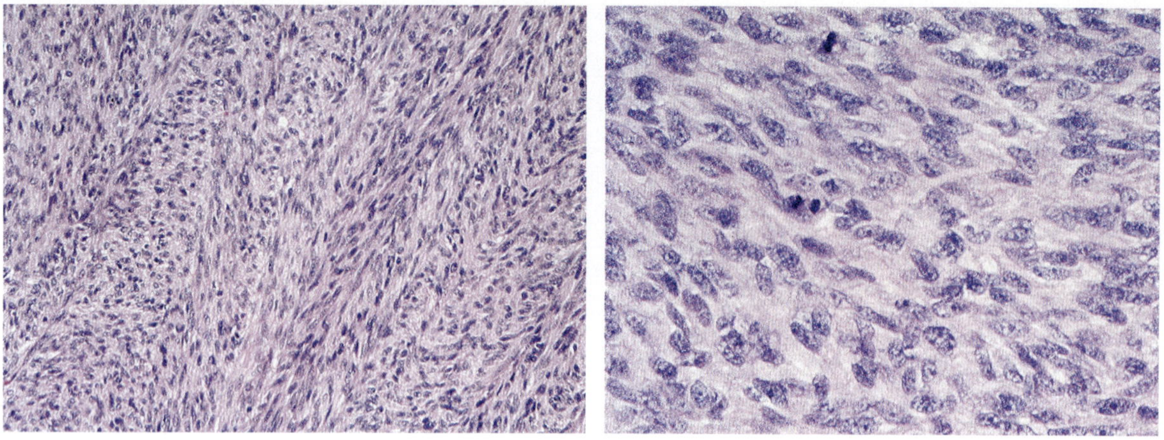

A B

FIGURE 6.34 Fibrosarcomatous change in dermatofibrosarcoma protuberans with long, intersecting fascicles of tumor cells with cytologic atypia and a high mitotic rate **(A** and **B)**. **(A,** Low power, H&E; **B,** high power, H&E.)

dermatofibrosarcoma protuberans seem to be the adequacy of surgical margin and the presence of fibrosarcomatous change. When fibrosarcomatous change occurs, local recurrence can be expected in approximately 50% to 60% of patients, and 5% to 15% of patients develop distant metastases.[57,61] Among 18 patients, all of whom were treated with wide local excision, however, Goldblum and colleagues[62] did not find an increased risk of distant metastasis within 5 years of clinical follow-up.

Adult Fibrosarcoma

Over the past several decades, the term *fibrosarcoma* has been used for a variety of sarcoma subtypes that, using modern ancillary techniques, we now recognize as distinct entities. Most commonly, areas of fibrosarcoma-like herringbone patterns may be observed in malignant peripheral nerve sheath tumor and monophasic fibrous synovial sarcoma. For this reason, the diagnosis of adult fibrosarcoma has become rare, representing a diagnosis of exclusion.

Clinical Features

Adult fibrosarcoma is seen most commonly in middle-aged to older adults. The deep soft tissues of the extremities and trunk/retroperitoneum are the most common anatomic sites (Fig. 6.35).[66] Most patients present with painless soft tissue swelling.

Fibrosarcoma of bone occurs over a broad age range, and, in contrast to osteosarcoma, there is no predilection for the second decade of life. Men and women appear to be affected equally. Most cases involve the bones around the knee and pelvis. More specifically, the most common anatomic locations in decreasing order of frequency are the distal femur, proximal tibia, ilium, and mandible. Clinical symptoms include pain and soft tissue swelling over the affected bone.[67]

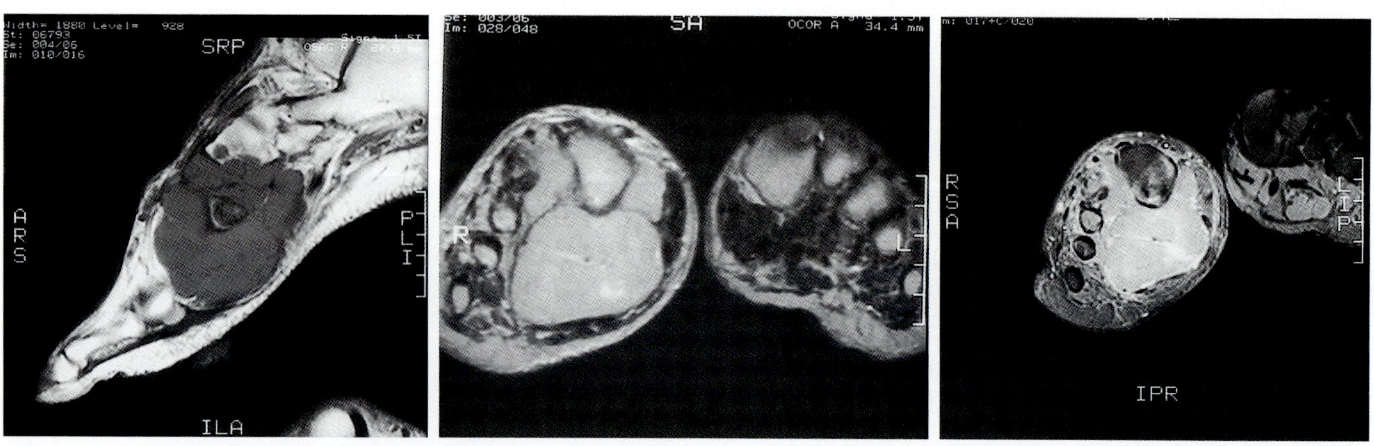

A B C

FIGURE 6.35 Fibrosarcoma. Sagittal T1-weighted **(A)**, coronal T2-weighted **(B)**, and coronal fat-suppressed T1-weighted, gadolinium-enhanced **(C)** magnetic resonance images of the foot show a large, enhancing soft tissue mass arising in the plantar soft tissues of the foot and extending medial and lateral to the first metatarsal shaft.

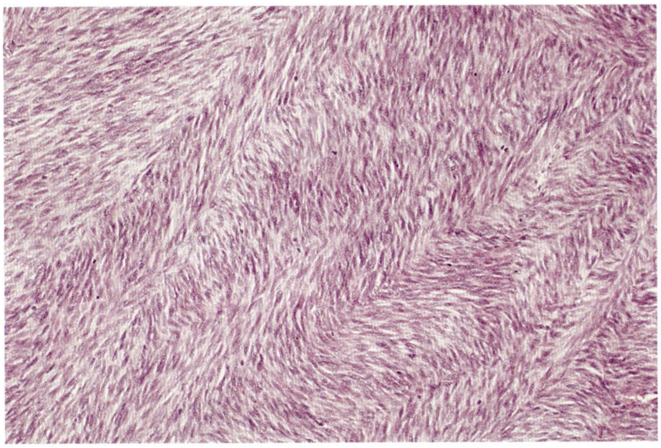

FIGURE 6.36 Classic fibrosarcoma with cellular intersecting fascicles creating the "herringbone" pattern. (H&E.)

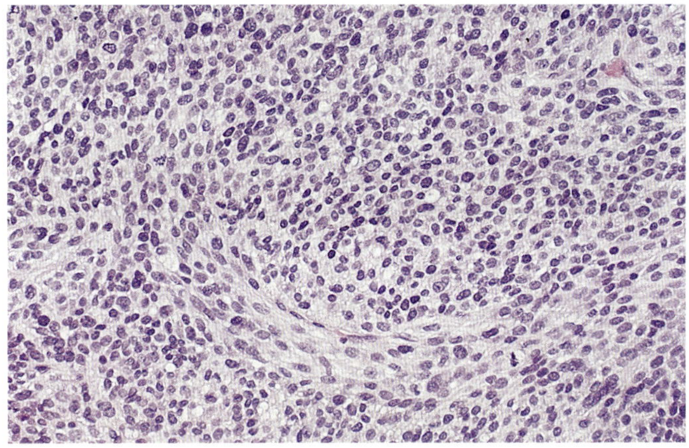

FIGURE 6.38 Rare examples of fibrosarcoma are composed of more rounded tumor cells resembling Ewing's sarcoma. The presence of even focal spindling of the tumor cells excludes the diagnosis of Ewing's sarcoma. (H&E.)

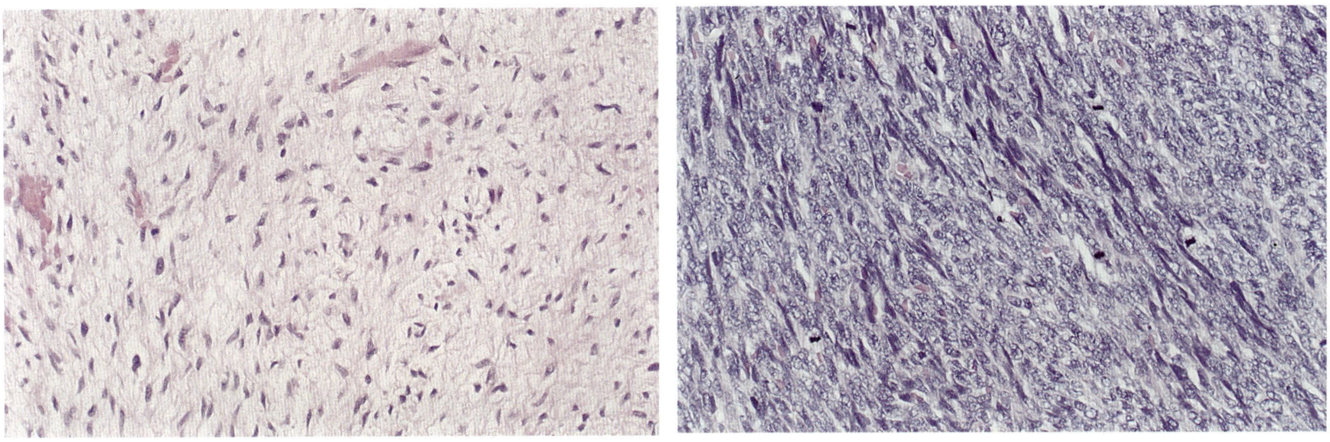

A B

FIGURE 6.37 Fibrosarcomas range from low-grade, less cellular and more collagenized lesions **(A)** to higher grade, hypercellular forms with a high mitotic index **(B)**. Although the neoplastic cells appear obviously malignant, significant nuclear pleomorphism, as observed in so-called malignant fibrous histiocytoma, is not present. (**A** and **B**, H&E.)

Fibrosarcomas may arise from pre-existing bone conditions, including fibrous dysplasia, Paget's disease, irradiated bone, and chronic osteomyelitis.

Pathologic Findings

Histology

Microscopically, adult fibrosarcomas are typically hypercellular, high-grade lesions composed of fascicles of spindle cells arranged in a herringbone pattern (Fig. 6.36). Collagen production may be abundant in less cellular, lower grade lesions, making distinction from desmoid tumor or desmoplastic fibroma difficult (Fig. 6.37). Cytologically the cells of fibrosarcoma range from typical, elongated, fibroblastic nuclei to short, blunted nuclei that may focally resemble Ewing's sarcoma. The presence of even a minor spindled component excludes the latter (Fig. 6.38), however. Marked nuclear pleomorphism and tumor giant cells are absent in adult fibrosarcoma. Osteoclast-type giant cells may be seen but are rarely numerous. Mitotic figures are usually abundant and often atypical, especially in the higher grade forms. The absence of osseous matrix production in fibrosarcoma is the only reliable feature separating it from fibroblastic osteosarcoma.

Ancillary Studies

Ultrastructurally, fibrosarcomas show features of fibroblasts with dilated and prominent rough endoplasmic reticulum and only rarely contain intermediate filaments. Immunohistochemically, diffuse positivity for vimentin is the only consistent finding; focal positivity for smooth muscle actin is observed occasionally. The latter may reflect a minor degree of myofibroblastic differentiation. Cytokeratin and S-100 protein are typically negative.

Prognosis and Therapy

Adverse prognostic factors include large tumor size, histologic grade, and localization within deep soft tissue. The risk of local recurrence seems related to the adequacy of surgical resection. Wide surgical resection is the therapy of choice. High-grade lesions arising within bone may be treated similar to osteosarcoma with preoperative chemotherapy and limb-salvage resection, when feasible.

Angioleiomyoma (Vascular Leiomyoma)

Clinical Features

Angioleiomyoma occurs in adults 30 to 50 years old. Men are affected more frequently than women. The most common anatomic site is the extremities, especially the lower extremities (Fig. 6.39).[68,69] Less frequently, angioleiomyomas occur in the head and neck and trunk regions. In contrast to most soft tissue tumors, angioleiomyomas are frequently painful subcutaneous or deep dermal lesions.

Pathologic Findings

Histology

Most angioleiomyomas are well-circumscribed lesions, generally measuring less than 2 cm in greatest dimension. The tumors are composed predominantly of interlacing fascicles of mature, well-differentiated smooth muscle cells with uniform ovoid to cigar-shaped nuclei and abundant tapering eosinophilic cytoplasm (Fig. 6.40). Vascular channels (angiomatoid component) range from slit-like and inconspicuous to dilated and cavernous to thick and muscular walled (Fig. 6.41). Mitotic figures usually are not identified. Similar to other smooth muscle tumors, areas of hyalinization and dystrophic microcalcifications are seen frequently.[68]

Ancillary Studies

As expected, angioleiomyomas show immunoexpression for vimentin, smooth muscle actin, and desmin. HMB45 and S-100 protein are usually negative. Although data are limited, no reproducible chromosomal abnormality has been observed in angioleiomyoma.[70,71]

Prognosis and Therapy

Angioleiomyoma is a completely benign lesion. Simple excision is the therapy of choice, and local recurrence is extraordinarily rare. Distant metastasis has not been documented.

Leiomyoma of Deep Soft Tissues and Bone

Clinical Features

Leiomyoma of deep soft tissue usually arises in young to middle-aged adults; there is no sex predilection.[72] The

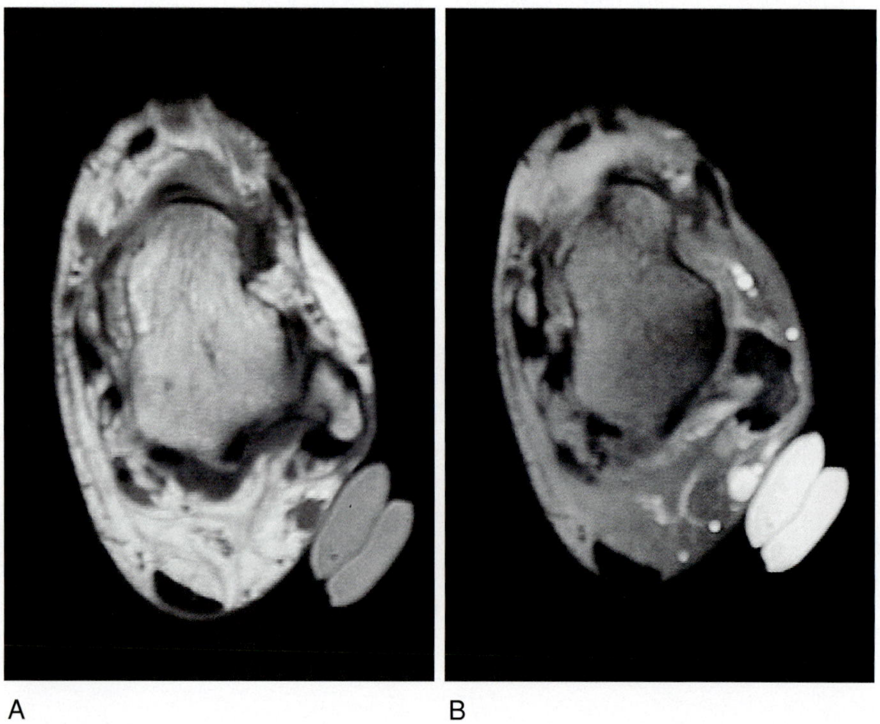

FIGURE 6.39 Angioleiomyoma. Axial proton density **(A)** and fat-suppressed, gadolinium-enhanced T1-weighted **(B)** magnetic resonance images of the ankle reveal a small, subcutaneous lesion posterior to the fibula. The lesion enhances intensely after the administration of gadolinium. The lobulated, hyperintense masses overlying the area are vitamin E capsules placed on the skin at the time of magnetic resonance imaging.

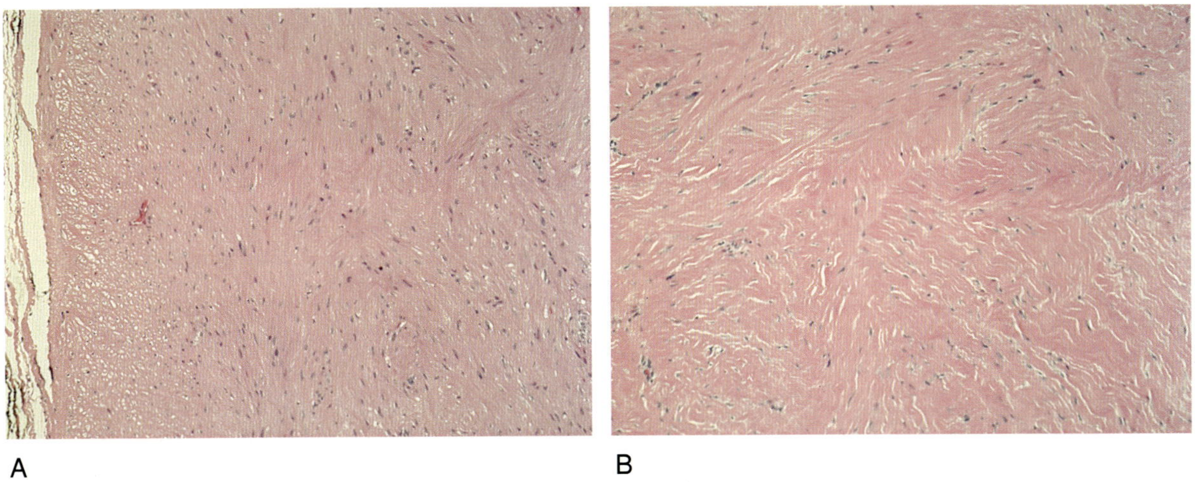

FIGURE 6.40 Angioleiomyomas are well-circumscribed lesions predominantly composed of benign, mature-appearing smooth muscle cells **(A** and **B)**. **(A,** Low power, H&E; **B,** high power, H&E.)

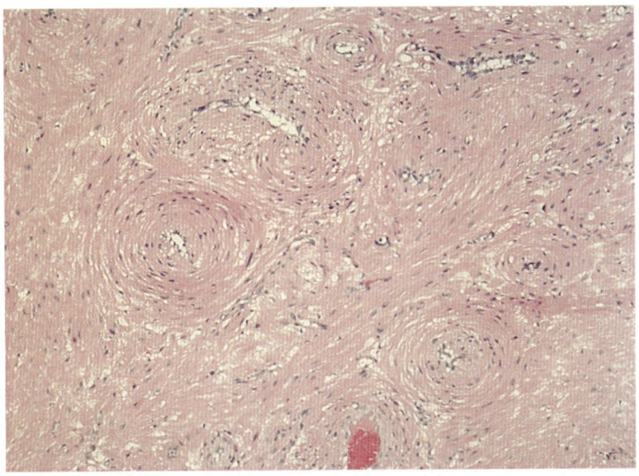

FIGURE 6.41 The finding of blood vessels, ranging from inconspicuous and slit-like to large and muscular-walled, is diagnostic of angioleiomyoma. (H&E.)

extremities are the most common anatomic location, followed by the pelvis and retroperitoneum. Diagnosis of the latter depends on tumors being clearly distinct from the uterus.[73] Painless soft tissue swelling is the most common clinical complaint. Intra-abdominal tumors may be associated with intestinal obstruction and/or urinary symptoms.[74]

Leiomyoma arising in bone is an extraordinarily rare, controversial lesion. We have never encountered a bona fide example. The skull and craniofacial region, especially the mandible, is the most common reported anatomic site.[75] Patients typically present with pain. Radiographically, leiomyomas of bone are usually lytic and geographic, with or without a sclerotic rim.

Pathologic Findings

Histology

Leiomyomas of deep soft tissue are typically well-circumscribed lesions that may range from small tumors (2 cm) to huge abdominal masses, measuring 37 cm in greatest dimension.[74] They typically are composed of well-differentiated and mature smooth muscle cells, containing ovoid to blunt-ended, cigar-shaped nuclei and abundant tapering eosinophilic cytoplasm, arranged in interlacing fascicles and bundles, often intersecting at perpendicular angles (Fig. 6.42). Virtually no nuclear pleomorphism is present, although some nuclei may appear enlarged with a smudgy chromatin pattern (ancient change). Mitotic activity is typically scant, with fewer than one mitosis per 50 high-power fields.[72,73] Degenerative changes, most prominent centrally within the lesion, are observed frequently and include extensive hyalinization, dystrophic microcalcifications, and myxoid areas (Fig. 6.43).

Fine Needle Aspiration Biopsy

FNAB of leiomyomas yields variably cellular smears with tumor cells arranged in loose clusters, tissue bundles, and fascicles. The neoplastic cells display uniform and elongated, cigar-shaped nuclei with blunted-to-pointed ends and abundant, variably vacuolated, dense cytoplasm.[76] Distinguishing low-grade leiomyosarcoma from leiomyoma may be difficult to impossible based on cytologic features alone. Although mitotic counts are essential for this separation in histologic specimens, their usefulness in cytologic preparations is severely limited. Nevertheless, we regard the presence of even a single mitotic figure in a deep soft tissue smooth muscle tumor as suggestive of malignancy.

Ancillary Studies

As expected, the ultrastructural features of leiomyoma are those of smooth muscle differentiation and include intracytoplasmic filaments with densities, cellular junctions, and basement membrane. Electron microscopy is generally not necessary to establish the diagnosis.

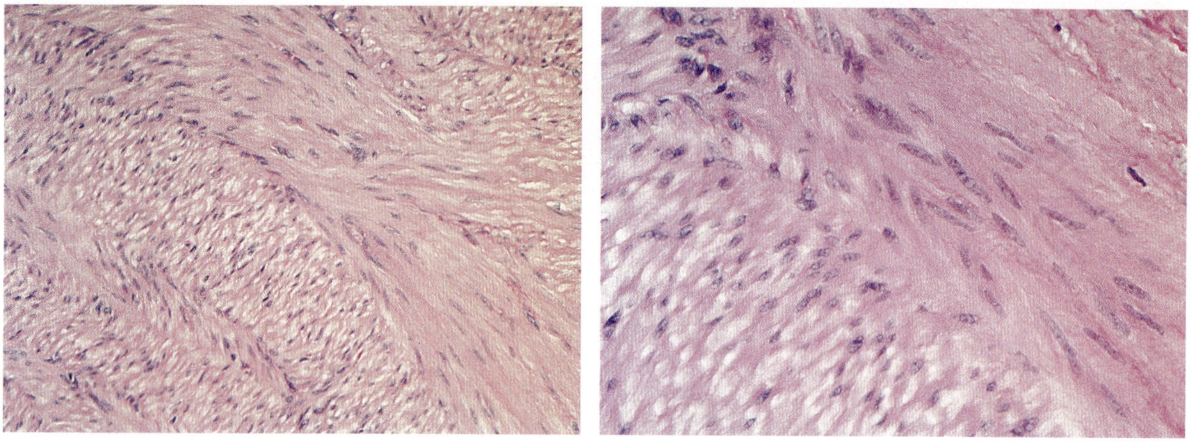

A B

FIGURE 6.42 Deep soft tissue leiomyomas are composed of well-differentiated, mature-appearing smooth muscle cells, containing ovoid to blunt-ended, cigar-shaped nuclei and abundant tapering eosinophilic cytoplasm, arranged in interlacing fascicles and bundles, often intersecting at perpendicular angles **(A** and **B)**. **(A,** Low power, H&E; **B,** high power, H&E.)

Immunohistochemically the tumor cells appear diffusely positive for vimentin and show at least focal positivity for actin, smooth muscle actin, and desmin. S-100 protein is typically negative. Intra-abdominal and retroperitoneal leiomyomas are frequently positive for estrogen and progesterone receptors, whereas tumors that arise in the deep somatic soft tissues of the extremities and trunk do not express these markers.[73,74]

Prognosis and Therapy

Complete excision of leiomyoma, regardless of anatomic site, usually results in cure. Local recurrence rarely is observed.

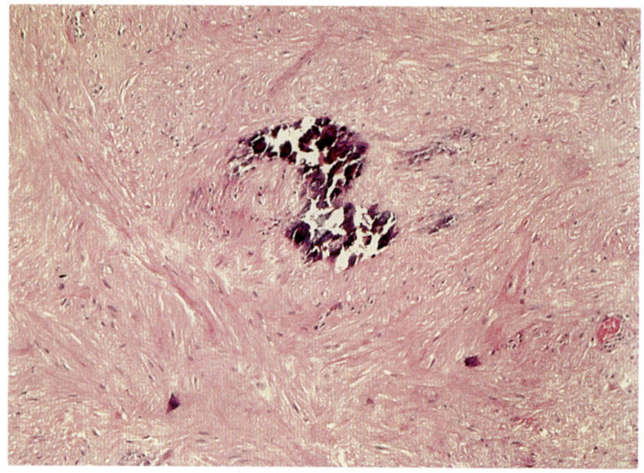

FIGURE 6.43 Hyalinization and dystrophic microcalcifications are frequent findings in deep soft tissue leiomyoma. (H&E.)

Leiomyosarcoma of Deep Soft Tissues and Bone

Leiomyosarcomas of soft tissue occur as three different forms—cutaneous, large blood vessel type (e.g., inferior vena cava), and deep somatic soft tissues.[77] For the purpose of this discussion, we focus on tumors occurring in deep soft tissues and include a brief discussion of the skeletal form.

Clinical Features

Leiomyosarcoma involving deep soft tissues generally occurs in middle-aged to older adults. The most common anatomic site is the retroperitoneum; many intra-abdominal forms seem to arise from large blood vessels, principally the inferior vena cava.[78] Large intramuscular veins of the extremities, principally of the lower limb, are a less frequent site of origin. When leiomyosarcomas arise within the retroperitoneum, women are affected more commonly than men. In other sites, this female predilection is not observed.[77] Leiomyosarcoma is seen rarely in children; the most common anatomic sites are the extremities followed by the trunk.[79] Most patients present with evidence of soft tissue swelling or mass effect.

Although leiomyosarcoma of bone may be found in patients over a broad age range, it is seen most commonly in patients older than age 20. There is no gender bias.[80] The bones around the knee (distal femur and proximal tibia) are the most common anatomic sites, followed in frequency by the craniofacial region. Most patients complain of localized pain with or without soft tissue swelling. A few cases develop as a complication of radiation therapy.[80] The radiographic features for leiomyosarcoma of bone are those of a lytic, poorly marginated defect usually within the metaphysis. Most cases show cortical destruction, periosteal reaction, and frequently soft tissue mass. Mineralization within the tumor is distinctly absent.

Pathologic Findings

Histology

At low power, leiomyosarcomas may appear deceptively circumscribed, exhibiting a whorled appearance. Fascicles and bundles of well-demarcated smooth muscle cells intersect at perpendicular angles (Fig. 6.44). Less frequent patterns include storiform arrangements, hemangiopericytoma-like vascular patterns, nuclear palisading (mimicking nerve sheath tumors), and myxoid changes (Fig. 6.45).[81] Large lesions frequently exhibit areas of hyalinization, dystrophic microcalcifications, or coagulative tumor necrosis (Fig. 6.46). Cytologically, individual tumor cells are spindled with elongated to cigar-shaped nuclei and abundant eosinophilic cytoplasm. Nuclear pleomorphism is variable, ranging from minimal to marked, indistinguishable from so-called malignant fibrous histiocytoma (Fig. 6.47). In low-grade tumors, mitotic figures may be scarce but tend to be found easily in higher grade cases. Unusual cytomorphologic features include epithelioid cytology, granular cytoplasmic changes, extensive cytoplasmic vacuolation, and abundant osteoclast-like giant cells.[82] Collections of rhabdoid cells are seen in approximately 5% of cases and may be associated with more aggressive clinical behavior.[83]

The distinction between low-grade leiomyosarcoma and leiomyoma may be difficult. Based on solid data and reported biologic outcome, we regard the presence of atypia and any level of mitotic activity as diagnostic of leiomyosarcoma.[72,77] By light microscopy, high-grade, pleomorphic leiomyosarcoma

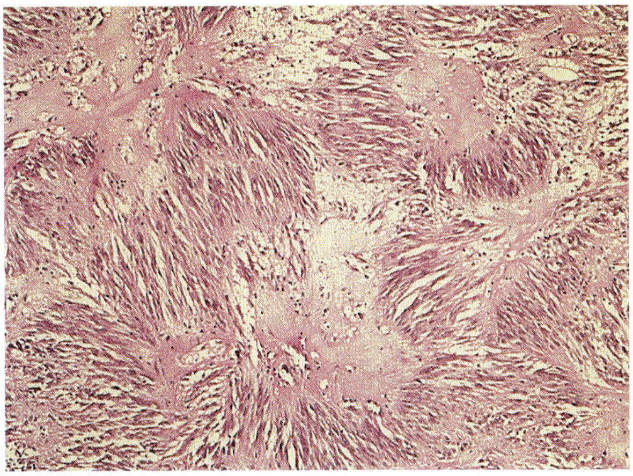

FIGURE 6.45 Rarely, leiomyosarcoma may exhibit nuclear palisading, mimicking a nerve sheath tumor. (H&E.)

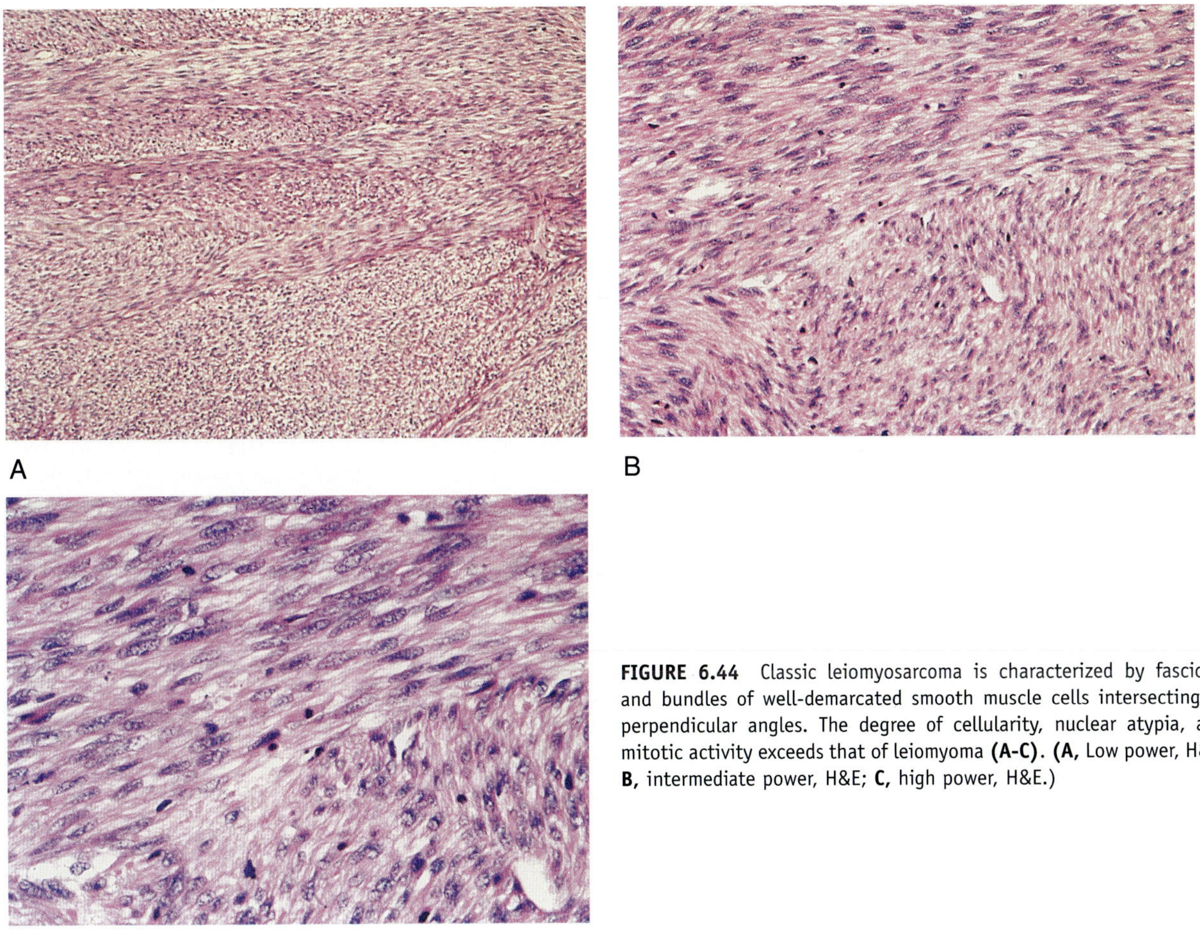

A

B

C

FIGURE 6.44 Classic leiomyosarcoma is characterized by fascicles and bundles of well-demarcated smooth muscle cells intersecting at perpendicular angles. The degree of cellularity, nuclear atypia, and mitotic activity exceeds that of leiomyoma **(A-C)**. **(A,** Low power, H&E; **B,** intermediate power, H&E; **C,** high power, H&E.)

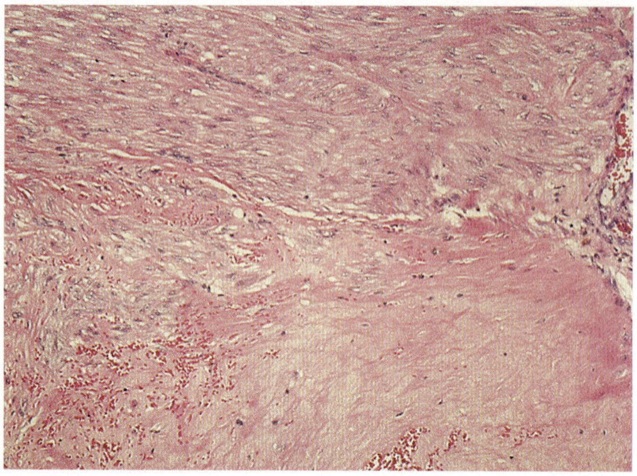

FIGURE 6.46 Areas of hyalinization are common in leiomyosarcoma. (H&E.)

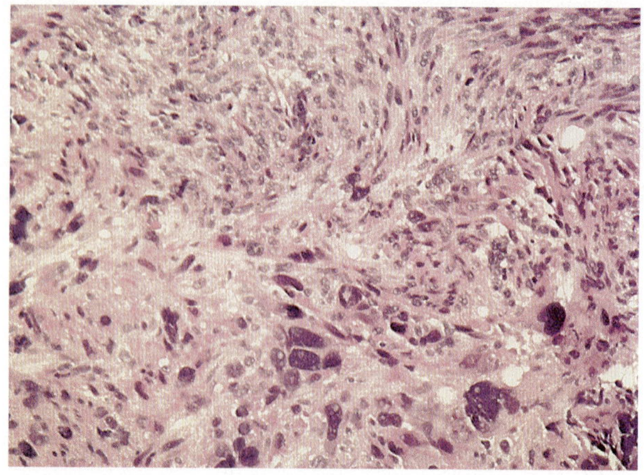

FIGURE 6.47 Occasionally, leiomyosarcoma may be composed of markedly pleomorphic tumor cells, resembling malignant fibrous histiocytoma (pleomorphic leiomyosarcoma). (H&E.)

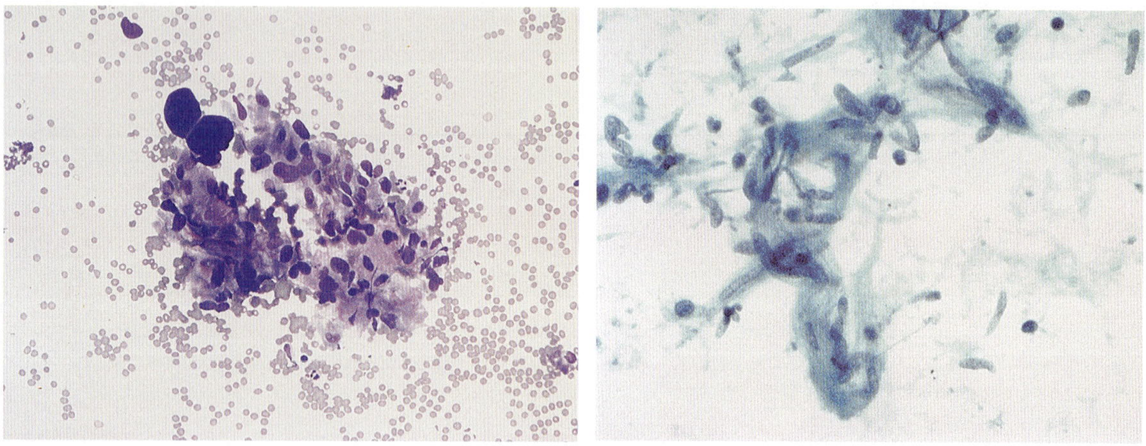

A B

FIGURE 6.48 In contrast to other sarcomas, fine needle aspiration biopsy of leiomyosarcoma generally yields cellular smears predominantly composed of cohesive clusters and aggregates of tumor cells. Nuclear atypia is variable, ranging from the typical, cigar-shaped nuclei to multinucleated tumor giant cells **(A** and **B)**. **(A,** Diff-Quik; **B,** Papanicolaou.)

may be indistinguishable from so-called malignant fibrous histiocytoma. To establish the diagnosis of pleomorphic leiomyosarcoma, we require the presence, at least focally, of definite leiomyosarcomatous fascicles and positivity for one or more muscle markers (e.g., actin, smooth muscle actin, or desmin).[84]

Fine Needle Aspiration Biopsy

FNAB specimens of leiomyosarcoma are variably cellular and, in contrast to other spindle cell sarcomas, are arranged more often in loose clusters, tissue bundles, and fascicles. Individually dispersed tumor cells are less commonly evident (Fig. 6.48). Tao and Davidson[76] documented that the presence of closely packed spindle-shaped tumor cells in "parallel side-by-side arrangements" suggests a diagnosis of leiomyosarcoma. The neoplastic cells typically have elongated, cigar-shaped, hyperchromatic nuclei with blunted-to-pointed ends and are surrounded by abundant dense to sometimes vacuolated cytoplasm. Solitary "stripped" or naked nuclei are observed commonly. Rarely, an epithelioid pattern may predominate, mimicking a carcinoma (Fig. 6.49). High-grade pleomorphic examples often are composed of discohesive solitary tumor cells displaying marked nuclear pleomorphism and accompanied by anaplastic tumor giant cells (Fig. 6.50). Without immunohistochemistry, pleomorphic leiomyosarcoma may be indistinguishable from other pleomorphic sarcomas, but this distinction does not influence therapy. In these cases, we typically render the diagnosis of pleomorphic sarcoma, not otherwise specified.[85]

Ancillary Studies

Ultrastructurally, leiomyosarcomas generally show at least focal evidence of smooth muscle differentiation, including abundant intermediate filaments with densities, pinocytotic vesicles, and

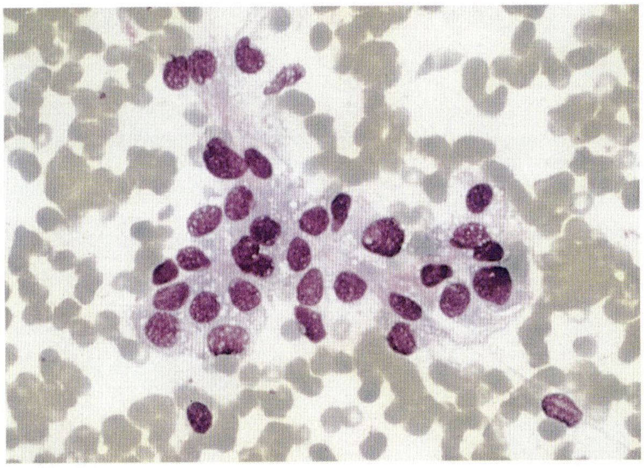

FIGURE 6.49 Rare examples of leiomyosarcoma may exhibit a predominantly epithelioid morphology, suggesting the diagnosis of carcinoma. (Diff-Quik.)

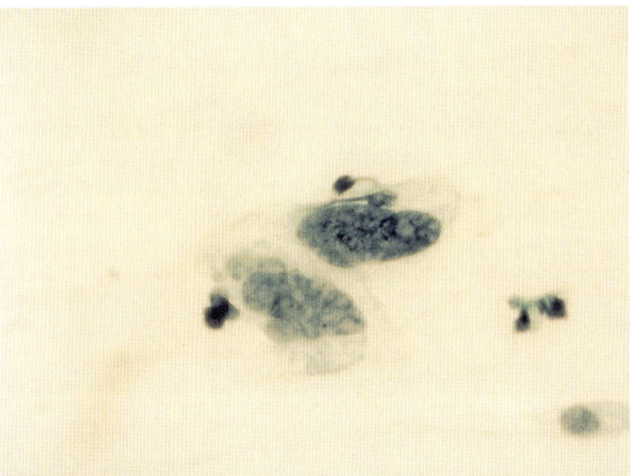

FIGURE 6.50 Some high-grade leiomyosarcomas consist virtually entirely of pleomorphic tumor cells. These cases are difficult to subtype specifically by fine needle aspiration biopsy and probably are best diagnosed as pleomorphic sarcoma, not otherwise specified. (Papanicolaou.)

cellular junctions. These structures may be difficult to demonstrate in more poorly differentiated examples.

Immunohistochemically, leiomyosarcomas are always positive for vimentin and generally express one or more markers of smooth muscle differentiation, including actin, smooth muscle actin, desmin, and h-caldesmon. Less frequently, focal positivity may be observed with S-100 protein, CD117, cytokeratin (rarely diffuse), and EMA.[79-81] Cytogenetic analyses of leiomyosarcomas have revealed complex karyotypic changes, but no specific chromosomal abnormality has been identified yet.[86]

Prognosis and Therapy

Adverse prognostic indicators for soft tissue leiomyosarcoma include localization within the retroperitoneum and large tumor size (>10 cm). In the extremities, older age (>62 years), FNCLCC grade 3, tumor size greater than 4 cm, localization in deep soft tissues, and disruption portend a worse clinical outcome.[77] Small, superficially located tumors arising within the extremities are more amenable to surgical resection and less likely to recur locally. Leiomyosarcomas arising in children are almost always low-grade neoplasms, generally curable by complete resection.[79]

The prognosis of primary leiomyosarcoma of bone tends to be poor. The most important prognostic indicator appears to be histologic grade, and most are high-grade neoplasms. Approximately 50% of patients with high-grade leiomyosarcoma of bone develop metastases within 5 years of diagnosis; additionally, approximately 40% of patients die as a result of this disease.[80] Wide surgical resection, including limb-salvage resection or amputation, is the therapy of choice for deep soft tissue and bone leiomyosarcomas. The role of chemotherapy at this time has not been well established.

Schwannoma (Neurilemoma)

Nerve sheath tumors, especially benign forms, are fairly common neoplasms occurring in virtually all anatomic compartments and sites. Outside of neurofibromatosis, most deep-seated, benign nerve sheath lesions are schwannomas (neurilemomas); neurofibromas generally present as solitary cutaneous masses and rarely are observed within the deep soft tissues of the extremities, thorax, or abdomen.

Clinical Features

Schwannomas may arise at any age, but most occur between ages 20 and 50 years.[87] There is no gender bias. Most tumors are solitary and develop on the peripheral nerves of the extremities and head and neck region (Fig. 6.51). Other common anatomic sites include the posterior mediastinum and retroperitoneum (Fig. 6.52).[88] The majority of schwannomas are solitary and sporadic; approximately 3% are multiple and associated with neurofibromatosis type 2, and 2% are multiple (schwannomatosis) and not associated with neurofibromatosis type 2.[89] Patients typically present with slow-growing tumors often associated with pain and neurologic symptoms. Schwannomas arising in the sinonasal tract and nasopharynx may be associated with headache, nasal obstruction, epistaxis, rhinorrhea, or otitis media.[90]

Neurofibromatosis type 2 is much rarer than the more common neurofibromatosis type 1 disease. Both types are inherited as an autosomal dominant trait, however, and have a high rate of penetrance. The gene for neurofibromatosis type 2 is located on chromosome 22. Most patients present in adolescence or as young adults, complaining of loss of hearing and/or tinnitus, secondary to the development of bilateral acoustic (vestibular) schwannomas. These patients are also at risk of developing cutaneous schwannomas, gliomas, meningiomas, and ependymomas. Patients with multiple schwannomas in the absence of bilateral acoustic schwannomas now are considered to have a separate disorder, schwannomatosis.

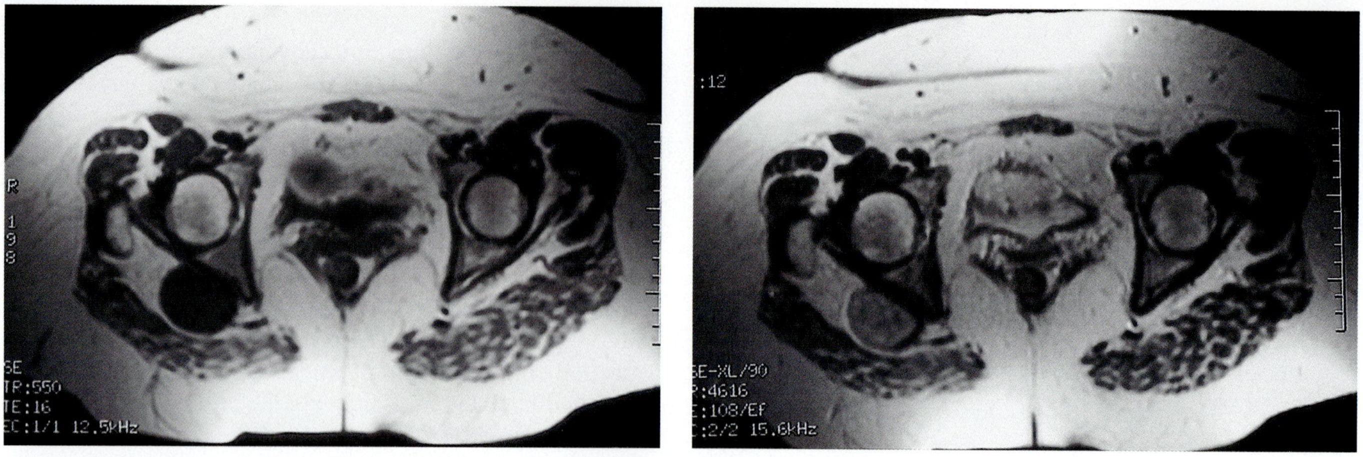

A

B

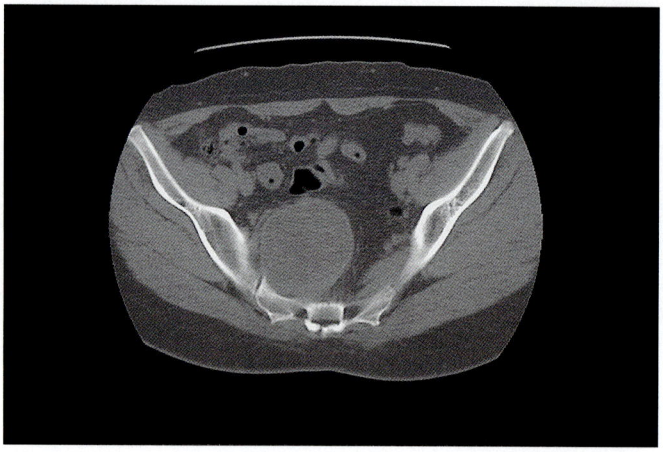

C

FIGURE 6.51 Schwannoma. Axial T1-weighted **(A)** and T2-weighted **(B)** magnetic resonance images reveal a well-defined, rounded soft tissue mass posterior to the right ischium arising from the sciatic nerve. In another patient, computed tomographic scan of the pelvis **(C)** shows a large, homogeneous soft tissue mass anterior to the sacroiliac joint on the right.

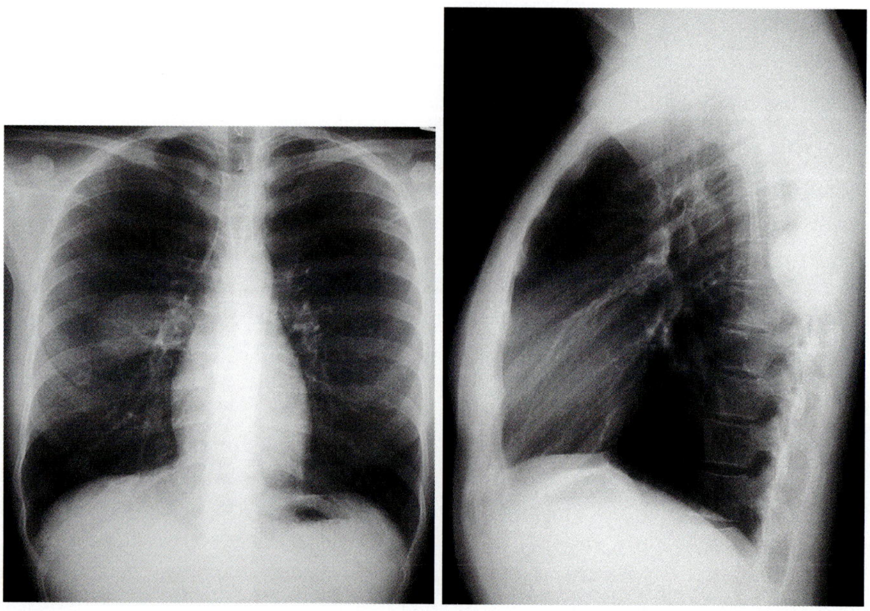

A B

FIGURE 6.52 Schwannoma. Posteroanterior **(A)** and lateral **(B)** radiographs of the chest show a rounded soft tissue mass in the posterior right hemithorax arising from the seventh intercostal nerve.

Primary schwannoma of bone is an extraordinarily rare lesion and is found in patients over a broad age range. Females are afflicted slightly more often than males. The most common anatomic location is the mandible, possibly related to the presence of the mental nerve.[91] Other common locations include the distal femur, scapula, ribs, sacrum, and skull. Most patients are asymptomatic at diagnosis. Radiographically, intraosseous schwannomas have a distinctly benign, lytic appearance, with sharply defined margins and focal sclerosis. In the long bones, metaphyseal localization is common. Nonosseous schwannomas secondarily involving bone (pressure necrosis), especially when originating from spinal nerve roots, are far more common than their skeletal counterparts.

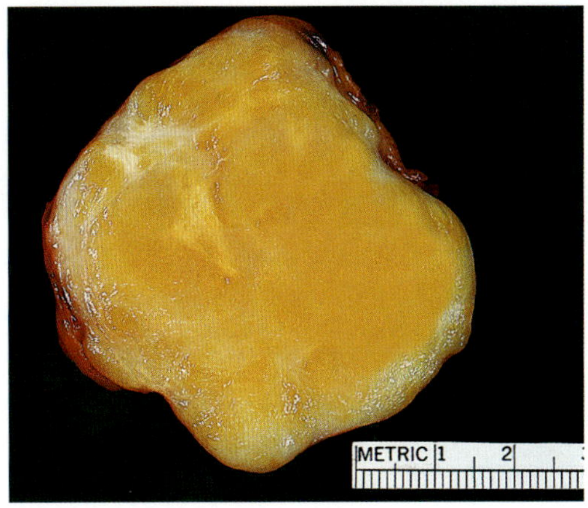

FIGURE 6.53 Schwannomas appear grossly well circumscribed with variable amounts of yellow and white discoloration, depending on the lipid content.

Pathologic Findings

Histology

Schwannomas are well-circumscribed, encapsulated masses that usually arise as eccentric, sometimes dumbbell-shaped lesions of peripheral nerve (Fig. 6.53). As previously mentioned, they are only rarely cutaneous and almost always solitary. Residual nerve fibers may be seen at the periphery of the tumor adjacent to the capsule. Encapsulation may be less evident or lacking altogether in schwannomas arising in the sinonasal tract and nasopharynx.[90] Microscopically, the histologic hallmark of schwannomas is the presence of alternating Antoni A (cellular and compact spindle cell proliferation arranged in bundles and intersecting fascicles) and Antoni B (hypocellular spindle cell proliferation arranged haphazardly within a loose matrix) regions. In the Antoni A areas, the spindle cells often align in a linear fashion, producing the so-called Verocay bodies. Microcystic change and inflammatory cells are usually evident in the Antoni B zones. Another helpful feature is the presence of hyalinized blood vessels and variable numbers of lipid-laden macrophages (Fig. 6.54). Cytologically, the Schwann cell nuclei are generally small and hyperchromatic and have a wavy-to-serpentine appearance. Atypia in the form of ancient change is often present and may be widespread, but the degree of atypia exceeds the expected mitotic activity, which in degenerative schwannomas is virtually absent (Fig. 6.55). As a general rule, the diagnosis of malignancy should be avoided in any spindle cell tumor with moderate-to-marked atypia but a correspondingly low mitotic rate.

An additional diagnostic pitfall is "cellular" schwannoma, a tumor consisting predominantly (or exclusively) of Antoni A areas and lacking diagnostic Verocay bodies (Fig. 6.56).[88] Mitotic activity may be high, and focal necrosis is observed occasionally. Helpful diagnostic clues include circumscription, the presence of hyalinized blood vessels, and strong and diffuse S-100 protein positivity. Cellular schwannomas are seen more commonly in the paravertebral region of the mediastinum, retroperitoneum, and pelvis.[88]

Less frequently, schwannomas undergo cystic changes; the cysts are likely a degenerative phenomenon but may be lined by more rounded-appearing Schwann cells, imparting a pseudoglandular appearance (Fig. 6.57). Rarely, epithelial glands and neuroblastoma-like rosettes also have been documented.[92]

Compared with neurofibromas, malignant transformation of schwannomas is an extraordinarily rare event. Such tumors are commonly epithelioid, most often resembling malignant peripheral nerve sheath tumor or angiosarcoma, and frequently fatal.[93,94] The presence of large epithelioid cells with abundant eosinophilic cytoplasm within otherwise classic schwannoma may represent a precursor lesion for malignant transformation.[93]

Fine Needle Aspiration Biopsy

In most cases, FNAB is extraordinarily useful for the differential diagnosis of benign nerve sheath tumor versus malignant peripheral nerve sheath tumor. Cytologic smears from schwannomas are often cellular; however, the cells usually are arranged as cohesive cellular tissue aggregates or ropy bundles, containing the cytoplasmic processes of the individual Schwann cells (Fig. 6.58).[95] Morphologically, the tumor cells are spindled with wavy-to-serpentine nuclei and may show significant atypia (ancient change) (Fig. 6.59). Mitotic activity is virtually never observed. Nuclear palisading is a helpful but uncommon finding in cytologic preparations (Fig. 6.60).

Ancillary Studies

The ultrastructural features of schwannoma are essentially those of Schwann cells, consisting of plump, spindled cells with long cytoplasmic processes. The tumor cell bodies and processes are coated by a distinct external basal lamina associated with long spacing collagen (Luse bodies).

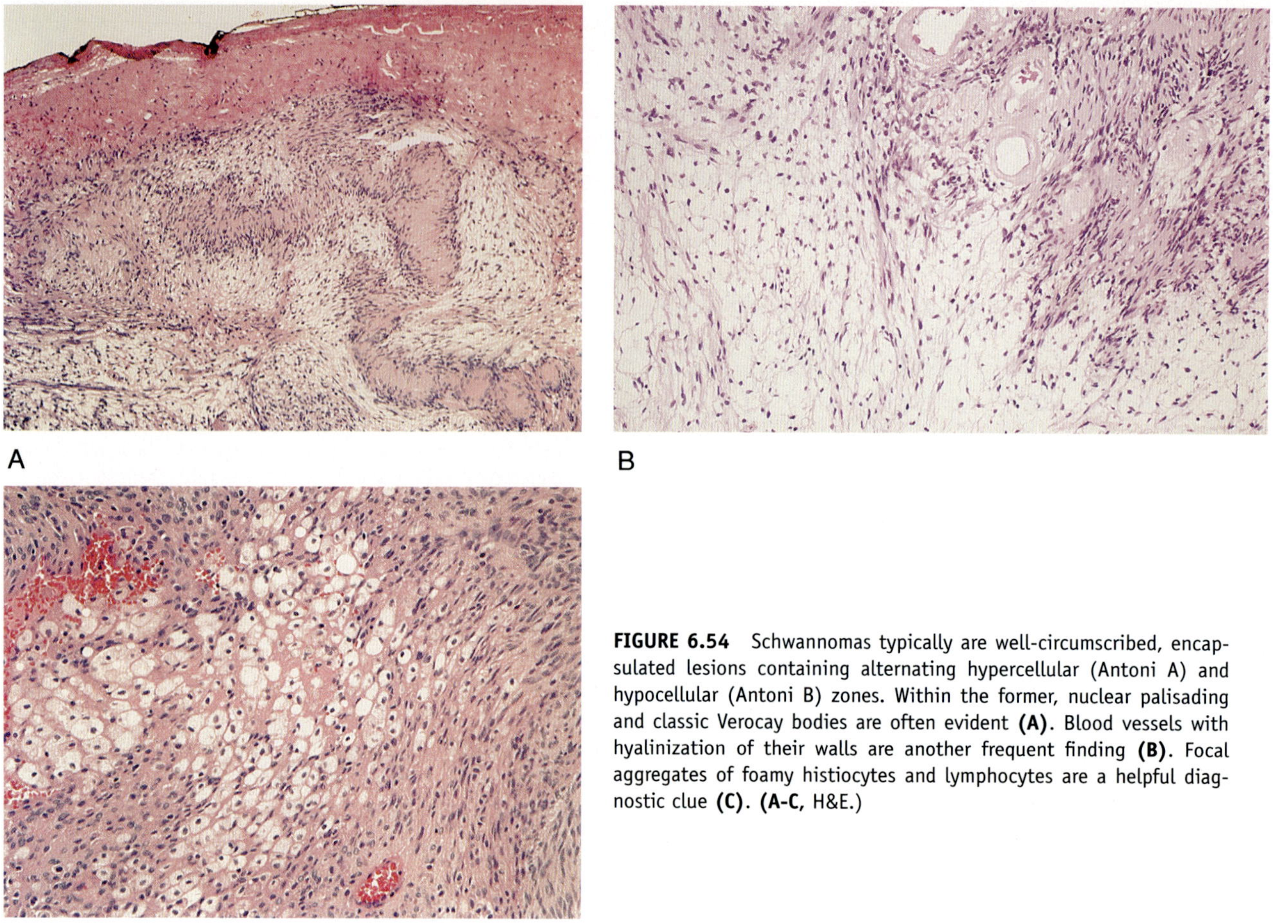

A

B

C

FIGURE 6.54 Schwannomas typically are well-circumscribed, encapsulated lesions containing alternating hypercellular (Antoni A) and hypocellular (Antoni B) zones. Within the former, nuclear palisading and classic Verocay bodies are often evident **(A)**. Blood vessels with hyalinization of their walls are another frequent finding **(B)**. Focal aggregates of foamy histiocytes and lymphocytes are a helpful diagnostic clue **(C)**. **(A-C,** H&E.)

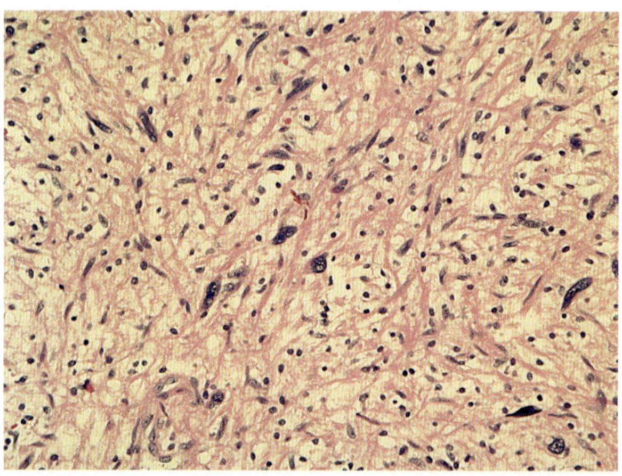

FIGURE 6.55 Ancient change in schwannomas with enlarged Schwann cell nuclei that appear smudgy and hyperchromatic. These atypical features are of no prognostic significance. (H&E.)

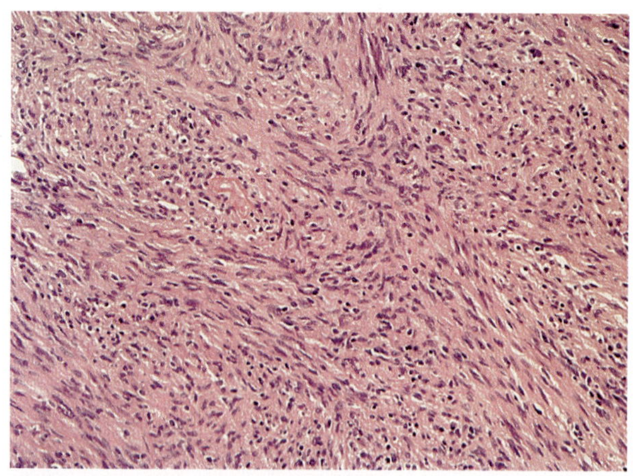

FIGURE 6.56 Cellular schwannomas essentially consist of only Antoni A. The presence of encapsulation and hyalinized blood vessels helps establish the diagnosis. (H&E.)

Strong and diffuse nuclear and cytoplasmic staining for S-100 protein is a hallmark of schwannoma; patchy and focal staining for S-100 protein is more typical of malignant peripheral nerve sheath tumor.[97] Among cases of malignant peripheral nerve sheath tumor, up to 50% may be negative for S-100 protein. For these reasons, a spindle cell lesion with "borderline" malignant features that is strongly and diffusely S-100 protein positive is probably not malignant. Such a tumor is far more likely to represent schwannoma than a malignant peripheral nerve sheath tumor. Anaplastic and malignant tumors that are strongly and diffusely S-100 protein positive are far more likely to represent melanoma than malignant peripheral nerve sheath tumor. Schwannomas also express Leu-7 and occasionally glial fibrillary acidic protein. CD34

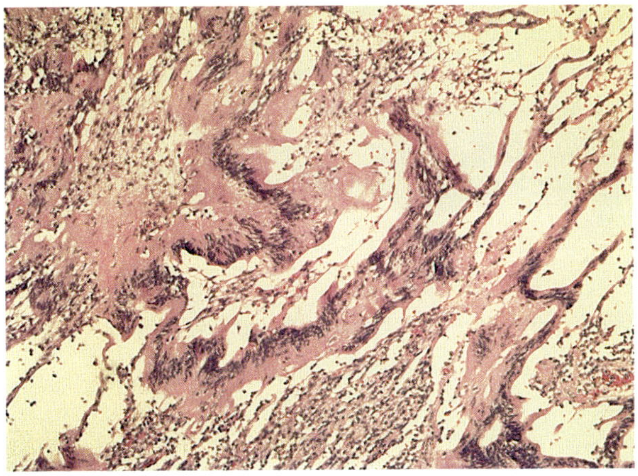

FIGURE 6.57 Cystic changes in schwannomas sometimes are characterized by palisading of Schwann cell nuclei along the cyst wall lining, creating a pseudoglandular appearance. (H&E.)

decorates a population of scattered, probably reactive "non-schwannian" cells, most obvious in the Antoni B regions.[98]

Clonal chromosomal aberrations are observed frequently in schwannoma. Documented recurrent aberrations include loss of 22q material, loss of a sex chromosome, and trisomy 7.[99]

Prognosis and Therapy

Schwannomas are benign lesions and generally cured by local excision. Local recurrence is rare and appears slightly more likely to occur (<5% of cases) in the cellular variant.[88] Metastasis has not been documented.

Psammomatous Melanotic Schwannoma

Psammomatous melanotic schwannoma is a rare tumor that most commonly arises from posterior spinal nerve roots, alimentary tract, and, less frequently, bone.[100,101] Most patients are 15 to 40 years old at diagnosis. Up to 55% of patients have Carney's syndrome—myxomas, spotty cutaneous pigmentation, and endocrine overactivity (Cushing's syndrome).[100] Common complaints include pain and neurologic deficits. Microscopically, the tumors are well circumscribed but incompletely encapsulated and show heavy brown-black melanin pigmentation. Individual cells range from epithelioid/polygonal to spindled and may exhibit whorls and nuclear palisading. Nuclei are ovoid to round and vesicular

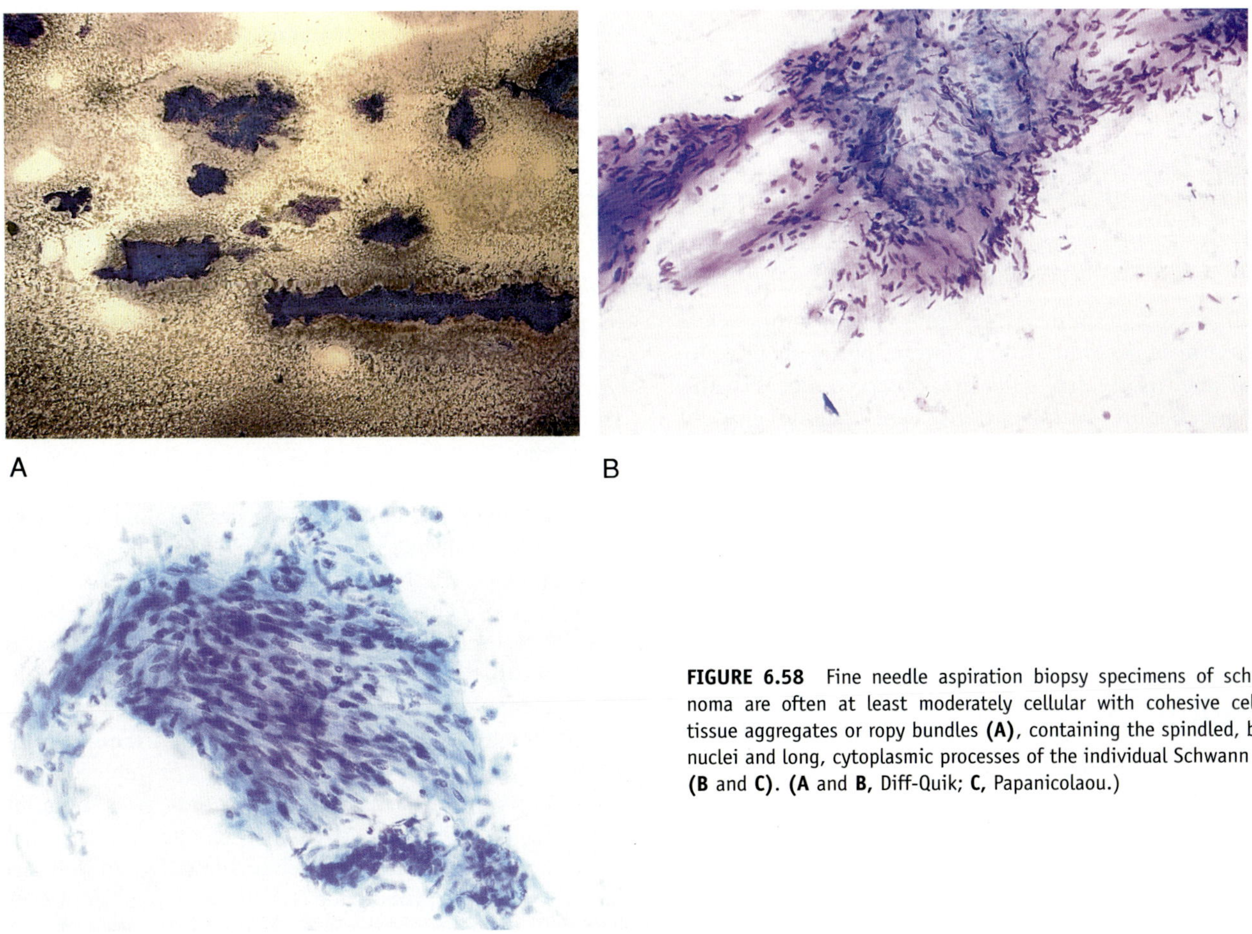

A

B

C

FIGURE 6.58 Fine needle aspiration biopsy specimens of schwannoma are often at least moderately cellular with cohesive cellular tissue aggregates or ropy bundles **(A)**, containing the spindled, bland nuclei and long, cytoplasmic processes of the individual Schwann cells **(B** and **C)**. **(A** and **B,** Diff-Quik; **C,** Papanicolaou.)

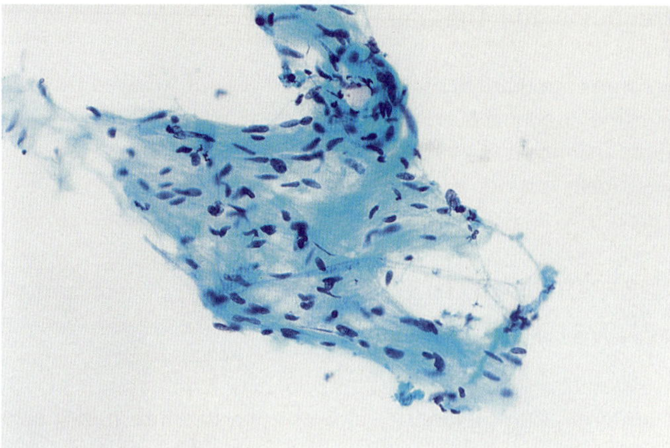

A

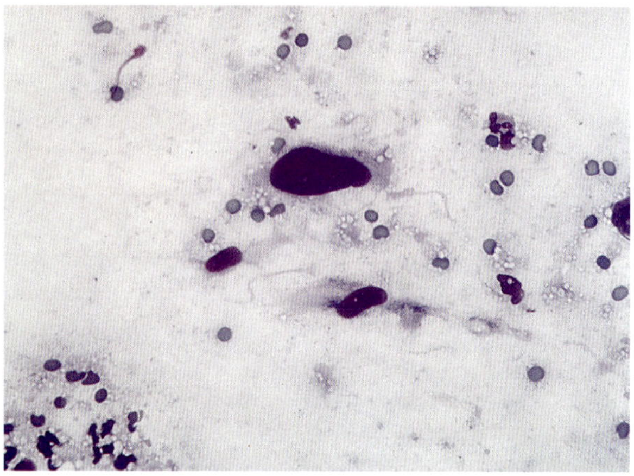

B

FIGURE 6.59 Cytologically, schwannomas generally show spindled to slightly wavy, uniform, and hyperchromatic nuclei **(A)**. Occasional examples exhibit larger cells with a smudgy chromatin pattern, so-called ancient change **(B)**. **(A,** Papanicolaou; **B,** Diff-Quik.)

and often have a prominent nucleolus. Significant nuclear pleomorphism is generally not a feature, although binucleated and multinucleated cells are observed occasionally. Psammoma bodies (calcifications) are usually present (Fig. 6.61). Surgical resection is the recommended therapy. The clinical behavior cannot be predicted based solely on histology. In the series of 31 patients reported by Carney,[100] 21 were alive without evidence of disease, 2 developed local recurrences, 3 developed distant metastases, and 7 died. Three patients were lost to follow-up.

Neurofibroma

Clinical Features

Neurofibromas arise as fusiform expansions of the nerve. In deep-seated lesions arising from major nerve trunks, the residual nerve may be identified easily, but in the more common superficial form, residual nerve is usually not clinically demonstrable. Neurofibromas may exist as one of

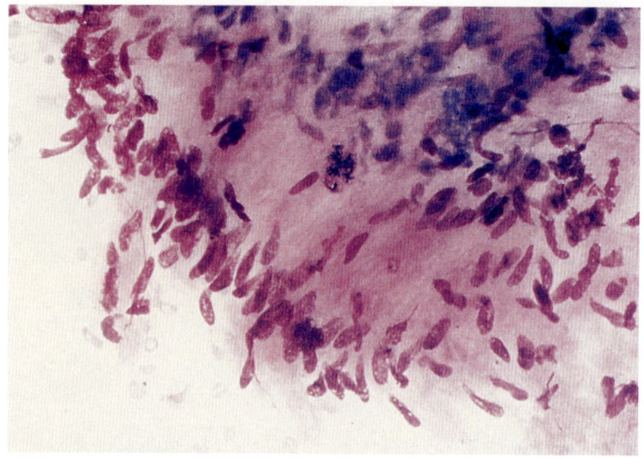

FIGURE 6.60 Nuclear palisading is a helpful but rare finding in cytologic preparations of schwannomas. (Diff-Quik.)

three forms—localized (solitary), diffuse, or plexiform. The localized form is the most common and typically arises as sporadic, solitary, and cutaneous/subcutaneous lesions in young adults. These tumors may be found at virtually any anatomic site (Fig. 6.62). A few solitary neurofibromas arise in patients with neurofibromatosis type 1. Diffuse neurofibromas are observed most commonly as plaque-like skin lesions involving the head and neck regions of children and young adults. It has been estimated that about 10% of cases may be associated with neurofibromatosis type 1.[102] As the name implies, diffuse neurofibromas grow as diffuse and infiltrative masses, entrapping but not destroying residual adnexal structures. Plexiform neurofibromas are virtually pathognomonic of neurofibromatosis type 1. Most patients present in early childhood. Plexiform neurofibromas produce a tortuous, worm-like expansion of peripheral nerves and frequently involve large nerve trunks (Fig. 6.63). When the latter produces gross enlargement of an extremity, it is called *elephantiasis neuromatosa*. The most common neurofibroma seen in neurofibromatosis type 1 is the solitary form; however, because it most frequently is observed sporadically, it is the least specific for the disease.

Neurofibromatosis (von Recklinghausen's disease) exists as two principal forms—type 1 or peripheral variant (café au lait macules, multiple neurofibromas, freckling in the axilla, optic gliomas, iris hamartomas, osseous dysplastic lesions) and type 2 or central variant (bilateral acoustic schwannomas).[103] Neurofibromatosis type 1 is far more common than type 2. Both types are inherited in an autosomal dominant pattern with a high penetrance. We have already discussed neurofibromatosis type 2 with schwannomas. The neurofibromatosis type 1 gene is a tumor-suppressor gene located on chromosome 17.[104] In addition, patients with neurofibromatosis are at increased risk of developing a sarcoma. Determining the exact incidence of malignant change is difficult, but the incidence seems to range from 2% to 7%.[105,106] Patients with neurofibromatosis type 1 are at increased risk of developing other tumors, such as adenocarcinomas and pheochromocytomas.

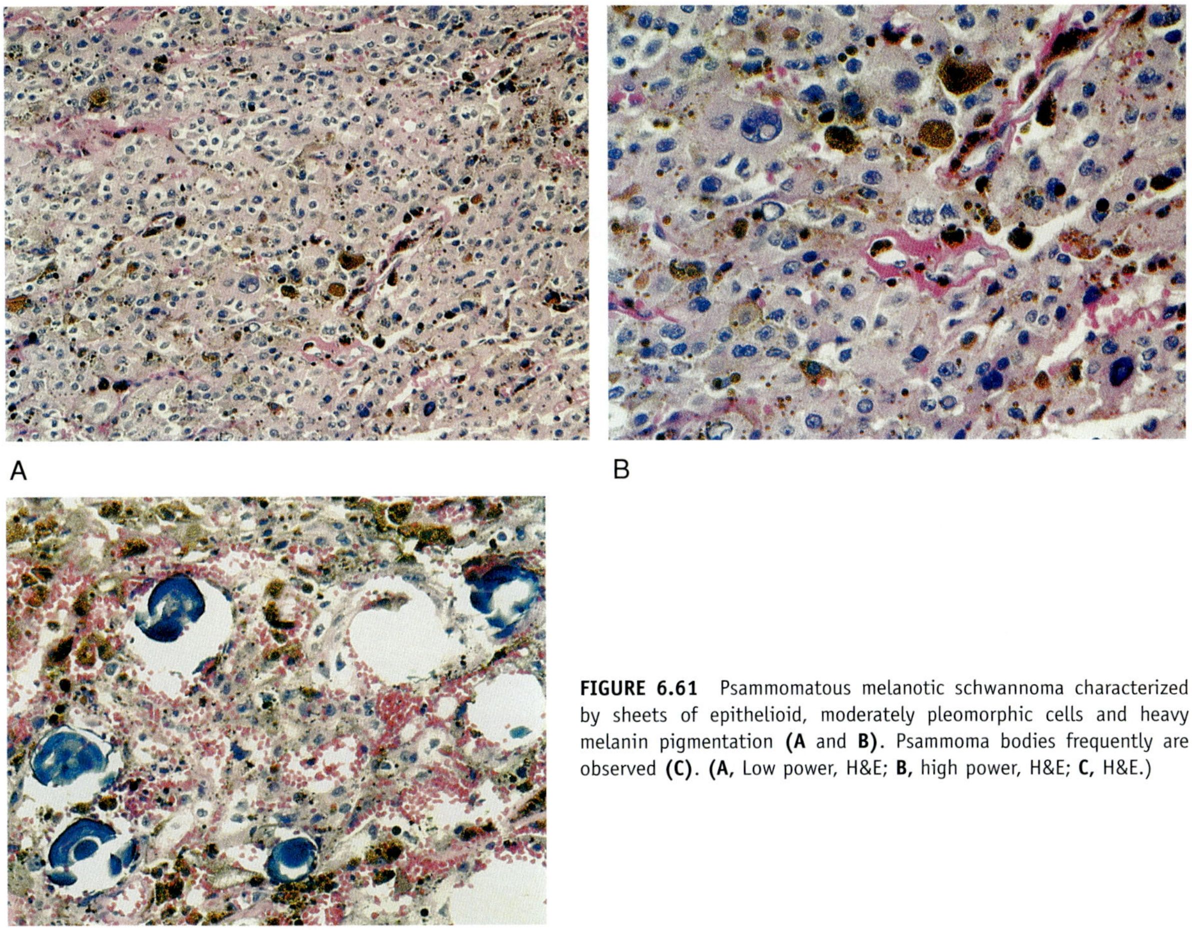

A B C

FIGURE 6.61 Psammomatous melanotic schwannoma characterized by sheets of epithelioid, moderately pleomorphic cells and heavy melanin pigmentation **(A** and **B)**. Psammoma bodies frequently are observed **(C)**. (**A,** Low power, H&E; **B,** high power, H&E; **C,** H&E.)

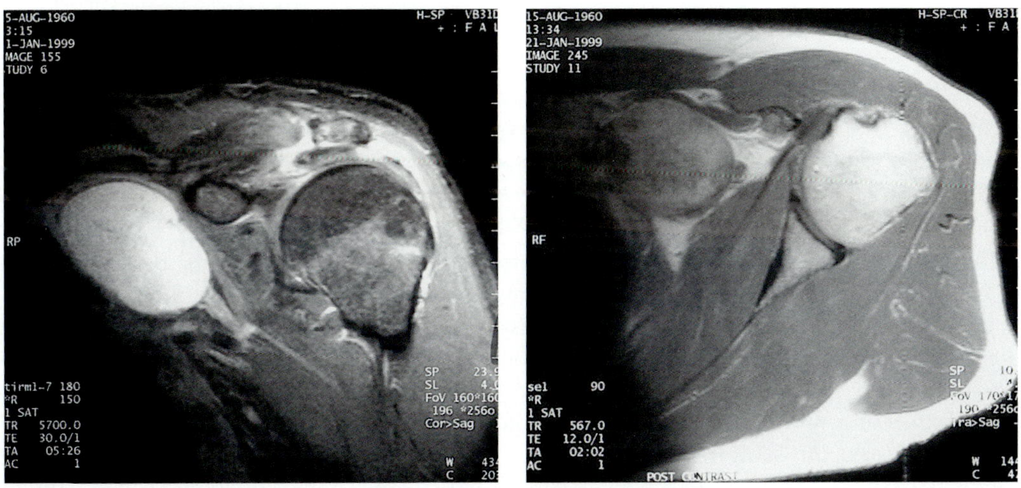

A B

FIGURE 6.62 Neurofibroma. Coronal short tau inversion recovery (STIR) **(A)** and axial T1-weighted, fat-suppressed, gadolinium-enhanced **(B)** magnetic resonance images reveal a well-defined soft tissue mass in the axilla, anterior to the subscapularis muscle.

Pathologic Findings

Histology

Neurofibromas may present as one of three forms: solitary and circumscribed (most common), diffuse, and plexiform. Histologically, neurofibromas are unencapsulated and generally arise as fusiform expansions of peripheral nerve, although this is often not evident in cutaneous tumors. The microscopic appearance depends on the relative volume of cellular elements and mucinous stroma. In contrast to schwannomas, which are composed of mostly Schwann cells, neurofibromas show a greater mixture of cellular elements, including Schwann cells, fibroblasts, and inflammatory cells. Most neurofibromas are composed of haphazardly arranged Schwann

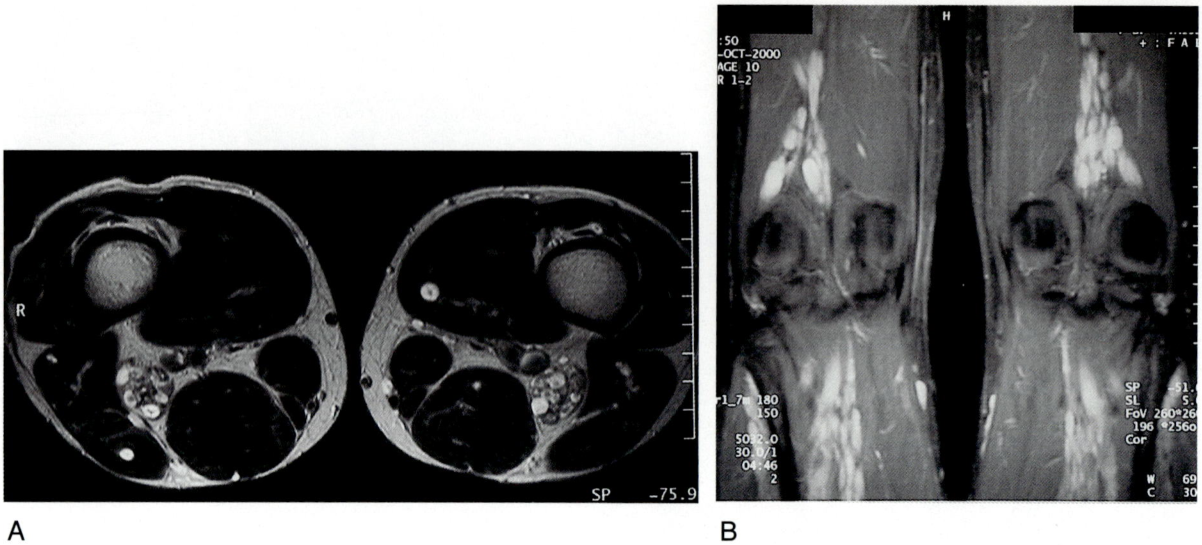

FIGURE 6.63 Plexiform neurofibroma. Axial T2-weighted **(A)** and coronal short tau inversion recovery (STIR) **(B)** magnetic resonance images reveal extensive, vermiform masses extending along the deep neurovascular bundles in the posterior thighs bilaterally.

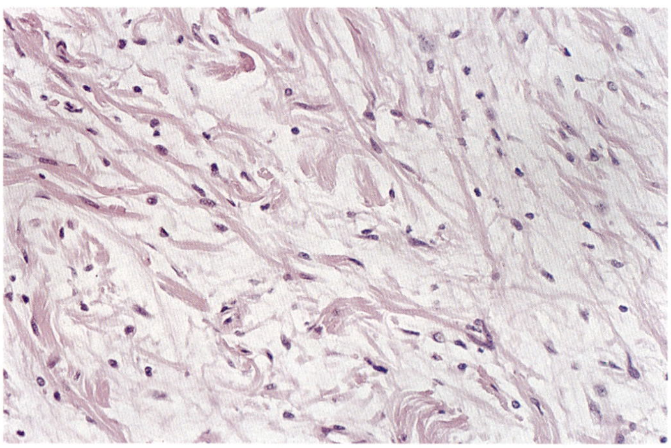

FIGURE 6.64 Most cases of solitary neurofibroma show haphazardly scattered Schwann cells accompanied by variable amounts of wire-like strands of collagen, embedded in a partially myxoid stroma. (H&E.)

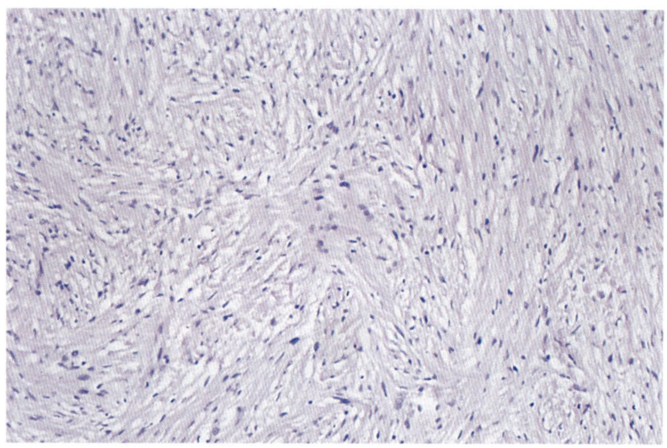

FIGURE 6.65 More cellular cases of solitary neurofibroma appear more compact and may exhibit storiform patterns. (H&E.)

cells accompanied by variable amounts of wire-like strands of collagen, embedded in at least a partially myxoid stroma (Fig. 6.64). Chronic inflammatory cells and histiocytes often are distributed randomly throughout the tumor. More cellular tumors appear more compact with less myxoid matrix, often exhibiting prominent whorls and storiform patterns (Fig. 6.65). As in schwannomas, degenerative features (ancient change) characterized by enlarged and hyperchromatic Schwann cell nuclei (often having a "smudged" appearance) may be evident (Fig. 6.66).[107] Mitotic figures are virtually absent.

Compared with the localized or solitary type, diffuse neurofibromas have a more uniform matrix of fine fibrillary collagen and diffusely infiltrate and entrap pre-existing adnexal structures (Fig. 6.67). The Schwann cells are generally shorter but remain uniform. Wagner-Meissner bodies or clusters are a characteristic feature. The main differential diagnosis is dermatofibrosarcoma protuberans; correlation with clinical findings and judicious use of immunohistochemistry help avoid a misdiagnosis.

Plexiform neurofibromas produce tortuous expansion of multiple nerve branches, ranging from simply an increase in endoneurial contents to areas resembling solitary neurofibroma (Fig. 6.68). Over time, the contents of these expanded nerve fibers spill out into the adjacent skin and soft tissues, creating the appearance of a combined plexiform/diffuse neurofibroma (Fig. 6.69).[102]

Neurofibromas may exhibit nuclear atypia that is of no clinical significance. Infrequent mitotic activity (<1 mitotic figure per 10 high-power fields) in otherwise normal-appearing (or even cellular) neurofibromas is of no clinical relevance. Conservative surgical resection is adequate treatment.[107] Diffuse nuclear atypia, increased cellularity (closely packed tumor cells), and mitotic activity exceeding

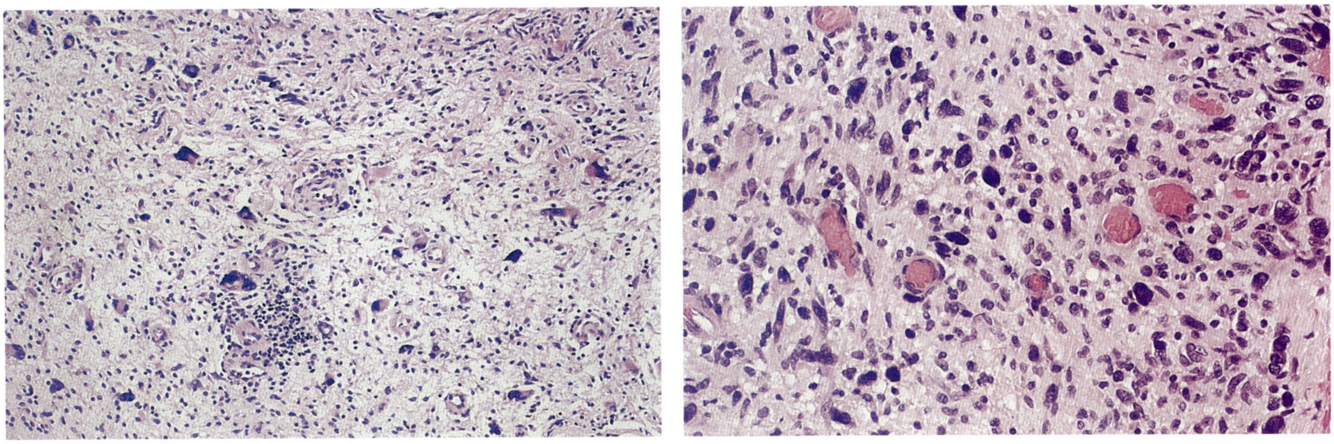

A B

FIGURE 6.66 Ancient change, similar to that observed in schwannoma, may be focal or widespread within a given tumor. Although the nuclei appear enlarged and atypical, the smudgy chromatin pattern and virtual absence of mitotic activity help establish the diagnosis **(A** and **B)**. **(A,** low power, H&E; and **B,** high power, H&E.)

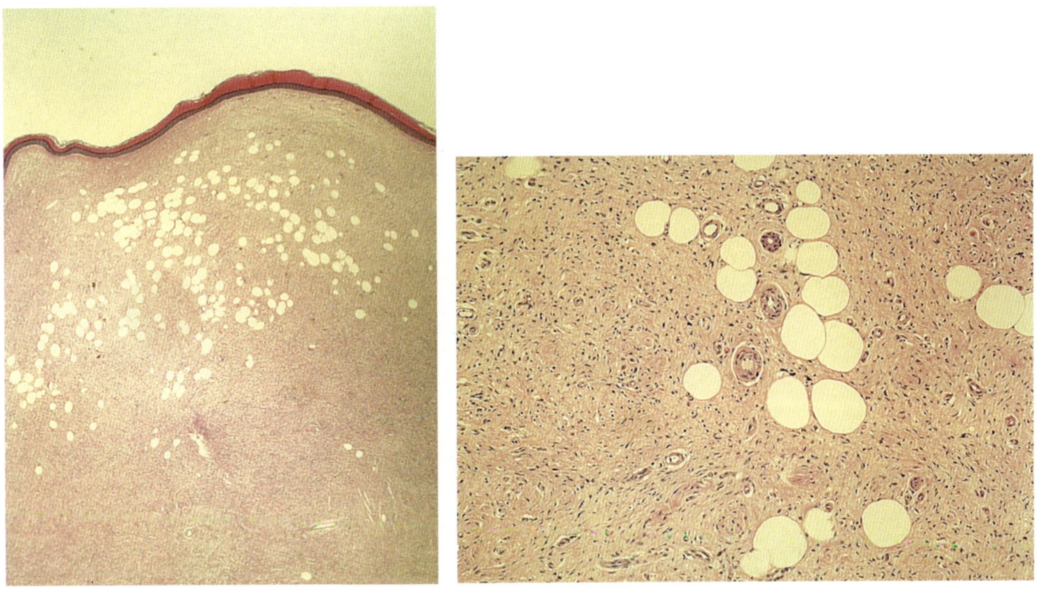

A B

FIGURE 6.67 Diffuse neurofibroma replaces the dermis with a more uniform matrix of fine fibrillary collagen, entrapping pre-existing adnexal structures. Note the resemblance to dermatofibrosarcoma protuberans **(A** and **B)**. **(A,** Low power, H&E; **B,** high power, H&E.)

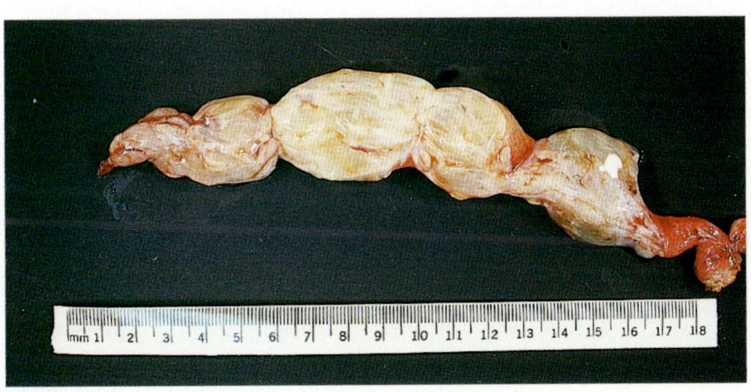

FIGURE 6.68 Plexiform neurofibroma produces tortuous expansion of a large peripheral nerve. Note the myxoid stromal changes.

one mitotic figure per 10 high-power fields, especially if accompanied by necrosis, indicate malignant change (Fig. 6.70). When a neurofibroma shows some but not all of these atypical features, some have proposed the designation of "neurofibroma with atypical features."[102]

Fine Needle Aspiration Biopsy

FNAB of neurofibromas rarely is performed because most such cases, outside of the clinical setting of neurofibromatosis, arise as cutaneous lesions, easily amenable to superficial tissue

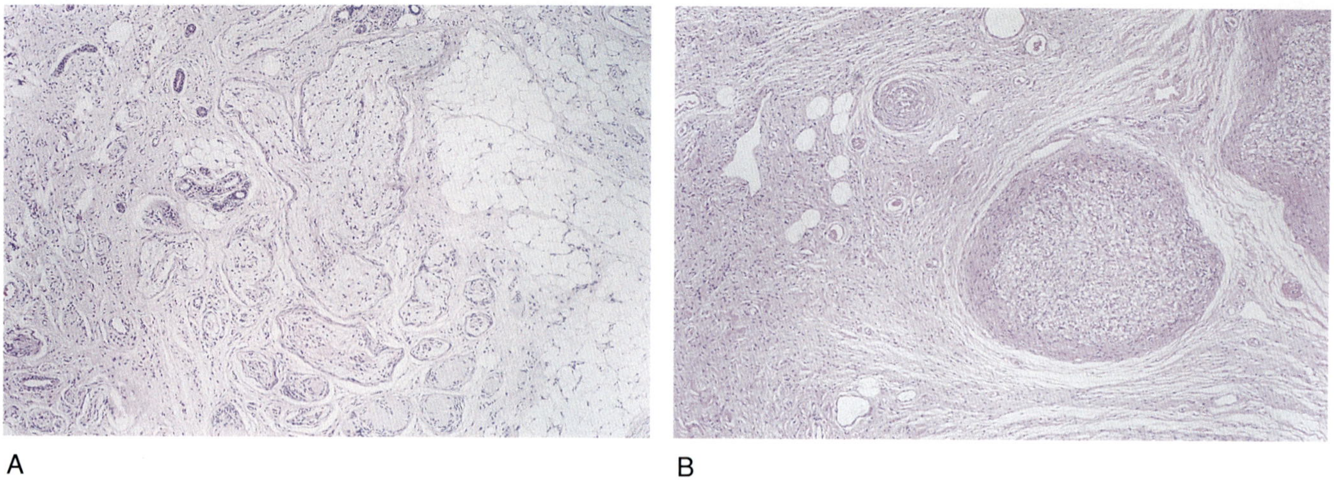

FIGURE 6.69 Plexiform neurofibromas cause an increase in endoneurial contents, expanding individual nerve fibers and ultimately spilling out into the adjacent soft tissues (**A** and **B**). (**A** and **B**, H&E.)

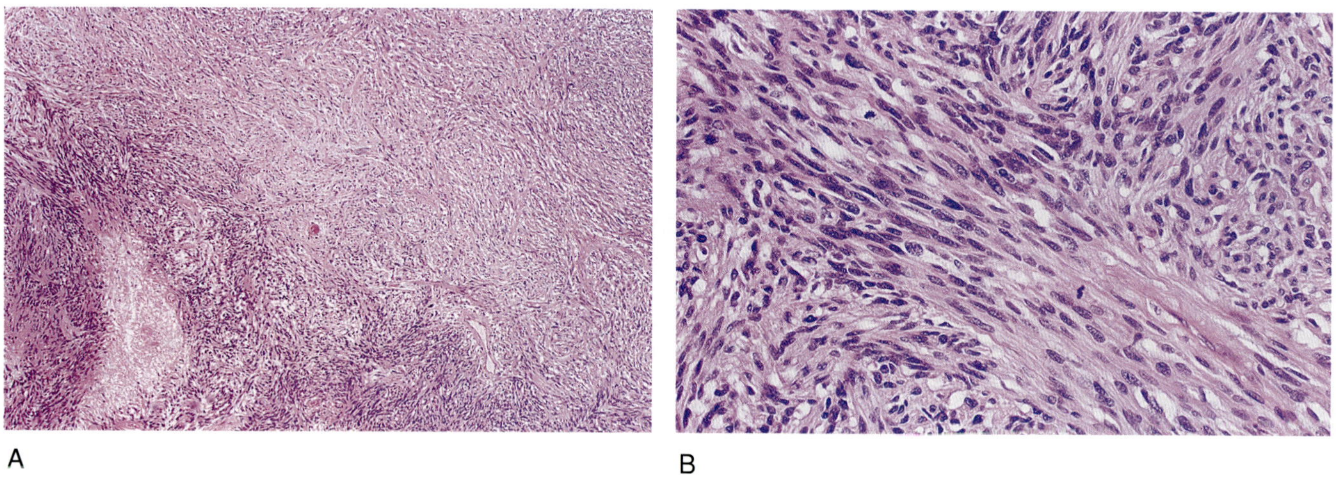

FIGURE 6.70 Malignant change in neurofibroma characterized by hypercellularity, necrosis, and increased mitotic activity (**A** and **B**). (**A**, Low power, H&E; **B**, high power, H&E.)

biopsy and resection. Consequently, most benign nerve sheath tumor aspirates represent schwannomas. In FNAB specimens, schwannomas and neurofibromas are generally indistinguishable from each other. Smears are typically cellular and composed of variably sized cohesive tissue fragments containing a metachromatic-to-myxoid stroma.[108] Individual cells appear spindled with ovoid-to-spindled nuclei and abundant cytoplasmic processes. Nucleoli are generally not seen. Ancillary studies on cell block material help establish the diagnosis.

Ancillary Studies

Ultrastructurally, neurofibromas contain a variety of cell types, reflected in the electron microscopic findings. Typical Schwann cells (as previously described) are admixed with perineural cells, fibroblasts (often with less prominent rough endoplasmic reticulum), and a collagenous stroma.

In contrast to schwannoma, S-100 protein decorates some but not all of the cells, in keeping with the observation that neurofibromas contain a variety of other cell types. Nuclear immunopositivity for p53 is usually negative in neurofibromas. Conversely, most malignant peripheral nerve sheath tumors, especially high-grade forms, appear positive for p53 (>20% nuclear staining).[109,110] In difficult cases, p53 expression may be a useful adjunct to distinguish neurofibroma from malignant peripheral nerve sheath tumor.

Clonal chromosomal aberrations have been documented in neurofibroma but appear less common than is seen in schwannoma. No recurrent or diagnostic abnormalities have been described.[99]

Prognosis and Therapy

Solitary neurofibromas in patients without neurofibromatosis are cured by local excision. For patients with neurofibromatosis, surgery is limited to lesions that are persistently painful or in anatomic locations that could compromise function. The risk of malignant transformation is difficult to predict but is more likely to occur in patients who have had the disease for many years.

Malignant Peripheral Nerve Sheath Tumor

The term *malignant peripheral nerve sheath tumor* encompasses the older designations of *neurofibrosarcoma* and *malignant schwannoma*. The diagnosis of malignant peripheral nerve sheath tumor usually requires at least one of the following clinical settings: (1) origin from a peripheral nerve, usually a large nerve trunk; (2) origin from a pre-existing benign nerve sheath tumor, usually a neurofibroma; or (3) occurrence in a patient with neurofibromatosis. Rarely, the diagnosis may be rendered outside of these clinical settings, if classic morphologic features are evident.

Clinical Features

Most cases of malignant peripheral nerve sheath tumor occur in patients 20 to 50 years old, but patients with neurofibromatosis may develop malignant peripheral nerve sheath tumors at an earlier age. In the Mayo Clinic series, the average age of patients without neurofibromatosis was 40 years and of patients with neurofibromatosis was 29 years.[111] Approximately 10% of cases involve children. Among patients with neurofibromatosis, there appears to be a male predilection, whereas the sporadic form of malignant peripheral nerve sheath tumor affects men and women equally. Most patients present with a soft tissue mass with or without associated pain. Neurologic deficits often occur from tumors involving large nerve trunks. Between 21% and 52% of patients have neurofibromatosis type 1.[111,112] Most malignant peripheral nerve sheath tumors arise from large peripheral nerve trunks (Fig. 6.71). Among patients with

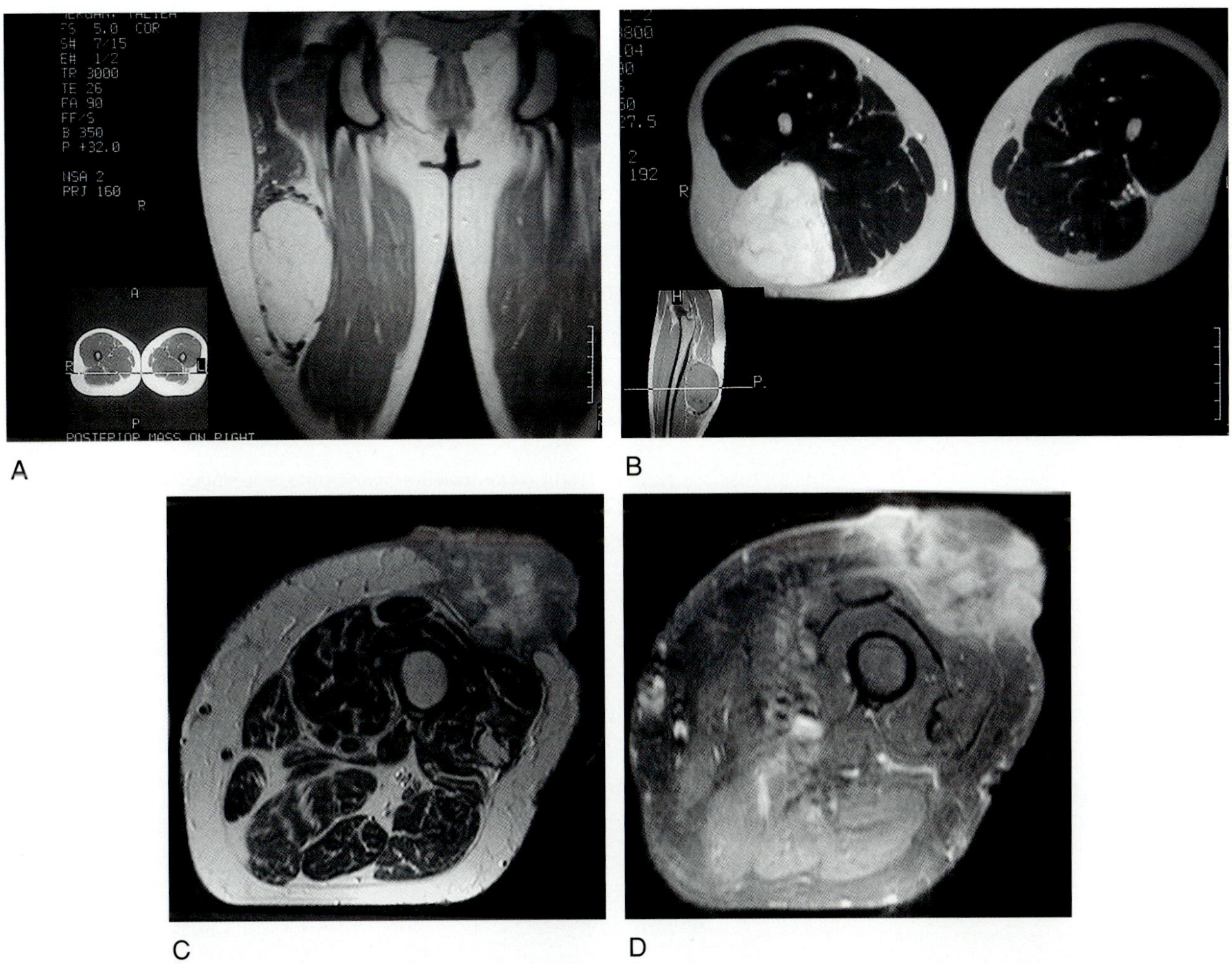

FIGURE 6.71 Malignant peripheral nerve sheath tumor. Coronal proton density **(A)** and axial T2-weighted **(B)** magnetic resonance images show a well-defined, hyperintense mass arising in the superficial aspect of the lateral portion of the hamstrings compartment of the right thigh. In another patient, axial T2-weighted **(C)** and gadolinium-enhanced, fat-suppressed T1-weighted **(D)** magnetic resonance images show a large, heterogeneous mass arising in the soft tissues of the anterolateral aspect of the left thigh. The mass enhances intensely but inhomogeneously after administration of gadolinium. The lesion is centered approximately at the level of the skin.

neurofibromatosis, usually after a 10- to 20-year latent period, 2% to 7% develop malignant peripheral nerve sheath tumors.[105,106,111]

Malignant peripheral nerve sheath tumor arising in bone is an extraordinarily rare event. Tumors may occur with or without an association with neurofibromatosis.[114,115] Data are too limited to draw any definite demographic conclusions.

Pathologic Findings

Histology

Compared with other spindle cell tumors, the morphologic diversity of malignant peripheral nerve sheath tumor is impressive. Most appear as obvious infiltrative, high-grade sarcomas, resembling fibrosarcoma, composed of long, sweeping fascicles and herringbone patterns (Fig. 6.72). Malignant peripheral nerve sheath tumors show far greater histologic and cytologic variability than fibrosarcoma, however. In the appropriate clinical context, densely cellular fascicles alternating with hypocellular myxoid zones ("marbled appearance"), nuclear palisading, geographic necrosis, and heterologous differentiation (e.g., metaplastic bone) strongly suggest the diagnosis of malignant peripheral nerve sheath tumor.[111-113] Additional helpful morphologic features less commonly observed include giant rosettes, glandular differentiation, perineural and intraneural spread, and condensation of tumor cells in a perivascular distribution.[112] A hemangiopericytoma-like vascular pattern is not unusual (Fig. 6.73). Cytologically the tumor cells are usually spindled, wavy to comma-shaped, and obviously malignant. Marked nuclear pleomorphism with tumor giant cells, resembling malignant fibrous histiocytoma, sometimes occurs and may be more common in patients with neurofibromatosis (Fig. 6.74).

By themselves, none of the aforementioned histologic features is pathognomonic of malignant peripheral nerve sheath tumor. Rhythmic nuclear palisading, creating a tiger

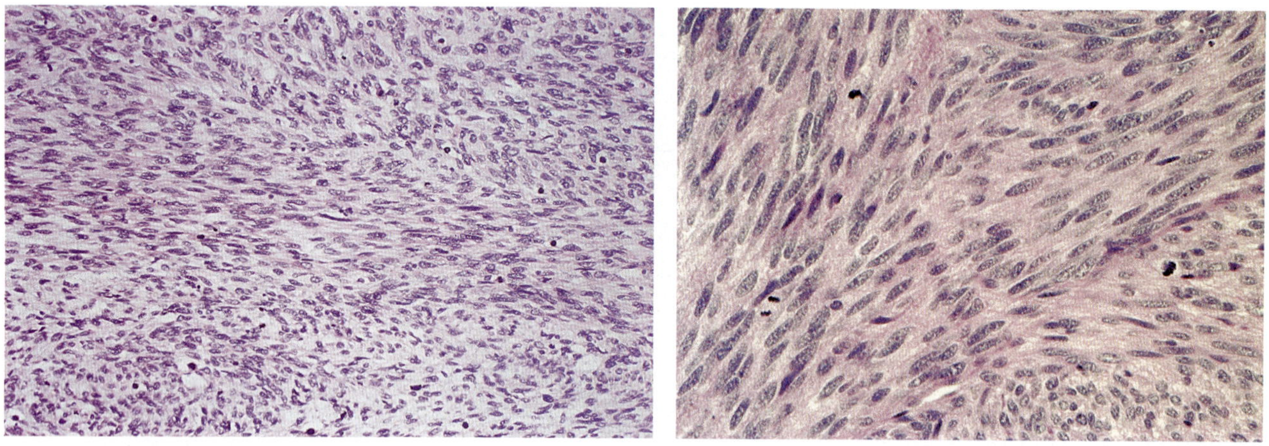

A B

FIGURE 6.72 Most examples of malignant peripheral nerve sheath tumor resemble fibrosarcoma, appearing as obviously high-grade sarcomas and composed of long, sweeping fascicles and occasionally exhibiting herringbone patterns (**A** and **B**). (**A,** Low power, H&E; **B,** high power, H&E.)

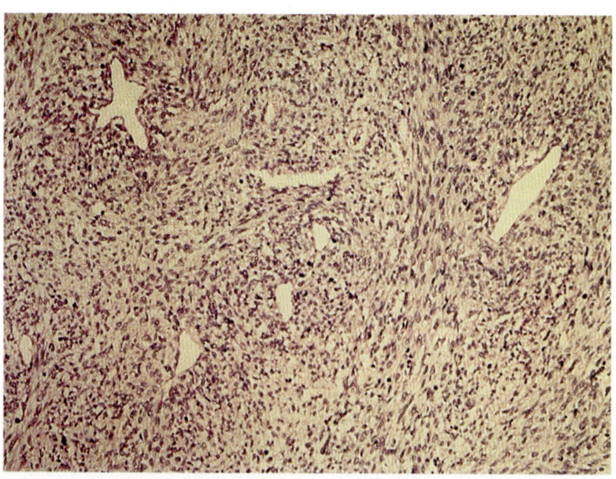

FIGURE 6.73 As in many sarcomas, a hemangiopericytoma-like vascular pattern may be observed in malignant peripheral nerve sheath tumor. (H&E.)

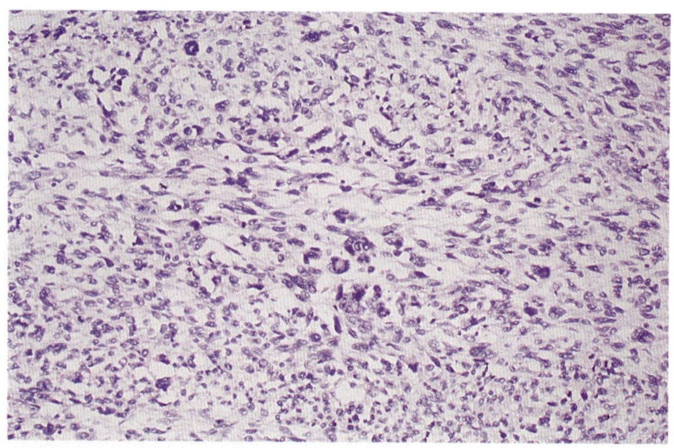

FIGURE 6.74 Occasional cases of malignant peripheral nerve sheath tumor appear anaplastic with multinucleated tumor giant cells, resembling malignant fibrous histiocytoma. (H&E.)

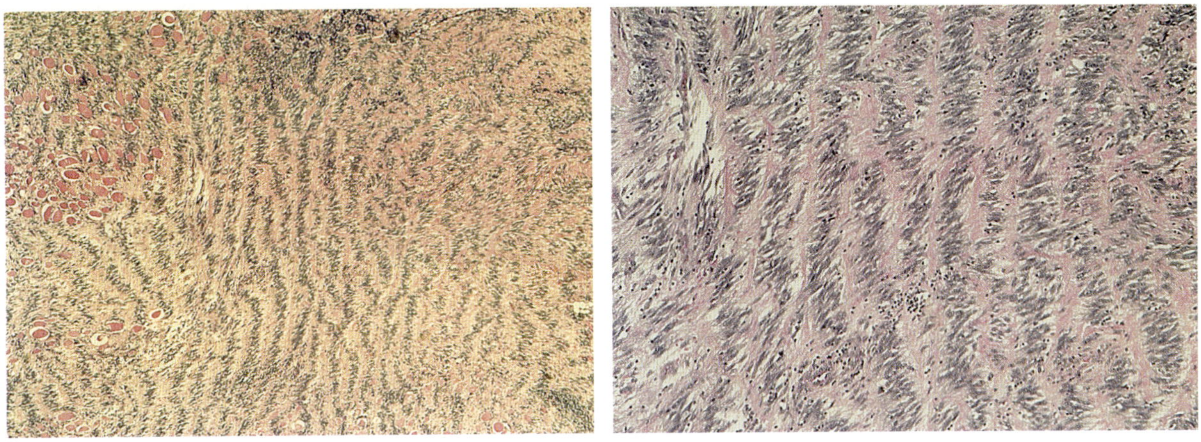

A B

FIGURE 6.75 A helpful diagnostic feature for malignant peripheral nerve sheath tumor is the presence of rhythmic nuclear palisading. This finding tends to be uncommon and is not entirely specific because it may be seen rarely in smooth muscle tumors **(A** and **B)**. **(A,** Low power, H&E; **B,** high power, H&E.)

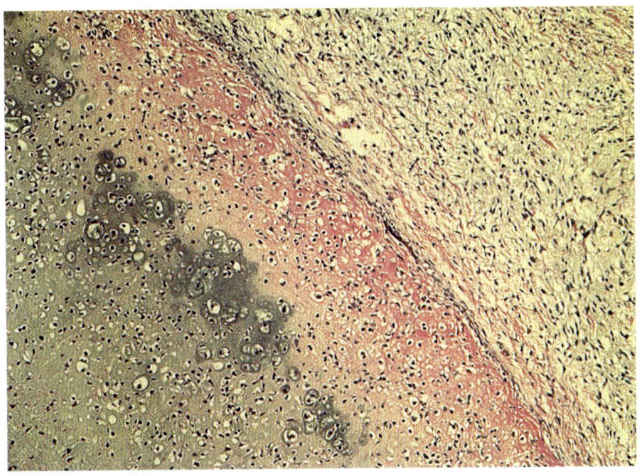

FIGURE 6.76 Malignant peripheral nerve sheath tumor with osseous and cartilaginous metaplasia. (H&E.)

stripe appearance, occurs in relatively few cases (Fig. 6.75). Approximately 10% to 20% of cases contain heterologous elements, including glandular differentiation, rhabdomyosarcoma, and bone or cartilaginous metaplasia (Fig. 6.76).[111-113] Malignant peripheral nerve sheath tumors with neuroepithelial features, resembling Ewing's sarcoma, are observed rarely, most commonly in children.[116] The diagnosis of malignant peripheral nerve sheath tumor is based mostly on clinical grounds, accounting for the significant degree of morphologic diversity.

The epithelioid variant of malignant peripheral nerve sheath tumor deserves special consideration because of its unusual histologic features and immunohistochemical properties. Morphologically the tumors consist of cords and nodules of polygonal to epithelioid-appearing tumor cells that closely resemble a melanoma or carcinoma (Fig. 6.77).[117] In contrast to nonepithelioid forms, epithelioid malignant peripheral nerve sheath tumor shows diffuse and strong positivity for S-100 protein; however, in contrast to melanoma, HMB 45 is uniformly negative.

Fine Needle Aspiration Biopsy

In FNAB specimens, malignant peripheral nerve sheath tumors are virtually always recognized as malignant. In the absence of a specific clinical scenario, rendering a specific diagnosis of malignant peripheral nerve sheath tumor is usually not possible, however, because the cytologic findings are nonspecific. Smears are highly cellular and composed of mostly individually dispersed tumor cells. In most cases, the cells appear spindled, displaying ovoid-to-elongated, comma-to-serpentine shapes and containing hyperchromatic nuclei and scant-to-tapering cytoplasm. Nuclear-to-cytoplasmic ratios are higher than those observed with schwannoma. Multinucleated tumor giant cells are observed frequently (Fig. 6.78).[118] Rarely, malignant peripheral nerve sheath tumor may exhibit a more epithelioid/polygonal cell morphology.

Ancillary Studies

The ultrastructural features of malignant peripheral nerve sheath tumor depend largely on the degree of differentiation (or tumor grade). Low-grade, well-differentiated cases show features of Schwann cell differentiation with cellular processes covered by basal lamina. In high-grade forms, the characteristic basal lamina may be poorly developed and incomplete, making interpretation of schwannian differentiation more difficult.

There is no reliable immunohistochemical marker diagnostic of malignant peripheral nerve sheath tumor. As expected, all cases express vimentin. Immunohistochemical detection of S-100 protein is a useful technique, helping to confirm nerve sheath differentiation. However, up to 50% of cases of classic malignant peripheral nerve sheath tumor are negative for S-100 protein.[97,112,119] When positive, the staining pattern is typically focal and patchy, in contrast to the

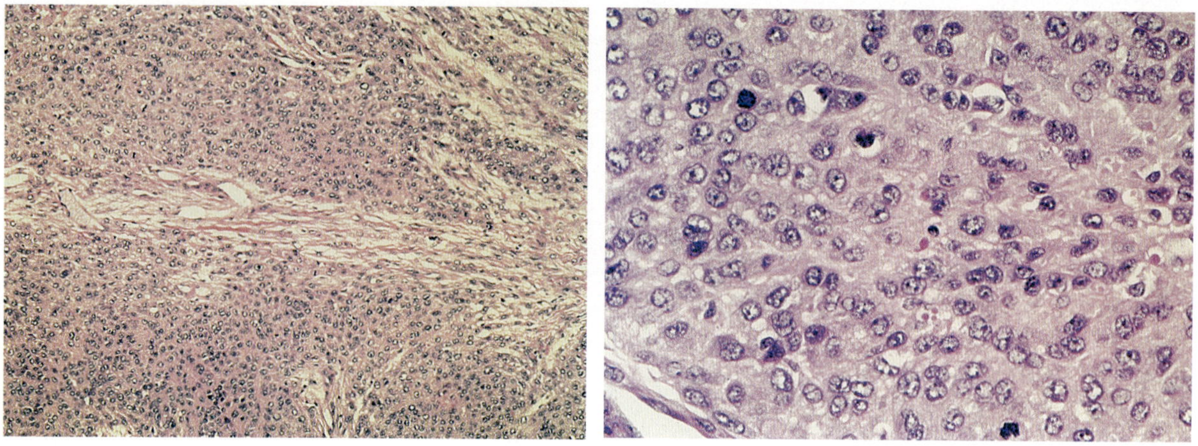

A B

FIGURE 6.77 Epithelioid malignant peripheral nerve sheath tumor is characterized by nests and cords of frankly malignant epithelioid tumor cells, resembling melanoma or carcinoma **(A** and **B)**. **(A,** Low power, H&E; **B,** high power, H&E.)

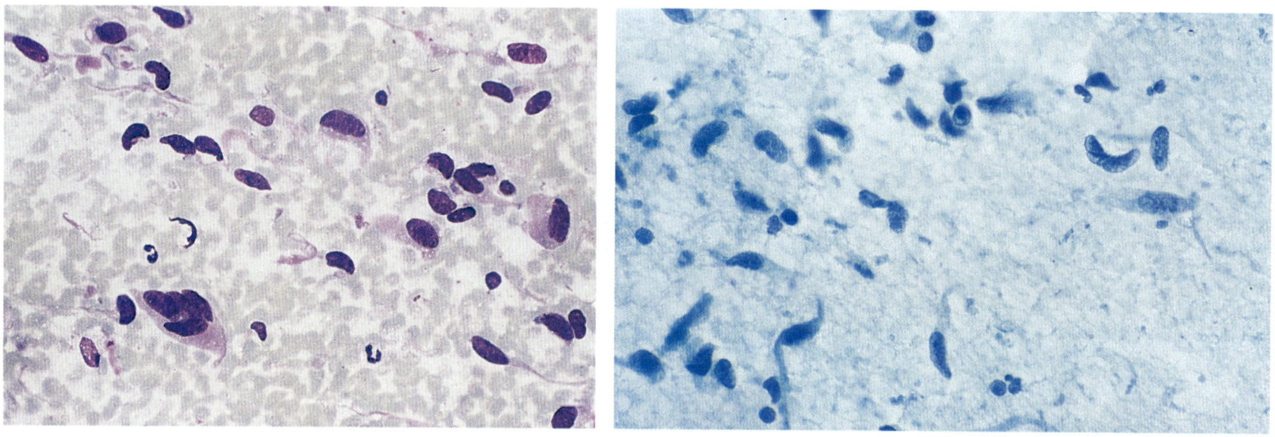

A B

FIGURE 6.78 Fine needle aspiration biopsy of malignant peripheral nerve sheath tumor generally shows mostly discohesive and obviously malignant spindle to serpentine-shaped tumor cells. Note the multinucleated tumor giant cell in **A (A** and **B)**. **(A,** Diff-Quik; **B,** Papanicolaou.)

more diffuse staining observed with schwannoma. For these reasons, immunohistochemical staining for S-100 protein is more useful for distinguishing benign from malignant peripheral nerve sheath tumors than in differentiating malignant peripheral nerve sheath tumors from other spindle cell sarcomas.[97] Less commonly, malignant peripheral nerve sheath tumors express cytokeratins, EMA, desmin, glial fibrillary acidic protein, and HMB 45, reflecting their potential for divergent differentiation.[119,120] As already mentioned, the epithelioid variant of malignant peripheral nerve sheath tumor shows diffuse and strong positivity for S-100 protein but is uniformly negative for specific melanoma markers, such as HMB 45.[117] By cytogenetic analysis, malignant peripheral nerve sheath tumors show complex karyotypes with numerous clonal chromosomal aberrations, none of which appear specific for these tumors.[99]

Prognosis and Therapy

Ducatman and colleagues[111] evaluated 120 cases of malignant peripheral nerve sheath tumors and found no significant correlation between survival and either histologic grade or mitotic rate. Tumor size (>5 cm) and the presence of neurofibromatosis adversely affected overall prognosis. Survival also appeared to be improved after a total rather than a subtotal resection of the tumor.[111] Meis and associates[112] reported 78 cases of malignant peripheral nerve sheath tumors in children and, by multivariate analysis, found tumor size, age 7 years or older, tumor necrosis equal to or greater than 25%, and the presence of neurofibromatosis to be "independent adverse prognostic factors." Wide surgical resection with negative margins is the preferred therapy.

REFERENCES

Nodular Fasciitis

1. Bernstein KE, Lattes R: Nodular (pseudosarcomatous) fasciitis, a non-recurrent lesion: Clinicopathologic study of 134 cases. Cancer 1982;49:1668.
2. Allen PW: Nodular fasciitis. Pathology 1972;4:9.
3. Lauer DH, Enzinger FM: Cranial fasciitis of childhood. Cancer 1980;45:401.
4. Daroca PJ Jr, Pulitzer DR, LoCicero J: Ossifying fasciitis. Arch Pathol Lab Med 1982;106:682.
5. Stanley MW, Skoog L, Tani EM, et al: Nodular fasciitis: Spontaneous resolution following diagnosis by fine-needle aspiration. Diagn Cytopathol 1993;9:322.
6. Montgomery EA, Meis JM: Nodular fasciitis: Its morphologic spectrum and immunohistochemical profile. Am J Surg Pathol 1991;15:942.
7. Sawyer JR, Sammartino G, Baker GF, et al: Clonal chromosome aberrations in a case of nodular fasciitis. Cancer Genet Cytogenet 1994;76:154.

Proliferative Fasciitis and Myositis

8. Chung EB, Enzinger FM: Proliferative fasciitis. Cancer 1975;36:1450.
9. Enzinger FM, Dulcey F: Proliferative myositis: Report of thirty-three cases. Cancer 1967;20:2213.
10. Meis JM, Enzinger FM: Proliferative fasciitis and myositis of childhood. Am J Surg Pathol 1992;16:364.
11. Lundgren L, Kindblom LG, Williams J, et al: Proliferative myositis and fasciitis: A light and electron microscopic, cytologic, DNA-cytometric and immunohistochemical study. APMIS 1992;100:437.
12. el Jabbour JN, Bennett MH, Burke MM, et al: Proliferative myositis: An immunohistochemical and ultrastructural study. Am J Surg Pathol 1991;15:654.
13. Dembinski A, Bridge JA, Neff JR, et al: Trisomy 2 in proliferative fasciitis. Cancer Genet Cytogenet 1992;60:27.
14. Ohjimi Y, Iwasaki H, Ishiguro M, et al: Trisomy 2 found in proliferative myositis cultured cell. Cancer Genet Cytogenet 1994;76:157.

Fibroma of Tendon Sheath

15. Chung EB, Enzinger FM: Fibroma of tendon sheath. Cancer 1979;44:1945.
16. Pulitzer DR, Martin PC, Reed RJ: Fibroma of tendon sheath: A clinicopathologic study of 32 cases. Am J Surg Pathol 1989;13:472.
17. Dal Cin P, Sciot R, De Smet L, et al: Translocation 2;11 in a fibroma of tendon sheath. Histopathology 1998;332:433.

Nuchal-Type Fibroma

18. Michal M, Fetsch JF, Hes O, et al: Nuchal-type fibroma: A clinicopathologic study of 52 cases. Cancer 1999;85:156.
19. Balachandran K, Allen PW, MacCormac LB: Nuchal fibroma: A clinicopathologic study of nine cases. Am J Surg Pathol 1995;19:313.
20. Shek TWH: Extranuchal nuchal fibroma. Am J Surg Pathol 1996;20:902.
21. Zamecnik M, Michal M: Nuchal-type fibroma is positive for CD34 and CD99. Am J Surg Pathol 2001;25:970.

Elastofibroma

22. Jarvi O, Hopsu-Havu V, Wartiovaara J, et al: Elastofibroma dorsi: A degenerative pseudotumor. Cancer 1969;23:42.
23. Nagamine N, Nohara Y, Ito E: Elastofibroma in Okinawa: A clinicopathologic study of 170 cases. Cancer 1982;50:1794.
24. Giebel GD, Bierhoff E, Vogel J: Elastofibroma and pre-elastofibroma: A biopsy and autopsy study. Eur J Surg Oncol 1996;22:93.
25. Naylor MF, Nascimento AG, Sherrick AD, et al: Elastofibroma dorsi: Radiologic findings in 12 patients. AJR Am J Roentgenol 1996;167:683.
26. Kransdorf MJ, Meis JM, Montgomery E: Elastofibroma: MR and CT appearance with radiologic-pathologic correlation. AJR Am J Roentgenol 1992;159:575.
27. Harigopal M, Seshan SV, DeLellis RA, et al: Aspiration cytology of elastofibroma dorsi: Case report with ultrastructural and immunohistochemical findings. Diagn Cytopathol 2002;26:310.
28. Mojica WD, Kuntzman T: Elastofibroma dorsi: Elaboration of cytologic features and review of its pathogenesis. Diagn Cytopathol 2000;23:393.
29. Fukuda Y, Miyake H, Masuda Y, et al: Histogenesis of unique elastinophilic fibers of elastofibroma: Ultrastructural and immunohistochemical studies. Hum Pathol 1987;18:424.
30. McComb EN, Feely MG, Neff JR, et al: Cytogenetic instability, predominantly involving chromosome 1, is characteristic of elastofibroma. Cancer Genet Cytogenet 2001;98:142.

Superficial and Deep Fibromatoses

31. Mikkelsen OA: Dupuytren's disease: Initial symptoms, age of onset and spontaneous course. Hand 1977;9:11.
32. Allen RA, Woolner LB, Ghormley RK: Soft tissue tumors of the sole with special reference to plantar fibromatosis. J Bone Joint Surg Am 1955;37:14.
33. Billig R, Baker R, Immergut M, et al: Peyronie's disease. Urology 1975;6:409.
34. Ling RS: The genetic factor in Dupuytren's disease. J Bone Joint Surg Br 1963;45:709.
35. Wever ID, Dal Cin P, Fletcher CDM, et al: Cytogenetic, clinical, and morphologic correlations in 78 cases of fibromatosis: A report from the CHAMP Study Group. Mod Pathol 2000;13:1080.
36. Merchant NB, Lewis JJ, Woodruff JM, et al: Extremity and trunk desmoid tumors: A multifactorial analysis of outcome. Cancer 1999;86:2045.
37. Burke AP, Sobin LH, Shekita KM, et al: Intra-abdominal fibromatosis: A pathologic analysis of 130 tumors with comparison of clinical subgroups. Am J Surg Pathol 1990;14:335.
38. Raab SS, Silverman JF, McLeod DL, et al: Fine needle aspiration biopsy of fibromatoses. Acta Cytol 1993;37:323.
39. Yantiss RK, Spiro IJ, Compton CC, et al: Gastrointestinal stromal tumor versus intra-abdominal fibromatosis of the bowel wall: A clinically important differential diagnosis. Am J Surg Pathol 2000;24:947.

Solitary Fibrous Tumor

40. Suster S, Nascimento AG, Miettinen M, et al: Solitary fibrous tumors of soft tissue: A clinicopathologic and immunohistochemical study of 12 cases. Am J Surg Pathol 1995;19:1257.
41. Nielsen GP, O'Connell JX, Dickersin R, et al: Solitary fibrous tumor of soft tissue: A report of 15 cases, including 5 malignant examples with light microscopic, immunohistochemical, and ultrastructural data. Mod Pathol 1997;10:1028.
42. Alawi F, Stratton D, Freedman PD: Solitary fibrous tumor of the oral soft tissues: A clinicopathologic and immunohistochemical study of 16 cases. Am J Surg Pathol 2001;25:900.
43. Vallat-Decouvelaere AV, Dry SM, Fletcher CDM: Atypical and malignant solitary fibrous tumors in extrathoracic locations: Evidence of their comparability to intra-thoracic tumors. Am J Surg Pathol 1998;22:1501.
44. Clayton AC, Salomao DR, Keeney GL, et al: Solitary fibrous tumor: A study of cytologic features of six cases diagnosed by fine-needle aspiration. Diagn Cytopathol 2001;25:172.
45. Hasegawa T, Hirose T, Seki K, et al: Solitary fibrous tumor of the soft tissue: An immunohistochemical and ultrastructural study. Am J Clin Pathol 1996;106:325.

Hemangiopericytoma

46. Guillou L, Fletcher JA, Fletcher CDM, et al: Extrapleural solitary fibrous tumour and haemangiopericytoma. In Fletcher CDM, Unni KK, Mertens F (eds): Pathology and Genetics: Tumours of Soft Tissue

and Bone. World Health Organization Classification of Tumours. Lyon, France: IARC Press, 2002, pp 86–93.

47. Enzinger FM, Smith BH: Hemangiopericytoma: An analysis of 106 cases. Hum Pathol 1976;7:61.
48. Wold LW, Unni KK, Cooper KL, et al: Hemangiopericytoma of bone. Am J Surg Pathol 1982;6:53.
49. Folpe AL, Devaney K, Weiss SW: Lipomatous hemangiopericytoma: A rare variant of hemangiopericytoma that may be confused with liposarcoma. Am J Surg Pathol 1999;23:1201.
50. Chhieng D, Cohen JM, Waisman J, et al: Fine-needle aspiration cytology of hemangiopericytoma: A report of five cases. Cancer 1999;87:190.

Collagenous Fibroma

51. Evans HL: Desmoplastic fibroma: A report of seven cases. Am J Surg Pathol 1995;19:1077.
52. Nielsen GP, O'Connell JX, Dickersin R, et al: Collagenous fibroma (desmoplastic fibroblastoma): A report of seven cases. Mod Pathol 1996;9:781.
53. Hasegawa T, Shimoda T, Hiroshashi S, et al: Collagenous fibroma (desmoplastic fibroblastoma): Report of four cases and review of the literature. Arch Pathol Lab Med 1998;122:455.
54. Sciot R, Samson I, van den Berghe H, et al: Collagenous fibroma (desmoplastic fibroblastoma): Genetic link with fibroma of tendon sheath. Mod Pathol 1999;12:565.

Benign Fibrous Histiocytoma

55. Fletcher CDM: Benign fibrous histiocytoma of subcutaneous and deep soft tissue: A clinicopathologic analysis of 21 cases. Am J Surg Pathol 1990;14:801.
56. Clark BE, Xipell JM, Thomas DP: Benign fibrous histiocytoma of bone. Am J Surg Pathol 1985;9:806.

Dermatofibrosarcoma Protuberans

57. Browne WB, Antonescu CR, Leung DHY, et al: Dermatofibrosarcoma protuberans: A clinicopathologic analysis of patients treated and followed at a single institution. Cancer 2000;88:2711.
58. McKee PH, Fletcher CDM: Dermatofibrosarcoma protuberans presenting in infancy and childhood. J Cutan Pathol 1991;18:241.
59. Fletcher CDM, Theaker JM, Flanagan A, et al: Pigmented dermatofibrosarcoma protuberans (Bednar tumor): Melanocytic colonization or neuroectodermal differentiation? A clinicopathological and immunohistochemical study. Histopathology 1988; 13:631.
60. Harvell JD, Kilpatrick SE, White WL: Histogenetic relations between giant cell fibroblastoma and dermatofibrosarcoma protuberans: CD34 staining showing the spectrum and a simulator. Am J Dermatopathol 1998;20:339.
61. Mentzel T, Beham A, Katenkamp D, et al: Fibrosarcomatous ("high-grade") dermatofibrosarcoma protuberans: Clinicopathologic and immunohistochemical study of a series of 41 cases with emphasis on prognostic significance. Am J Surg Pathol 1998;22:576.
62. Goldblum JR, Reith JD, Weiss SW: Sarcomas arising in dermatofibrosarcoma protuberans: A reappraisal of biologic behavior in eighteen cases treated by wide local excision with extended clinical follow up. Am J Surg Pathol 2000;24:1125.
63. Domanski HA, Gustafson P: Cytologic features of primary, recurrent, and metastatic dermatofibrosarcoma protuberans. Cancer 2002; 96:351.
64. Dal Cin P, Polito P, Van Eyken P, et al: Anomalies of chromosomes 17 and 22 in giant cell fibroblastoma. Cancer Genet Cytogenet 1997;97:165.
65. Cin PD, Sciot R, de Wever I, et al: Cytogenetic and immunohistochemical evidence that giant cell fibroblastoma is related to dermatofibrosarcoma protuberans. Genes Chromosomes Cancer 1996;15:73.

Adult Fibrosarcoma

66. Pritchard DJ, Soule E, Taylor WF, et al: Fibrosarcoma—a clinicopathologic and statistical study of 199 tumors of the soft tissues of the extremities and trunk. Cancer 1974;33:888.
67. Bertoni F, Capanna R, Calderoni P, et al: Primary central (medullary) fibrosarcoma of bone. Semin Diagn Pathol 1984;1:185.

Angioleiomyoma

68. Hachisuga T, Hashimoto H, Enjoji M: Angioleiomyoma: A clinicopathologic reappraisal of 562 cases. Cancer 1984;54:126.
69. Duhig D, Ayer JP: Vascular leiomyoma: A study of sixty-one cases. Arch Pathol Lab Med 1959;68:424.
70. Heim S, Mandahl N, Kristoffersson U, et al: Structural chromosome aberrations in a case of angioleiomyoma. Cancer Genet Cytogenet 1986;20:325.
71. Hennig Y, Caselitz J, Stern C, et al: Karyotype evolution in a case of uterine angioleiomyoma. Cancer Genet Cytogenet 1999;108:79.

Leiomyoma and Leiomyosarcoma

72. Kilpatrick SE, Mentzel T, Fletcher CDM: Leiomyoma of deep soft tissue: Clinicopathologic analysis of a series. Am J Surg Pathol 1994;18:576.
73. Billings SD, Folpe AL, Weiss SW: Do leiomyomas of deep soft tissue exist? An analysis of highly differentiated smooth muscle tumors of deep soft tissue supporting two distinct subtypes. Am J Surg Pathol 2001;25:1134.
74. Paal E, Miettinen M: Retroperitoneal leiomyomas: A clinicopathologic and immunohistochemical study of 56 cases with a comparison to retroperitoneal leiomyosarcomas. Am J Surg Pathol 2001;25:1355.
75. Vaillo-Vinagre A, Ballestin-Carcavila C, Madero-Garcia S, et al: Primary angioleiomyoma of the iliac bone: Clinical pathological study of one case with flow cytometric DNA content and S-phase fraction analysis. Skeletal Radiol 2000;29:181.
76. Tao LC, Davidson DD: Aspiration biopsy cytology of smooth muscle tumors: A cytologic approach to the differentiation between leiomyosarcoma and leiomyoma. Acta Cytol 1993;37:300.
77. Farshid G, Pradham M, Goldblum J, et al: Leiomyosarcoma of somatic soft tissues: A tumor of vascular origin with multivariate analysis of outcome in 42 cases. Am J Surg Pathol 2002;26:14.
78. Hines OJ, Nelson S, Quinones-Baldrich WJ, et al: Leiomyosarcoma of the inferior vena cava: Prognosis and comparison with leiomyosarcoma of other anatomic sites. Cancer 1999;85:1077.
79. de Saint Aubain Somerhausen N, Fletcher CDM: Leiomyosarcoma of soft tissue in children: Clinicopathologic analysis of 20 cases. Am J Surg Pathol 1999;23:755.
80. Antonescu CR, Erlandson RA, Huvos AG: Primary leiomyosarcoma of bone: A clinicopathologic, immunohistochemical, and ultrastructural study of 33 patients and a literature review. Am J Surg Pathol 1997;21:1281.
81. Rubin BP, Fletcher CDM: Myxoid leiomyosarcoma of soft tissue, an underrecognized variant. Am J Surg Pathol 2000;24:927.
82. Mentzel T, Calonje E, Fletcher CDM: Leiomyosarcoma with prominent osteoclast-type giant cells: Analysis of eight cases closely mimicking the so-called giant cell variant of malignant fibrous histiocytoma. Am J Surg Pathol 1994;18:258.
83. Oshiro Y, Shiratsuchi H, Oda Y, et al: Rhabdoid features in leiomyosarcoma of soft tissue: With special reference to aggressive behavior. Mod Pathol 2000;13:1211.
84. Oda Y, Miyajima K, Kawaguchi K, et al: Pleomorphic leiomyosarcoma: Clinicopathologic and immunohistochemical study with special emphasis on its distinction from ordinary leiomyosarcoma and malignant fibrous histiocytoma. Am J Surg Pathol 2001;25:1030.
85. Kilpatrick SE, Geisinger KR: Soft tissue sarcomas: The usefulness and limitations of fine-needle aspiration biopsy. Am J Clin Pathol 1998;110:50.

86. Mandahl N, Fletcher CD, Dal Cin P, et al: Comparative cytogenetic study of spindle cell and pleomorphic leiomyosarcomas of soft tissues: A report from the CHAMP Study Group. Cancer Genet Cytogenet 2000;116:66.

Schwannoma

87. Das Gupta TK, Brasfield RD, Strong EW, et al: Benign solitary schwannomas (neurilemomas). Cancer 1969;24:355.
88. White W, Shiu MH, Rosenblum MK, et al: Cellular schwannoma: A clinicopathologic study of 57 patients and 58 tumors. Cancer 1990;66:1266.
89. Antinheimo J, Sankila R, Carpen O, et al: Population based analysis of sporadic and type 2 neurofibromatosis–associated meningiomas and schwannomas. Neurology 2000;54:71.
90. Hasegawa SL, Mentzel T, Fletcher CDM: Schwannomas of the sinonasal tract and nasopharynx. Mod Pathol 1997;10:777.
91. de la Monte SM, Dorfman HD, Chandra R, et al: Intraosseous schwannoma: Histologic features, ultrastructure, and review of the literature. Hum Pathol 1984;15:551.
92. Goldblum JR, Beals TF, Weiss SW: Neuroblastoma-like neurilemoma. Am J Surg Pathol 1994;18:266.
93. McMenamin ME, Fletcher CDM: Expanding the spectrum of malignant change in schwannomas: Epithelioid malignant change, epithelioid malignant peripheral nerve sheath tumor, and epithelioid angiosarcoma: A study of 17 cases. Am J Surg Pathol 2001;25:13.
94. Woodruff JM, Selig AM, Crowley K, et al: Schwannoma (neurilemoma) with malignant transformation: A rare, distinctive peripheral nerve sheath tumor. Am J Surg Pathol 1994;18:882.
95. Dahl I, Hagmar S, Idvall I: Benign solitary neurilemoma (schwannoma): A correlative cytological and histological study of 28 cases. Acta Pathol Microbiol Immuno Scand [A] 1984;92:91.
96. Ryd W, Mugal S, Ayyash K: Ancient neurilemoma: A pitfall in the cytologic diagnosis of soft tissue tumors. Diagn Cytopathol 1986;2:244.
97. Weiss SW, Langloss JM, Enzinger FM: Value of S-100 protein in the diagnosis of soft tissue tumors with particular reference to benign and malignant Schwann cell tumors. Lab Invest 1983;49:299.
98. Khalifa MA, Montgomery EA, Ismiil N, et al: What are the CD34+ cells in benign peripheral nerve sheath tumors? Double immunostaining study of CD34 and S-100 protein. Am J Clin Pathol 2000;114:123.
99. Mertens F, Dal Cin P, de Wever I, et al: Cytogenetic characterization of peripheral nerve sheath tumours: A report of the CHAMP study group. J Pathol 2000;190:31.
100. Carney JA: Psammomatous melanotic schwannoma: A distinctive, heritable tumor with special associations, including cardiac myxoma and the Cushing syndrome. Am J Surg Pathol 1990;14:206.
101. Myers JL, Bernreutter W, Dunham W: Melanotic schwannoma of bone: Clinicopathologic, immunohistochemical, and ultrastructural features of a rare primary bone tumor. Am J Clin Pathol 1990;93:424.

Neurofibroma

102. Weiss SW, Goldblum JR: Benign tumors of peripheral nerves. In Enzinger and Weiss's Soft Tissue Tumors, 4th ed. St. Louis: Mosby, 2001, p 111.
103. NIH Consensus Development Conference Statement: Neurofibromatosis conference statement. Arch Neurol 1988;45:575.
104. Collins FS, Ponder BAJ, Seizinger BR: The von Recklinghausen neurofibromatosis region on chromosome 17: Genetic and physical maps come into focus. Am J Hum Genet 1989;44:1.
105. Sorensen SA, Mulvihill JJ, Nielsen A: A long term follow-up of von Recklinghausen neurofibromatosis: Survival and malignant neoplasms. N Engl J Med 1986;314:1010.
106. Zoller MET, Rembeck B, Oden A: Malignant and benign tumors in patients with neurofibromatosis type 1 in a defined Swedish population. Cancer 1997;79:2125.
107. Lin BTY, Weiss LM, Medeiros LJ: Neurofibroma and cellular neurofibroma with atypia: A report of 14 tumors. Am J Surg Pathol 1997;21:1443.
108. Resnick JM, Fanning CV, Caraway NP, et al: Percutaneous needle biopsy diagnosis of benign neurogenic neoplasms. Diagn Cytopathol 1997;16:17.
109. McCarron KF, Goldblum JR: Plexiform neurofibroma with and without associated malignant peripheral nerve sheath tumor: A clinicopathologic and immunohistochemical analysis of 54 cases. Mod Pathol 1998;11:612.
110. Halling KC, Scheithauer BW, Halling AC, et al: p53 expression in neurofibroma and malignant peripheral nerve sheath tumor: An immunohistochemical study of sporadic and NF1-associated tumors. Am J Clin Pathol 1996;106:282.

Malignant Peripheral Nerve Sheath Tumor

111. Ducatman BS, Scheithauer BW, Plepgras DG, et al: Malignant peripheral nerve sheath tumors: A clinicopathologic study of 120 cases. Cancer 1986;57:2006.
112. Meis JM, Enzinger FM, Martz KL, et al: Malignant peripheral nerve sheath tumors (malignant schwannomas) in children. Am J Surg Pathol 1992;16:694.
113. Ducatman BS, Scheithauer BW: Malignant peripheral nerve sheath tumors with divergent differentiation. Cancer 1984;54:1049.
114. Wesche WA, Khare V, Rao BN, et al: Malignant peripheral nerve sheath tumor of bone in children and adolescents. Pediatr Dev Pathol 1999;2:159.
115. Bullock MJ, Bedard YC, Bell RS, et al: Intraosseous malignant peripheral nerve sheath tumor: Report of a case and review of the literature. Arch Pathol Lab Med 1995;119:367.
116. Abe S, Imamura T, Park P, et al: Small round-cell type of malignant peripheral nerve sheath tumor. Mod Pathol 1998;11:747.
117. Laskin WB, Weiss SW, Bratthauer GL: Epithelioid variant of malignant peripheral nerve sheath tumor (malignant epithelioid schwannoma). Am J Surg Pathol 1991;15:1136.
118. McGee RS, Ward WG, Kilpatrick SE: Malignant peripheral nerve sheath tumor: A fine needle aspiration biopsy study. Diagn Cytopathol 1997;17:298.
119. Wick MR, Swanson PE, Scheithauer BW, et al: Malignant peripheral nerve sheath tumor: An immunohistochemical study of 62 cases. Am J Clin Pathol 1987;87:425.
120. Johnson TL, Lee MW, Meis JM, et al: Immunohistochemical characterization of malignant peripheral nerve sheath tumors. Surg Pathol 1991;4:121.

CHAPTER 7

Giant Cell Tumors of Bone and Soft Tissue

The collective term *giant cell tumors of bone and soft tissue*, when used in this chapter, refers to lesions that contain multinucleated giant cells resembling osteoclasts, which, because of their number, often are reflected in the nomenclature of the tumor. In other words, the osteoclast-type giant cells are almost universally present and are considered part of the diagnostic criteria for these tumors. These lesions include giant cell tumors of bone and soft tissue; giant cell reparative granuloma; localized tenosynovial giant cell tumor (giant cell tumor of tendon sheath); diffuse tenosynovial giant cell tumor (pigmented villonodular synovitis); plexiform fibrohistiocytic tumor; and malignant fibrous histiocytoma, giant cell type (Table 7.1). Virtually any bone or soft tissue lesion may contain osteoclast-type giant cells, sometimes misleading or obscuring the diagnosis. Certain tumors, not discussed in this chapter, are more likely to contain them, however, and these are listed in Table 7.2.

Osteoclast-type giant cells likely are formed by the fusion of multiple mononuclear osteoclast precursors. Morphologically, osteoclast-type giant cells are large cells containing multiple, uniform-appearing, round-to-ovoid nuclei that are distributed randomly throughout their cytoplasm. Although individual osteoclast-type giant cells may vary in size and number of nuclei present, there should be little to no cytologic and nuclear variability from one giant cell to the next. This latter feature helps distinguish these benign-appearing giant cells from "malignant" giant cells. When examining lesions rich in osteoclast-type giant cells, it is necessary to pay particular attention to the background stromal cells because their morphologic appearance (not the osteoclast-type giant cells), coupled with clinical and radiographic correlation, establishes the diagnosis.

Giant Cell Tumor

Clinical Features

Giant cell tumor, also known as *osteoclastoma*, is a benign but locally aggressive neoplasm generally arising in adults between the ages of 20 and 40 years.[1,2] There seems to be a slight female predominance, especially among children and adolescents who develop the disease. Most patients complain initially of pain and swelling, rarely associated with fracture.

TABLE 7.1 Bone and Soft Tissue Tumors in Which Osteoclast-Type Giant Cells Are Definitionally Part of the Lesion

Bone	Soft Tissue
Giant cell tumor	Giant cell tumor
Giant cell reparative granuloma	Tenosynovial giant cell tumor, localized type
Brown tumor (hyperparathyroidism)	Tenosynovial giant cell tumor, diffuse type
MFH, giant cell type	MFH, giant cell type
	Plexiform fibrohistiocytic tumor

MFH, malignant fibrous histiocytoma.

TABLE 7.2 Bone and Soft Tissue Tumors Commonly Containing "Incidental" Osteoclast-Type Giant Cells That May Confound the Diagnosis

Bone	Soft Tissue
Simple bone cyst	Nodular fasciitis
Aneurysmal bone cyst	Myositis ossificans
Benign fibrous histiocytoma	Benign fibrous histiocytoma
MFH*	MFH*
Osteosarcoma	Osteosarcoma
Chondroblastoma	
Chondromyxoid fibroma	
Metaphyseal fibrous defect	

*MFHs other than the giant cell type.
MFH, malignant fibrous histiocytoma.

The most common anatomic locations are the bones around the knee, the distal femur and proximal tibia (Fig. 7.1), followed by the distal radius and sacrum (Fig. 7.2); however, giant cell tumor also may involve the pelvic bones and vertebral bodies (but not the dorsal elements) (Fig. 7.3). The small bones of the digits rarely are involved (Fig. 7.4).[3] Although almost always solitary, rare multicentric forms have been reported.[4] Radiographically, giant cell tumors form geographic, lytic lesions that, in the long bones, are almost always epiphyseal-centered with or without focal extension into the metaphysis. A sclerotic rim is usually absent. Giant cell tumors frequently destroy the cortex and extend into soft tissues, but a periosteal reaction is rarely seen. When giant cell tumors extend into or locally recur in soft tissues, a peripheral shell of ossification often is observed (Fig. 7.5).

Rarely, giant cell tumor may occur solely within extraskeletal superficial and deep soft tissues. In contrast to giant cell tumor of bone that more commonly is associated with the lower extremities, soft tissue giant cell tumor most commonly arises from the upper extremity, usually the arm or hand.[5] Most giant cell tumors of soft tissue occur above the superficial fascia, localized to the dermis or in the subcutaneous adipose tissue.

Pathologic Findings

Histology

The most striking histologic feature of giant cell tumor is the presence of innumerable osteoclast-type giant cells. These giant cells may be quite large and have variable numbers of nuclei, up to 100 per cell. The background stromal cells are slightly spindled to ovoid, often containing nuclei closely resembling those observed in the osteoclast-type giant cells. Significant nuclear atypia is not observed in either the giant cells or the background stromal cells (Fig. 7.6). Mitotic figures within the stromal cells may be numerous but are of no concern in the appropriate clinical and radiographic context. Focal necrosis is a common finding in giant cell tumor, usually leaving behind residual "tombstones" or "ghost" giant cells (Fig. 7.7). Other areas may lack the typical osteoclast-type giant cells and include abundant fibrous tissue and spindled cells arranged in short fascicles and storiform patterns, resembling metaphyseal fibrous defect. Xanthomatous changes, including abundant

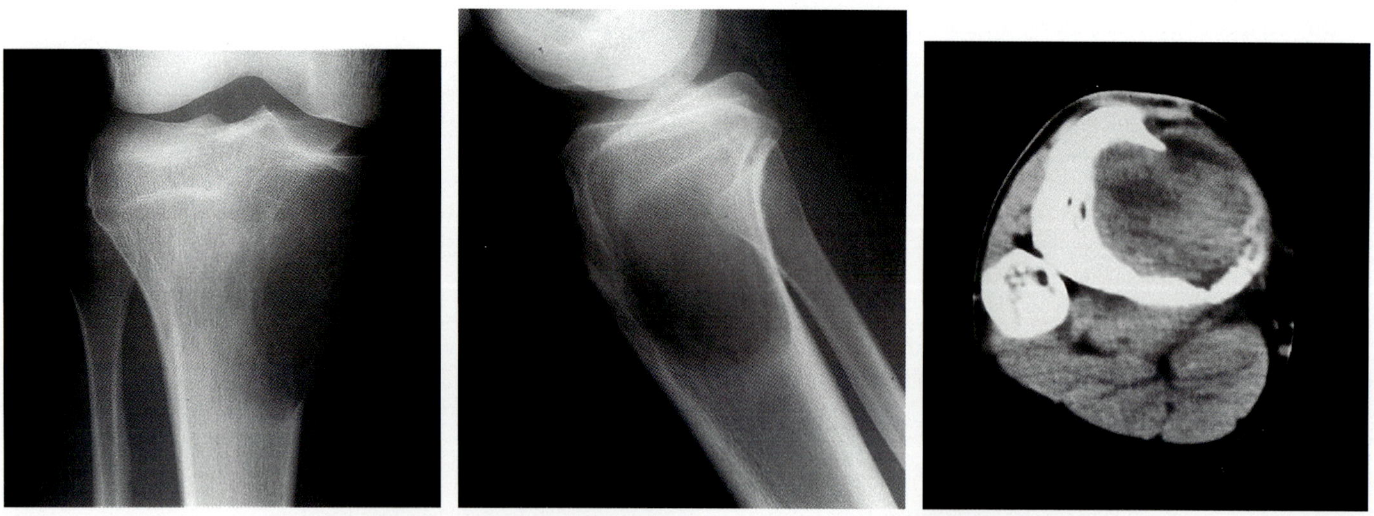

A B C

FIGURE 7.1 Giant cell tumor of the tibia. Anteroposterior **(A)** and lateral **(B)** radiographs of the proximal tibia show a well-demarcated, purely lytic lesion in the proximal tibia. The lesion extends to the subchondral bone of the tibia, and there is no associated periosteal new bone production. An axial computed tomographic scan from the same patient shows the lytic proximal tibia lesion with dissolution of the anteromedial tibial cortex **(C)**.

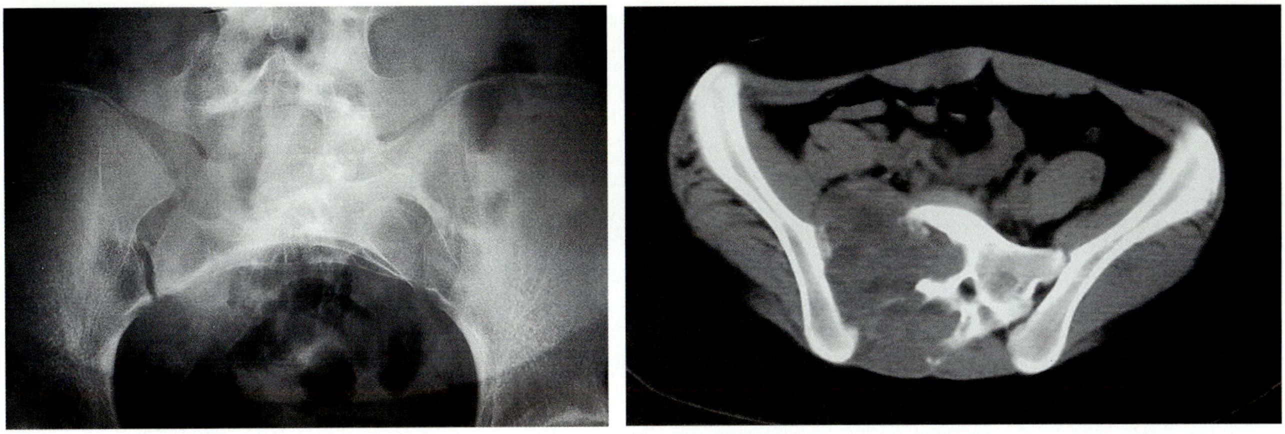

A B

FIGURE 7.2 Giant cell tumor of the sacrum. An anteroposterior radiograph of the sacrum reveals a lytic lesion in the right sacral ala. The superior margin of the right sacral ala is destroyed **(A)**. An axial computed tomographic scan shows the extensive lytic lesion in the right sacral ala. The tumor extends into the soft tissues anteriorly and posteriorly and extends into the spinal canal **(B)**.

foamy histiocytes, also may be present (Fig. 7.8). Reactive-appearing bone formation is common and often is seen at the periphery of the lesion, especially in giant cell tumors of bone that have extended into soft tissues (Fig. 7.9). Similar findings also are observed in the soft tissue variant of giant cell tumor. Hyaline cartilage and chondroid matrix are never present in giant cell tumor. Secondary aneurysmal bone cyst–like changes may be seen in bone and soft tissue giant cell tumors.

Fine Needle Aspiration Biopsy

The diagnosis of giant cell tumor of bone is rendered easily by fine needle aspiration biopsy. Cytologic smears are generally cellular and comprise aggregates of uniform-appearing, ovoid to slightly spindled stromal cells and numerous osteoclast-type giant cells. The stromal cells have high nuclear-to-cytoplasmic ratios, but the nuclei show evenly distributed chromatin and inconspicuous-to-small nucleoli. Significant nuclear atypia is

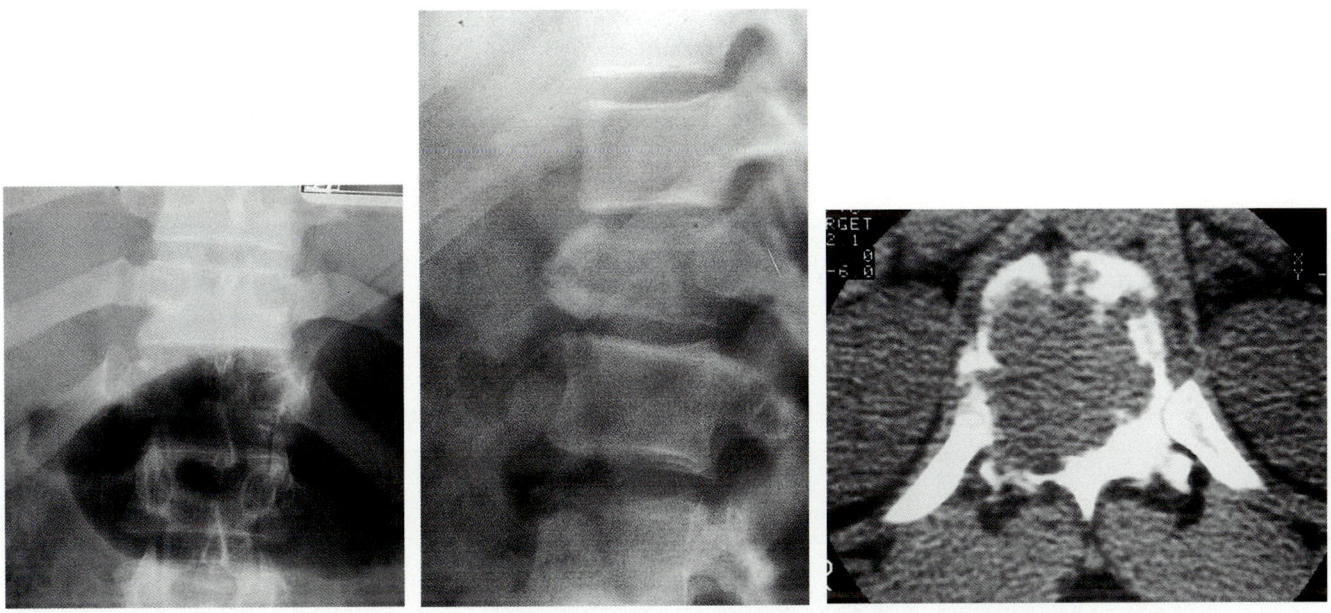

A B C

FIGURE 7.3 Giant cell tumor of the vertebral body. Anteroposterior **(A)** and lateral **(B)** radiographs of the spine reveal a destructive lesion of the T12 vertebral body associated with a mild compression fracture. An axial computed tomographic scan shows the extensive lytic lesion of the T12 vertebra, centered in the vertebral body centrum but extending into the spinal canal and producing erosion of the right lamina **(C)**.

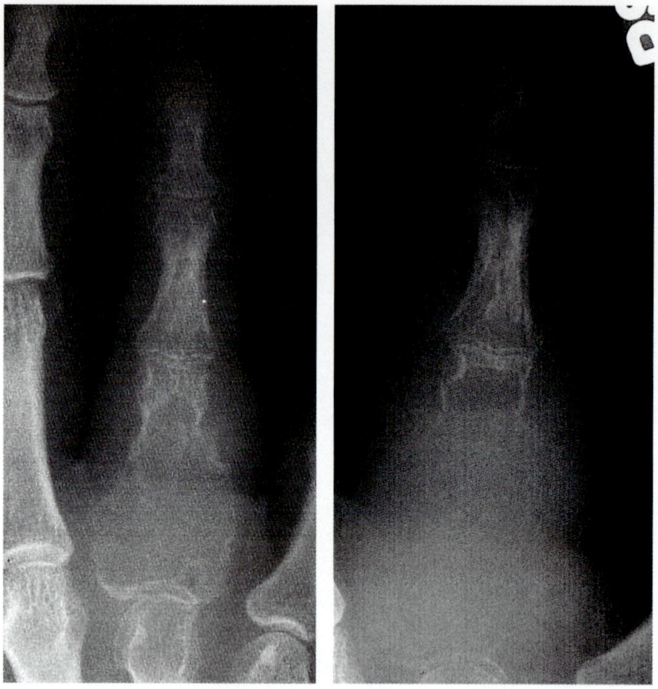

A B

FIGURE 7.4 Aggressive giant cell tumor. A posteroanterior radiograph of the ring finger reveals an extensive lytic lesion of the proximal phalanx of the affected digit. No matrix calcification is identified **(A)**. Two months later, the extent of bone destruction has progressed dramatically **(B)**.

not observed and if present should suggest the diagnosis of giant cell–rich osteosarcoma (Fig. 7.10). Similarly, matrix material rarely is observed in cytologic smears.

Ancillary Studies

Ultrastructurally, the osteoclast-type giant cells and the mononuclear cells appear virtually identical, characterized by histiocytic features including increased mitochondria, sparse rough endoplasmic reticulum, and lysosomes. The osteoclast-type giant cells also reveal a ruffled cytoplasmic border.

Immunohistochemically, the mononuclear cells and osteoclast-type giant cells of giant cell tumor show positivity for CD68 and tartrate-resistant acid phosphatase but appear negative for S-100 protein and desmin. Smooth muscle actin positivity also is observed in the mononuclear stromal cells.[5]

To date, a specific and reproducible translocation in giant cell tumor has not been found. The most frequent chromosomal aberrations are telomeric alterations, most commonly affecting chromosomes 11p, 13p, 14p, 15p, 19q, 20q, and 21p.[6] Cases associated with aneurysmal bone cysts have shown rearrangements of 16q22 or 17p13.[7]

Prognosis and Therapy

Giant cell tumors of bone and soft tissue should be considered at least low-grade malignant lesions with the potential, albeit rare, of metastasis. There are no histologic features predictive of prognosis. Minimal curettage and bone grafting lead to local recurrence in 40% to 50% of cases. More extensive curettage, often involving chemical cauterization, reduces the risk of local recurrence to approximately 10% to 20%. Of patients with giant cell tumor, 1% to 3% develop pulmonary metastasis (Fig. 7.11). This usually ominous sign leads to death in only a few patients, however. Most pulmonary lesions from a "benign metastasizing giant cell tumor" tend to grow slowly and may remain stationary.[8] Reports of spontaneous resolution also have been documented.[9] Some authors advocate surgical resection for these lesions.

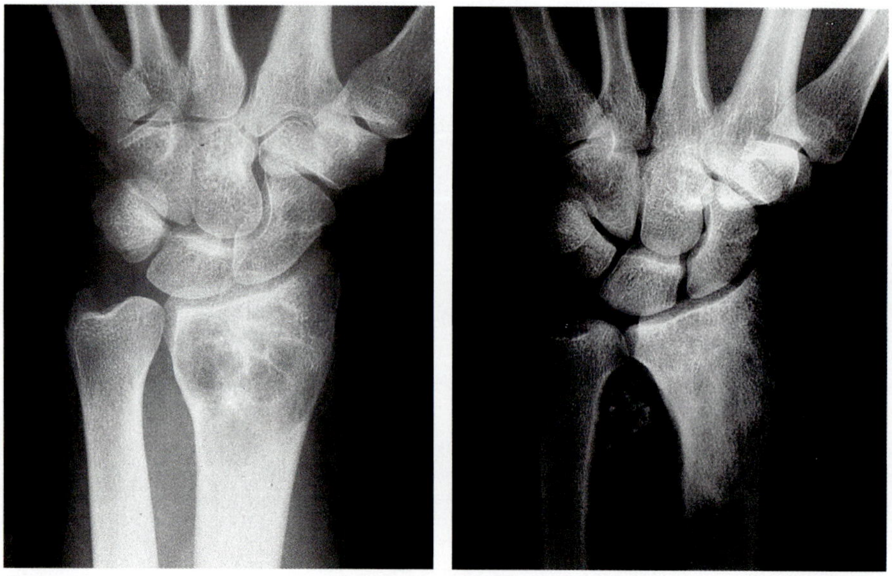

A B

FIGURE 7.5 Giant cell tumor with soft tissue recurrence. A posteroanterior radiograph of the wrist shows a well-demarcated lytic lesion in the distal radius. The lesion is subchondral in location **(A)**. Two years later, after operative curettage of the radial lesion, recurrence of the tumor in the interosseous soft tissues has produced a peripherally calcified mass **(B)**.

TABLE 7.3 Clinical Variants of Giant Cell Reparative Granuloma

	Digits (Giant Cell Reaction)	Jaw	Hyperparathyroidism (Brown Tumor)
Age (yr)*	5-20	5-20	30-60
Gender	F > M	F > M	F > M
Location†	Phalanges Metatarsals Metacarpals	Mandible Maxilla	Mandible Clavicle Ribs Pelvis
Inherited syndromes	None	Cherubism	MEN syndromes

*Most common age range.
†Most common anatomic locations.
MEN, multiple endocrine neoplasia.

usually in the skull. Hyperparathyroidism and Paget's disease are discussed in greater detail in Chapter 16.

Clinical Features

Giant cell reparative granuloma usually arises as a lytic lesion within the jaws or digits of female patients 5 to 20 years of age.[11,12] In the jaw, giant cell reparative granuloma most commonly localizes to the anterior portion of the mandible (central giant cell lesion), although involvement of the maxilla and interosseous sinuses occasionally occurs. Most cases represent asymptomatic incidental findings or come to clinical attention because of painless swelling of the affected bone. Rarely, giant cell reparative granuloma may arise within the soft tissues of the gingiva without bony involvement (peripheral giant cell lesion). Cherubism is an autosomal dominant disorder manifesting in childhood and associated with bilateral and symmetric giant cell reparative granulomas of the mandible. Patients usually present with symmetric swelling of the face and jaw in early childhood. Regression of the lesions generally begins in adolescence.[13] When giant cell reparative granuloma involves the hands or feet, the phalanges, metacarpals, or metatarsal bones may be involved. Most patients present with pain and, occasionally, soft tissue swelling.[11]

Microscopically similar lesions have been described in the vertebral spine and ethmoid bones, referred to as a "solid variant of aneurysmal bone cyst."[14] Giant cell reparative granuloma simply may reflect a spectrum of aneurysmal bone cyst.

Radiographically, giant cell reparative granulomas, regardless of origin, are characteristically lytic and expansile but usually well circumscribed without cortical erosion (Figs. 7.12 and 7.13). Less commonly, giant cell reparative granulomas appear more aggressive, especially in the tubular bones, with destruction of the cortex and extension into soft tissues. In the jawbones, resorption of teeth also may occur.

Pathologic Findings

Histology

Morphologically, giant cell reparative granulomas of all clinical types are associated with numerous, randomly distributed, osteoclast-type giant cells admixed with a uniform population of ovoid-to-spindled stromal cells. In contrast to conventional giant cell tumor, the background stroma tends to be more fibrotic and hypervascular. Pigmented histiocytes are often present (Fig. 7.14). Foci of osteoid and reactive bone usually are observed (Fig. 7.15). The histologic features

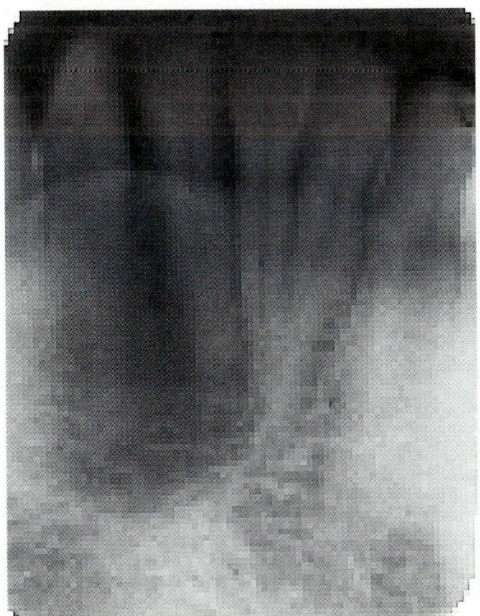

A

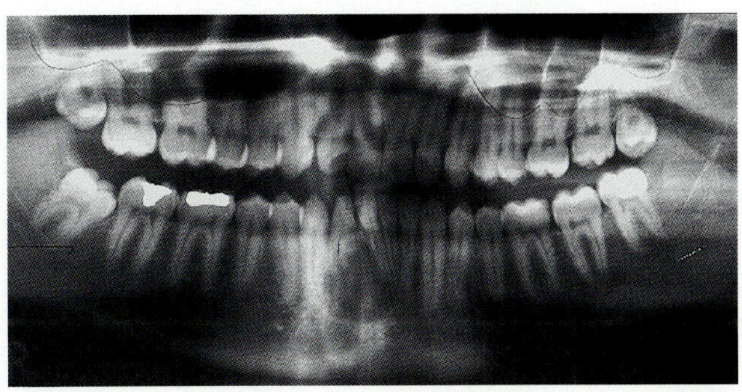

B

FIGURE 7.12 Giant cell reparative granuloma. Occlusal **(A)** and panorama **(B)** radiographs of the mandible show a lytic lesion of the mandible. The roots of the affected teeth are displaced by the lesion, but there is no aggressive bone destruction. (Courtesy of Donald A. Tyndall, DDS, MSPH, PhD, UNC-CH School of Dentistry.)

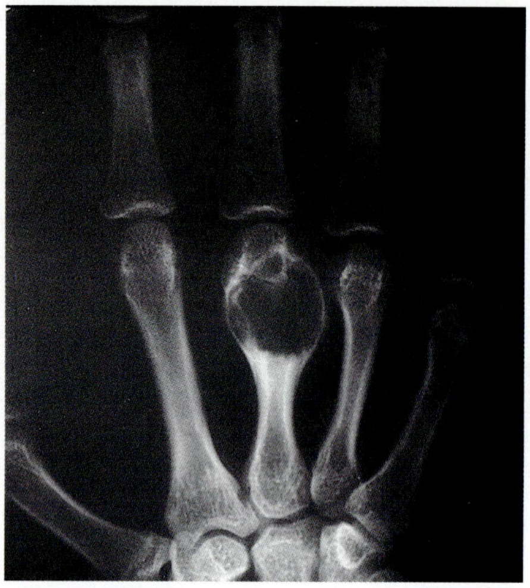

FIGURE 7.13 Giant cell reparative granuloma. A posteroanterior radiograph of the hand shows a well-demarcated, expansile, and lytic lesion of the distal right third metacarpal.

closely resemble those seen in aneurysmal bone cyst, including occasional blood-filled cysts, and are essentially identical to brown tumor of hyperparathyroidism (Fig. 7.16). Clinical and radiographic correlation is essential to establishing the diagnosis of giant cell reparative granuloma.

Fine Needle Aspiration Biopsy

Fine needle aspiration biopsy of giant cell reparative granulomas is usually moderately cellular and composed of aggregates and solitary, benign-appearing spindle cells accompanied by osteoclast-type giant cells. The spindle cell component appears fibroblastic and has more abundant cytoplasm than the background stromal cells of conventional giant cell tumor. Additionally, the number of giant cells is typically less than that observed with conventional giant cell tumor (Fig. 7.17).

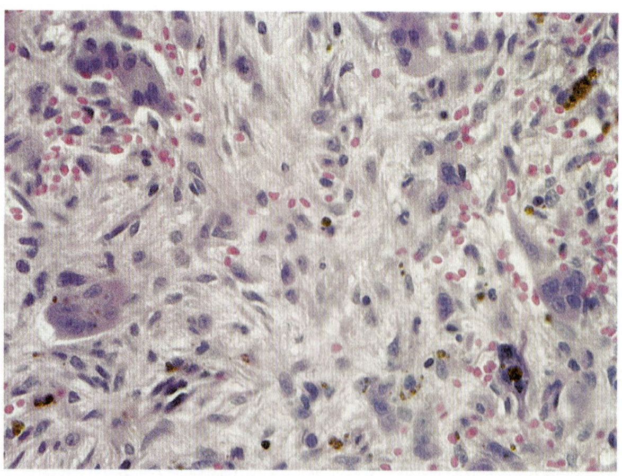

FIGURE 7.14 Giant cell reparative granuloma comprises randomly distributed giant cells within a largely fibrotic and hypervascular stroma. Note the hemosiderin-laden macrophages. (H&E.)

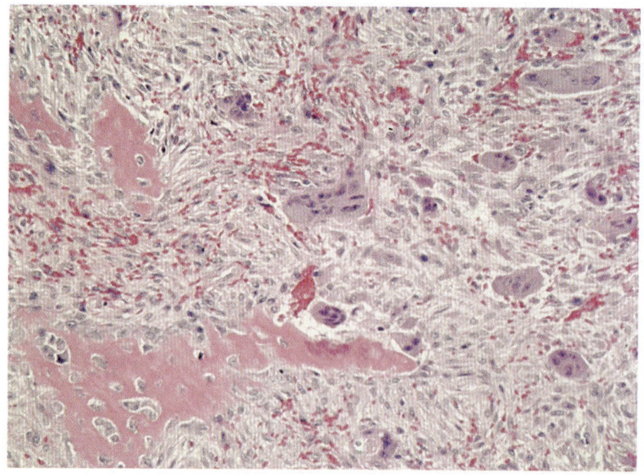

FIGURE 7.15 Similar to giant cell tumor, giant cell reparative granuloma frequently has foci of reactive-appearing bone. (H&E.)

Ancillary Studies

The ultrastructural features of giant cell reparative granuloma reveal myofibroblastic differentiation in the stromal cells, including intermediate filaments. The osteoclast-type giant cells are essentially identical to cells observed in giant cell tumor.

Cytogenetic analysis has revealed a t(X;4)(q22;q31.3) arrangement in a single case of giant cell reparative granuloma.[15] A case of the "solid" variant of aneurysmal bone cyst was found to have a chromosome 16 rearrangement.[16]

Prognosis and Therapy

Giant cell reparative granuloma of the jaws or digits generally is cured by simple curettage. Local recurrence may occur in 20% of cases, however. In the phalanges, amputation rarely is

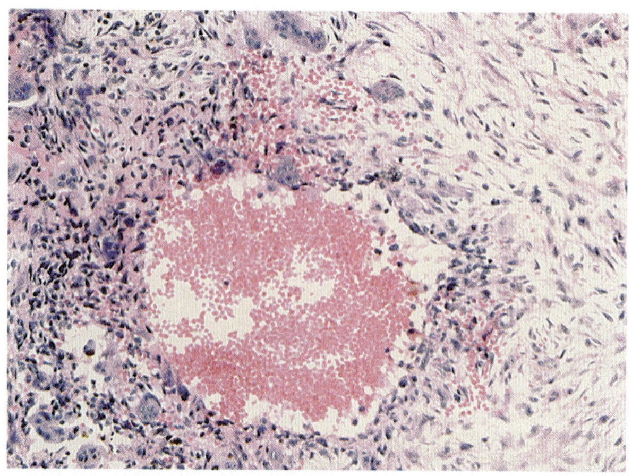

FIGURE 7.16 Blood-filled cysts, resembling aneurysmal bone cyst, are relatively common in giant cell reparative granuloma. (H&E.)

required for adequate local control. Distant metastasis is never seen. There are no reliable clinical or histologic features in giant cell reparative granuloma predictive of clinical behavior.

Diffuse Tenosynovial Giant Cell Tumor (Pigmented Villonodular Synovitis)

Diffuse tenosynovial giant cell tumor most commonly involves joint spaces but also may extend into extra-articular soft tissues. For this reason, the tumor is known by a variety of designations, at least partly dependent on origin: pigmented villonodular bursitis, extra-articular pigmented villonodular synovitis, and proliferative synovitis.

Clinical Features

Diffuse tenosynovial giant cell tumor most commonly affects patients 20 to 40 years old. Although virtually any joint may be affected, diffuse tenosynovial giant cell tumor most commonly involves the knee; other joints that may be involved include the ankle and foot, hip, and shoulder.[17,18] Diffuse tenosynovial giant cell tumor may involve the intra-articular spaces and extra-articular (bursa and tendon sheaths) soft tissues.[19] Most examples of the extra-articular form are likely the result of intra-articular extension. Among extra-articular examples, the wrist and the knee are the most common anatomic sites.[19] Clinical symptoms may be of long duration (e.g., several years) and include localized pain and tenderness, joint effusion, hemarthrosis, and limitation of motion. Usually only one joint is affected, although the process rarely may be polyarticular. Many patients with polyarticular disease have a familial history of diffuse tenosynovial giant cell tumor, leading some authors to propose that the process may have a genetic component.

Because of its tendency to involve intra-articular spaces, magnetic resonance imaging is more useful than conventional radiographs for identifying diffuse tenosynovial giant cell tumor. Radiographically, most examples appear as soft tissue masses within and sometimes extending outside of the joint space. Frequently the process is associated with single-to-multiple, well-defined cortical bone defects, often involving both sides of the joint (Fig. 7.18). Rarely, these defects may be large, extending into the metaphysis, mimicking a primary bone neoplasm. Juxta-articular osteoporosis is generally not associated with the diffuse form of tenosynovial giant cell tumor.

Pathologic Findings

Histology

Histologic features of diffuse tenosynovial giant cell tumor are virtually identical to those seen in the localized form. Instead of producing a discrete solitary mass, the diffuse form of tenosynovial giant cell tumor forms a "diffuse" multinodular, infiltrative, and, when intra-articular, expansile process of the synovial fronds. A collagenous capsule surrounding the tumor is absent. Morphologically, diffuse tenosynovial giant cell tumor comprises sheets of uniform-appearing, mononuclear histiocyte–like cells admixed with numerous but randomly distributed, osteoclast-type giant cells and lymphocytes (Fig. 7.19). Xanthomatous changes

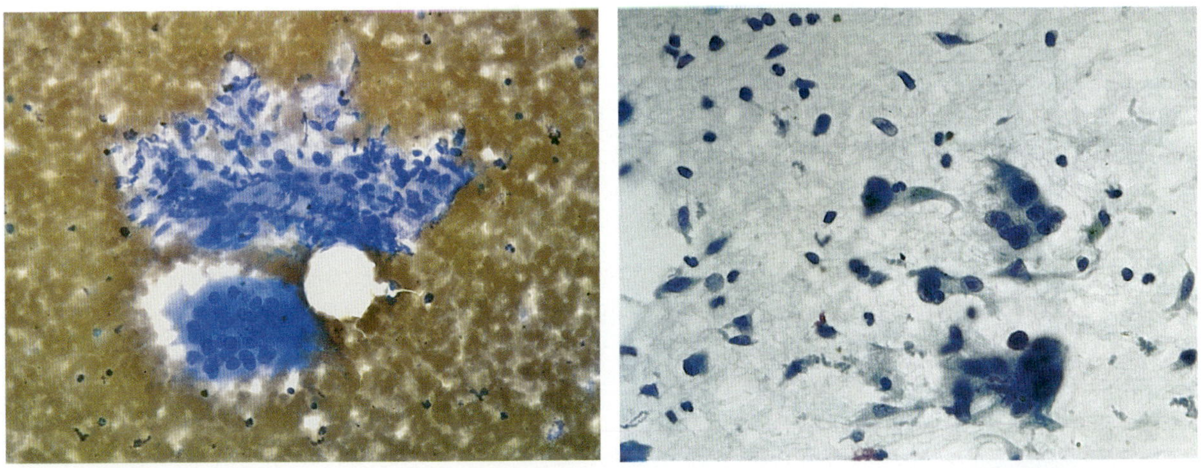

A B

FIGURE 7.17 Fine needle aspiration biopsy specimen of giant cell reparative granuloma with scattered osteoclast-type giant cells and aggregates and solitary fibroblast-like cells. Compared with giant cell tumor, the stromal cells in giant cell reparative granuloma generally display more abundant cytoplasm and greater variability. (**A,** Diff-Quik; **B,** Papanicolaou.)

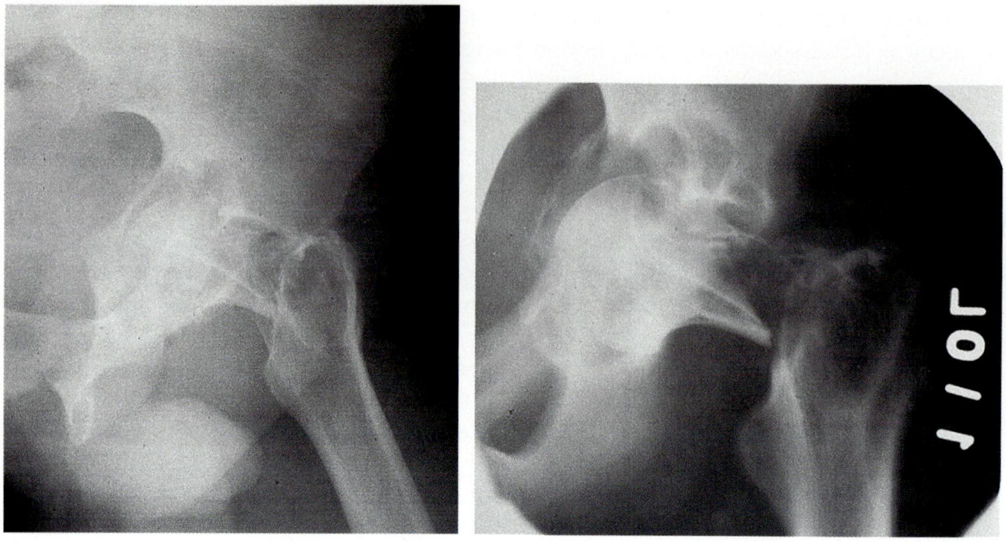

A B

FIGURE 7.18 Diffuse tenosynovial giant cell tumor (pigmented villonodular synovitis). Anteroposterior **(A)** and tomographic **(B)** images of the hip show destruction of bone in the femoral head and in the adjacent acetabulum. A pathologic fracture has developed through the femoral neck.

with aggregates of foamy histiocytes and cholesterol crystal clefts also frequently are present (Fig. 7.20). Hemosiderin-pigment deposition is observed at least focally in all cases (Fig. 7.21). Similar to the localized form, mitotic activity may be significant, sometimes exceeding 5 mitoses per 10 high-power fields. The background stroma ranges from areas with little to no collagenization to foci of significant hyalinization and less cellularity. In the more hyalinized areas, aggregates of the histiocytoid cells may exhibit a pseudoglandular appearance (Fig. 7.22).

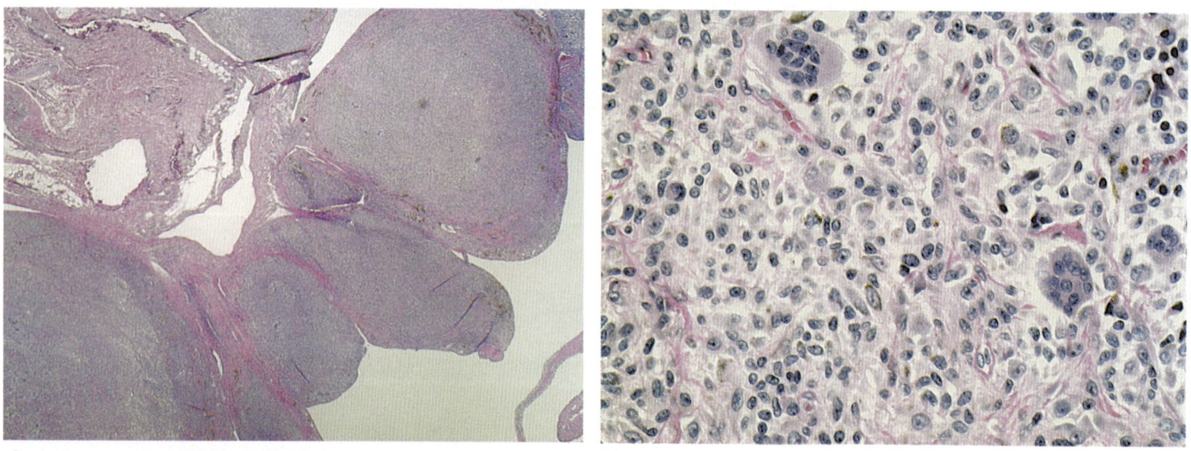

A B

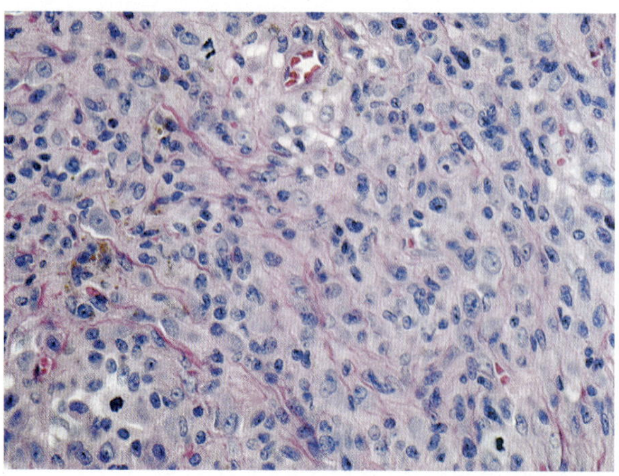

C

FIGURE 7.19 Diffuse tenosynovial giant cell tumor shows a multinodular, diffuse thickening of the synovial fronds **(A)**. Scattered osteoclast-type giant cells are admixed with a uniform-appearing population of "histiocytoid" cells within a variably collagenous background **(B)**. Osteoclast-type giant cells may not be present throughout all fields and, in some cases, may be sparse **(C)**. **(A,** Low power, H&E; **B** and **C,** H&E.)

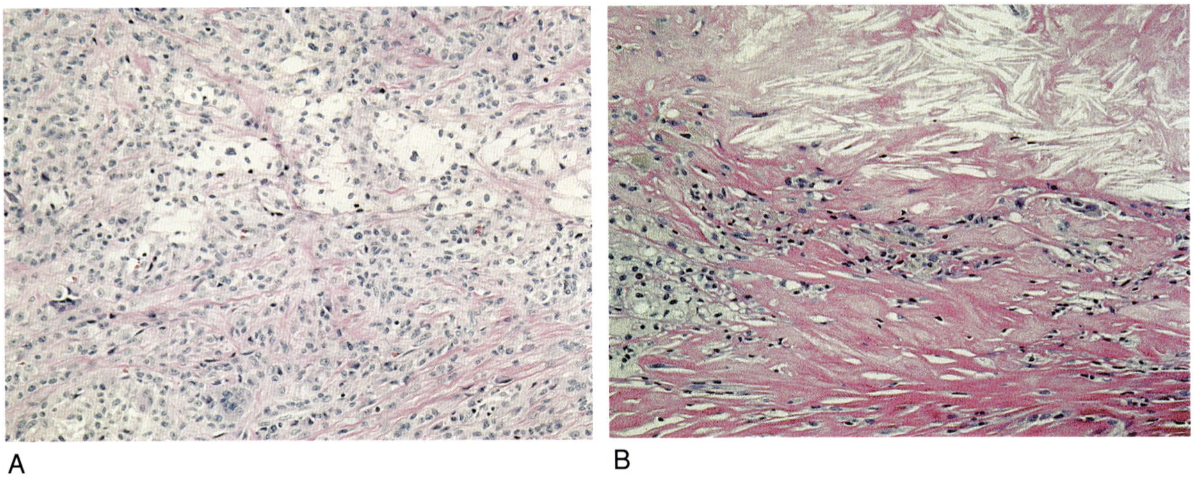

FIGURE 7.20 Aggregates of foamy histiocytes and foci of cholesterol clefts are common findings in diffuse tenosynovial giant cell tumor **(A and B)**. **(A** and **B,** H&E.)

Fine Needle Aspiration Biopsy

Cytologic smears from the diffuse form of tenosynovial giant cell tumor tend to be highly cellular and composed of aggregates and discohesive, bland-appearing, mononuclear histiocyte–like cells admixed with osteoclast-type giant cells and foamy histiocytes (Fig. 7.23).[20] Hemosiderin-pigment laden histiocytes also generally are observed (Fig. 7.24). Significant nuclear atypia is not a feature and, if present, should suggest a malignant diagnosis.

Ancillary Studies

Ultrastructurally, most mononuclear cells have features suggestive of histiocyte differentiation, containing numerous lysosomes, mitochondria, and a ruffled cell membrane. Phagocytosis of erythrocytes and hemosiderin also is observed. Other cells with fibroblastic and myofibroblastic features are seen less commonly.[21]

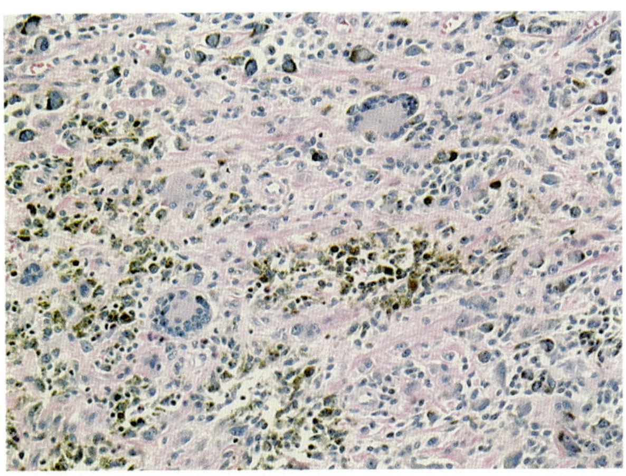

FIGURE 7.21 A histologic hallmark of diffuse tenosynovial giant cell tumor is the presence of randomly distributed, hemosiderin-laden macrophages. These cells also may be seen in the localized form but tend to be less prominent. (H&E.)

Immunohistochemically the osteoclast-type giant cells and many of the background mononuclear cells show features supportive of histiocytic differentiation, tending to express CD68, vimentin, and, less commonly, factor 13A.[19,22] Actin and desmin positivity has been reported in some of the mononuclear cells.[19]

Cytogenetic analysis has revealed abnormalities of chromosome 1p, trisomy 5, and trisomy 7.[23,24] The diffuse form of giant cell tumor may be aneuploid in 50% of cases, whereas localized giant cell tumors are virtually always diploid.[17]

Prognosis and Therapy

For the most part, diffuse tenosynovial giant cell tumor should be considered a locally aggressive but nonmetastasizing lesion. Less than complete excision or partial synovectomy results in local recurrence rates up to 50%. For the intra-articular form, complete total synovectomy is recommended; arthroscopic

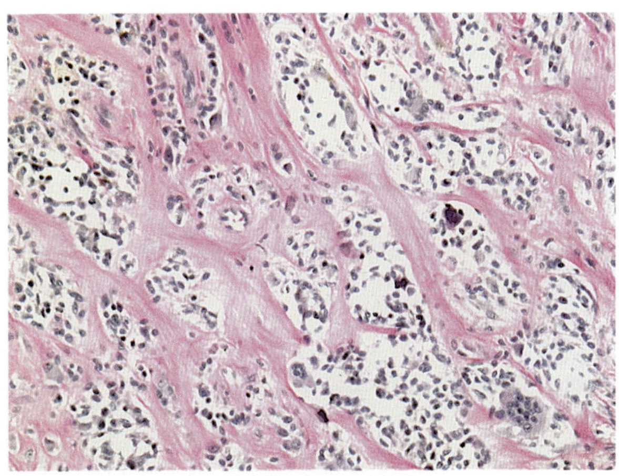

FIGURE 7.22 In more hyalinized areas, aggregates of histiocytoid cells displaying a pseudoglandular appearance may confound the diagnosis of diffuse tenosynovial giant cell tumor. (H&E.)

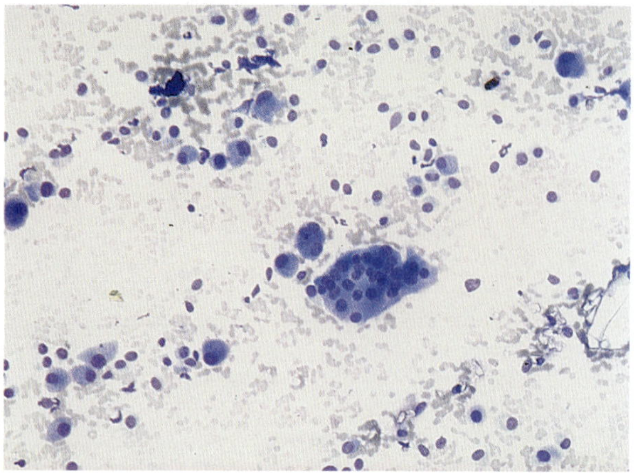

A

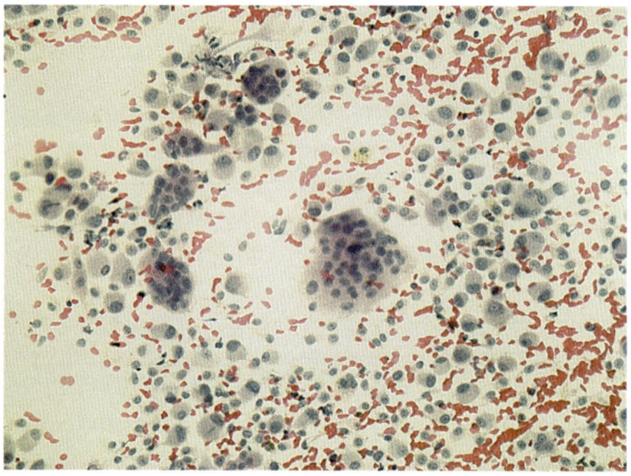

B

FIGURE 7.23 Fine needle aspiration biopsy specimens of diffuse tenosynovial giant cell tumor tend to be highly cellular with numerous discohesive, polygonal-to-histiocytoid cells accompanied by randomly distributed, osteoclast-type giant cells. Minimal nuclear atypia is present **(A and B)**. **(A,** Diff-Quik; **B,** Papanicolaou.)

surgery is inadequate. For extra-articular forms, wide excision with negative margins is the therapy of choice.[19] Amputation is sometimes necessary for adequate control of the disease. There are no morphologic features that are helpful in predicting prognosis.

The existence of a "malignant" form of tenosynovial giant cell tumor is controversial and likely rarely exists. The designation most commonly has been used when frankly malignant (sarcoma-like) areas are seen in conjunction with a usual-appearing localized or diffuse tenosynovial giant cell tumor. Patients with malignant tenosynovial giant cell tumor tend to be older (>40 years) than patients with conventional diffuse tenosynovial giant cell tumor. Histologic features include a diffuse infiltrative pattern comprising cells with enlarged nucleoli, macronucleoli, abundant eosinophilic cytoplasm, spindling, and significant mitotic activity (>10 mitoses per 10 high-power fields).[19,25] Necrosis and stromal myxoid change frequently are observed.[19] In these cases, wide excision or amputation may be required.

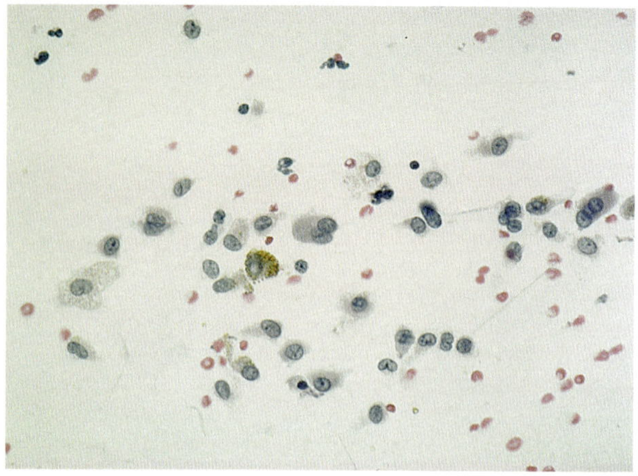

FIGURE 7.24 Scattered pigmented histiocytes frequently are found. (Papanicolaou.)

Localized Tenosynovial Giant Cell Tumor (Giant Cell Tumor of Tendon Sheath)

Tenosynovial giant cell tumor, localized type, also is called *nodular tenosynovitis* and *giant cell tumor of tendon sheath*. By definition, localized tenosynovial giant cell tumor forms a discrete mass composed of round-to-polygonal, synovial-like cells admixed with variable numbers of chronic inflammatory cells and osteoclast-type giant cells.

Clinical Features

Although localized giant cell tumor may occur at any age, it is observed most commonly between 30 and 50 years and shows a slight predilection for females. Most tumors occur in the hands, especially the fingers, but tumors also are seen in decreasing order of frequency in the toes, ankle and foot, knee, and wrist.[26] Finger and toe lesions often arise adjacent to interphalangeal joint spaces. Localized giant cell tumor is typically a slow-growing process, and in many patients, the lesions have been present for several years. Clinical symptoms may include pain, soft tissue swelling, and limitation of movement. Radiographically the classic clinical presentation is a well-circumscribed soft tissue mass adjacent to an underlying joint (Fig. 7.25). Cortical erosion of the underlying bone may be present (Fig. 7.26). These bony changes are observed more commonly in localized giant cell tumors of the toes than in tumors involving the fingers.

Pathologic Findings

Histology

Localized giant cell tumor typically presents as an exophytic mass that may or may not be connected to the underlying

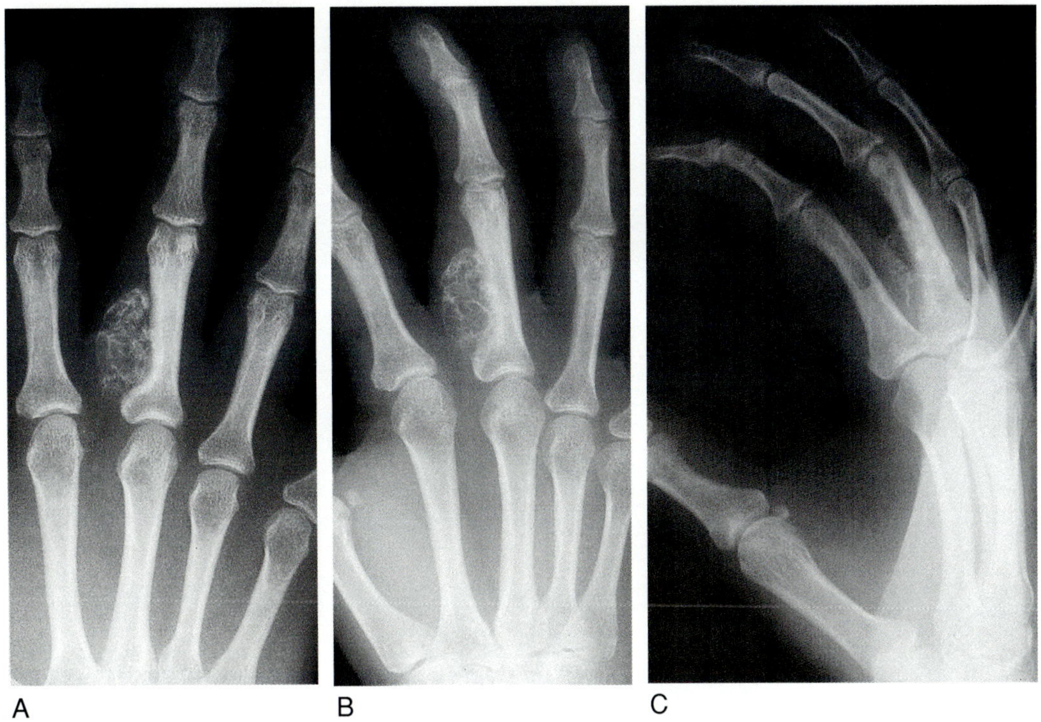

FIGURE 7.25 Localized tenosynovial giant cell tumor (giant cell tumor of tendon sheath). Anteroposterior **(A)**, oblique **(B)**, and lateral **(C)** radiographs of the long finger show a peripherally calcified lesion in the soft tissues adjacent to the proximal phalanx of the long finger. There is pressure erosion along the radial aspect of the proximal phalanx.

synovium. Most tumors are lobulated and at least partially encapsulated. Dense collagenous septa divide the tumor into variably sized lobules. Within the lobules, uniform-appearing, mononuclear histiocyte–like cells are admixed with variable numbers of osteoclast-type giant cells, foamy histiocytes, and chronic inflammatory cells. The background stroma may be significantly collagenized and hyalinized. Similar to the diffuse form, areas with little to no osteoclast-type giant cells also may be observed (Fig. 7.27). Hemosiderin-pigment deposition usually is focally present but is typically less prominent than in the diffuse form. Mitotic activity may exceed 3 mitotic figures per 10 high-power fields but should not cause any concern if other classic morphologic features are present.

Fine Needle Aspiration Biopsy

Fine needle aspiration biopsy rarely is performed in localized giant cell tumors because of their superficial location. Most are excised easily. Cytologic smears tend to be hypercellular and comprise an admixture of clusters and solitary mononuclear histiocyte–like cells, osteoclast-type giant cells, foamy histiocytes, and scattered lymphocytes (Fig. 7.28). In the appropriate clinical and radiographic context, the diagnosis is rendered easily on fine needle aspiration biopsy material.

Ancillary Studies

Ultrastructural studies reveal virtually identical findings to those seen in the diffuse form of giant cell tumor, and the findings in the osteoclast-type giant cells and some of the mononuclear cells suggest a histiocytic lineage.[21] These cells are admixed with fibroblasts. Likewise, immunohistochemical results are similar to results observed in the diffuse form.[22]

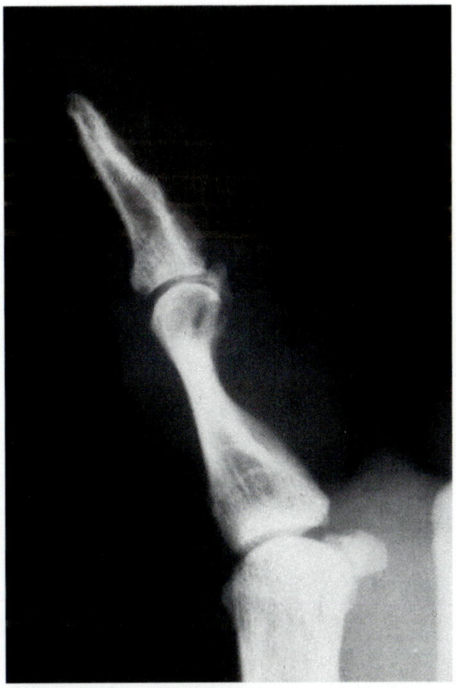

FIGURE 7.26 Localized tenosynovial giant cell tumor (giant cell tumor of tendon sheath). A lateral radiograph of the thumb reveals an extraosseous mass along the anterior surface of the thumb producing a prominent cortical erosion of the subjacent surface of the proximal phalanx.

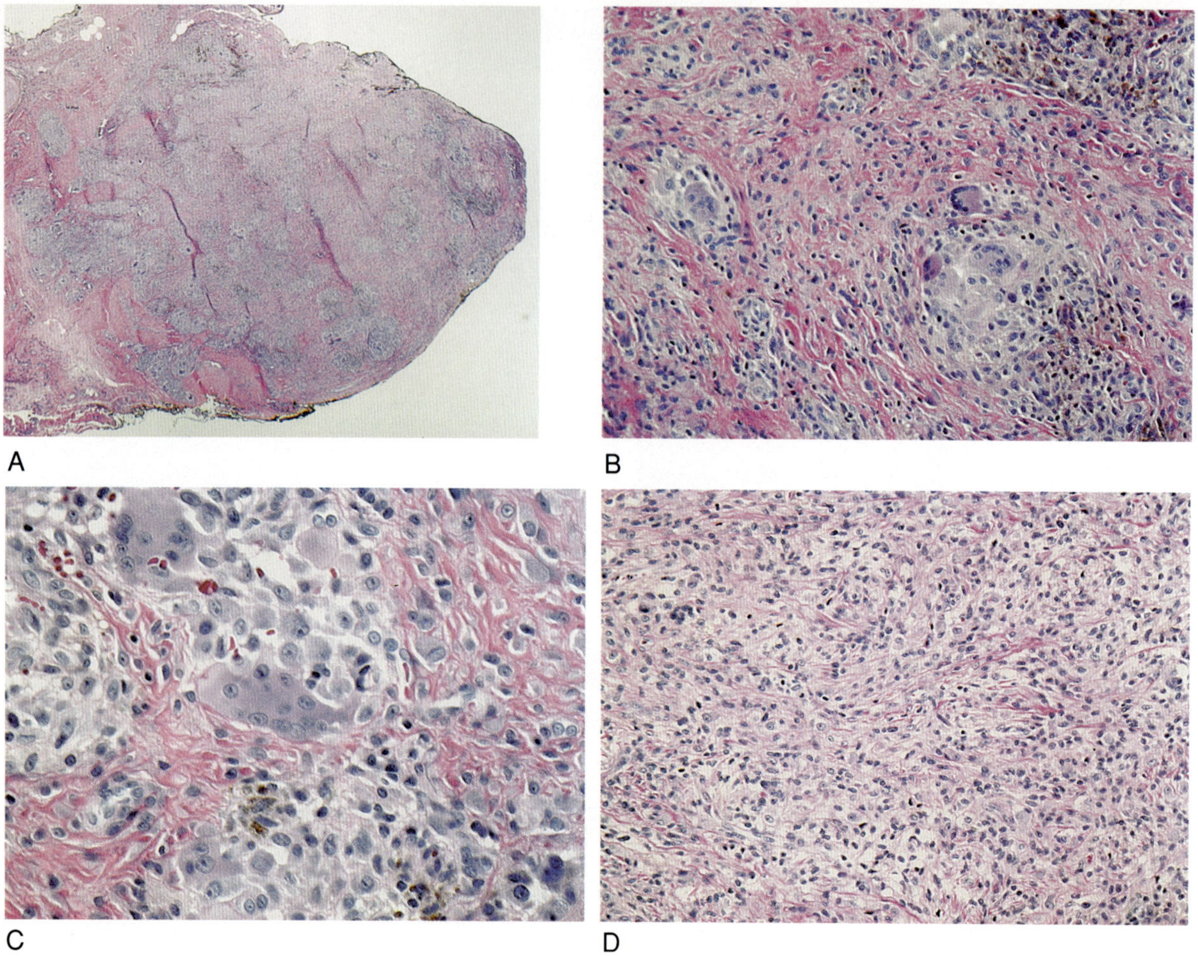

FIGURE 7.27 Localized tenosynovial giant cell tumor showing a solitary, well-circumscribed nodule histologically identical to one of the nodules of the diffuse form. Aggregates of uniform-appearing, mononuclear "histiocytoid" cells are accompanied by scattered osteoclast-type giant cells. The background stroma shows variable collagenization and hemosiderin pigment deposition **(A-C)**. Areas with virtually no giant cells may be seen **(D)**. (**A,** Low power, H&E; **B,** intermediate power, H&E; **C,** high power, H&E; **D,** H&E.)

Cytogenetic analysis has yielded variable results. The most common abnormality seems to represent rearrangements involving 1p11-13. Gains of chromosomes 5 and 7, typically seen in the diffuse form, have not been observed in localized giant cell tumors.[23]

Prognosis and Therapy

Despite being a benign lesion, localized giant cell tumor may recur in 20% of cases. Local recurrence is more likely to occur in patients who have undergone simple enucleation. For this reason, recommended therapy consists of removal of circumferential tissue around the tumor proper. Metastasis does not occur with localized giant cell tumor. There are no reliable histologic features predictive of locally aggressive clinical behavior.

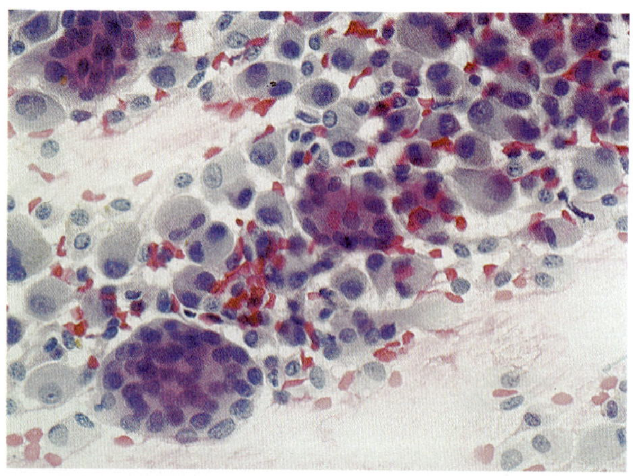

FIGURE 7.28 Fine needle aspiration biopsy of localized giant cell tumor is virtually identical to that observed with the diffuse form. Mostly discohesive, uniform-appearing, polygonal-to-histiocytoid cells with minimal nuclear atypia are accompanied by variable numbers of osteoclast-type giant cells. (Papanicolaou.)

Plexiform Fibrohistiocytic Tumor

Clinical Features

Plexiform fibrohistiocytic tumor is a rare, low-grade sarcoma usually arising in infants and children and less commonly affecting adults. The tumor occurs in females more often than males. At the time of diagnosis, most patients complain of a small (<3 cm), painless soft tissue mass localized to the dermis or subcutaneous fat or both. The upper extremities, especially the hands and wrists, are involved in two thirds of cases followed by, in decreasing order of frequency, the lower extremities and trunk.[27,28] Plexiform fibrohistiocytic tumor is rare in the head and neck region.

Pathologic Findings

Histology

Plexiform fibrohistiocytic tumor has a distinctive biphasic histologic appearance, being composed of variably sized histiocytic nodules admixed with infiltrative fibroblastic fascicles, creating a plexiform arrangement. The histiocytic nodules typically are well demarcated from the spindle cell component and consist of clusters of mononuclear cells and randomly distributed, osteoclast-type giant cells (Fig. 7.29). The fibroblastic component closely resembles a cellular fibromatosis or nodular fasciitis with a uniform spindle cell population arranged in fascicles and vague storiform patterns, accompanied by variable amounts of collagen deposition (Fig. 7.30). In

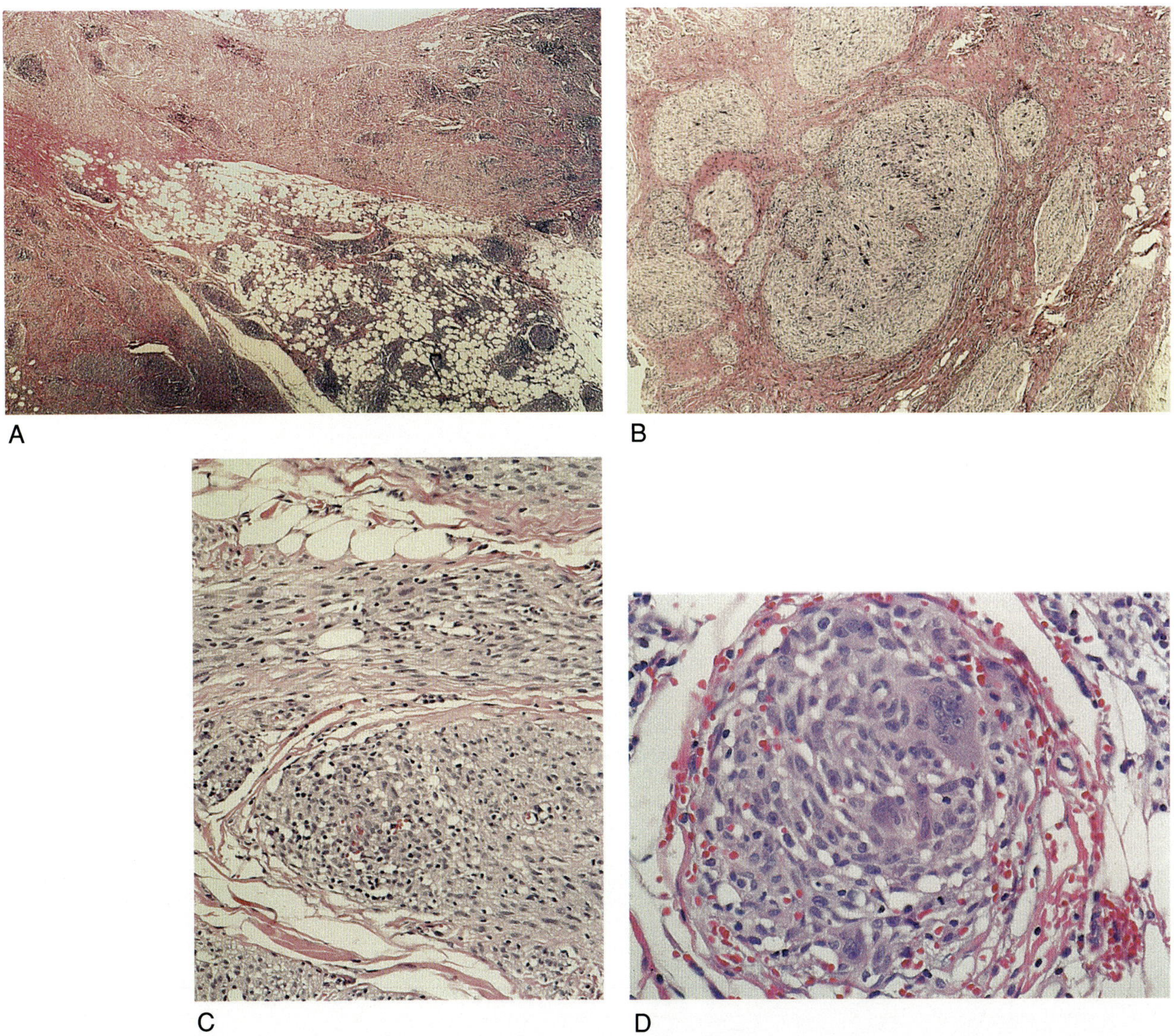

FIGURE 7.29 Plexiform fibrohistiocytic tumor is a markedly infiltrative tumor with a biphasic appearance, consisting of variably sized nodules of histiocytoid cells and osteoclast-type giant cells accompanied by moderately cellular fascicles of fibroblast-like cells. Aggregates of lymphocytes and extravasated red blood cells also may be present **(A-D)**. (**A** and **B,** Low power; **C,** intermediate power; **D,** high power; H&E.)

any given tumor, the proportion of both components is variable, including cases dominated by the histiocytic nodules (fibrohistiocytic subtype), fibroblastic fascicles (fibroblastic subtype), or equal proportions of both components (mixed subtype).[28] Nuclear pleomorphism and cellular atypia are minimal; mitotic activity rarely exceeds 3 mitotic figures per 10 high-power fields. Variable numbers of extravasated red blood cells and lymphoid aggregates may be observed.

Fine Needle Aspiration Biopsy

The cytologic features of plexiform fibrohistiocytic tumor rarely have been described.[29] Smears are typically highly cellular and consist of mostly discohesive, bland-appearing, spindle-shaped cells with round-to-ovoid nuclei, inconspicuous-to-small nucleoli, and variable amounts of tapering cytoplasm. Histiocytes and lymphocytes may be present (Fig. 7.31). Variable numbers of osteoclast-type giant cells are seen. The cytologic features closely resemble other myofibroblastic lesions, especially nodular fasciitis. It is doubtful that the diagnosis of primary plexiform fibrohistiocytic tumor can be rendered on cytologic material alone.

Ancillary Studies

Ultrastructural findings of the spindle and mononuclear cells of plexiform fibrohistiocytic tumor reveal features of myofibroblasts and histiocytes, including lysosomes, dilated rough endoplasmic reticulum, numerous mitochondria, and bundles of intermediate filaments. Although likely nonspecific, intracisternal crystalline inclusions of uncertain significance also have been documented.[30]

Immunohistochemical cytoplasmic staining for vimentin and CD68 often is observed in the osteoclast-type giant cells and mononuclear cells within the histiocytic clusters. The spindle cells within the fibroblastic fascicles commonly express smooth muscle actin and muscle-specific actin, reflecting myofibroblastic differentiation. Desmin and S-100 protein are uniformly negative.[30,31] No reproducible cytogenetic abnormalities have been observed in plexiform fibrohistiocytic tumor.

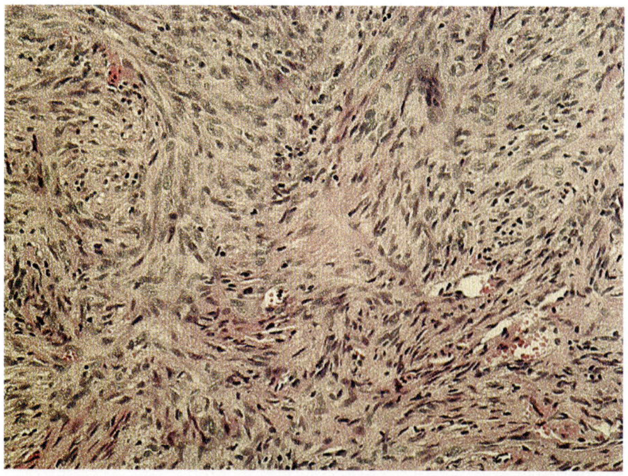

FIGURE 7.30 Plexiform fibrohistiocytic tumor may be dominated by an infiltrative fibroblastic component, composed of uniform-appearing spindled cells arranged in fascicles and storiform patterns, resembling a cellular nodular fasciitis or a cellular fibromatosis. (H&E.)

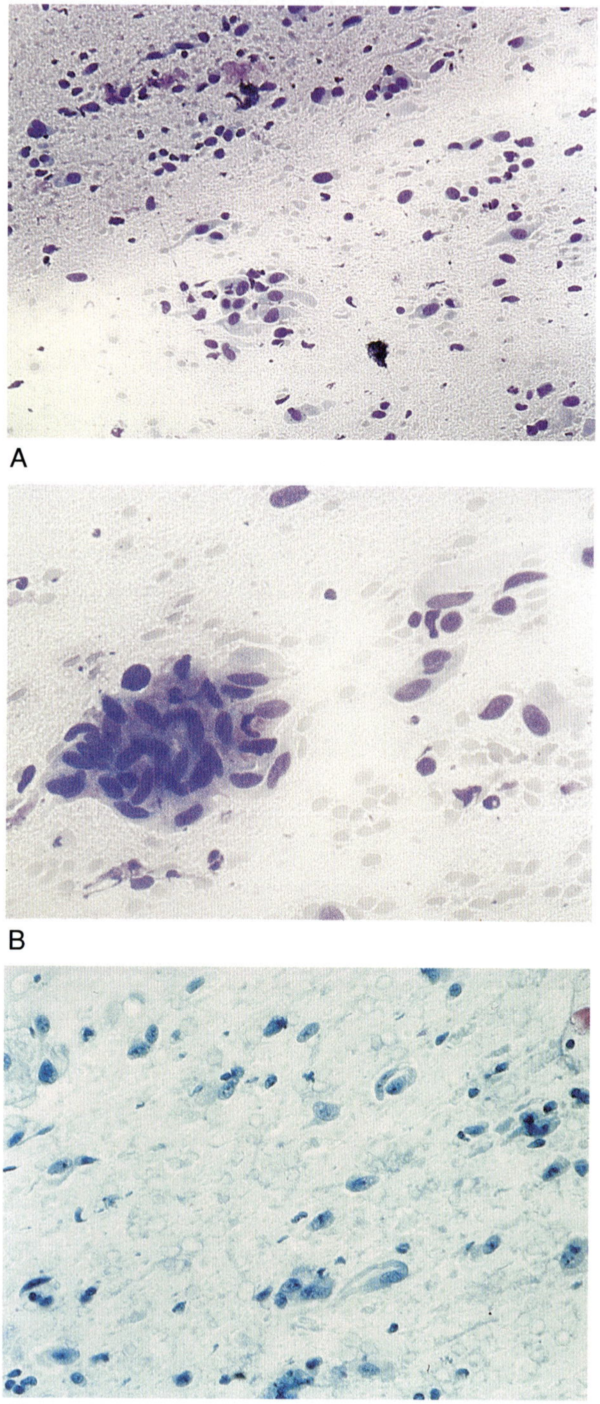

A

B

C

FIGURE 7.31 Fine needle aspiration biopsy of plexiform fibrohistiocytic tumor yields cellular smears dominated by the spindle cell "fibroblastic" component with scattered lymphocytes. The cytologic features are nondiagnostic and may mimic closely nodular fasciitis **(A-C)**. (**A,** Low power, Diff-Quik; **B,** high power, Diff-Quik; **C,** Papanicolaou.)

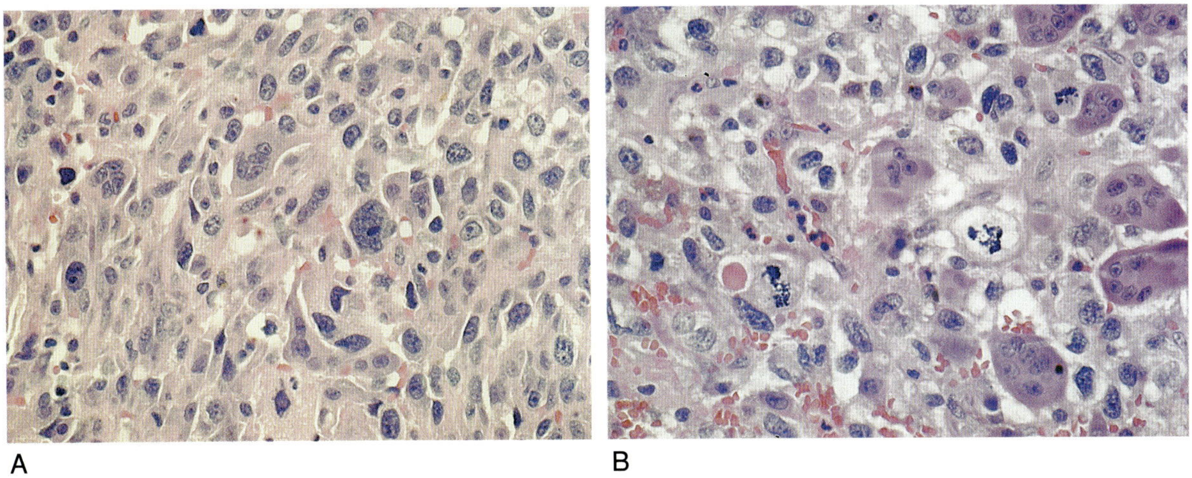

FIGURE 7.32 The key to the diagnosis of giant cell malignant fibrous histiocytoma is the presence of significant atypia and mitotic activity, including atypical mitoses, in the background stromal cells. The diagnosis remains one of exclusion, however, because other sarcoma subtypes (e.g., leiomyosarcoma) and sarcomatoid carcinoma may be rich in osteoclast-type giant cells (**A** and **B**). (**A** and **B**, H&E.)

Prognosis and Therapy

Plexiform fibrohistiocytic tumor should be regarded as a low-grade sarcoma. Wide local excision with negative margins is recommended. Local recurrence rates range from 12% to 40%, but regional (lymph node) and systemic metastases occur in fewer than 5% of patients.[27,28,30] There are no clinical or pathologic features predictive of prognosis.

Malignant Fibrous Histiocytoma, Giant Cell Type

Giant cell malignant fibrous histiocytoma also is called *malignant giant cell tumor of soft tissues*.[32,33] Similar to other forms of so-called malignant fibrous histiocytoma, giant cell malignant fibrous histiocytoma now is regarded as a diagnosis of exclusion because its morphologic pattern may be observed in a variety of other tumor subtypes (e.g., leiomyosarcoma, osteosarcoma, and sarcomatoid carcinoma). In the past, examples of the recently recognized giant cell tumor of soft tissues were included in this category as well.[33] For these reasons, the diagnosis of giant cell malignant fibrous histiocytoma should be reserved for undifferentiated pleomorphic sarcomas with abundant osteoclast-type giant cells. Using the aforementioned definition, the diagnosis of giant cell malignant fibrous histiocytoma is rare. Most cases affect older patients and arise as deep-seated tumors involving the extremities or trunk. Painless soft tissue swelling is the most frequent complaint. Morphologically the tumor cells appear spindled to ovoid, showing marked nuclear pleomorphism and abundant mitotic activity. Randomly distributed but abundant osteoclast-type giant cells are evident (Fig. 7.32). Immunohistochemical cytoplasmic staining for smooth muscle actin or desmin may be focally present, but diffuse staining for both markers supports the diagnosis of leiomyosarcoma. The presence of even focal osteoid and bone production by the malignant cells establishes the diagnosis of osteosarcoma. For therapeutic purposes, giant cell malignant fibrous histiocytoma should be considered a high-grade sarcoma, requiring wide or radical resection and, when necessary, chemotherapy or radiation therapy or both.

REFERENCES

Giant Cell Tumor and Malignant Giant Cell Tumor

1. Hutter RVP, Worcester JN, Francis KC: Benign and malignant giant cell tumor of bone: A clinicopathologic analysis of the natural history of the disease. Cancer 1962;15:653.
2. McDonald DJ, Sim FH, McLeod RA, et al: Giant cell tumor of bone. J Bone Joint Surg Am 1986;68:235.
3. Biscaglia R, Bacchini P, Bertoni F: Giant cell tumor of the bones of the hand and foot. Cancer 2000;88:2022.
4. Peimer CA, Schiller AL, Mankin HJ, et al: Multicentric giant-cell tumor of bone. J Bone Joint Surg Am 1980;62:652.
5. Folpe AL, Morris RJ, Weiss SW: Soft tissue giant cell tumor of low malignant potential: A proposal for the reclassification of malignant giant cell tumor of soft parts. Mod Pathol 1999;12:894.
6. Bridge JA, Neff JR, Mouron BJ: Giant cell tumor of bone: Chromosomal analysis of 48 specimens and review of the literature. Cancer Genet Cytogenet 1992;58:2.
7. Sciot R, Dorfman H, Brys P, et al: Cytogenetic-morphologic correlations in aneurysmal bone cyst, giant cell tumor of bone, and combined lesions: A report from the CHAMP study group. Mod Pathol 2000;13:1206.
8. Tubbs WS, Brown LR, Beabout JW, et al: Benign giant-cell tumor of bone with pulmonary metastasis: Clinical findings and radiologic appearance of metastases in 13 cases. AJR Am J Roentgenol 1992;158:331.
9. Kay RM, Eckhardt JJ, Seeger LL, et al: Pulmonary metastasis of benign giant cell tumor of bone: Six histologically confirmed cases, including one of spontaneous resolution. Clin Orthop 1994;302:219.
10. Rock MG, Sim FH, Unni KK, et al: Secondary malignant giant-cell tumor of bone: Clinicopathological assessment of nineteen patients. J Bone Joint Surg Am 1986;68:1073.

Giant Cell Reparative Granuloma

11. Yamaguchi T, Dorfman HD: Giant cell reparative granuloma: A comparative clinicopathologic study of lesions in gnathic and extragnathic sites. Int J Surg Pathol 2001;9:189.
12. Waldron CA, Shafer WG: The central giant cell reparative granuloma of the jaws: An analysis of 38 cases. Am J Clin Pathol 1966;45:437.
13. Yamaguchi T, Dorfman HD, Eising S: Cherubism: Clinicopathologic features. Skeletal Radiol 1999;28:350.
14. Sannerkin NG, Mott MG, Roylance J: An unusual intraosseous lesion with fibroblastic, osteoclastic, osteoblastic, aneurysmal and fibromyxoid elements: A "solid" variant of aneurysmal bone cyst. Cancer 1983;51:2278.
15. Buresh CJ, Seemayer TA, Nelson M, et al: t(X;4)(q22;q31.3) in giant cell reparative granuloma. Cancer Genet Cytogenet 1999;115:80.
16. Dal Cin P, Kozakewich HP, Goumnerova L, et al: Variant translocations involving 16q22 and 17p13 in solid and extraosseous forms of aneurysmal bone cyst. Genes Chromosomes Cancer 2000;28:233.

Diffuse and Localized Tenosynovial Giant Cell Tumors

17. Abdul-Karim FW, El-Naggar AK, Joyce MJ, et al: Diffuse and localized tenosynovial giant cell tumor and pigmented villonodular synovitis: A clinicopathologic and flow cytometric DNA analysis. Hum Pathol 1992;23:729.
18. Schwartz HS, Unni KK, Pritchard DJ: Pigmented villonodular synovitis: A retrospective review of large affected joints. Clin Orthop 1989;247:243.
19. De Saint Aubain Somerhausen N, Fletcher CD: Diffuse-type giant cell tumor: Clinicopathologic and immunohistochemical analysis of 50 cases with extraarticular disease. Am J Surg Pathol 2000;24:479.
20. Gonzalez-Campora R, Salas Herrero E, Otal-Salaverri C, et al: Diffuse tenosynovial giant cell tumor of soft tissues: Report of a case with cytologic and cytogenetic findings. Acta Cytol 1995;39:770.
21. Alguacil-Garcia A, Unni KK, Goellner JR: Giant cell tumor of tendon sheath and pigmented villonodular synovitis: An ultrastructural study. Am J Clin Pathol 1978;69:6.
22. O'Connell JX, Fanburg JC, Rosenberg AE: Giant cell tumor of tendon sheath and pigmented villonodular synovitis: Immunophenotype suggests a synovial origin. Hum Pathol 1995;26:771.
23. Sciot R, Rosai J, Dal Cin P, et al: Analysis of 35 cases of localized and diffuse giant cell tumor: Report from the CHAMP study group. Mod Pathol 1999;12:576.
24. Fletcher JA, Henkle C, Atkins L, et al: Trisomy 5 and trisomy 7 are nonrandom aberrations in pigmented villonodular synovitis: Confirmation of trisomy 7 in uncultured cells. Genes Chromosomes Cancer 1992;4:264.
25. Bertoni F, Unni KK, Beabout JW, et al: Malignant giant cell tumor of the tendon sheaths and joints (malignant pigmented villonodular synovitis). Am J Surg Pathol 1997;21:153.
26. Ushijima M, Hashimoto H, Tsuneyoshi M, et al: Giant cell tumor of the tendon sheath (nodular tenosynovitis): A study of 207 cases to compare the large joint group with the common digit group. Cancer 1986;15:875.

Plexiform Fibrohistiocytic Tumor

27. Enzinger FM, Zhang R: Plexiform fibrohistiocytic tumor presenting in children and young adults: An analysis of 65 cases. Am J Surg Pathol 1988;12:818.
28. Remstein ED, Arndt CAS, Nascimento AG: Plexiform fibrohistiocytic tumor: Clinicopathologic analysis of 22 cases. Am J Surg Pathol 1999;22:662.
29. Angervall L, Kindblom LG, Lindholm K, et al: Plexiform fibrohistiocytic tumor: Report of a case involving preoperative aspiration cytology and immunohistochemical and ultrastructural analysis of surgical specimens. Pathol Res Pract 1992;188:350.
30. Hollowood K, Holley MP, Fletcher CDM: Plexiform fibrohistiocytic tumour: Clinicopathological, immunohistochemical and ultrastructural analysis in favour of myofibroblastic lesion. Histopathology 1991;19:503.
31. Zelger B, Weinlich G, Steiner H, et al: Dermal and subcutaneous variants of plexiform fibrohistiocytic tumor. Am J Surg Pathol 1997;21:235.

Malignant Giant Cell Fibrous Histiocytoma

32. Angervall L, Hagmar B, Kindblom LG, et al: Malignant giant cell tumor of soft tissues: A clinicopathologic, cytologic, ultrastructural, angiographic, and microangiographic study. Cancer 1981;47:736.
33. Guccion JG, Enzinger FM: Malignant giant cell tumor of soft parts: An analysis of 32 cases. Cancer 1972;29:1518.

CHAPTER 8

Myxoid Tumors of Bone and Soft Tissue

Myxoid tumors of bone and soft tissue include lesions characterized by the production of an abundant extracellular myxoid (mucopolysaccharide) matrix. Although a variety of different tumors may show at least focal myxoid changes, Table 8.1 summarizes the lesions that definitionally exhibit myxoid morphology. This group of tumors encompasses a wide spectrum of benign, borderline malignant, and fully malignant lesions. Although these tumors have relatively specific clinical and pathologic features, considerable morphologic overlap exists between the various histologic subtypes in this group. Although immunohistochemistry and cytogenetics have yielded some valuable insights, light microscopy coupled with clinical and, if available, radiographic correlation is the most reliable means for diagnosing these tumors. Virtually all of the myxoid lesions express vimentin, and most show variable expression of actin, reflecting myofibroblastic differentiation. The mucinous matrix among the various myxoid tumors may exhibit differing staining properties; these are summarized in Table 8.2.

TABLE 8.1 Myxoid Tumors of Bone and Soft Tissue

Bone Origin	Soft Tissue Origin
Myxoma of the jaw	Intramuscular myxoma
Chondromyxoid fibroma	Juxta-articular myxoma
Chordoma	Deep aggressive angiomyxoma
	Ossifying fibromyxoid tumor
	Mixed tumor/myoepithelioma and parachordoma
	Low-grade fibromyxoid sarcoma
	Myxofibrosarcoma
	Myxoid and round cell liposarcoma
	Myxoid chondrosarcoma
	Myxoinflammatory fibroblastic sarcoma

TABLE 8.2 Mucinous Stromal Characteristics of Various Myxoid Tumors

	Vascularity	Matrix	Staining Characteristics
Intramuscular myxoma	Hypovascular	Hyaluronic acid	Alcian blue, mucicarmine positive, hyaluronidase sensitive
Myxoid liposarcoma	Hypervascular	Hyaluronic acid	Alcian blue, mucicarmine positive, hyaluronidase sensitive
Myxofibrosarcoma (myxoid MFH)	Hypervascular	Hyaluronic acid	Alcian blue, mucicarmine positive, hyaluronidase sensitive
Extraskeletal myxoid chondrosarcoma	Hypovascular	Chondroitin sulfate	Alcian blue, mucicarmine positive, hyaluronidase resistant
Chordoma	Hypovascular	Chondroitin sulfate	Alcian blue, mucicarmine positive, hyaluronidase resistant

MFH, malignant fibrous histiocytoma.

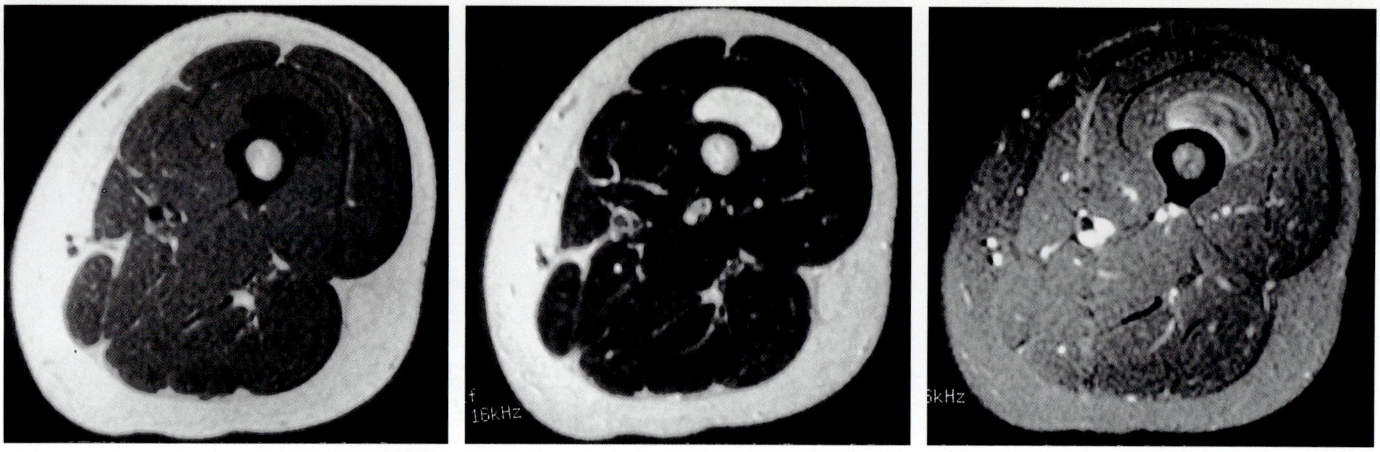

A B C

FIGURE 8.1 Myxoma. Axial T1-weighted **(A)**, T2-weighted **(B)**, and fat-suppressed T1-weighted gadolinium-enhanced **(C)** magnetic resonance images show a well-defined lesion within the vastus intermedius muscle and abutting the shaft of the femur. On the T1-weighted image **(A)**, the lesion is hypointense to adjacent muscle. On the T2-weighted image **(B)**, the lesion is hyperintense to muscle, and the lesion enhances heterogeneously after intravenous administration of gadolinium **(C)**.

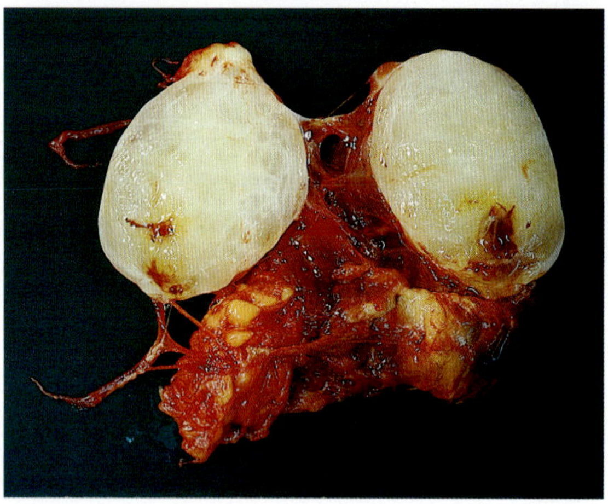

FIGURE 8.2 Cross section of intramuscular myxoma with well-circumscribed borders and a mostly homogeneous, mucinous cut surface.

Similar to immunohistochemistry, special stains are rarely necessary for histologic subtyping. When correlated with clinical and radiographic features, fine needle aspiration biopsy (FNAB) is a useful and accurate tool in the diagnosis and management of myxoid lesions, especially myxoid sarcomas. Chondromyxoid fibroma usually exhibits a prominent myxoid stroma, but we discuss it with the other chondroid lesions (see Chapter 13) because the differential diagnosis more often includes these entities.

Intramuscular Myxoma

Clinical Features

Intramuscular myxoma is observed most commonly in adults older than age 40. There is a female predilection. The most frequent anatomic sites are the deep skeletal muscles of the extremities, principally the thigh, shoulder, buttocks, and arm. Most patients present with complaints of painless soft tissue swelling.[1,2] Magnetic resonance imaging reveals features typical of myxoid lesions with bright signal intensity (hyperintense to skeletal muscle) on T2-weighted images and low signal intensity on T1-weighted images (Fig. 8.1).[3,4] Most tumors appear less than 10 cm in greatest dimension and are well circumscribed (Fig. 8.2).

Myxomas are associated rarely with other lesions. Mazabraud's syndrome presents as polyostotic fibrous dysplasia and intramuscular soft tissue myxomas.

Pathologic Findings

Histology

Most intramuscular myxomas are composed of uniformly bland, spindled-to-stellate tumor cells embedded in an abundant, hypocellular myxomatous stroma. Focally, pseudocystic spaces may be present. A distinctive feature of intramuscular myxoma is the absence of significant vascularity (Fig. 8.3). The myxoid stroma also may appear vacuolated. Despite the presence of a fibrous capsule surrounding the tumor, entrapped skeletal muscle fibers may be identified within the tumor proper (Fig. 8.4). Myxomas may contain areas of increased cellularity, increased collagen deposition, and hypervascularity, leading to a mistaken diagnosis of myxofibrosarcoma (Fig. 8.5).[1] Compared with myxofibrosarcoma, intramuscular myxomas lack significant nuclear pleomorphism, and necrosis is not present. Mitoses are virtually never seen.

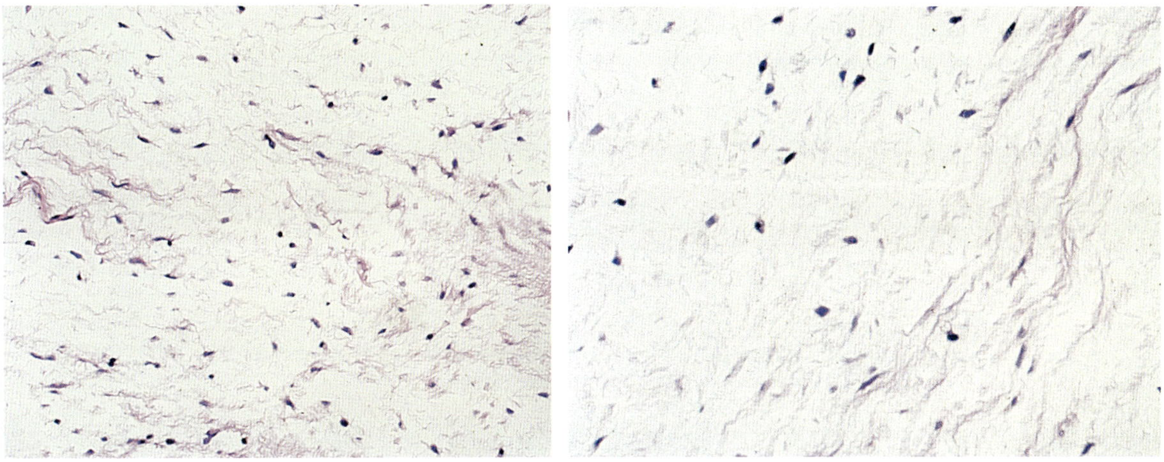

A B

FIGURE 8.3 Intramuscular myxoma characterized by a hypocellular, hypovascular myxoid stroma. Individual tumor cells appear uniform, spindled to stellate, lacking significant nuclear atypia **(A** and **B)**. **(A** and **B,** H&E.)

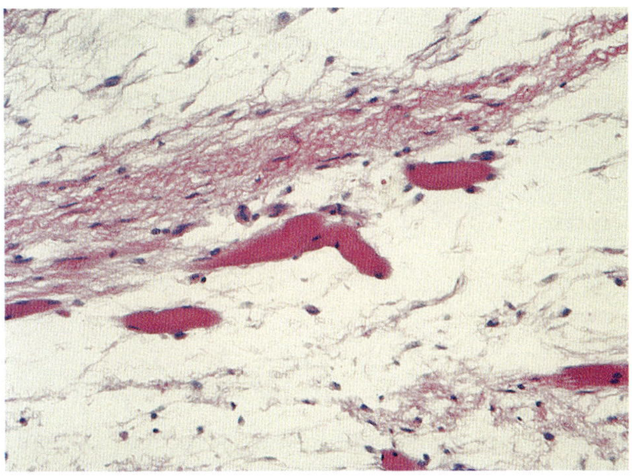

FIGURE 8.4 Intramuscular myxoma with entrapped skeletal muscle fibers. **(A,** Low power, H&E; **B,** high power, H&E.)

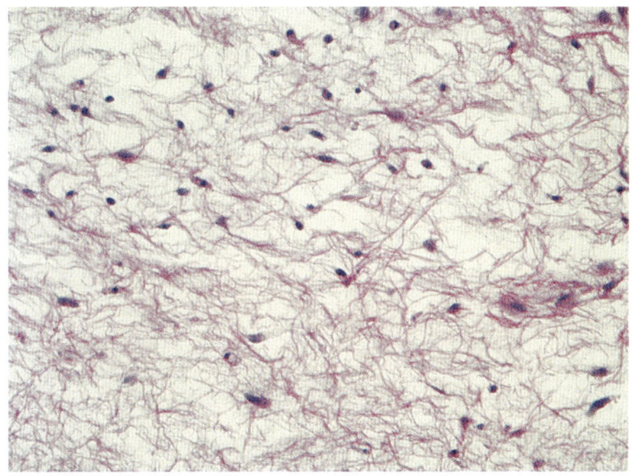

FIGURE 8.5 Intramuscular myxoma with abundant collagen deposition. (H&E.)

Fine Needle Aspiration Biopsy

FNAB yields hypocellular smears with a film of magenta-appearing granular material covering the entire slide. Individual tumor cells appear uniform, spindled to stellate with spindled-to-ovoid nuclei and inconspicuous nucleoli. The spindle cells often exhibit long cytoplasmic processes that may be intertwined to form *fibrillary tangles* (Fig. 8.6).[4] Significant nuclear atypia is never seen and, if present, should suggest the possibility of low-grade myxofibrosarcoma. A comparison of intramuscular myxoma with some of the more common myxoid sarcomas is summarized in Table 8.3.

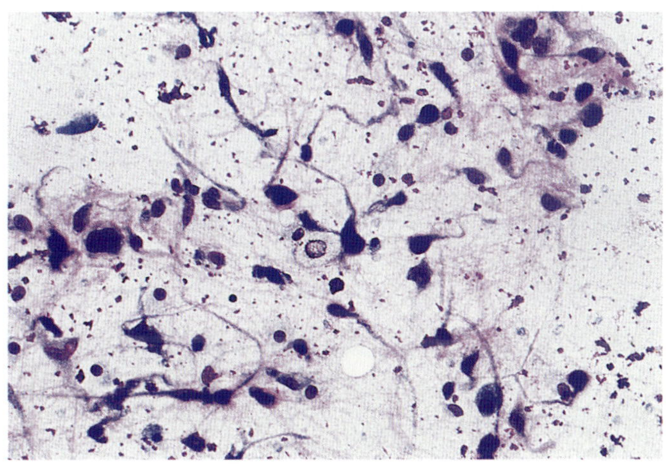

FIGURE 8.6 Fine needle aspiration biopsy sample of intramuscular myxoma shows mostly uniform tumor cells with long cytoplasmic processes and a background myxoid, granular film. (Diff-Quik.)

Ancillary Studies

Ultrastructurally, tumor cells show features of fibroblasts/myofibroblasts with prominent secretory activity. These

TABLE 8.3 Clinical and Cytologic Features of Some Common Adult Myxoid Tumors

	Clinical Aspects		Pathologic Features		
	Age Range (Yr)*	**Anatomic Site†**	**Usual Cytologic Features**	**Nuclear Pleomorphism**	**Immunohistochemical/ Molecular Profile**
Intramuscular myxoma	40-60	Deep soft tissues, extremities	Myxoid granular film, hypocellular, spindled cells with long, cytoplasmic processes	Absent	Vimentin positive, S-100 negative/ normal karyotype
Myxofibrosarcoma	50-80	Dermal/ subcutaneous, extremities	Myxoid granular film, individually dispersed tumor cells, variable vascularity	Usually significant, often marked	Vimentin positive/ complex karyotype (nondiagnostic)
Myxoid/round cell liposarcoma	40-70	Deep soft tissues, extremities	Myxoid stromal fragments, individually dispersed ovoid tumor cells, arborizing blood vessels, round cell component composed of larger, sometimes epithelioid cells	Minimal; if round cell component is present, may be significant	Vimentin positive, S-100 variable/ t(12;16)(q13;p11) CHOP-TLS
Myxoid chondrosarcoma	40-70	Deep soft tissues, extremities	Myxoid stromal fragments, spindled-to-round tumor cells arranged in anastomosing cords, nests, and clusters; absence of vascularity	Minimal to absent	Vimentin positive, S-100 variable/ t(9;22)(q21-31;q12) EWS-CHN(TEC)

*Common ages at tumor presentation.
†Most common anatomic location.

findings include dilated rough endoplasmic reticulum, Golgi complexes, intermediate filaments, and occasional intracytoplasmic lipid droplets.[5]

Immunohistochemistry is not generally helpful in the diagnosis of myxoma. As expected, the tumor cells show diffuse and strong positivity for vimentin, but occasional focal positivity for desmin, actin, and CD34 is observed. S-100 protein is uniformly negative. Cytogenetic analysis in most cases reveals a normal, diploid karyotype.[6]

Prognosis and Therapy

Intramuscular myxoma generally is cured by local excision. Histology does not predict clinical outcome.[1]

Juxta-articular Myxoma

Clinical Features

Juxta-articular myxoma may affect patients over a wide age range but most commonly is observed in middle-aged men. The most common anatomic location is the soft tissues of the knee, followed in decreasing order of frequency by the elbow, shoulder, and ankle joints. Most lesions arise predominantly within subcutaneous adipose tissue with variable involvement of the dermis, joint space, and surrounding musculature. Common presenting complaints include soft tissue swelling, pain, and tenderness of the affected joint.[7] The imaging characteristics are similar to those observed with intramuscular myxoma; however, juxta-articular myxoma is more commonly cystic.[8]

Pathologic Findings

Histology

Morphologically, juxta-articular myxoma manifests as a combination of intramuscular myxoma and ganglion cyst–like features. Nodules of hypocellular and hypovascular myxoid material are composed of randomly distributed but uniform-appearing, spindled to stellate–appearing cells (Fig. 8.7). Areas of increased cellularity may be present, but significant atypia and atypical mitotic figures are never seen (Fig. 8.8). Variably thickened fibrous tissue walls form the ganglion-like

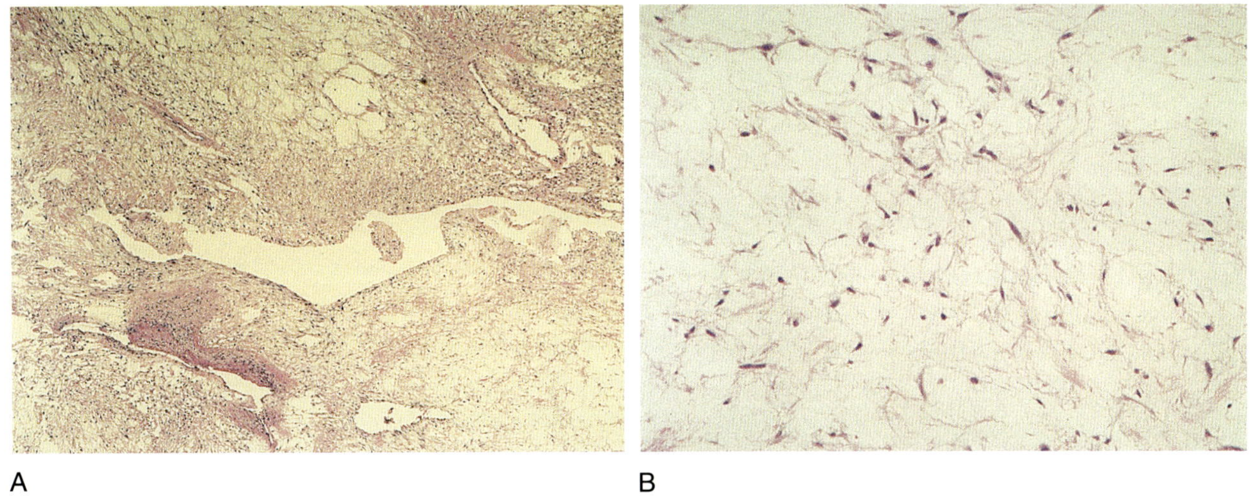

FIGURE 8.7 Juxta-articular myxoma shows a combination of ganglion-like cystic spaces and hypocellular myxoma regions. Individual tumor cells appear bland (**A** and **B**). (**A**, Low power, H&E; **B**, high power, H&E.)

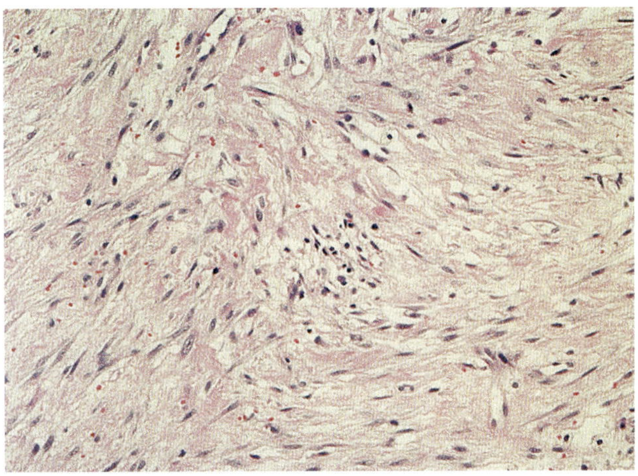

FIGURE 8.8 Juxta-articular myxoma with a more cellular and collagenous region, resembling nodular fasciitis. (H&E.)

cystic spaces. Areas of chronic inflammation and hemorrhage with hemosiderin pigment deposition are frequent in recurrent lesions.

Ancillary Studies

Ultrastructurally, the lesional cells of juxta-articular myxoma show features similar to those observed with intramuscular myxoma, displaying differentiation toward fibroblasts and myofibroblasts. The immunohistochemical findings are similar with uniform positivity for vimentin, focal positivity for desmin and actin, but negativity for S-100 protein.

Cytogenetic analysis of a single case of juxta-articular myxoma has revealed two distinct, cytogenetically abnormal clonal cell populations: inv(2)(p15q36) and +7, t(8;22)(q11-12), suggesting that juxta-articular myxomas may represent a neoplastic process.[9]

Prognosis and Therapy

Juxta-articular myxoma is a benign but potentially locally aggressive lesion. In the largest series to date, local recurrence occurred in one third of cases.[7] Wide resection is the treatment of choice; radical resection and radiation therapy are not justified. Malignant transformation has not been documented.

Myxoma of the Jaw

Myxoma of the jaw is a rare but locally aggressive myxomatous lesion generally afflicting adolescents and young adults. Females are affected slightly more often than males.[10] Tumors are localized to the mandible in two thirds of cases and in the maxilla in the remainder. Radiographically, most tumors exhibit a unilocular-to-multilocular appearance with bone destruction and ill-defined margins, simulating a malignancy. A few tumors are associated with an unerupted tooth.[10] Myxoma of the jaw appears histologically similar to intramuscular myxoma but is often more cellular. Variable amounts of stromal collagen are present (Fig. 8.9).[11] Similar to other forms of myxoma, FNAB yields hypocellular smears with an abundant myxoid film containing scattered, bland but uniform-appearing, ovoid to slightly spindled cells.[12] Immunohistochemically, myxomas of the jaw are positive for vimentin and actin but generally negative for desmin and S-100 protein.[11] Because of its tendency for bone destruction and invasion into surrounding structures, myxoma of the jaw is associated with a relatively high recurrence rate and requires wide resection. The maxillary form may behave more aggressively than the mandibular form and sometimes spreads into the maxillary sinus.

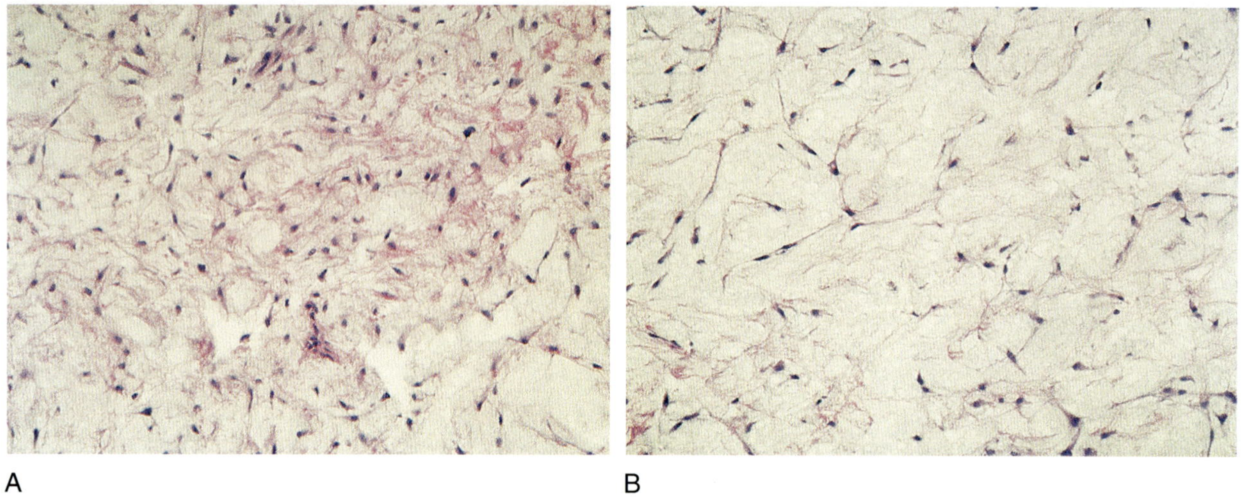

FIGURE 8.9 Myxoma of the jaw often appears more cellular and collagenous than intramuscular myxoma but lacks significant cellular atypia (**A** and **B**). (**A** and **B**, H&E.)

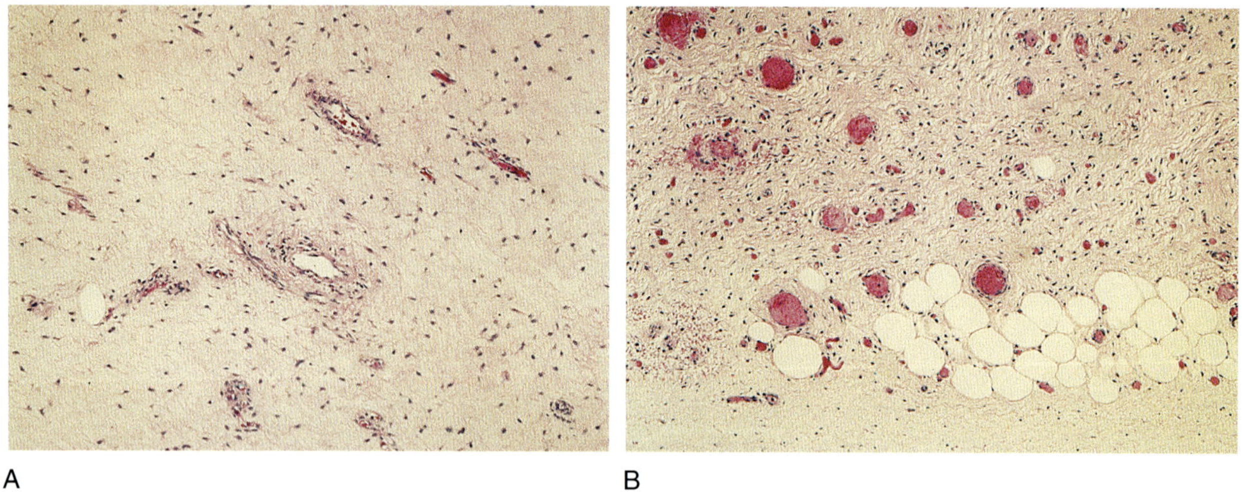

FIGURE 8.10 Aggressive angiomyxoma showing a population of mostly uniform-appearing, stellate-to-ovoid tumor cells randomly distributed in a slightly myxoid stroma with variably sized blood vessels (**A**). The tumor is infiltrative, often entrapping adjacent structures, including adipose tissue (**B**). (**A** and **B**, H&E.)

Aggressive (Deep) Angiomyxoma

Clinical Features

Aggressive angiomyxoma is observed almost exclusively in middle-aged to older women, involving the deep soft tissues of the pelvis, perineum, vulva, buttock, and inguinal and retroperitoneal regions.[13,14] Rare cases have been reported in the scrotal region of men.[15] Most patients present with complaints of a slow-growing, painless mass. Initial physical examinations often significantly underestimate the size of the lesion.[13] Consequently, most cases of aggressive angiomyxoma are fairly large masses at initial diagnosis. Radiographically, aggressive angiomyxomas are large infiltrative masses, often exhibiting unusual growth patterns with "translevator extension" and involvement of adjacent perineal structures. High signal intensity on T2-weighted magnetic resonance images, reflecting the abundant myxomatous stroma, is typical.[16]

Pathologic Findings

Histology

Despite its bland histologic characteristics, aggressive angiomyxoma is a markedly infiltrative lesion, frequently entrapping skeletal muscle, adipose tissue, and regional structures. As the name implies, aggressive angiomyxoma is more vascular than conventional myxoma, and numerous blood vessels of variable sizes and shapes are present.[13] Typically the tumor shows relatively low cellularity and comprises a mostly uniform, spindled-to-stellate population of tumor cells, embedded in a partially collagenous, myxoid matrix (Fig. 8.10). The myxoid matrix is often negative for special mucin stains

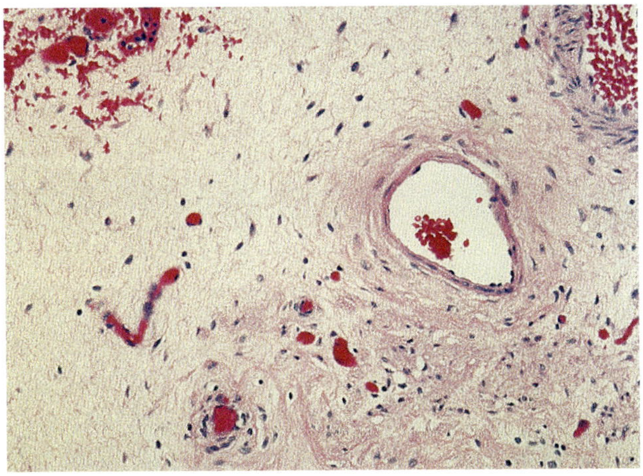

FIGURE 8.11 Aggressive angiomyxoma showing aggregates of well-developed smooth muscle adjacent to a large blood vessel. (H&E.)

and may represent a mostly edematous phenomenon.[13] Individual tumor cells reveal mostly uniform and ovoid nuclei, inconspicuous-to-small nucleoli and are surrounded by scant pale eosinophilic cytoplasm. Multinucleated cells rarely are observed. Significant nuclear pleomorphism is never present. Mitotic activity is generally less than one mitotic figure per 10 high-power fields. A characteristic finding is the presence of bundles and fascicles of bland, smooth muscle cells primarily oriented around blood vessels (Fig. 8.11).

Fine Needle Aspiration Biopsy

FNAB of aggressive angiomyxoma is usually nondiagnostic, revealing hypocellular smears with randomly distributed, bland-appearing, stellate-to-spindle cells containing bipolar cytoplasmic processes. These stromal cells lie within a background of watery, myxoid film.[17]

Ancillary Studies

The ultrastructural features of aggressive angiomyxoma show evidence of fibroblastic and myofibroblastic differentiation. Immunohistochemically the neoplastic cells usually appear positive for vimentin, desmin, actin, smooth muscle actin, and estrogen and progesterone receptors; approximately half of tumors express CD34.[13] Similar to conventional intramuscular myxoma, S-100 protein is uniformly negative.

Only a few examples of aggressive angiomyxoma have been investigated with cytogenetic analysis. The most common abnormality involves structural rearrangements of chromosome 12, especially 12q13-15.[18]

Prognosis and Therapy

With wide resection, the local recurrence rate of aggressive angiomyxoma ranges from 36% to 72%.[13,14] Local control usually can be achieved by re-excision. Distant metastases do not occur.

Ossifying Fibromyxoid Tumor

Clinical Features

Ossifying fibromyxoid tumor is a rare neoplasm most commonly arising in middle-aged to older adults. Men are affected more commonly than women. The most common anatomic locations are the extremities, but it also has been reported in the head and neck, trunk, and retroperitoneum.[19] Most patients report the presence of painless soft tissue swelling, often of long duration.

Pathologic Findings

Histology

Ossifying fibromyxoid tumors are usually well-circumscribed, multinodular lesions composed of a uniform population of round to ovoid–shaped tumor cells arranged in anastomosing cords and nests, embedded in a fibromyxoid stroma. An incomplete shell of mature metaplastic bone is observed in the periphery of the tumors in most cases (Fig. 8.12).[19] Significant nuclear pleomorphism is not present (Fig. 8.13). Mitotic activity is infrequent.

Rare examples of ossifying fibromyxoid tumors may show "atypical" or "malignant" features, including increased cellularity, increased mitotic activity, and osteoid/bone deposition by the neoplastic cells more centrally within the lesion (Fig. 8.14).[20] Whether these cases are examples of low-grade osteosarcoma is unclear.

Ancillary Studies

The ultrastructural features of ossifying fibromyxoid tumor include intracytoplasmic dense core granules, intermediate filaments, prominent rough endoplasmic reticulum, and scattered mitochondria.[21] Immunohistochemically, ossifying fibromyxoid tumors are virtually always positive for vimentin and S-100 protein and often express neuron-specific enolase, synaptophysin, and actin.[21] Occasionally, positivity for desmin and glial fibrillary acidic protein may be observed. Rare examples have shown positivity for keratin.

Two cases of ossifying fibromyxoid tumor have been subjected to cytogenetic analysis. Both cases showed complex karyotypes, with one exhibiting a hypodiploid karyotype with structural rearrangements of chromosomes 6 and 14.[22,23]

Prognosis and Therapy

Local recurrence after excision has been documented in 27% of cases.[19] Although recurrent lesions may show increased cellularity and mitotic activity, no histologic findings in the

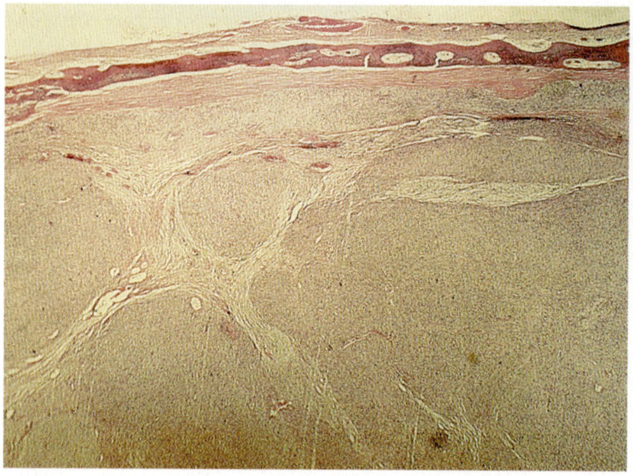

A

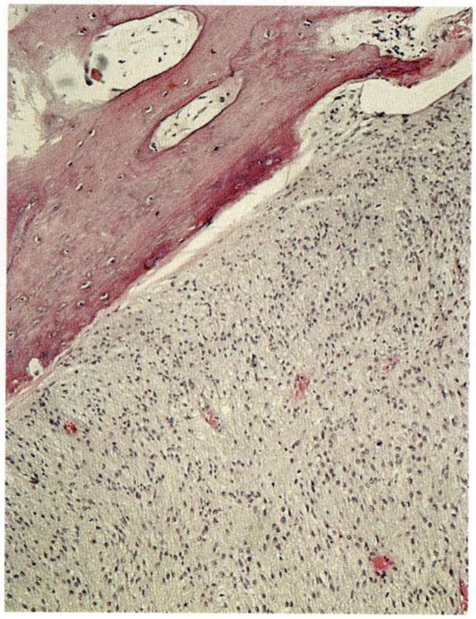

B

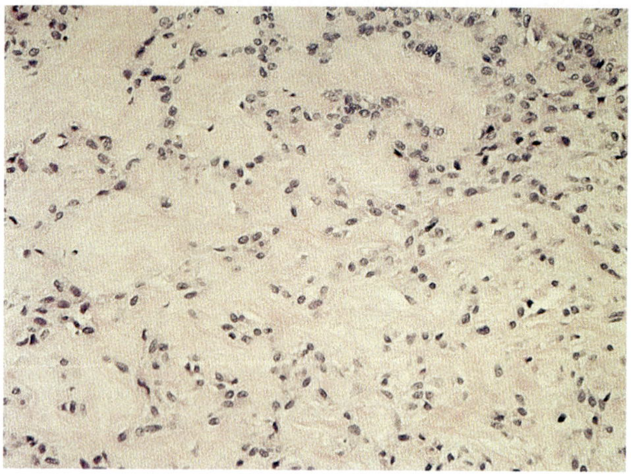

C

FIGURE 8.12 Ossifying fibromyxoid tumor is usually multinodular, well circumscribed, and characterized by an incomplete shell of mature, lamellar bone. Individual tumor cells are arranged solitarily or in nests and anastomosing cords within a myxoid stroma **(A-C)**. **(A,** Low power, H&E; **B,** intermediate power, H&E; **C,** high power, H&E.)

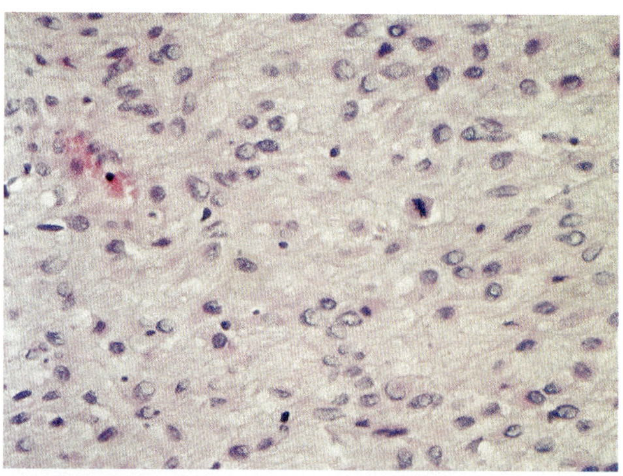

FIGURE 8.13 Cytologically, ossifying fibromyxoid tumor shows mostly uniform, round-to-ovoid tumor cells without significant nuclear pleomorphism and only occasional mitotic figures. (H&E.)

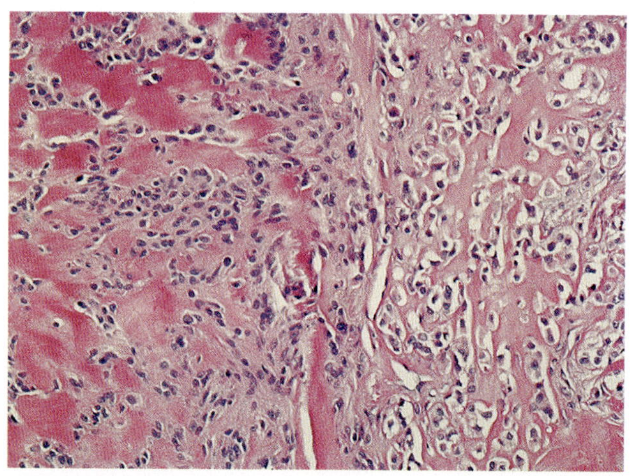

FIGURE 8.14 Atypical ossifying fibromyxoid tumor with more primitive, centrally located osteoid deposition, suggesting osteosarcoma. (H&E.)

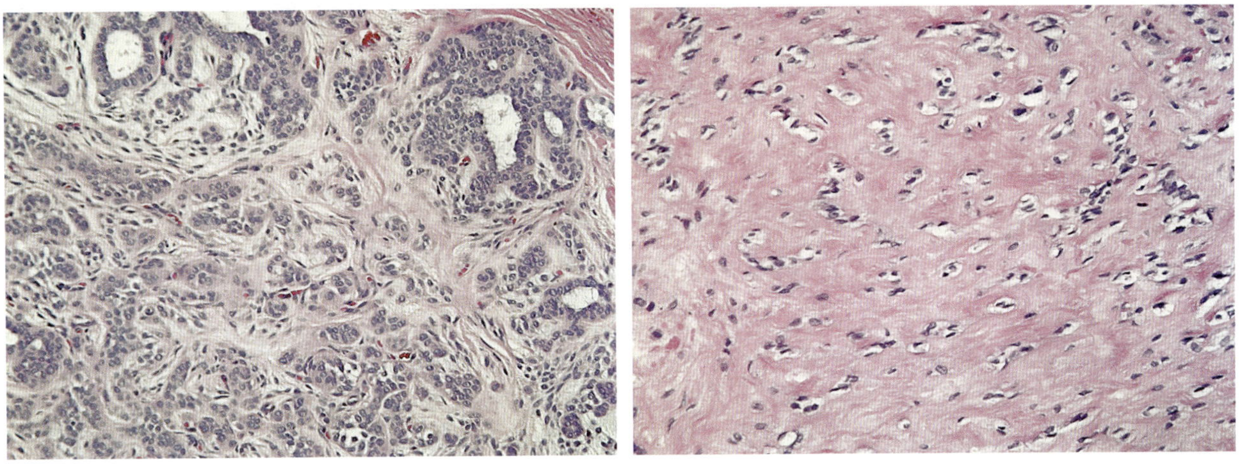

A B

FIGURE 8.15 Mixed tumor with epithelioid cells arranged in nests, ductules, and glandular patterns within a partially myxoid stroma **(A)**. Mixed tumor with cords of cells within a myxohyalinized stroma **(B)**. (**A** and **B**, H&E.)

primary lesion are predictive of clinical outcome. Pulmonary metastasis has been documented only in one example of atypical (malignant) ossifying fibromyxoid tumor.[20]

Mixed Tumor/Myoepithelioma/ Parachordoma

Mixed tumors are classically well-circumscribed lesions displaying epithelial and myoepithelial elements in varying proportions within a hyalinized-to-chondromyxoid stroma. Tumors composed virtually entirely of myoepithelial cells, closely resembling tumor cells observed in pleomorphic adenoma and lacking ductal differentiation, are called *myoepithelioma*.[24,25] Considered part of a morphologic spectrum, parachordomas closely resemble mixed tumors/myoepitheliomas but tend to exhibit extensive cytoplasmic vacuolation.[26]

Clinical Features

Mixed tumors/myoepitheliomas and parachordomas usually are found in adults (average age, 35 years).[24,26] Many patients (possibly 20%) are children younger than 10 years old. There may be a slight male predominance, but data are limited.

Most cases arise in the subcutaneous or deep subfascial soft tissues of the extremities (upper more than lower extremities). Less commonly, localization within the head and neck and trunk regions is observed. Most patients present with superficial-to-subfascial, painless swellings, ranging from a few weeks' to several years' duration. Localized pain rarely is reported. Rare examples have been described in bone.[27]

Pathologic Findings

Histology

Histologically, mixed tumors of soft tissue show the same morphologic spectrum observed in mixed tumors of the salivary gland. Varying proportions of uniform-appearing, epithelioid cells with eosinophilic-to-clear cytoplasm, arranged in nests, cords, and ductules accompanied by spindled cells, are embedded in a hyalinized-to-chondromyxoid matrix (Fig. 8.15).[24,25] Divergent differentiation, including squamous, adipocytic, and bone and cartilaginous metaplasia, may be observed (Fig. 8.16). From a strict histologic perspective, pure myoepitheliomas differ from mixed tumors in that the former often lack a definite ductal component (Fig. 8.17). Additionally the myoepithelial cells range from plasmacytoid to spindled forms. Rarely, mixed tumors may contain a population of cells with "rhabdoid" features (Fig. 8.18).[28] Parachordomas closely resemble (and are perhaps indistinguishable from) mixed tumors with the exception that cytoplasmic vacuolation is a prominent feature in the former.[26,29] Mitotic activity tends to be scant, usually fewer than two per 10 high-power fields. Similar to salivary lesions, dedifferentiation into frank carcinoma or sarcoma rarely is seen.

Ancillary Studies

Despite a broad morphologic spectrum, greater than 95% of cases express cytokeratin, vimentin, and S-100 protein.[24,25] Less commonly, positivity for calponin, smooth muscle actin, glial fibrillary acidic protein, desmin, and epithelial membrane antigen is observed.

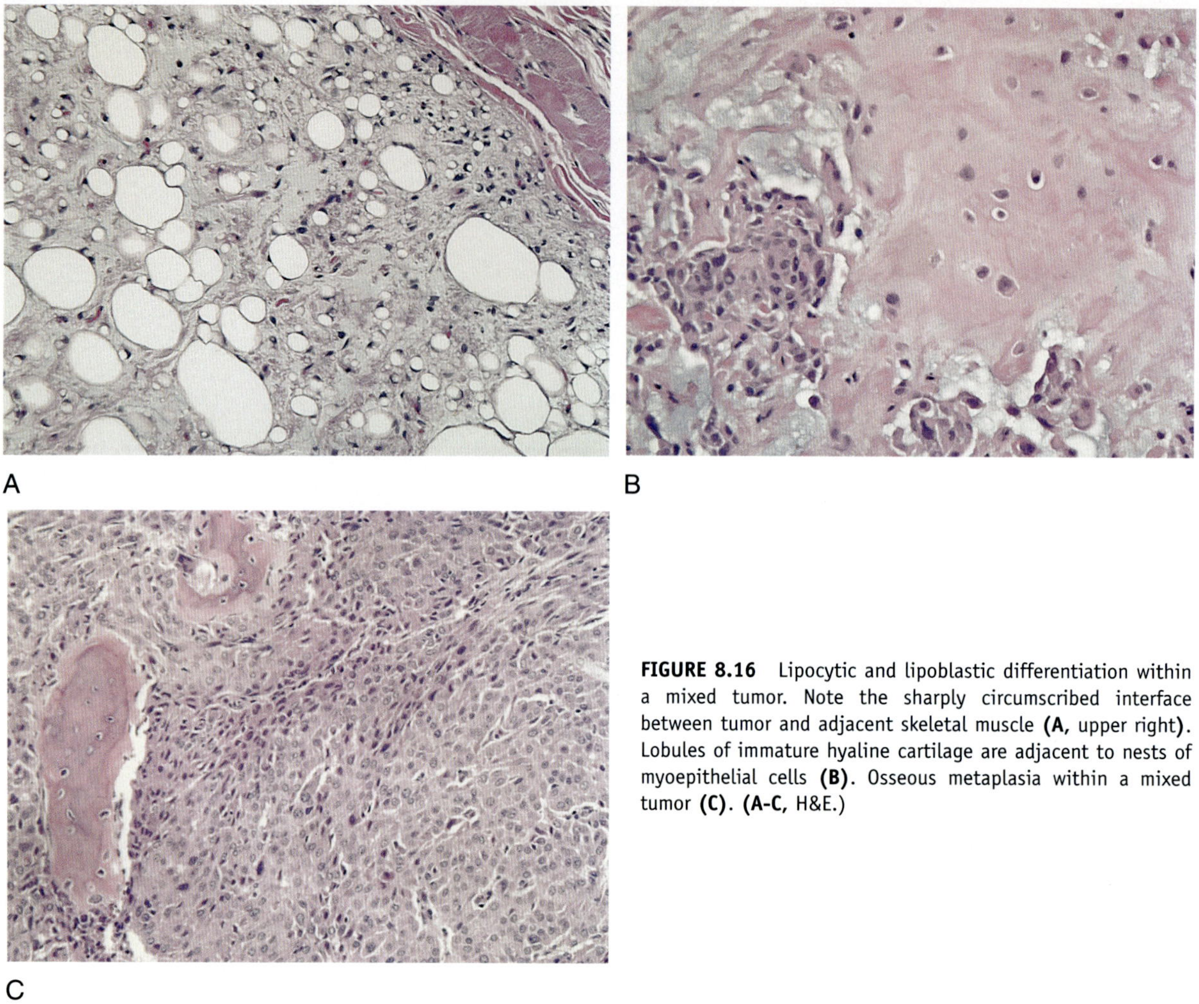

FIGURE 8.16 Lipocytic and lipoblastic differentiation within a mixed tumor. Note the sharply circumscribed interface between tumor and adjacent skeletal muscle **(A,** upper right**)**. Lobules of immature hyaline cartilage are adjacent to nests of myoepithelial cells **(B)**. Osseous metaplasia within a mixed tumor **(C)**. **(A-C,** H&E.)

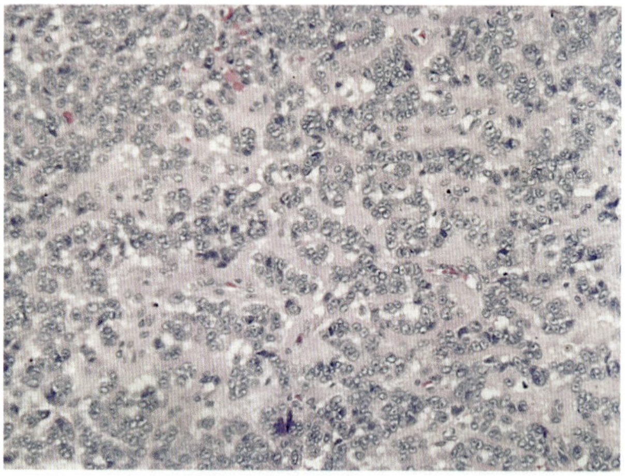

FIGURE 8.17 Less commonly, mixed tumors may be composed almost exclusively of myoepithelial cells (myoepitheliomas), most often round to polygonal and arranged in ill-defined nests and cords. (H&E.)

Prognosis and Therapy

Most mixed tumors/myoepitheliomas behave in a benign fashion and are cured after surgical resection. A few may recur locally, however, and even metastasize, resulting in death.[24] At present, no histologic features predict prognosis. Consequently, it is recommended that all cases be excised completely (negative margins).

Low-Grade Fibromyxoid Sarcoma

Clinical Features

Low-grade fibromyxoid sarcoma, also called *hyalinizing spindle cell tumor with giant rosettes*, is a rare, more recently described sarcoma typically arising in young to middle-aged adults. Men and women are affected roughly equally. The most common anatomic locations include the deep soft tissues of the lower extremities and trunk.[30,31] Most patients present with painless soft tissue swelling that may be of long duration.

Pathologic Findings

Histology

In most cases, low-grade fibromyxoid sarcoma consists of a mixture of collagenized regions transitioning between less

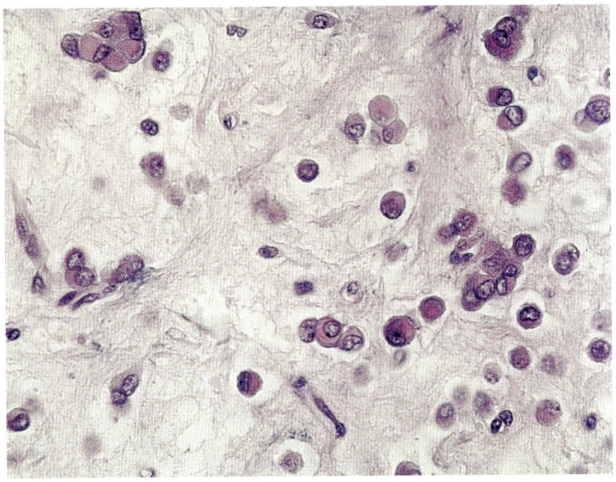

FIGURE 8.18 Rarely, mixed tumors may contain cells that exhibit "rhabdoid" features and intracytoplasmic hyaline inclusions. (H&E.)

cellular myxoid zones. The lesional cells are arranged in sweeping fascicles and whorling growth patterns.[30,31] Individual tumor cells are deceptively bland with round-to-ovoid, uniform nuclei; inconspicuous nucleoli; and pale eosinophilic tapering cytoplasm (Fig. 8.19). The background stroma appears variably collagenous but may show numerous curvilinear blood vessels, especially in the more myxoid zones.[31] Mitotic activity tends to be low, and significant nuclear pleomorphism is never observed. Tumors with increased cellularity and mitotic activity rarely are seen, mostly in recurrent lesions.[31] A less frequent pattern observed in low-grade fibromyxoid sarcoma is the presence of poorly formed collagenous rosettes. The latter consists of central cores of hyalinized collagen surrounded by more epithelioid-appearing tumor cells (Fig. 8.20). This unusual pattern initially resulted in the designation of *hyalinizing spindle cell tumor with giant rosettes*.[32] It now is believed that low-grade fibromyxoid sarcoma and hyalinizing spindle cell tumor giant rosettes are a spectrum of a similar neoplasm.[31]

Ancillary Studies

In conventional low-grade fibromyxoid sarcoma and hyalinizing spindle cell tumor with giant rosettes, the ultrastructural features are those of fibroblastic differentiation. The center of the rosettes is composed of banded collagen fibers; the epithelioid cells surrounding the rosettes appear similar to the spindle cells seen elsewhere in the tumor.[33]

Immunohistochemically the lesional cells show diffuse immunopositivity for vimentin. Smooth muscle actin, actin, and desmin are usually negative. S-100 protein, desmin, cytokeratin, and CD34 are generally negative. The rounded cells at the periphery of the rosettes may display a different immunophenotype with S-100 and Leu-7 positivity.[32,33]

Only three examples of low-grade fibromyxoid sarcoma have been subjected to cytogenetic analysis. No consistent chromosomal abnormality has been observed; however, two cases displayed supernumerary ring chromosomes.[34]

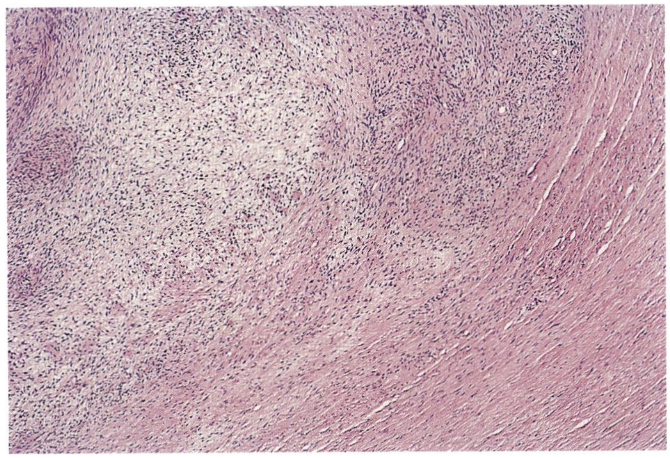

A

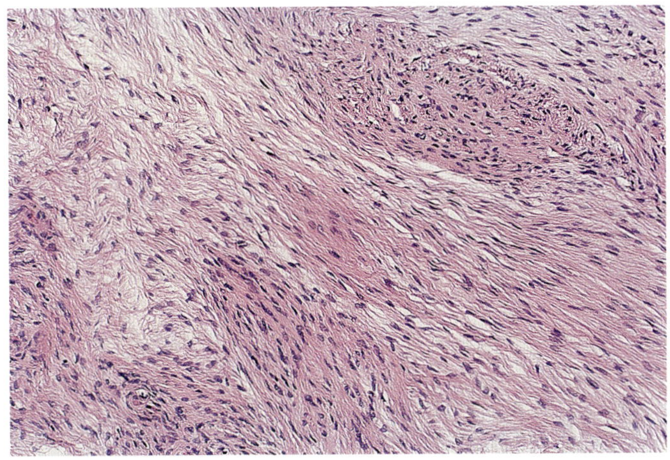

B

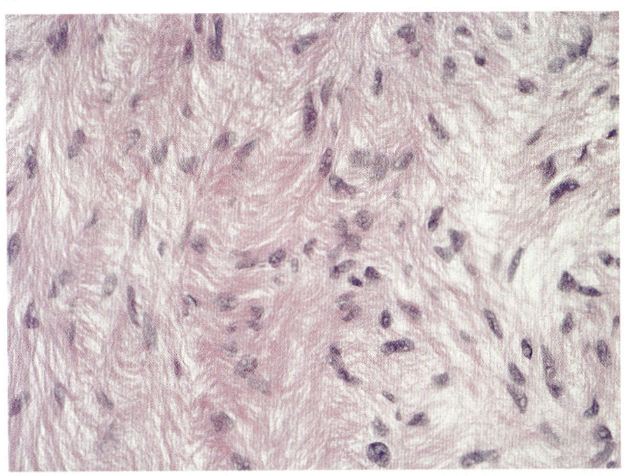

C

FIGURE 8.19 Low-grade fibromyxoid sarcoma characterized by alternating collagenous and myxoid zones with spindled cells arranged in fascicles and sheets. Individual tumor cells are remarkably bland and uniform **(A-C)**. **(A,** Low power, H&E; **B,** intermediate power, H&E; **C,** high power, H&E.)

Prognosis and Therapy

When low-grade fibromyxoid sarcoma initially was described, local recurrence and reported metastatic rates exceeded 75% and 50%, respectively.[30,31] Many of these

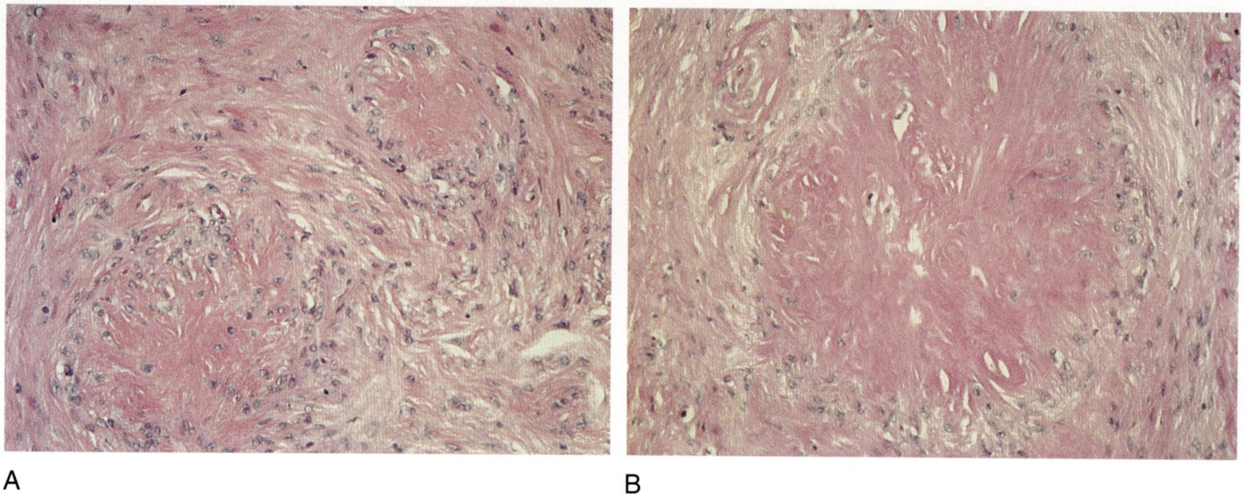

FIGURE 8.20 Rarely, low-grade fibromyxoid sarcoma may show giant collagenous rosettes (hyalinizing spindle cell tumor with giant rosettes) (**A** and **B**). (**A** and **B**, H&E.)

original tumors initially were not recognized as malignant, however, and treated accordingly. When recognized as malignant and excised completely, local recurrence occurs in less than 10% of patients; metastasis occurs in approximately 5% of patients.[31] Consequently, the risk of local recurrence and metastasis seems related to the adequacy of excision. Metastasis is infrequent, but extended, long-term clinical follow-up is recommended because it may occur several years after the initial diagnosis.

Myxofibrosarcoma (Myxoid Malignant Fibrous Histiocytoma)

Clinical Features

Myxofibrosarcoma is one of the most common adult sarcomas. Most patients are elderly, and men and women are affected equally.[35] Most examples arise in the dermal/subcutaneous tissues of the extremities, followed by the trunk (Fig. 8.21). Head and neck involvement rarely is observed.[35] A slowly enlarging, painless soft tissue mass is a common initial complaint.

Pathologic Findings

Histology

Myxofibrosarcomas are usually multinodular, infiltrative lesions with individual nodules separated by variably thickened fibrous bands (Fig. 8.22). A myxoid stroma should be at least focally (10%) present to establish the diagnosis. Within the myxoid matrix are scattered, thin-walled, curvilinear-shaped blood vessels and round-to-spindled, hyperchromatic tumor cells, displaying moderate-to-marked nuclear pleomorphism. The degree of cellularity is inversely proportional to the amount of myxoid stroma and tends to correlate with the grade of the tumor.[35] Low-grade lesions exhibit a prominent hypocellular, myxoid matrix throughout with scattered atypical spindled cells exhibiting mildly to moderately atypical, hyperchromatic nuclei. Solid areas are not observed, and mitoses are infrequent. At the opposite end, high-grade tumors are hypercellular, predominantly solid lesions with focal (at least 10%) myxoid areas identical to those observed in the low-grade form. The solid areas resemble pleomorphic malignant fibrous histiocytoma with markedly atypical cells arranged in fascicles and storiform patterns. Necrosis, hemorrhage, and atypical mitoses are seen frequently. Intermediate-grade tumors have features "intermediate" between the low-grade and high-grade forms. Compared with low-grade myxofibrosarcoma, they are usually more cellular and show more nuclear atypia but retain the myxoid stroma throughout, lacking the more solid cellular areas seen in the high-grade tumors (Fig. 8.23). In the intermediate-grade and high-grade lesions, the transition between the lower grade myxoid areas and the more cellular zones is often abrupt (Fig. 8.24).[35] So-called pseudolipoblasts, containing one or more mucin-filled cytoplasmic vacuoles, may be present, mimicking a liposarcoma (Fig. 8.25).

Fine Needle Aspiration Biopsy

Cytologic smears of myofibrosarcoma are characterized by variable amounts of a myxoid granular-to-filamentous background containing randomly distributed, mostly single, discohesive tumor cells and occasional loose cellular clusters. In general, the volume of the myxoid material is inversely proportional to the cellularity and grade of the tumor. In our experience, the curvilinear blood vessels typically seen in tissue sections are not usually present in cytologic smears.[36] Individual tumor cells display a plethora of cell shapes and sizes, ranging from round and polygonal to spindled and

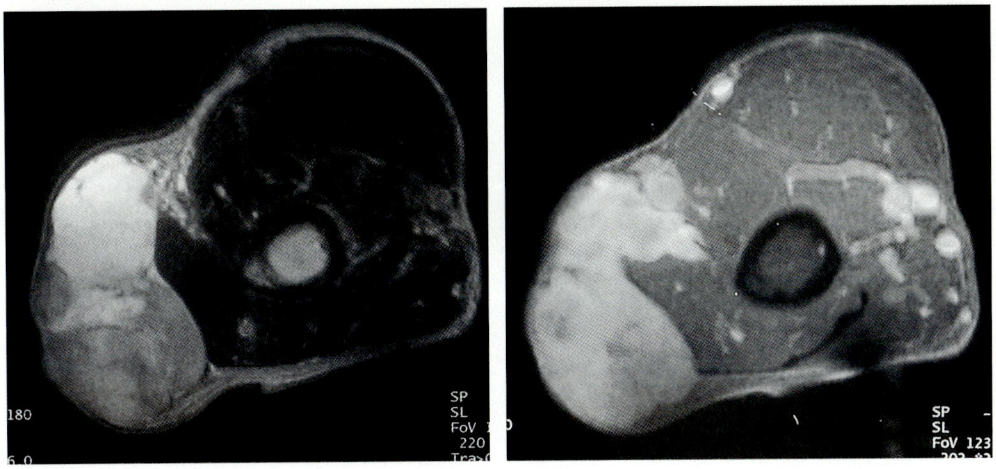

A B

FIGURE 8.21 Axial T2-weighted **(A)** and fat-suppressed T1-weighted **(B)** gadolinium-enhanced magnetic resonance images of the left upper arm show a large mass in the subcutaneous fat of the arm laterally and abutting and effacing the underlying musculature. The hyperintense anterior portion of the mass on the T2-weighted image reflects necrosis in the tumor. The mass enhances heterogeneously after intravenous administration of gadolinium.

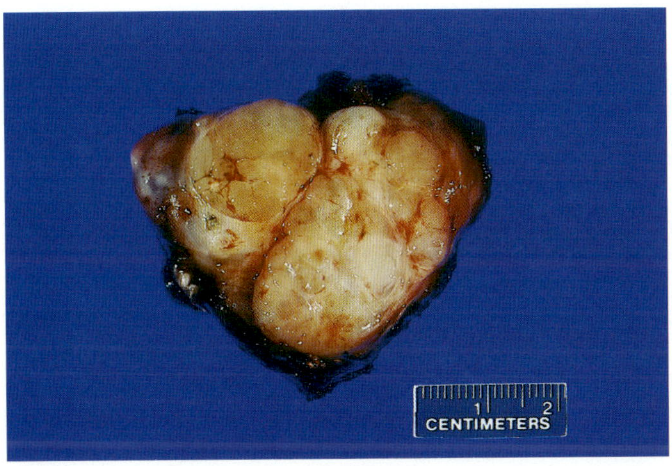

FIGURE 8.22 Myxofibrosarcoma appears grossly multinodular and variably myxoid.

stellate. Nuclei are frequently large, hyperchromatic, and pleomorphic, often containing prominent nucleoli; cytoplasm ranges from scant and wispy to dense and tapering, sometimes vacuolated. Multinucleated tumor giant cells occasionally are observed, more frequently in the high-grade examples. In most cases, low-grade and intermediate-grade myxofibrosarcomas are recognized more easily in FNAB preparations. Because of their less abundant myxoid stroma, higher grade cases appear more difficult to subtype specifically and are often indistinguishable from other adult pleomorphic sarcomas (e.g., malignant fibrous histiocytoma, pleomorphic liposarcoma) (Figs. 8.26 and 8.27).[36]

Ancillary Studies

Most tumor cells in myxofibrosarcoma show ultrastructural features consistent with fibroblastic differentiation, including prominent rough endoplasmic reticulum, scattered mitochondria, and Golgi apparatus.[35] Immunohistochemically, all myxofibrosarcomas express vimentin; in the more cellular areas, actin and smooth muscle actin sometimes are focally positive. CD68, Mac 387, and factor XIIIa are usually negative.[35]

Cytogenetic analysis of myxofibrosarcoma typically shows highly complex karyotypes and a variety of aberrations, including ring chromosomes and translocations. No reproducible chromosomal abnormality has been identified, however.[37]

Prognosis and Therapy

Local recurrence occurs in 50% of cases, regardless of histologic grade or depth of primary lesion.[35] Metastases generally are observed only in intermediate-grade and high-grade tumors and are more common in deep-seated tumors. Wide surgical resection is the recommended treatment.

Myxoid and Round Cell Liposarcoma

Myxoid liposarcoma is a relatively common, well-characterized soft tissue sarcoma generally regarded as having low-grade morphology and favorable clinical behavior. Conversely, round cell liposarcoma is a high-grade sarcoma associated with less favorable survival. In the past, these tumors were regarded as separate entities. Morphologic studies and cytogenetic analyses revealed, however, that myxoid and round cell liposarcoma represent end points of a spectrum of a similar entity.[38–40]

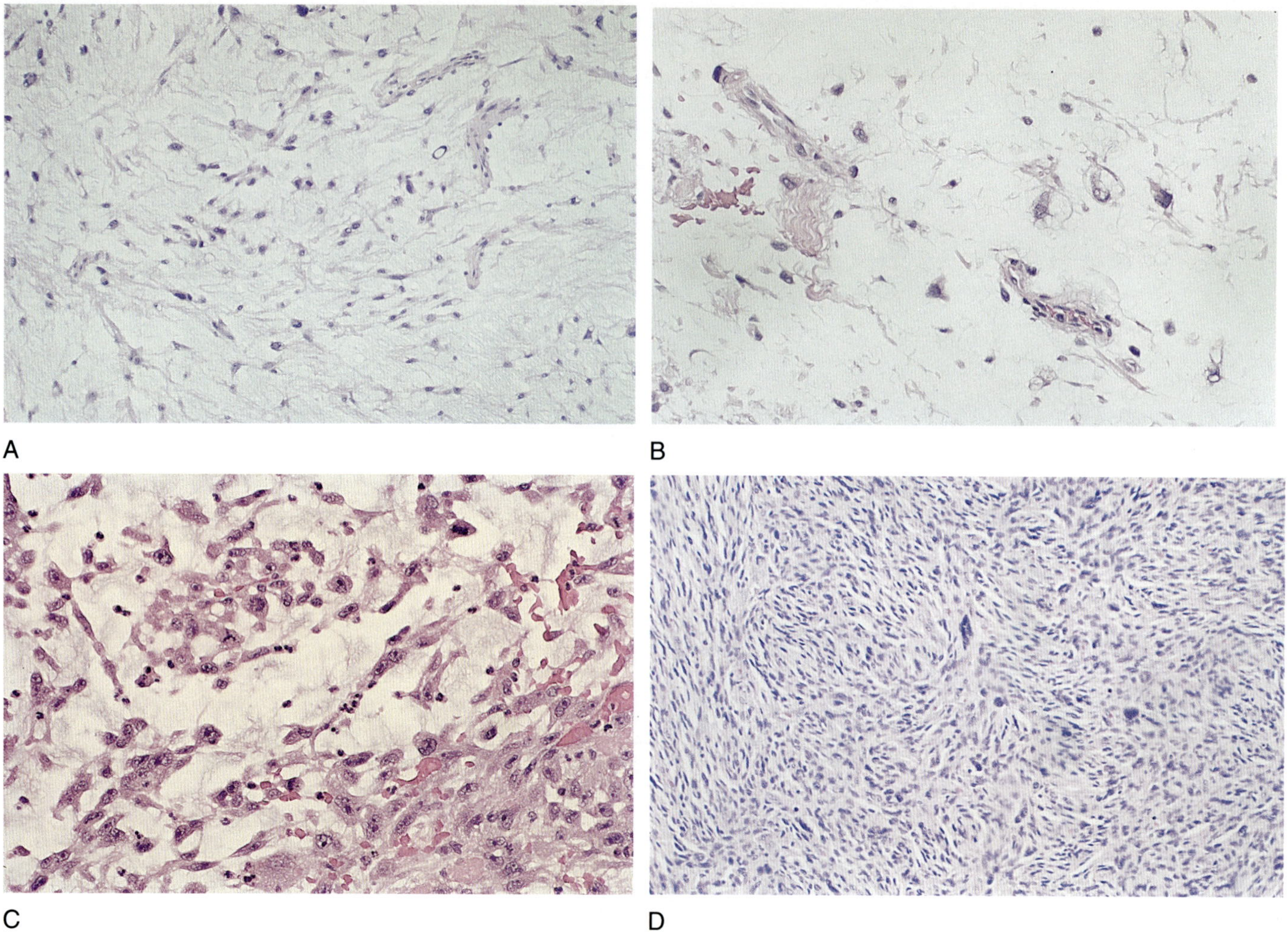

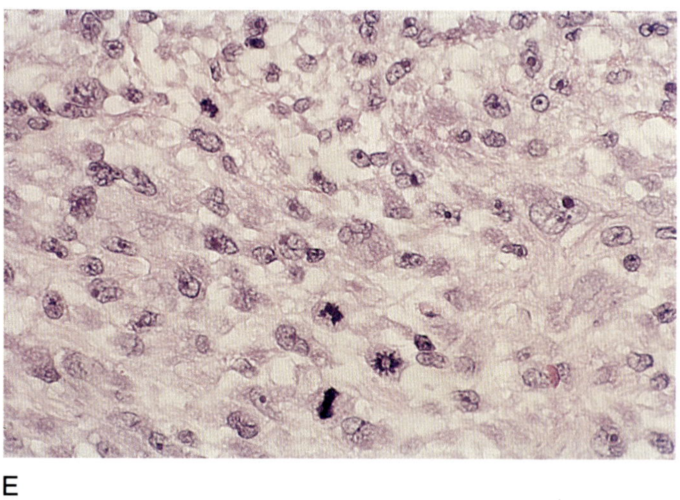

FIGURE 8.23 Low-grade myxofibrosarcoma appears hypocellular, but curvilinear blood vessels are prominent, and the tumor cells show at least moderate nuclear pleomorphism **(A** and **B)**. Compared with the low-grade form, intermediate-grade myxofibrosarcoma shows increased cellularity, greater nuclear atypia, and increased mitotic activity. Nevertheless, solid areas are not present, and the myxoid stroma remains obviously present throughout the lesion **(C)**. High-grade myxofibrosarcoma is characterized by solid areas, indistinguishable from other pleomorphic sarcomas, with marked nuclear atypia and numerous mitotic figures **(D** and **E)**. **(A,** Intermediate power, H&E; **B,** high power, H&E; **C,** H&E; **D,** low power, H&E; **E,** high power, H&E.)

Clinical Features

Most patients are middle-aged to older adults, and men are affected more commonly than women. The most common anatomic site is the deep subfascial tissues of the lower extremity, especially the thigh.[38] Rarely, myxoid liposarcoma arises within the retroperitoneum and intra-abdominal cavity. Myxoid liposarcoma is virtually never cutaneous/subcutaneous in origin. Painless soft tissue swelling is the most common clinical complaint.

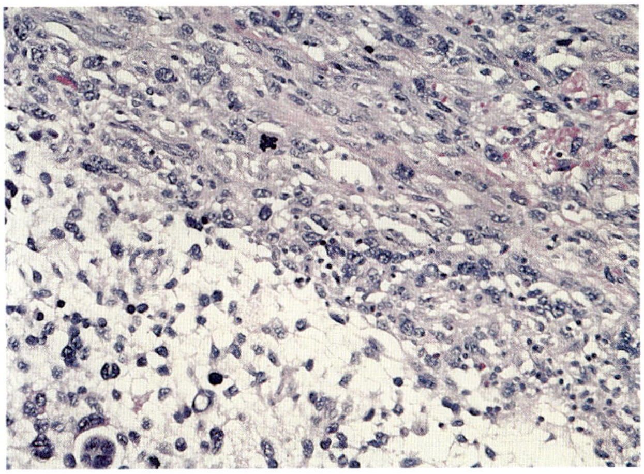

FIGURE 8.24 For proper grading and prognostication, adequate sampling of a myxofibrosarcoma is essential. Low-grade areas frequently show an abrupt transition with higher grade zones. (H&E.)

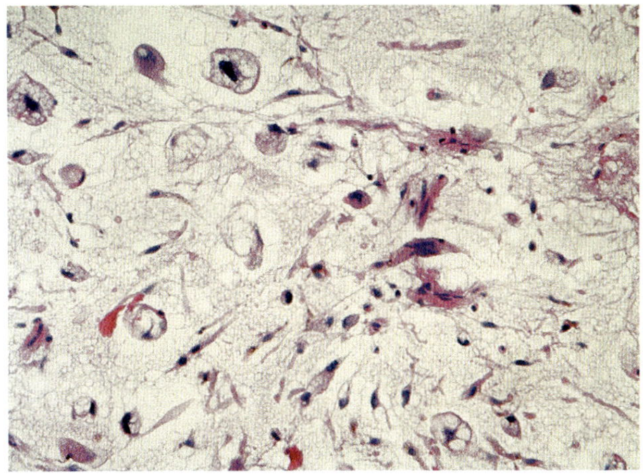

FIGURE 8.25 Myxofibrosarcoma often displays tumor cells with multivacuolated, mucin-filled cytoplasm, so-called *pseudolipoblasts*. The degree of nuclear pleomorphism greatly exceeds that observed in myxoid liposarcoma, however. (H&E.)

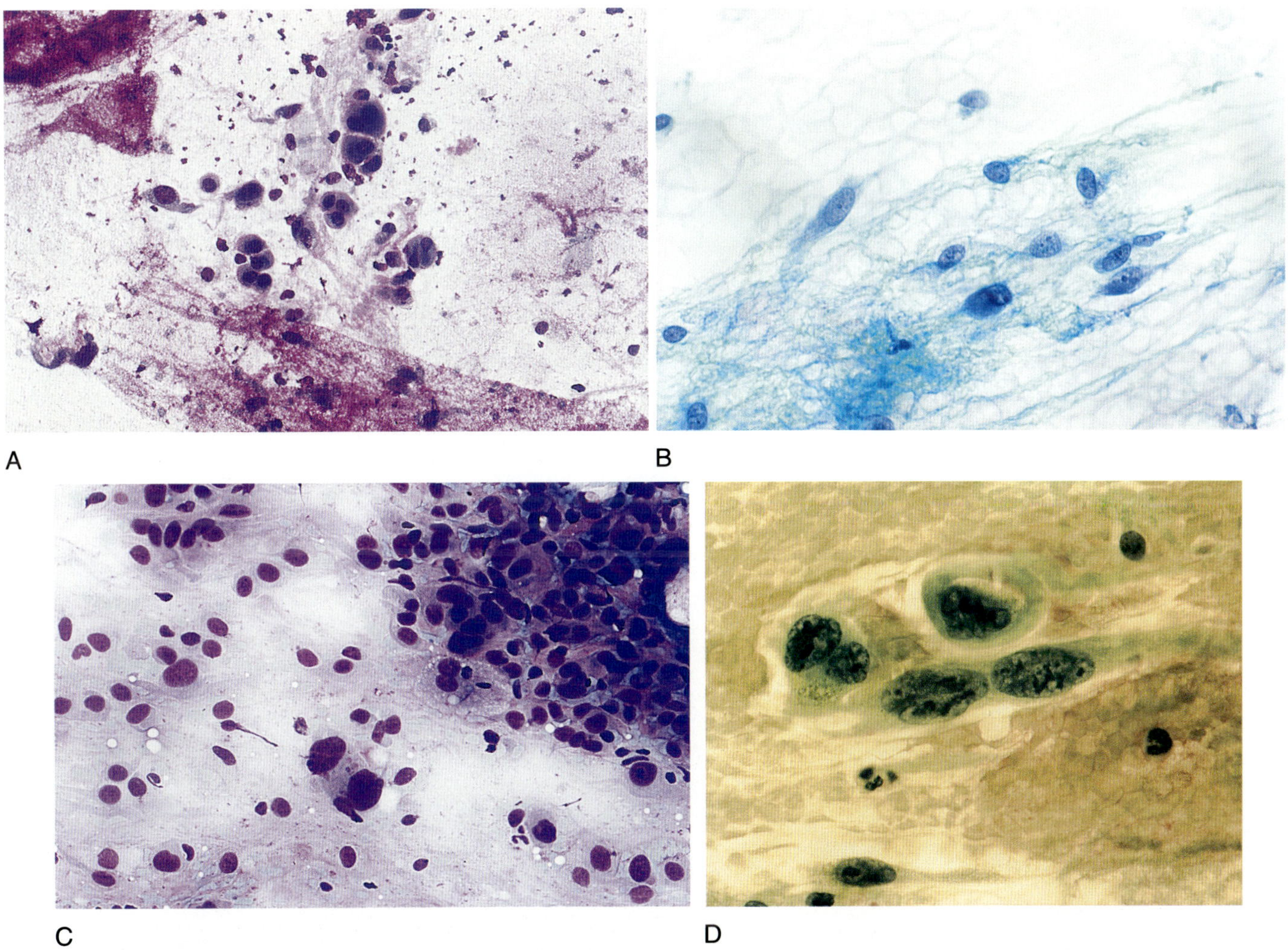

FIGURE 8.26 Fine needle aspiration biopsy of myxofibrosarcoma yields a diffuse, myxoid granular film, best observed in Romanowsky preparations, covering virtually the entire slide. The degree of cellularity and nuclear atypia correlates with the grade of the tumor and is inversely proportional to the amount of myxoid stroma. Lower grade samples appear less cellular and show mostly individual, ovoid-to-spindled tumor cells with moderate nuclear atypia **(A** and **B)**. High-grade myxofibrosarcoma shows highly cellular smears composed of markedly pleomorphic tumor cells and scattered multinucleated tumor giant cells **(C** and **D)**. **(A,** Diff-Quik; **B,** Papanicolaou; **C,** Diff-Quik; **D,** Papanicolaou.)

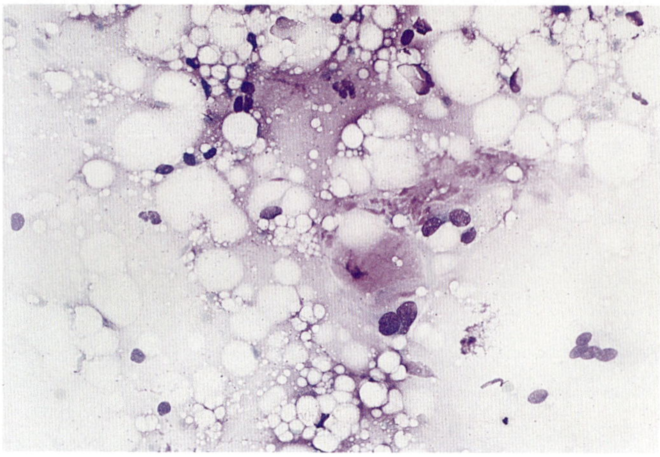

FIGURE 8.27 Because myxofibrosarcomas are highly infiltrative, we have rarely observed fine needle aspiration biopsy samples that were accompanied by abundant adipose tissue, closely resembling an atypical lipoma. (H&E.)

Pathologic Findings

Histology

In their pure form, myxoid liposarcomas are generally multilobulated lesions with at least focal areas containing a prominent plexiform and arborizing vascular network within a myxoid stroma. Cellularity ranges from slight to moderate, with cells appearing mostly uniform, ovoid to slightly spindled, with ovoid-to-round, hyperchromatic nuclei and inconspicuous nucleoli (Fig. 8.28). Signet ring cell lipoblasts often are observed, but multivacuolated lipoblasts tend to be uncommon (Fig. 8.29). Significant nuclear pleomorphism is not a feature of "pure" myxoid liposarcoma and should suggest the possibility of myxofibrosarcoma or round cell differentiation. In places, the myxoid stroma may show pseudocystic pooling, creating a "pulmonary edema" pattern (Fig. 8.30).

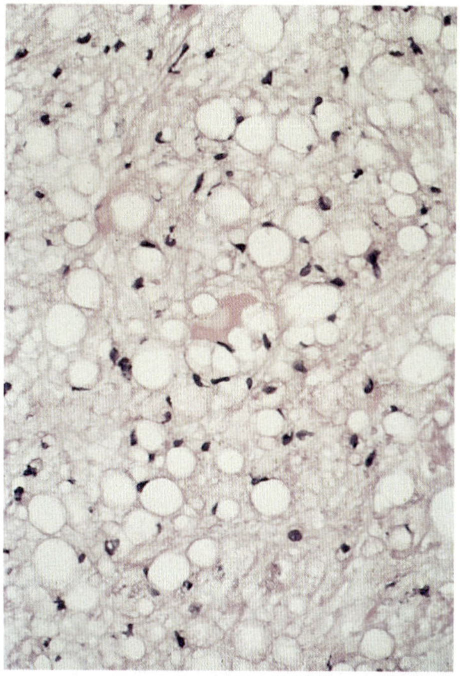

FIGURE 8.29 Signet ring cell lipoblasts commonly are observed in myxoid liposarcoma. (H&E.)

Round cell differentiation is characterized by a population of uniform but larger tumor cells with round, vesicular nuclei and small nucleoli, resembling the malignant cells of non-Hodgkin's lymphoma. In pure round cell forms, the tumor cells often are arranged in sheets and, less frequently, cords (Figs. 8.31 and 8.32). Occasionally the round cell nuclei may appear more epithelioid and show significant nuclear pleomorphism, suggesting the diagnosis of carcinoma. In mixed myxoid and round cell liposarcomas, round cell differentiation tends to predominate in perivascular areas and at the tumor–soft tissue interface.[38] Mixtures of myxoid and

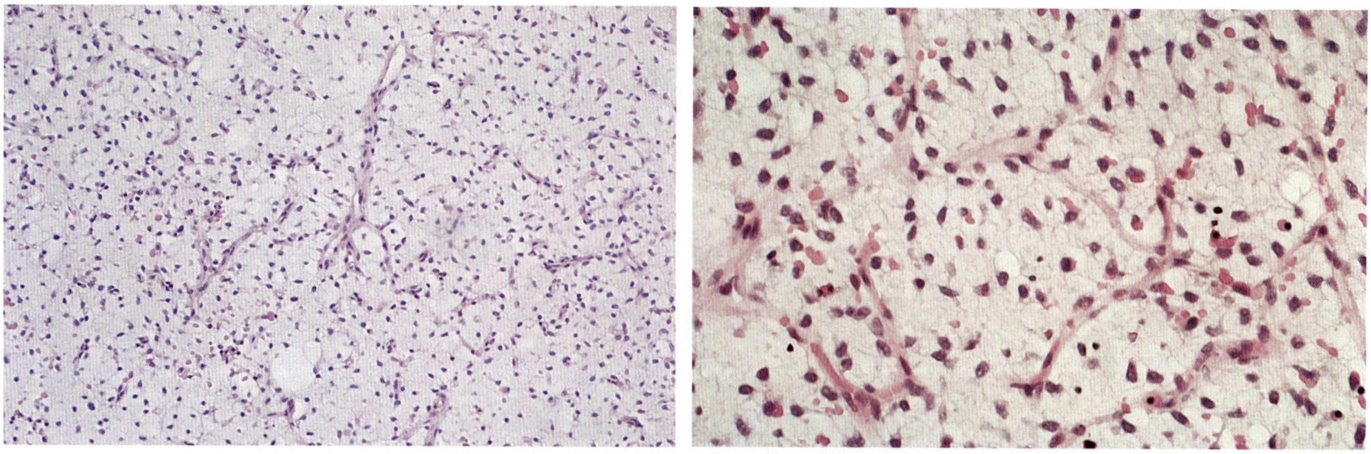

A B

FIGURE 8.28 Classic myxoid liposarcoma characterized by a randomly distributed population of uniform, ovoid tumor cells and a prominent hypervascular myxoid stroma with abundant arborizing vascular pattern **(A** and **B)**. **(A,** Low power, H&E; **B,** high power, H&E.)

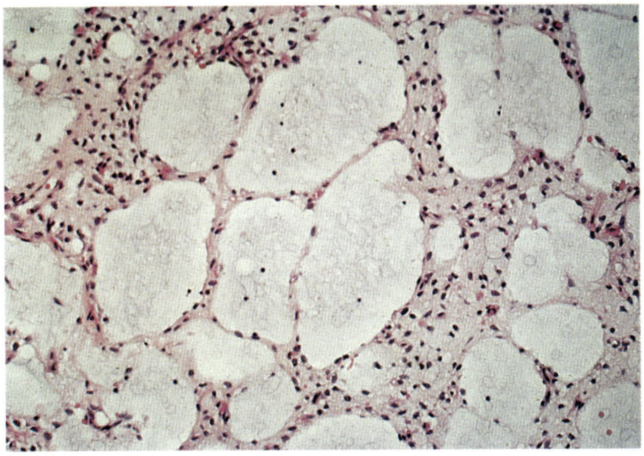

FIGURE 8.30 The myxoid stroma of myxoid liposarcoma sometimes becomes partially cystic with pools of mucin, mimicking a pulmonary edema pattern. (H&E.)

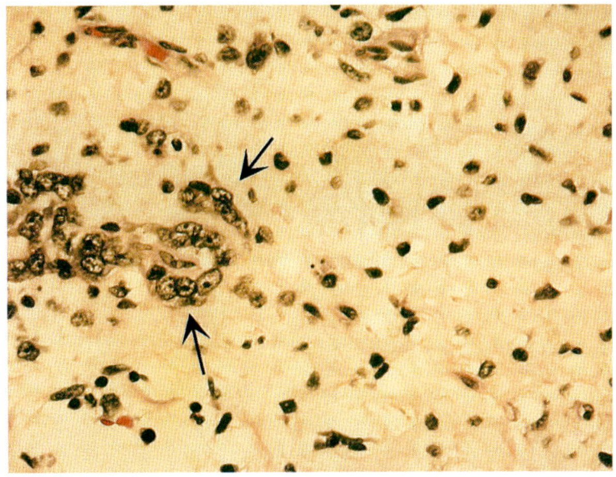

FIGURE 8.31 Mixed myxoid/round cell liposarcoma with cords of round cell differentiation *(arrows)* arising in a background of myxoid liposarcoma. (H&E.)

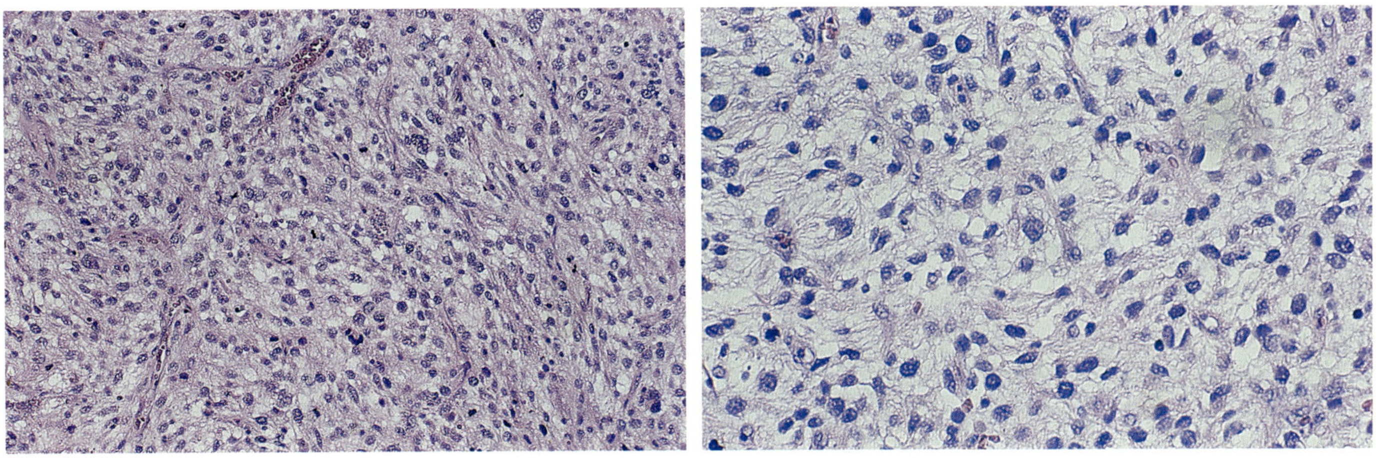

A

B

FIGURE 8.32 Pure round cell differentiation with a population of larger tumor cells. The myxoid stroma is still vaguely present, as is the arborizing vascular pattern **(A** and **B)**. **(A,** Low power, H&E; **B,** high power, H&E.)

round cell liposarcoma are common and have prognostic significance.[38,39]

Fine Needle Aspiration Biopsy

FNAB specimens of myxoid liposarcoma are characterized by scattered fragments of myxoid stroma, frequently containing arborizing, capillary-like blood vessels. In the absence of a round cell component, the tumor cells appear remarkably uniform and ovoid to slightly spindled (Fig. 8.33).[41] Nuclei are ovoid and hyperchromatic and contain inconspicuous nucleoli. Occasional univacuolated and rare multivacuolated lipoblasts accompany these cells (Fig. 8.34). When present, the round cell component is characterized by a significantly larger cell population composed of mostly round cells with hyperchromatic nuclei and occasional prominent nucleoli (Fig. 8.35). Cytoplasm is generally scant and only rarely vacuolated. The round tumor cells typically are dispersed solitarily and in small cellular clusters. Rarely the round cell component may have epithelioid features (small cohesive clusters of large tumor cells with round nuclei and hyperchromatic nuclei and surrounded by scant to eccentrically placed cytoplasm), mimicking the appearance of metastatic adenocarcinoma (Fig. 8.36).[41]

Ancillary Studies

The ultrastructural features reveal undifferentiated tumor cells and signet cell lipoblasts with a single, large lipid droplet, displacing the nucleus peripherally. Extracellular myxoid stromal material is evident.

Immunohistochemistry generally is not required to establish the diagnosis of myxoid liposarcoma. Vimentin and S-100 protein are usually positive. Cytogenetic analysis

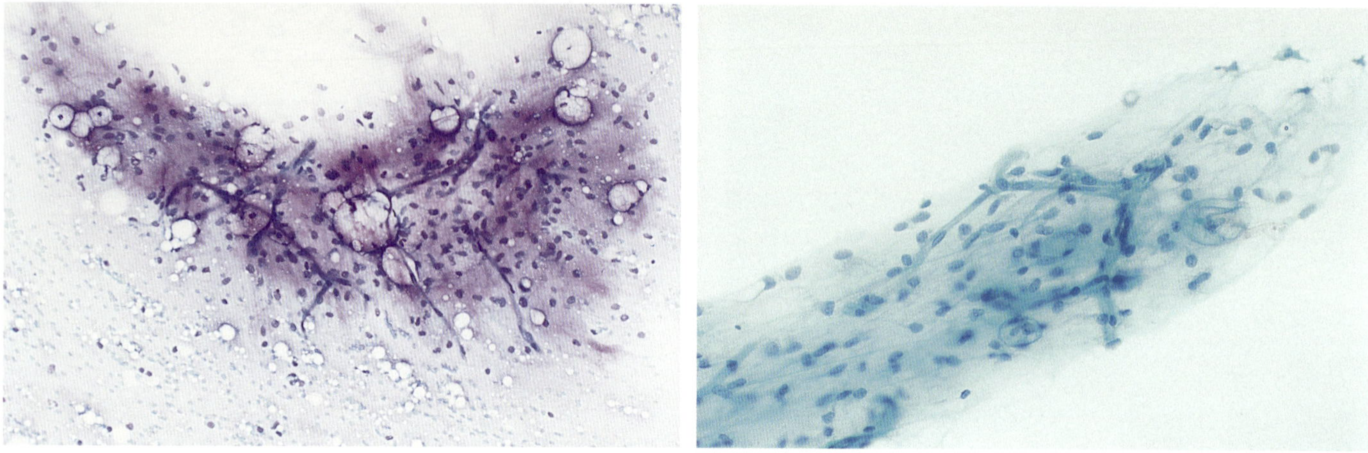

A B

FIGURE 8.33 Fine needle aspiration biopsy specimens of myxoid liposarcoma show myxoid stromal fragments with uniform-appearing ovoid tumor cells and arborizing blood vessels **(A** and **B)**. **(A,** Diff-Quik; **B,** Papanicolaou.)

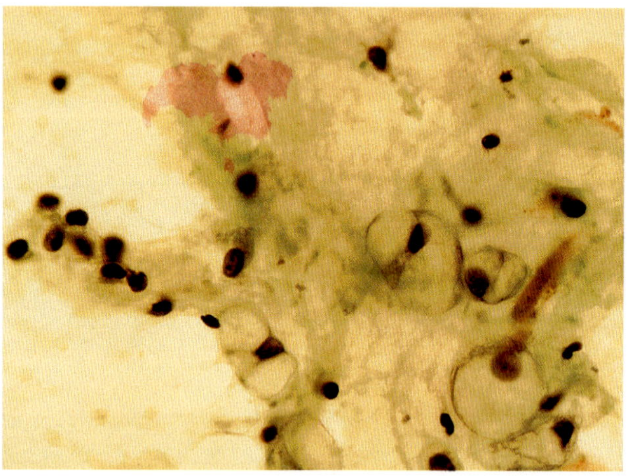

FIGURE 8.34 Multivacuolated and signet ring cell lipoblasts in myxoid liposarcoma. (Papanicolaou.)

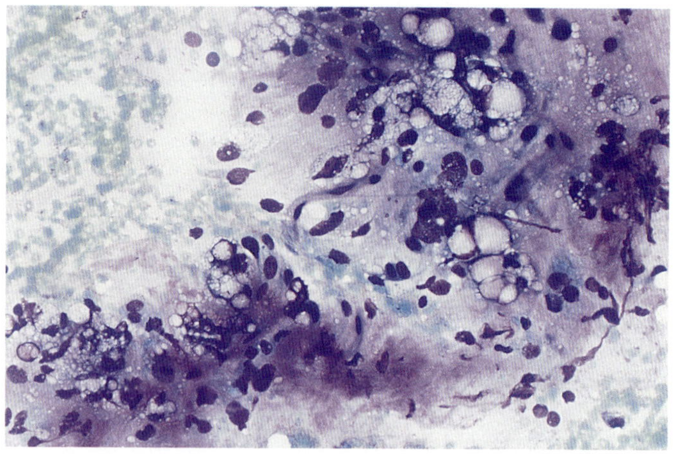

FIGURE 8.35 Mixed myxoid/round cell liposarcoma with a population of larger tumor cells (central) arising within a typical cytologic background of myxoid liposarcoma. (Diff-Quik.)

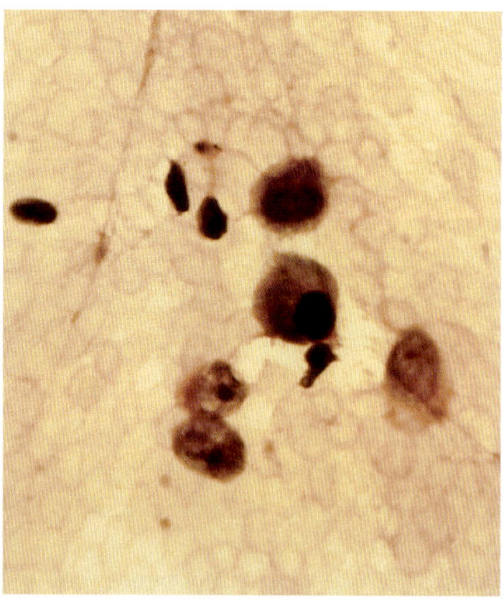

FIGURE 8.36 Round cell liposarcoma with epithelioid tumor cells containing vesicular nuclei and prominent nucleoli. (Papanicolaou.)

reveals the characteristic t(12;16)(q13;p11) with the CHOP-TLS fusion in more than 90% of cases of myxoid and round cell liposarcoma.[40]

Prognosis and Therapy

Unfavorable prognostic indicators include age greater than 45 years, round cell differentiation greater than 5%, and the presence of spontaneous tumor necrosis.[38,39] The prognostic significance of rare, hypercellular (non–round cell) regions in myxoid liposarcoma is unclear. Even pure myxoid liposarcomas may metastasize in 20% of patients.[38] Metastases may occur to unusual soft tissue locations, such as the chest wall or retroperitoneum. Wide surgical resection is the therapy of choice. Chemotherapy may be indicated for lesions with a significant round cell component or distant spread.

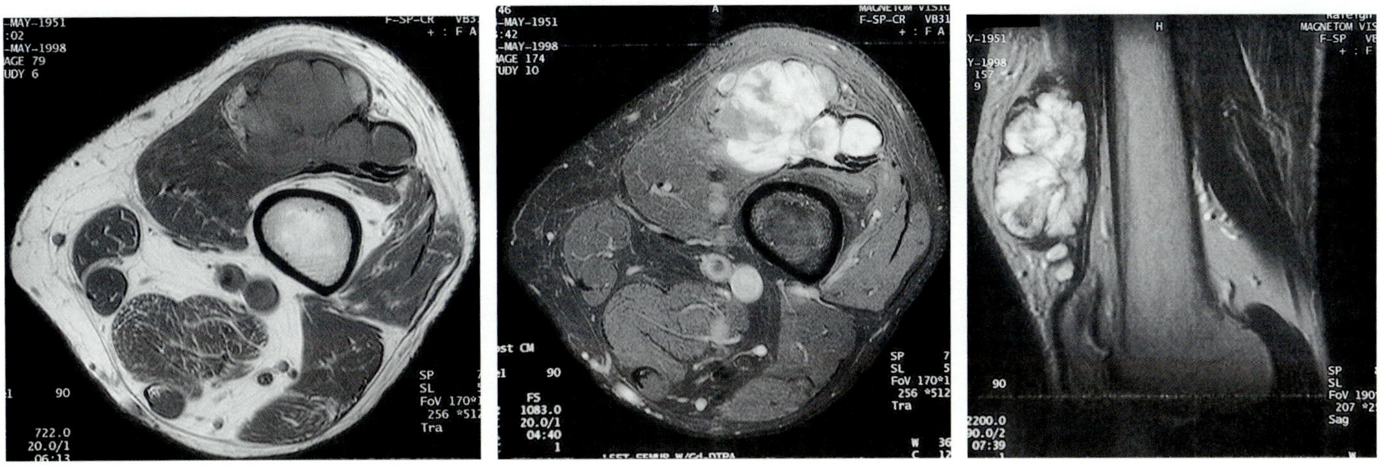

A B C

FIGURE 8.37 Extraskeletal myxoid chondrosarcoma. Axial T1-weighted **(A)**, fat-suppressed T1-weighted gadolinium-enhanced **(B)**, and sagittal short tau inversion recovery (STIR) **(C)** magnetic resonance images of the thigh show a mass in the distal quadriceps compartment, medial to the vastus medialis. The lesion is slightly hyperintense to muscle on the T1-weighted image **(A)** and enhances briskly after the administration of gadolinium **(B)**. On the sagittal image **(C)**, the lesion lies just anterior to the conjoined quadriceps tendon.

Extraskeletal Myxoid Chondrosarcoma (Chordoid Sarcoma)

Clinical Features

Extraskeletal myxoid chondrosarcoma is a rare sarcoma usually arising in older adults and more commonly affecting men.[42] Virtually all arise in the deep soft tissues of the lower extremities (usually proximal) and, less frequently, the trunk (Fig. 8.37). Most patients complain of an enlarging but painless, soft tissue mass. Rare primary skeletal cases have been reported.[43]

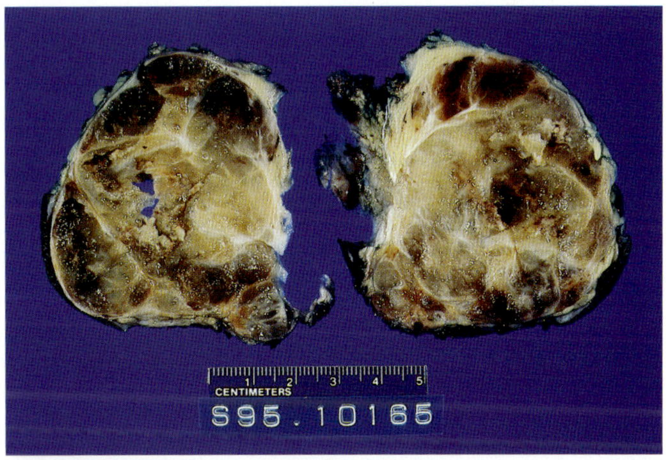

FIGURE 8.38 Myxoid chondrosarcoma is distinctly myxoid with variably sized lobules separated by fibrous septa.

Pathologic Findings

Histology

Morphologically, extraskeletal myxoid chondrosarcoma is abundantly myxoid and multilobular, with individual lobules frequently transversed by fibrous tissue septa (Fig. 8.38). Cellularity ranges from moderate to marked with a tendency in some nodules toward increased cellularity at the periphery. Most are hypovascular, at least compared with the other myxoid sarcomas. The tumor cells classically are arranged in anastomosing strands, rings, and nests and appear uniform, round to slightly spindled with hyperchromatic nuclei and inconspicuous nucleoli, and surrounded by clear, vacuolated-to-eosinophilic cytoplasm (Fig. 8.39).[42] Epithelioid cells with vesicular nuclei and abundant eosinophilic cytoplasm (rhabdoid features) occasionally are observed (Fig. 8.40). Mitotic activity tends to be fewer than one to two mitoses per 10 high-power fields. More cellular foci lacking the characteristic myxoid stroma may exhibit greater mitotic activity. Hyaline cartilage is seen rarely.

Fine Needle Aspiration Biopsy

Cytologic smears of extraskeletal myxoid chondrosarcoma reveal aggregates of myxoid stroma containing a population of mostly uniform-appearing, round-to-spindled tumor cells. Within the stromal fragments, the tumor cells are arranged in cords and small clusters or nests.[41] Blood vessels generally are not apparent. The nuclei of the tumor cells are remarkably uniform but range from round to ovoid and hyperchromatic with small-to-inconspicuous nucleoli, surrounded by a thin rim of scant to slightly vacuolated cytoplasm. The more spindle-shaped forms display a wispy-to-dense, tapering

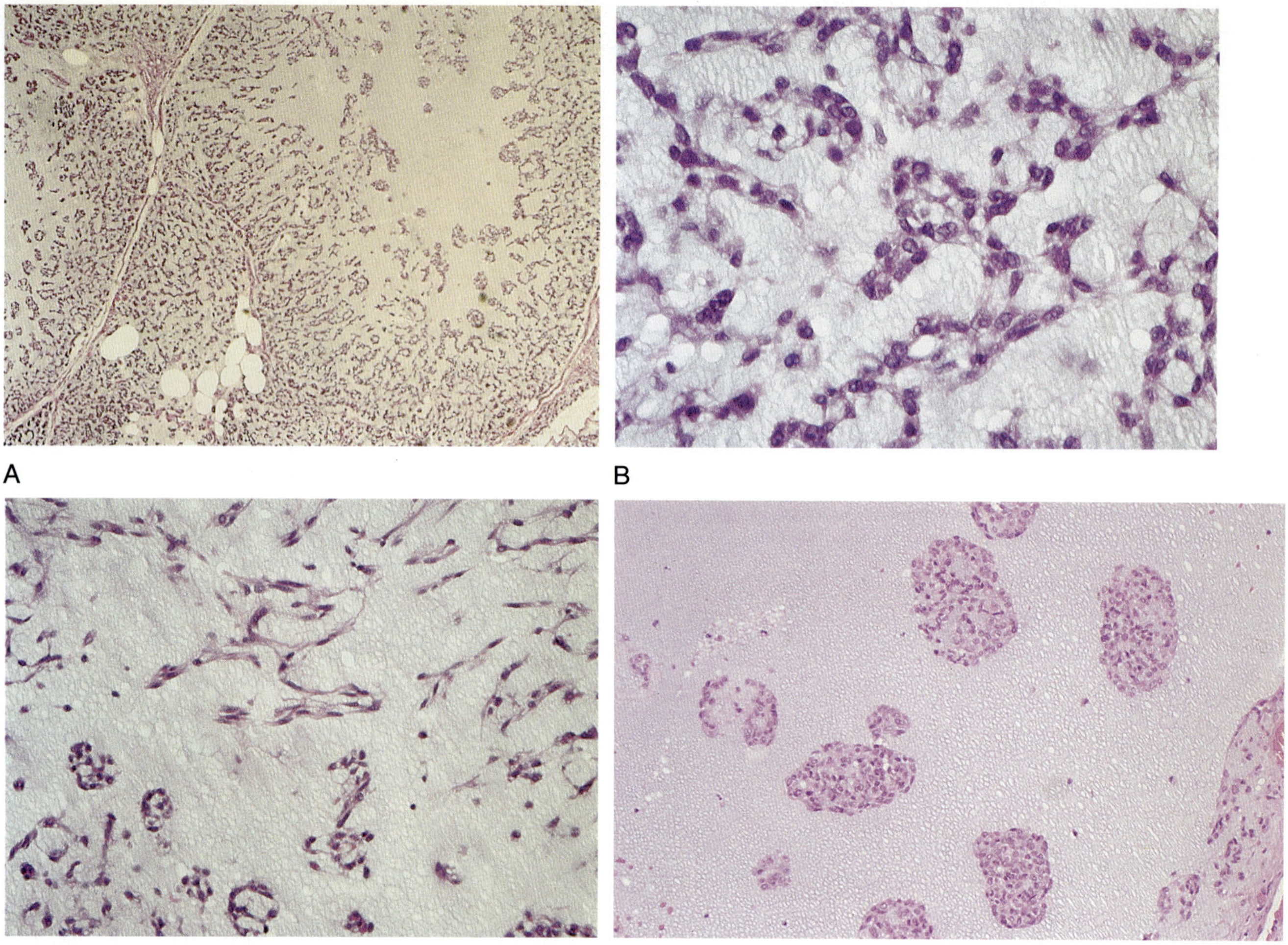

A B C D

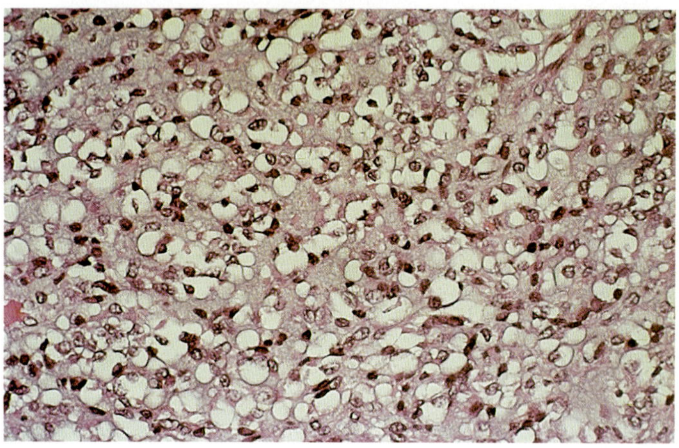

E

FIGURE 8.39 Myxoid chondrosarcoma appears multinodular, often exhibiting increased cellularity at the periphery of the nodules **(A)**. Individual tumor cells appear round to spindled and often are arranged in strands, cords, and nests **(B-D)**. Less commonly, the cells may appear markedly vacuolated **(E)**. **(A-E,** H&E.)

cytoplasm (Fig. 8.41). Similar to myxoid liposarcoma, significant nuclear pleomorphism is not a feature of myxoid chondrosarcoma. As in tissue biopsy specimens, definite hyaline cartilage differentiation is not generally present in cytologic preparations.[41]

Ancillary Studies

Ultrastructurally, extraskeletal myxoid chondrosarcoma is characterized by distinct cords of cells immersed in a glycosaminoglycan-rich matrix. Individual cells have numerous mitochondria and well-developed Golgi apparatus; less commonly, membrane-bound, dense-core granules compatible with neurosecretory granules are observed.[44]

Immunohistochemistry usually is not required to establish the diagnosis. Extraskeletal myxoid chondrosarcomas typically express vimentin, neuron-specific enolase, and synaptophysin.[44,45] S-100 protein positivity is observed in about half of tumors. Epithelial membrane antigen is expressed less frequently. Desmin, actin, smooth muscle actin, and cytokeratin are almost always negative. Cytogenetic analysis in most cases reveals t(9;22)(q22-31;q11-12) with the EWS-CHN (TEC) gene fusion product.[46]

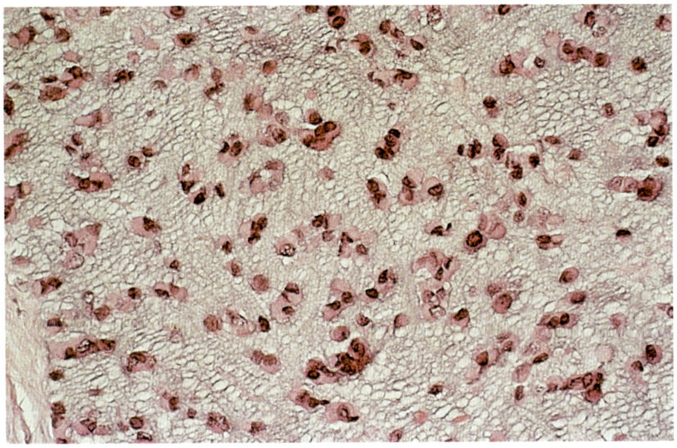

FIGURE 8.40 The tumor cells in myxoid chondrosarcoma occasionally exhibit "rhabdoid" features. (H&E.)

Prognosis and Therapy

Although classically considered a low-grade sarcoma, more recent evidence with long-term follow-up suggests local recurrence and metastatic rates approaching 50%.[42] Adverse prognostic indicators include older age of the patient, large tumor size (>10 cm), and localization in the proximal extremities or limb girdle. Whether tumor grade and high cellularity are correlated with clinical outcome is unclear because reports have produced conflicting data.[42,44] Wide surgical resection with negative margins is recommended.

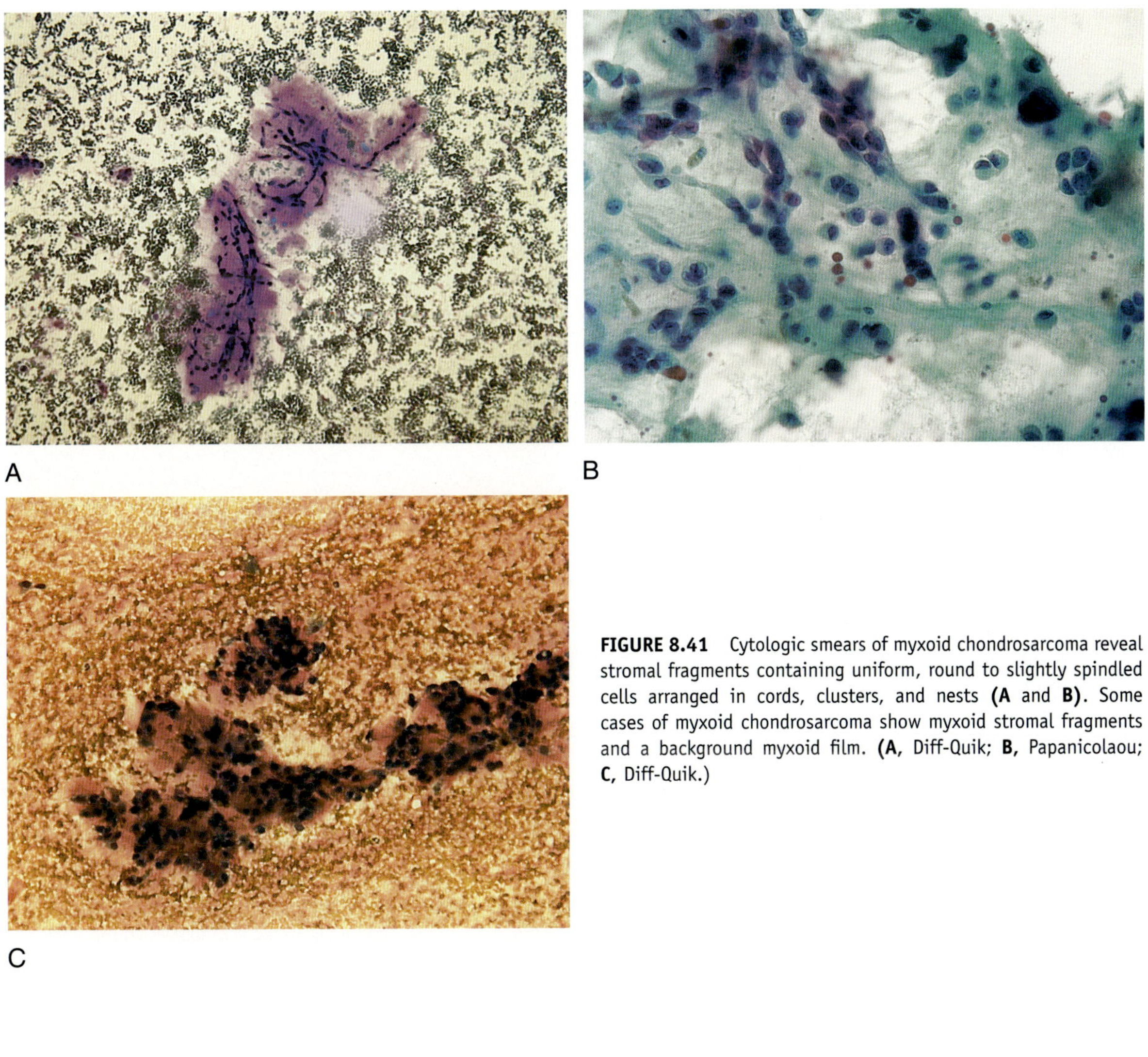

FIGURE 8.41 Cytologic smears of myxoid chondrosarcoma reveal stromal fragments containing uniform, round to slightly spindled cells arranged in cords, clusters, and nests **(A** and **B)**. Some cases of myxoid chondrosarcoma show myxoid stromal fragments and a background myxoid film. **(A,** Diff-Quik; **B,** Papanicolaou; **C,** Diff-Quik.)

Myxoinflammatory Fibroblastic Sarcoma (Inflammatory Myxohyaline Tumor of the Distal Extremities)

Myxoinflammatory fibroblastic sarcoma is a rare, more recently described sarcoma occurring primarily in adults. Men and women are affected roughly equally.[47,48] The tumor has an unusual predilection for the distal extremities, especially the hands and feet. Most patients report a slowly enlarging, painless soft tissue mass. Histologically, myxoinflammatory fibroblastic sarcomas are infiltrative and multinodular lesions. Varying amounts of myxohyalinized stroma and aggregates of acute and chronic inflammation are observed. Scattered large and bizarre, epithelioid tumor cells with vesicular nuclei, abundant eosinophilic cytoplasm, and prominent inclusion-like nucleoli, resembling Reed-Sternberg cells, are characteristic (Fig. 8.42). A few spindled cells also may be present. The atypical cells uniformly express vimentin but are negative for S-100 protein, desmin, actin, CD15, CD30, CD45, and epithelial membrane antigen. Focal CD68, CD34, and cytokeratin expression is observed in some cases.[47,48] Local recurrence rates range up to 67%.[48] This high rate may reflect the fact that most of these excisions were marginal or intralesional. Metastasis is rare, occurring in less than 5% of patients. Wide surgical resection with negative margins is recommended.

Chordoma

Clinical Features

Chordoma is a rare borderline to intermediate-grade malignant tumor that primarily presents in middle-aged to older adults. Men are affected more commonly than women. The most common anatomic location is the sacrum followed by the skull base (spheno-occipital/nasal) and mobile spine.[49,50] Among tumors arising in the spine, involvement of the cervical spine is observed more commonly than is involvement of the thoracolumbar region. Clinical symptoms vary depending on location. In the sacral region, localized pain is the most common presenting complaint. Bladder/bowel dysfunction may be seen. Nerve-related complaints (e.g., paresthesias) usually are observed in advanced cases. Complaints of headache, cranial nerve palsies, and pituitary dysfunction may accompany tumors arising at the skull base. Symptoms related to nerve root compression are common with chordomas involving the mobile spine. Chondroid chordoma is a rare form of chordoma with features of chordoma and chondrosarcoma arising almost exclusively at the skull base.[51]

Radiographically, chordomas form centrally located, lytic, and destructive lesions involving the axial skeleton. A concomitant soft tissue mass is usually present. With magnetic resonance imaging, chordomas appear hypointense on T1-weighted images and hyperintense on T2-weighted images (Fig. 8.43).

Pathologic Findings

Histology

Chordomas are multilobulated, myxoid lesions with individual lobules separated by variably sized fibrous tissue septa. Within the myxoid matrix, the tumor cells are solitary and free-floating or are arranged in anastomosing cords and sheets. Individual tumor cells appear mostly epithelioid with abundant eosinophilic-to-vacuolated cytoplasm. The latter may exhibit abundant vacuoles that displace the nucleus to the periphery, so-called *physaliferous cells*. Nuclear atypia ranges from slight to

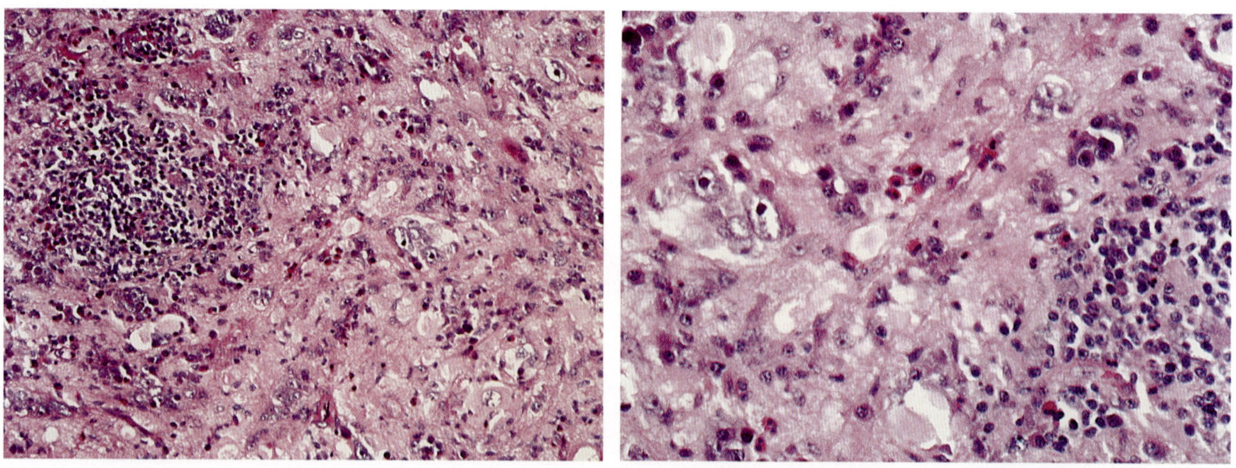

A B

FIGURE 8.42 Myxoinflammatory fibroblastic sarcoma with scattered, enlarged, and bizarre tumor cells with vesicular nuclei and inclusion-like nucleoli, accompanied by aggregates of lymphocytes, plasma cells, and eosinophils within a myxohyalinized stroma **(A** and **B)**. **(A,** Low power, H&E; **B,** high power, H&E.)

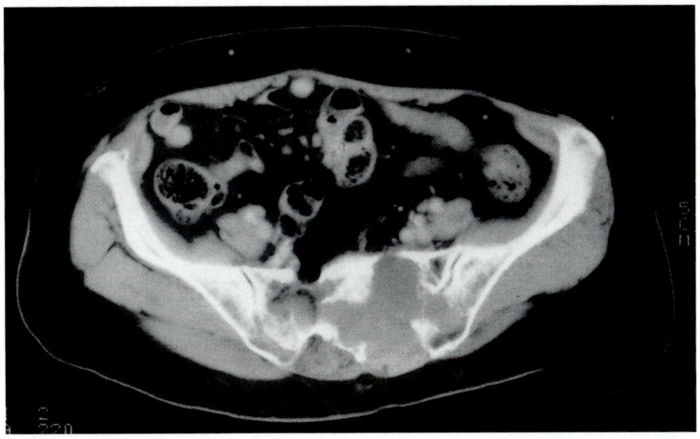

FIGURE 8.43 Chordoma. An axial computed tomography scan reveals an extensive destructive lesion invading the sacrum. The right and left sacral ala are involved, but destruction is more marked on the left. The tumor has crossed the posterior aspect of the left sacroiliac joint and invaded the posterior left ilium.

moderate (Fig. 8.44). Mitotic figures are scant. In chondroid chordoma, hyaline cartilage differentiation characterized by cells within distinct lacunae is observed. This unusual histologic subtype is seen almost exclusively, however, in the spheno-occipital region (Fig. 8.45).[51] Fewer than 5% of chordomas undergo dedifferentiation to a high-grade, pleomorphic sarcoma.

Fine Needle Aspiration Biopsy

FNAB generally yields slightly to moderately cellular smears within an extracellular granular film of myxoid background material. Individual neoplastic cells appear singly and in small clusters and strands. Most have round-to-ovoid nuclei surrounded by moderate amounts of dense-to-vacuolated cytoplasm. In some cells, the cytoplasmic vacuoles are sufficiently large so as to cause displacement and scalloping of the nucleus (classic physaliferous cell). Intranuclear inclusions occasionally are observed. Although most examples of chordoma lack

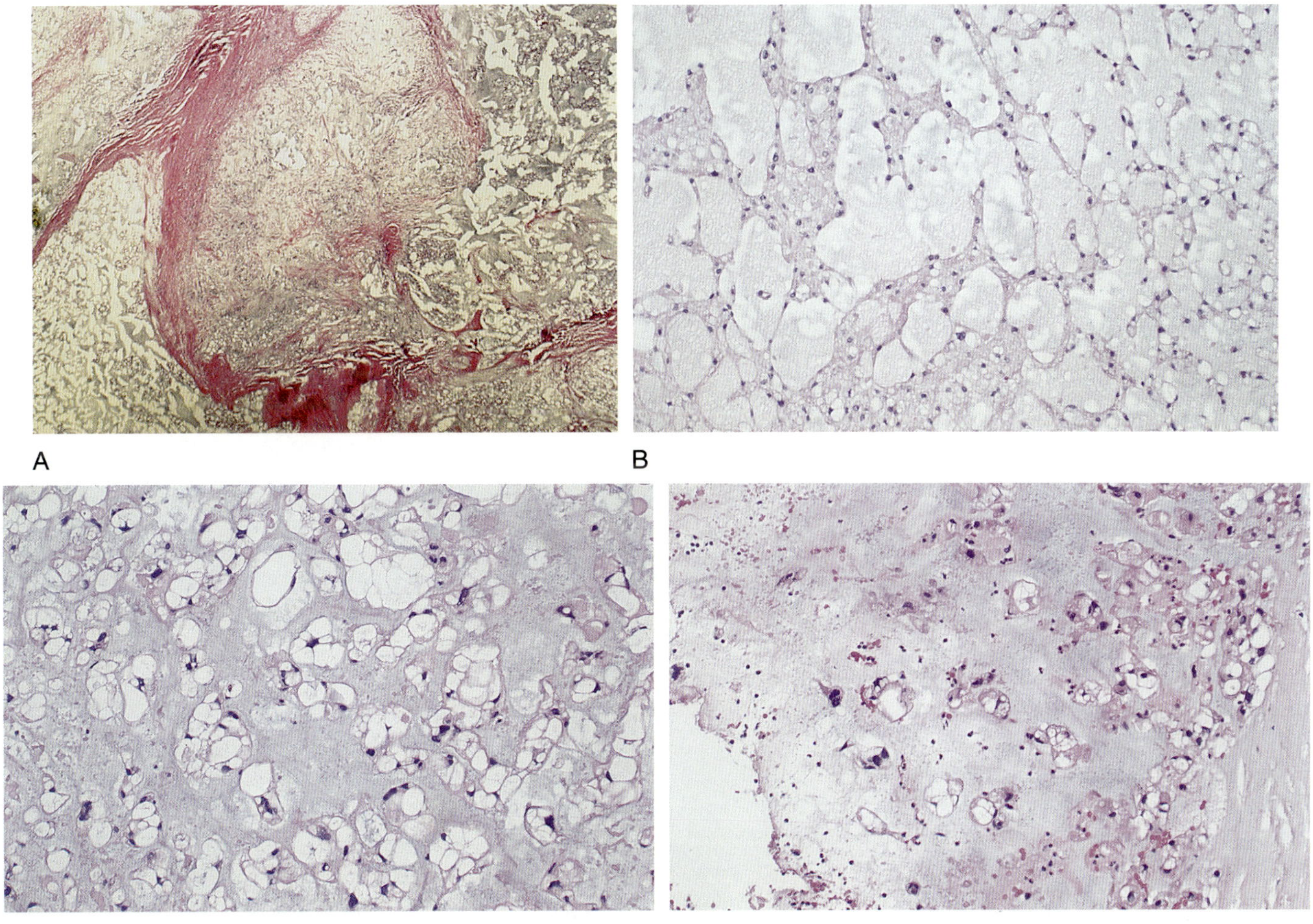

A B C D

FIGURE 8.44 At low power, chordomas reveal variably sized myxoid lobules separated by fibrous septa **(A)**. Individual tumor cells are arranged in cords or nests and have abundant eosinophilic-to-multivacuolated cytoplasm (physaliferous cells) **(B and C)**. Focal nuclear atypia may be present but has no prognostic significance **(D)**. **(A-D,** H&E.)

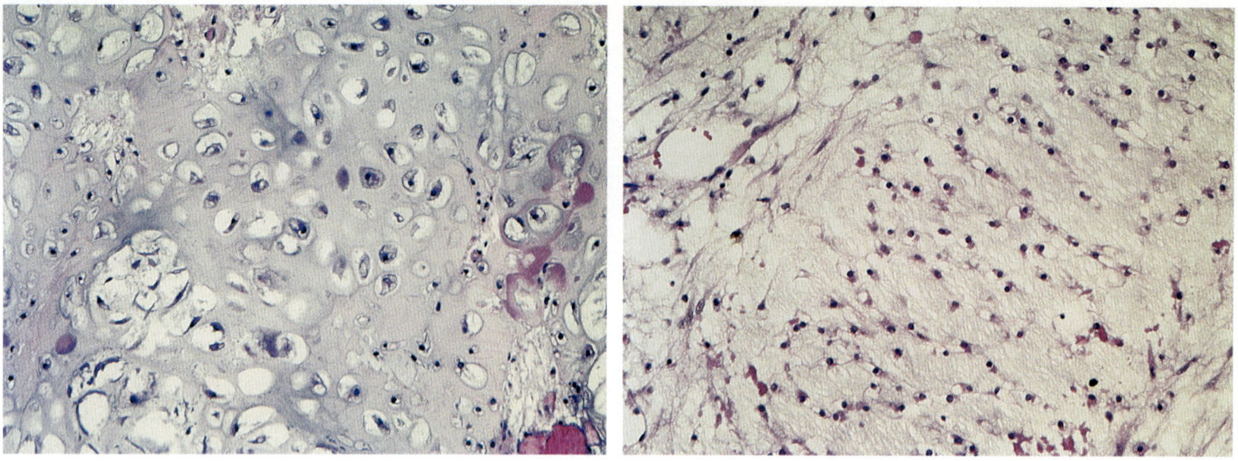

A B

FIGURE 8.45 Chondroid chordoma is defined as having definite hyaline cartilage differentiation **(A)**. Elsewhere, more typical features of chordoma are observed **(B)**. (**A** and **B**, H&E.)

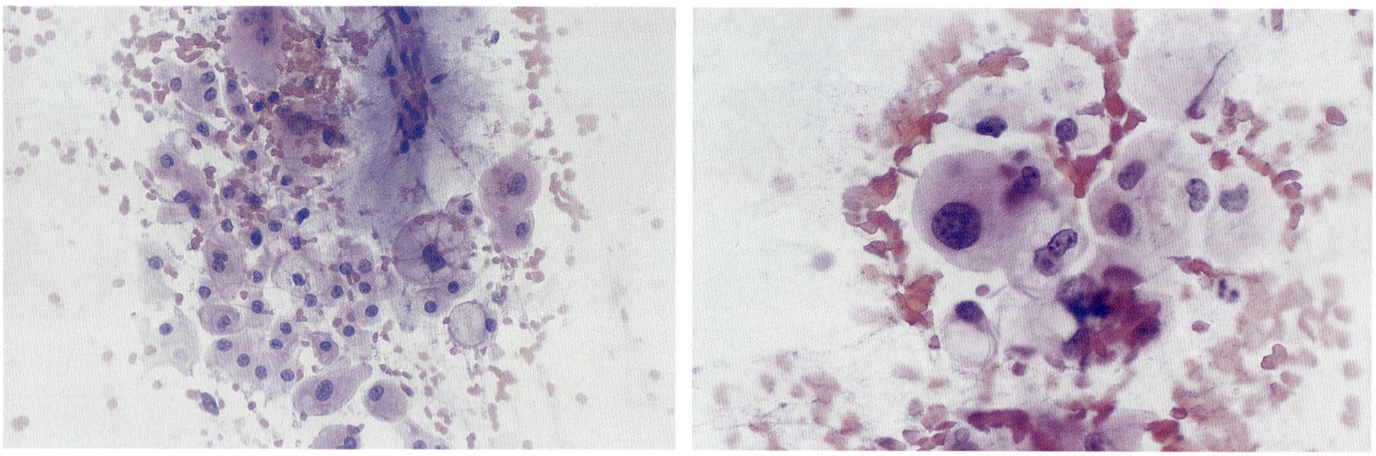

A B

FIGURE 8.46 Fine needle aspiration biopsy samples of chordoma show variably cellular smears composed of mostly clusters and solitary round tumor cells with dense-to-vacuolated cytoplasm **(A)**. Some cells may exhibit significant nuclear atypia **(B)**. (**A** and **B**, H&E.)

significant nuclear atypia, a few tumors exhibit bizarre-appearing anaplastic nuclei (Fig. 8.46).[52]

Ancillary Studies

Ultrastructurally, chordomas show evidence of epithelial differentiation, including the presence of well-developed desmosomes, intermediate filaments, and intracytoplasmic lumina with microvilli.[50] Abundant glycogen is often present.

Chordomas typically show immunoreactivity for cytokeratins, epithelial membrane antigen, vimentin, and, less commonly, S-100 protein. Chondroid chordomas are less consistently positive for these markers.[51] Dedifferentiated forms usually express only vimentin.[50]

Prognosis and Therapy

Among chordomas of the sacrum and mobile spine, adverse prognostic factors include large tumor size, inadequate surgical margins, tumor necrosis, and the development of local recurrence.[50] In the spheno-occipital region, there appears to be no significant difference in survival rates between classic chordoma and chondroid chordoma.[51] The survival of patients younger than 40 years old is significantly better than patients older than 40. Distant metastases are uncommon in chordomas; death is usually the result of complications of local spread. When possible, en bloc surgical resection is preferred and offers the best chance for cure. Radiation therapy may be used for unresectable lesions, but its benefit is unclear.[50]

REFERENCES

Intramuscular myxoma

1. Nielsen GP, O'Connell JX, Rosenberg AE: Intramuscular myxoma: a clinicopathologic study of 51 cases with emphasis on hypercellular and hypervascular variants. Am J Surg Pathol 1998;22:1222.
2. Enzinger FM: Intramuscular myxoma: A review and follow-up study of 34 cases. Am J Clin Pathol 1965;43:104.
3. Schwartz HS, Walker R: Recognizable magnetic resonance imaging characteristics of intramuscular myxoma. Orthopedics 1997;20:431.
4. Caraway NP, Staerkel GA, Fanning CV, et al: Diagnosing intramuscular myxoma by fine-needle aspiration: A multidisciplinary approach. Diagn Cytopathol 1994;11:255.
5. Hashimoto H, Tsuneyoshi M, Daimaru Y, et al: Intramuscular myxoma: A clinicopathologic, immunohistochemical, and electron microscopic study. Cancer 1986;58:740.
6. Meis-Kindblom JM, Sjogren H, Kindblom LG, et al: Cytogenetic and molecular genetic analyses of liposarcoma and its soft tissue simulators: Recognition of new variants and differential diagnosis. Virchows Arch 2001;439:141.

Juxta-Articular Myxoma

7. Meis JM, Enzinger FM: Juxta-articular myxoma: A clinical and pathologic study of 65 cases. Hum Pathol 1992;23:639.
8. King DG, Saifuddin A, Preston HV, et al: Magnetic resonance imaging of juxta-articular myxoma. Skeletal Radiol 1995;24:145.
9. Sciot R, Dal Cin P, Samson I, et al: Clonal chromosomal changes in juxta-articular myxoma. Virchows Arch 1999;434:177.

Myxoma of the Jaw

10. Kaffee I, Naor H, Buchner A: Clinical and radiological features of odontogenic myxoma of the jaws. Dentomaxillofac Radiol 1997;26:299.
11. Lo Muzio L, Nocini P, Favia G, et al: Odontogenic myxoma of the jaws: A clinical, radiologic, immunohistochemical, and ultrastructural study. Oral Surg Oral Med Oral Pathol Oral Radiol Endod 1996;82:426.
12. Kumar N, Jain S, Gupta S: Maxillary odontogenic myxoma: a diagnostic pitfall on aspiration cytology. Diagn Cytopathol 2002;27:111.

Aggressive Angiomyxoma

13. Fetsch JF, Laskin WB, Lefkowitz M, et al: Aggressive angiomyxoma: A clinicopathologic study of 29 female patients. Cancer 1996;78:79.
14. Steeper TA, Rosai J: Aggressive angiomyxoma of the female pelvis and perineum: Report of nine cases of a distinctive type of gynecologic soft-tissue neoplasm. Am J Surg Pathol 1983;7:463.
15. Iezzoni JC, Fechner RE, Wong LS, et al: Aggressive angiomyxoma in males: A report of four cases. Am J Clin Pathol 1995;104:391.
16. Outwater EK, Marchetto BE, Wagner BJ, et al: Aggressive angiomyxoma: Findings on CT and MR imaging. AJR Am J Roentgenol 1999;172:435.
17. Layfield LJ, Dodd LG: Fine-needle aspiration cytology findings in a case of aggressive angiomyxoma: A case report and review of the literature. Diagn Cytopathol 1997;16:425.
18. Nucci MR, Weremowicz S, Neskey DM, et al: Chromosomal translocation t(8;12) induces aberrant HMGIC expression in aggressive angiomyxoma of the vulva. Genes Chromosomes Cancer 2001;32:172.

Ossifying Fibromyxoid Tumor of Soft Parts

19. Enzinger FM, Weiss SW, Liang CY: Ossifying fibromyxoid tumor of soft parts: A clinicopathological analysis of 59 cases. Am J Surg Pathol 1989;13:817.
20. Kilpatrick SE, Ward WG, Mozes M, et al: Atypical and malignant variants of ossifying fibromyxoid tumor of soft parts: A clinicopathologic analysis of six cases. Am J Surg Pathol 1995;19:1039.
21. Matsumoto K, Yamamoto T, Min W, et al: Ossifying fibromyxoid tumor of soft parts: Clinicopathologic, immunohistochemical and ultrastructural study of four cases. Pathol Int 1999;49:742.
22. Nishio J, Iwasaki H, Ohjimi Y, et al: Ossifying fibromyxoid tumor of soft parts: Cytogenetic findings. Cancer Genet Cytogenet 2002;133:124.
23. Sovani V, Velagaleti GV, Filipowicz E, et al: Ossifying fibromyxoid tumor of soft parts: Report of a case with novel cytogenetic findings. Cancer Genet Cytogenet 2001;127:1.

Mixed Tumors/Myoepithelioma/Parachordoma

24. Kilpatrick SE, Hitchcock MG, Kraus MD, et al: Mixed tumors and myoepitheliomas of soft tissue: A clinicopathologic study of 19 cases with a unifying concept. Am J Surg Pathol 1997;21:13.
25. Michal M, Miettinen M: Myoepitheliomas of the skin and soft tissues: Report of 12 cases. Virchows Arch 1999;434:393.
26. Folpe AL, Agoff SN, Willis J, et al: Parachordoma is immunohistochemically and cytogenetically distinct from axial chordoma and extraskeletal myxoid chondrosarcoma. Am J Surg Pathol 1999;23:1059.
27. de Pinieux G, Beabout JW, Unni KK, et al: Primary mixed tumor of bone. Skeletal Radiol 2001;30:534.
28. Ferreiro JA, Nascimento AG: Hyaline-cell rich chondroid syringoma: A tumor mimicking malignancy. Am J Surg Pathol 1995;19:912.
29. Dabska M: Parachordoma: A new clinicopathologic entity. Cancer 1977;40:1586.

Low-Grade Fibromyxoid Sarcoma

30. Evans HL: Low-grade fibromyxoid sarcoma: A report of 12 cases. Am J Surg Pathol 1993;17:595.
31. Folpe AL, Lane KL, Paull G, et al: Low-grade fibromyxoid sarcoma and hyalinizing spindle cell tumor with giant rosettes: A clinicopathologic study of 73 cases supporting their identity and assessing the impact of high grade areas. Am J Surg Pathol 2000;24:1353.
32. Lane KL, Shannon RJ, Weiss SW: Hyalinizing spindle cell tumor with giant rosettes: A distinctive tumor closely resembling low-grade fibromyxoid sarcoma. Am J Surg Pathol 1997;21:1481.
33. Nielsen GP, Selig MK, O'Connell JX, et al: Hyalinizing spindle cell tumor with giant rosettes: A report of three cases with ultrastructural analysis. Am J Surg Pathol 1999;23:1227.
34. Mezzelani A, Sozzi G, Nessling M, et al: Low grade fibromyxoid sarcoma: A further low-grade soft tissue malignancy characterized by a ring chromosome. Cancer Genet Cytogenet 2000 15;122:144.

Myxofibrosarcoma

35. Mentzel T, Calonje E, Wadden C, et al: Myxofibrosarcoma: Clinicopathologic analysis of 75 cases with emphasis on the low-grade variant. Am J Surg Pathol 1996;20:391.
36. Kilpatrick SE, Ward WG: Myxofibrosarcoma of soft tissues: Cytomorphologic analysis of a series. Diagn Cytopathol 1999;20:6.
37. Clawson K, Donner LR, Dobin SM: Translocation (2;15)(p23;q21.2) and interstitial deletion of 7q in a case of low-grade myxofibrosarcoma. Cancer Genet Cytogenet 2001;127:140.

Myxoid and Round Cell Liposarcoma

38. Kilpatrick SE, Doyon J, Choong PFM, et al: The clinicopathologic spectrum of myxoid and round cell liposarcoma: A study of 95 cases. Cancer 1996;77:1450.
39. Smith TA, Easley KA, Goldblum JR: Myxoid/round cell liposarcoma of the extremities: A clinicopathologic study of 29 cases with particular attention to extent of round cell liposarcoma. Am J Surg Pathol 1996;20:171.
40. Tallini G, Akerman M, Dal Cin P, et al: Combined morphologic and karyotypic study of 28 myxoid liposarcomas: An implication of revised morphologic typing (a report from the CHAMP group). Am J Surg Pathol 1996;20:1047.
41. Kilpatrick SE, Ward WG, Bos GD: The value of fine-needle aspiration biopsy in the differential diagnosis of adult myxoid sarcoma. Cancer 2000;90:167.

Extraskeletal Myxoid Chondrosarcoma

42. Meis-Kindblom JM, Bergh P, Gunterberg B, et al: Extraskeletal myxoid chondrosarcoma: A reappraisal of its morphologic spectrum and prognostic factors based on 117 cases. Am J Surg Pathol 1999;23:636.
43. Kilpatrick SE, Inwards CY, Fletcher CDM, et al: Myxoid chondrosarcoma (chordoid sarcoma) of bone: A report of two cases and review of the literature. Cancer 1997;79:1903.
44. Oliveira AM, Sebo TJ, McGrory JE, et al: Extraskeletal myxoid chondrosarcoma: A clinicopathologic, immunohistochemical, and ploidy analysis of 23 cases. Mod Pathol 2000;13:900.
45. Goh YW, Spagnolo DV, Platten M, et al: Extraskeletal myxoid chondrosarcoma: A light microscopic, immunohistochemical, ultrastructural and immuno-ultrastructural study indicating neuroendocrine differentiation. Histopathology 2001;39:514.
46. Antonescu C, Argani P, Erlandson R, et al: Skeletal and extraskeletal myxoid chondrosarcoma: A comparative clinicopathologic, ultrastructural, and molecular study. Cancer 1998;83:1504.

Myxoinflammatory Fibroblastic Sarcoma

47. Montgomery EA, Devaney KO, Giordano T, et al: Inflammatory myxohyaline tumor of distal extremities with virocyte or Reed-Sternberg-like cells: A distinctive lesion with features simulating inflammatory conditions, Hodgkin's disease, and various sarcomas. Mod Pathol 1998;11:384.
48. Meis-Kindblom JM, Kindblom LG: Acral myxoinflammatory fibroblastic sarcoma: A low-grade tumor of the hands and feet. Am J Surg Pathol 1998;22:911.

Chordoma

49. Dahlin DC, McCarthy C: Chordoma: A study of fifty-nine cases. Cancer 1952;5:1170.
50. Bergh P, Kindblom LG, Gunterberg B, et al: Prognostic factors in chordoma of the sacrum and mobile spine: A study of 39 patients. Cancer 2000;88:2122.
51. Mitchell A, Scheithauer BW, Unni KK, et al: Chordoma and chondroid neoplasms of the spheno-occiput: An immunohistochemical study of 41 cases with prognostic and nosologic implications. Cancer 1993;72:2943.
52. Ronc R, Ramzy I, Duncan D: Anaplastic sacrococcygeal chordoma: Fine needle aspiration cytology findings and embryologic considerations. Acta Cytol 1986;30:183.

CHAPTER 9

Fatty Tumors of Bone and Soft Tissue

Fatty tumors of bone and soft tissue include tumors that, by definition, are at least partially composed of adipose tissue; this encompasses the various forms of lipoma and subtypes of liposarcoma listed in Table 9.1. In most cases, fatty tumors arise solely within extraskeletal soft tissues. Primary osseous conventional lipoma is the most common fatty tumor arising in bone but is extraordinarily rare in biopsy specimens.[1] Only rare case reports exist of skeletal well-differentiated liposarcoma, myxoid liposarcoma, and pleomorphic liposarcoma, primarily arising in the long tubular bones of the extremities.[2,3] For these reasons, we primarily focus on the clinical features of fatty tumors involving extraskeletal soft tissues, briefly discussing primary osseous lipoma when applicable. Myxoid/round cell liposarcoma is considered best in the context of other myxoid tumors and is described in Chapter 8. Pleomorphic liposarcoma and dedifferentiated liposarcoma are part of the differential diagnosis of "pleomorphic sarcomas" and are discussed along with malignant fibrous histiocytoma, pleomorphic rhabdomyosarcoma, and pleomorphic leiomyosarcoma. A variety of chromosomal aberrations have been discovered that seem to be relatively specific for many of these lipomatous tumors. These are summarized in Table 9.2.

Radiographic imaging, especially magnetic resonance imaging, is useful for suggesting that a neoplasm composition is "fatty," but it is not useful for histologic subtyping or for reliably separating lipoma from low-grade liposarcoma. The differential diagnosis of superficial and deep-seated fatty tumors

TABLE 9.1 Fatty Tumors of Soft Tissues

Lipoma
Lipomatosis
Angiolipoma
Chondroid lipoma
Myelolipoma
Spindle cell/pleomorphic lipoma
Myolipoma
Angiomyolipoma
Lipoblastoma/lipoblastomatosis
Lipofibromatosis
Well-differentiated liposarcoma (atypical lipoma)
Myxoid and round cell liposarcoma
Pleomorphic liposarcoma
Dedifferentiated liposarcoma

TABLE 9.2 Chromosomal Abnormalities of Lipomatous Tumors

Tumor	Chromosomal Abnormalities
Conventional and intramuscular lipoma	Aberrations (usually translocations) of 12q13-15 are most common; 6p21-23 translocations and aberrations (usually deletions) of 13q12-14 and 13q22 also frequently are seen
Lipoblastoma	Rearrangements of 8q11-13
Spindle cell/pleomorphic lipoma	Monosomy or partial loss of 13q12, 13q14-22, and/or 16q13
Angiolipoma	None (normal karyotype)
Hibernoma	Rearrangements of 11q13-21
Chondroid lipoma	t(11;16)(q13;p12-13)
Atypical lipoma/well-differentiated liposarcoma	Supernumerary ring and giant marker chromosomes, 12q14-15
Dedifferentiated liposarcoma	Same as atypical lipoma (above)
Myxoid/round cell liposarcoma	t(12;16)(q13;p11)

is one of the greater challenges in cytopathology. It encompasses the diagnoses of well-differentiated liposarcoma, lipoma (and various subtypes), and inadvertently sampled normal subcutaneous adipose tissue. Seemingly unremarkable adipose tissue may be observed in all of these entities. As a result, fine needle aspiration biopsy (FNAB) is adequate for ruling in the diagnosis of well-differentiated liposarcoma but probably inadequate for ruling out the diagnosis. The diagnosis of well-differentiated liposarcoma rests on the cytologic finding of atypical, enlarged hyperchromatic stromal cells or multivacuolated lipoblasts or both. Even in the event of benign cytologic findings, all deep-seated fatty tumors (by imaging studies or biopsy) of the extremities or retroperitoneum should be excised completely and sampled meticulously to exclude fully the possibility of well-differentiated liposarcoma.

Lipoma

Clinical Features

Lipoma is the most common mesenchymal soft tissue tumor of adults. It may occur at any age, but most, regardless of anatomic site, seem to arise in adults older than age 40. Lipomas are seen more commonly in obese patients and are rarely multifocal. Most conventional lipomas arise in subcutaneous fat (superficial), often involving the upper back, shoulders, or neck. The trunk and proximal extremities are affected less commonly. Because they often are detected at a later stage of development, subfascial and intramuscular (deep) lipomas may be quite large. A variety of anatomic locations may be observed, including the trunk and abdominal wall, extremities, and head and neck.[4,5] Most cases present as a painless soft tissue mass. Synovial lipoma (lipoma arborescens) is a rare villous lipomatous process of the synovium characterized by excess subsynovial fat.[6] Adult patients with synovial lipoma often complain of the gradual development of joint swelling. Lipomas arising adjacent to periosteum, usually the diaphysis of an extremity long bone, sometimes are called *parosteal lipomas*.[7] Intraosseous lipomas are extraordinarily rare tumors, usually arising in the metaphyseal regions of the long tubular bones of the lower extremities (e.g., femur, tibia). Intraosseous lipomas are often asymptomatic, incidental findings; some patients may complain of localized pain of the affected bone.[1]

Radiologically, most conventional lipomas appear well circumscribed and homogeneous with similar density to adjacent subcutaneous fat (Fig. 9.1). Variable fibrous strands may course through the tumor but generally are less prominent than that observed with well-differentiated liposarcoma.

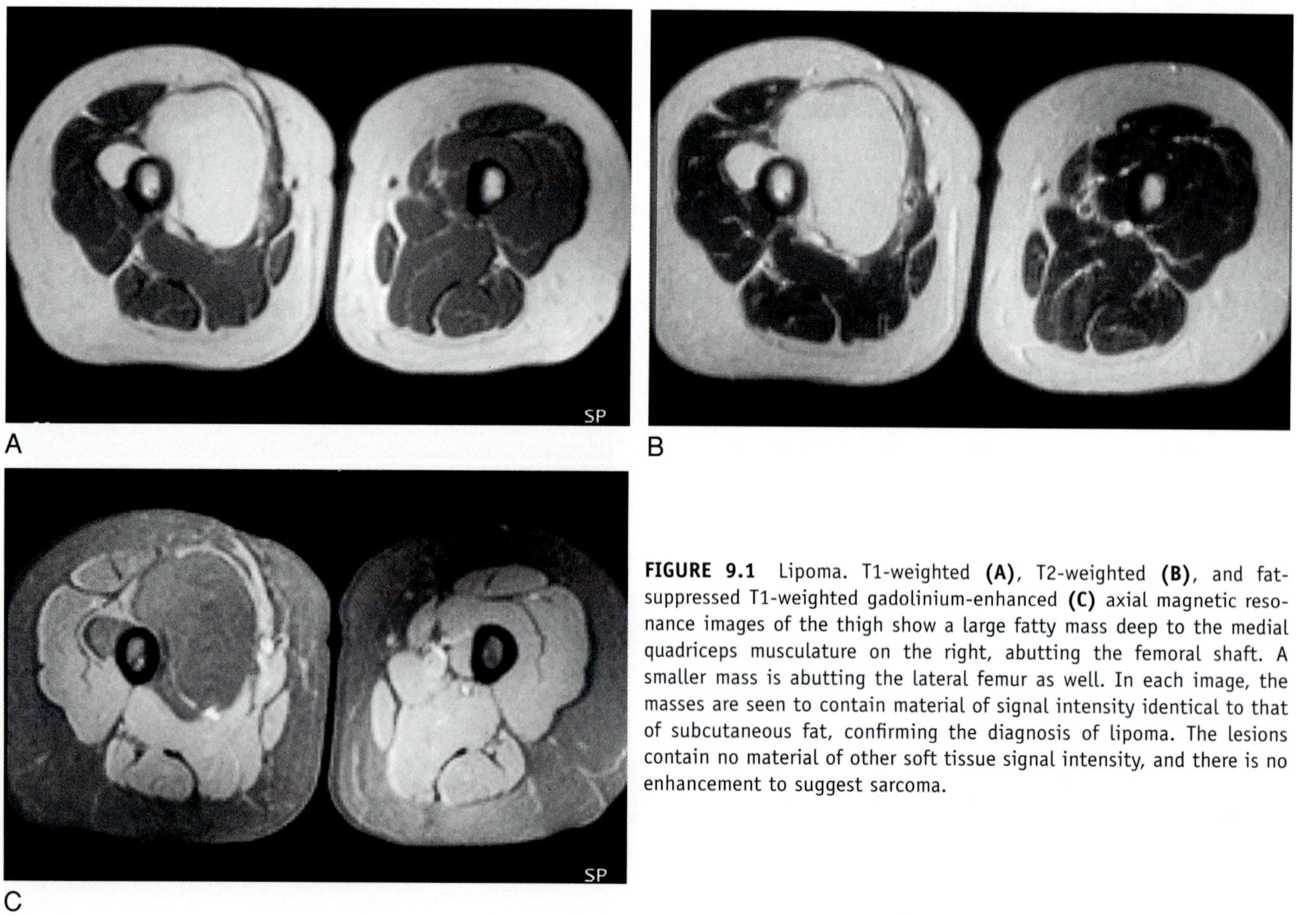

FIGURE 9.1 Lipoma. T1-weighted **(A)**, T2-weighted **(B)**, and fat-suppressed T1-weighted gadolinium-enhanced **(C)** axial magnetic resonance images of the thigh show a large fatty mass deep to the medial quadriceps musculature on the right, abutting the femoral shaft. A smaller mass is abutting the lateral femur as well. In each image, the masses are seen to contain material of signal intensity identical to that of subcutaneous fat, confirming the diagnosis of lipoma. The lesions contain no material of other soft tissue signal intensity, and there is no enhancement to suggest sarcoma.

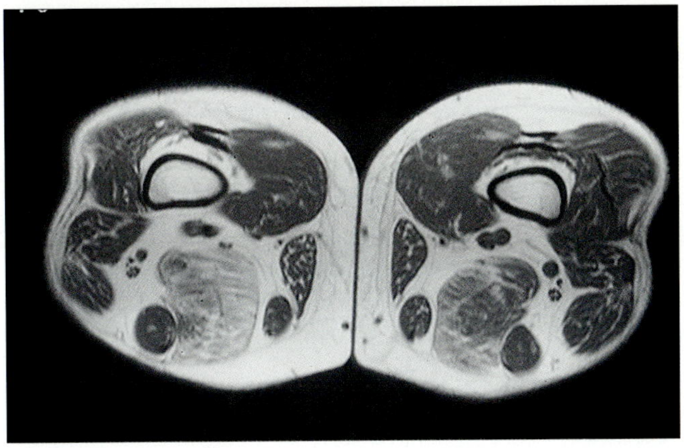

FIGURE 9.2 Intramuscular lipoma. A T1-weighted axial magnetic resonance image of the thighs shows diffuse fatty infiltration of the semimembranosus muscles bilaterally, particularly on the right.

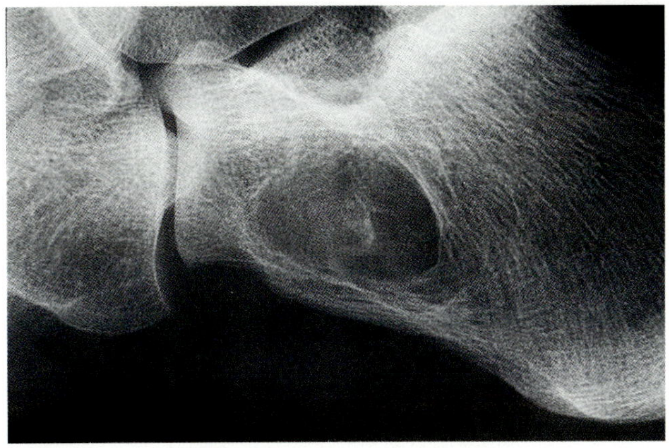

FIGURE 9.3 Intraosseous lipoma. A lateral radiograph of the hindfoot shows a well-defined, lytic lesion in the midcalcaneus containing a small calcification. Although the differential diagnosis of a focal lytic lesion in the calcaneus includes unicameral cyst, chondroblastoma, and intraosseous ganglion, the focal calcification, representing an area of necrosis, establishes the radiographic diagnosis of lipoma.

Intramuscular lipomas often show less circumscription and may be infiltrative (Fig. 9.2). Intraosseous lipomas usually produce well-circumscribed lytic lesions with an associated sclerotic rim (Fig. 9.3).[1]

Pathologic Findings

Histology

Superficial lipoma typically is lobulated with variably sized fibrous bands, thinly encapsulated, well vascularized, and composed of mature-appearing adipocytes mostly indistinguishable from the surrounding adipose tissue. Individual adipocytes show only slight variation in size and shape. Nuclei are peripherally placed, are bland, and may contain vacuoles (Lochkern) (Fig. 9.4). Less commonly, lipomas exhibit mixtures of additional mesenchymal elements, including abundant fibrous tissue (fibrolipoma), mucoid material (myxolipoma), and areas of bone (osteolipoma) and cartilage (chondrolipoma) differentiation. Secondary changes, such as fat necrosis, hemorrhage, and dystrophic calcifications, may be present. Intramuscular (deep) lipoma shows features similar to superficial lipoma but is often infiltrative, entrapping skeletal muscle fibers within the fat (Fig. 9.5).

Fine Needle Aspiration Biopsy

It is difficult to establish with certainty the diagnosis of lipoma by FNAB. Cytologic smears are variably cellular and typically composed of aggregates of adipose tissue indistinguishable from inadvertently sampled subcutaneous fat (Fig. 9.6). For this reason, we rarely render the diagnosis of lipoma by FNAB.

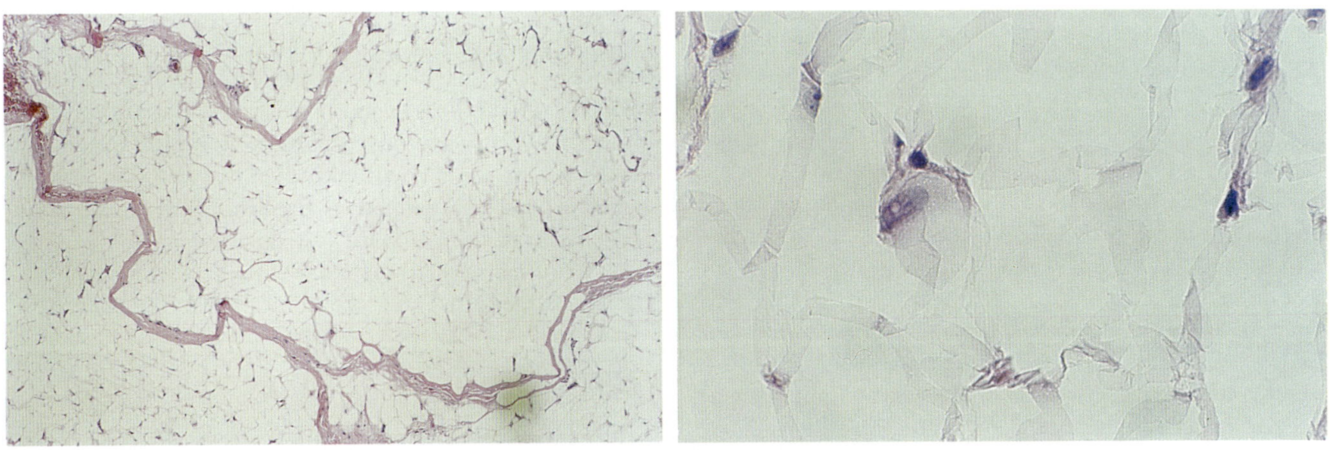

A B

FIGURE 9.4 Conventional lipoma is characterized by sheets of mostly uniform adipocytes separated by bands of fibrous tissue. Note the peripherally placed, bland-appearing nuclei with lacunae (**A** and **B**). (**A,** Low power; **B,** high power, H&E.)

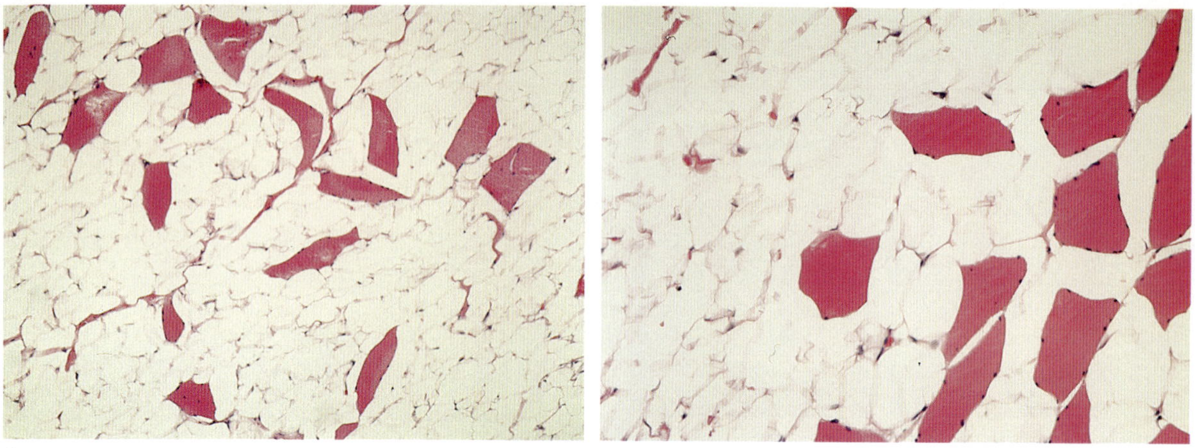

A B

FIGURE 9.5 Intramuscular lipoma with benign-appearing adipose tissue infiltrating skeletal muscle **(A** and **B)**. **(A,** Low power; **B,** high power, H&E.)

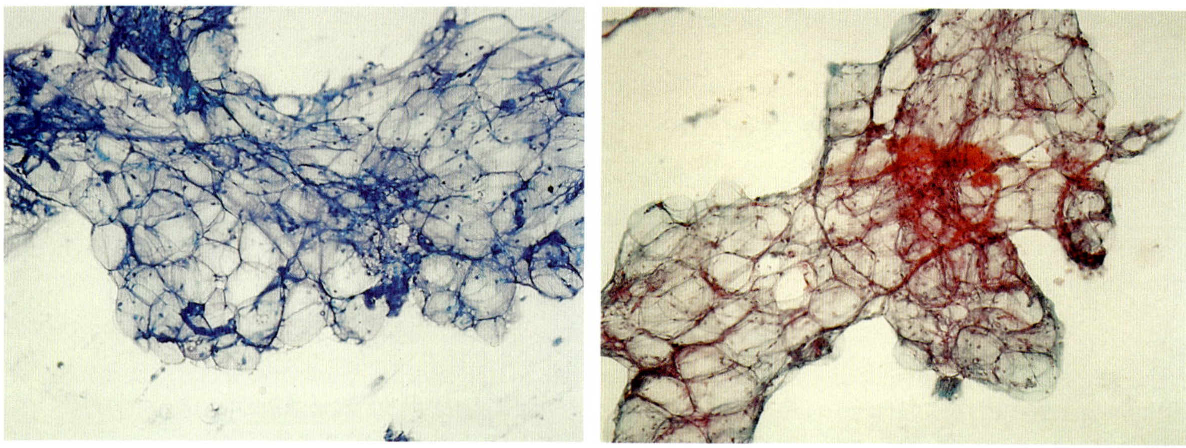

A B

FIGURE 9.6 Fine needle aspiration biopsy of lipoma is generally nondiagnostic, consisting of aggregates of adipose tissue indistinguishable from inadvertently sampled subcutaneous fat **(A** and **B)**. **(A,** Diff-Quik; **B,** Papanicolaou.)

The diagnosis of lipoma in a superficial, well-circumscribed, and mobile lesion with the gross consistency of adipose tissue may be rendered if the cytologic features are consistent. We believe, however, that deep-seated lipomatous tumors require excision and thorough sampling to exclude fully the diagnosis of well-differentiated liposarcoma.[8]

Ancillary Studies

The ultrastructural features of lipoma are essentially those of mature, normal white fat. The cytoplasm is occupied by a single large lipid vacuole compressing the nucleus to the periphery of the cell.[9]

Immunohistochemically, the mature adipocytes in lipoma show positivity for vimentin, S-100 protein, and leptin.[10] In general, immunohistochemical stains are of limited value, however, in the differential diagnosis of lipomatous tumors.

Cytogenetic analysis reveals clonal abnormalities in 75% of lipomas. The most common aberrations involve rearrangements of 12q13-15.[11] Less common abnormalities include translocations of 6p21-23 and interstitial deletions of 13q12-14 and 13q22.

Prognosis and Therapy

Superficial and deep lipomas are benign lesions. Local recurrence may occur and often is observed in deep intramuscular lipomas that are excised incompletely. For this reason, some authors have advocated total removal of the involved skeletal muscle or compartment to reduce the risk of local recurrence.[12] This radical approach should be tempered by the potential morbidity and loss of function to the patient.

Lipomatosis

Lipomatosis is a diffuse overgrowth of mature adipose tissue that may arise in a variety of different clinical settings. The process may be primary (arising in the absence of a pre-existing condition) or secondary to an underlying disease process or drug therapy. Additionally, lipomatosis may be a localized, diffuse process or may involve the entire body symmetrically. Most examples of diffuse lipomatosis occur in infants and children younger than age 2 years, affecting a significant portion of an extremity, head and neck region, trunk, pelvis, or intra-abdominal cavity.[13] Grossly enlarged digits also may occur. Symmetric lipomatosis has a predilection for Mediterranean middle-aged men often with a clinical history of liver disease or alcohol abuse or both, presenting as symmetric deposition of excess adipose tissue most notable on the upper back, shoulders, and neck. Localized pelvic lipomatosis is seen most frequently in African males. Involvement of the genitourinary region and gastrointestinal tract may lead to complaints of urinary frequency, perineal pain, hydronephrosis, or bowel obstruction.[14,15] Causes of secondary lipomatosis include steroid therapy (accumulation of excess adipose tissue in the face and upper back) and human immunodeficiency virus (HIV) lipodystrophy in acquired immunodeficiency syndrome patients (accumulation of excess fat around visceral organs, cervical fat pads, and excess breast tissue).[16]

Despite these different clinical settings, most patients with lipomatosis present with excess accumulation of adipose tissue in the affected areas, frequently resembling a lipomatous neoplasm. Regardless of cause, the morphologic features of lipomatosis include mature-appearing adipose tissue infiltrating various organ systems, especially skeletal muscle. Therapy is largely palliative with removal of excess fat. As expected, all primary forms of lipomatosis have a tendency to recur after resection. Lipomatosis secondary to steroid therapy usually regresses after reduction of drug levels. Recombinant growth hormone therapy has been used to treat HIV lipodystrophy.

Lipoblastoma/Lipoblastomatosis

Lipoblastoma/lipoblastomatosis may present as a lobulated, localized but well-circumscribed mass (lipoblastoma) or, alternatively, may be diffuse and infiltrative (lipoblastomatosis). The clinical and morphologic features within this spectrum are largely similar, however. Synonyms include *fetal lipoma* and *infantile lipoma*.

Clinical Features

Most cases present in infancy and early childhood, before age 5 years.[17,18] Rare congenital examples have been reported.[17,19] There seems to be a slightly male predilection. Lipoblastoma/lipoblastomatosis most commonly arises within the extremities but may be observed in the trunk and head and neck regions (Fig. 9.7). A few examples have been described involving visceral organs.[20,21] Most patients present with painless soft tissue swelling.

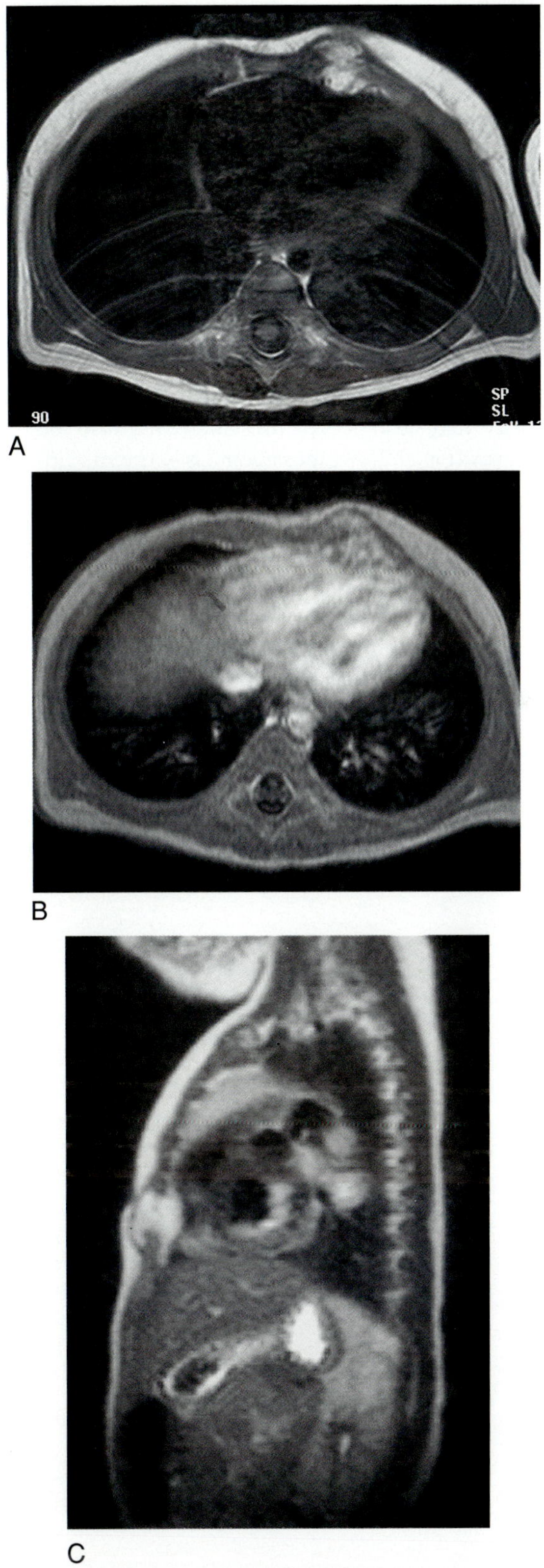

FIGURE 9.7 Lipoblastoma. T1-weighted axial **(A)**, T1-weighted gadolinium-enhanced axial **(B)**, and T1-weighted sagittal **(C)** magnetic resonance images show a chest wall lesion on the left, lying anterior to the heart. The mass is heterogeneous but composed largely of fat and enhances after administration of gadolinium. The adjacent ribs are displaced by the mass but not destroyed.

Pathologic Findings

Histology

A characteristic feature of lipoblastoma/lipoblastomatosis is the distinct lobulated appearance. Prominent bands of fibrous tissue, enclosing an admixture of mature and immature adipocytes, separate variably sized lobules.[17,18] Occasional lipoblasts may be observed. In general, the lobulation appears less prominent in the diffuse form (lipoblastomatosis). Myxoid degeneration is often at least focally present and rarely may be extensive. In these cases, the combination of myxoid stroma and prominent vascularity may lead to the mistaken diagnosis of myxoid liposarcoma (Fig. 9.8).[22] Liposarcoma is extraordinarily rare in children. As previously mentioned, lipoblastomatosis is associated with infiltration of adjacent structures, most notably skeletal muscle. Over time, lipoblastoma/lipoblastomatosis may undergo maturation, ultimately including mature, adult-appearing adipose tissue. Cellular atypia is not observed.[17]

Ancillary Studies

Ultrastructurally, lipoblastoma/lipoblastomatosis shows features of normal-developing "white" adipose tissue, ranging from more primitive lipoblasts to mature adipocytes. Immunohistochemistry is generally not useful for establishing the diagnosis of lipoblastoma/lipoblastomatosis. As in lipomas, individual fat cells appear positive for S-100 protein and vimentin. The most common cytogenetic abnormality observed in lipoblastoma/lipoblastomatosis is rearrangements of 8q11-13.[11]

Prognosis and Therapy

Surgical resection of the localized form (lipoblastoma) generally results in complete cure. Reported rates for local recurrence range from 9% to 22%.[17,18,23] Local recurrences are more likely to occur in the diffuse form (lipoblastomatosis) after incomplete excision. Diffuse lesions probably should be widely excised. Metastasis does not occur in either form of the disease.

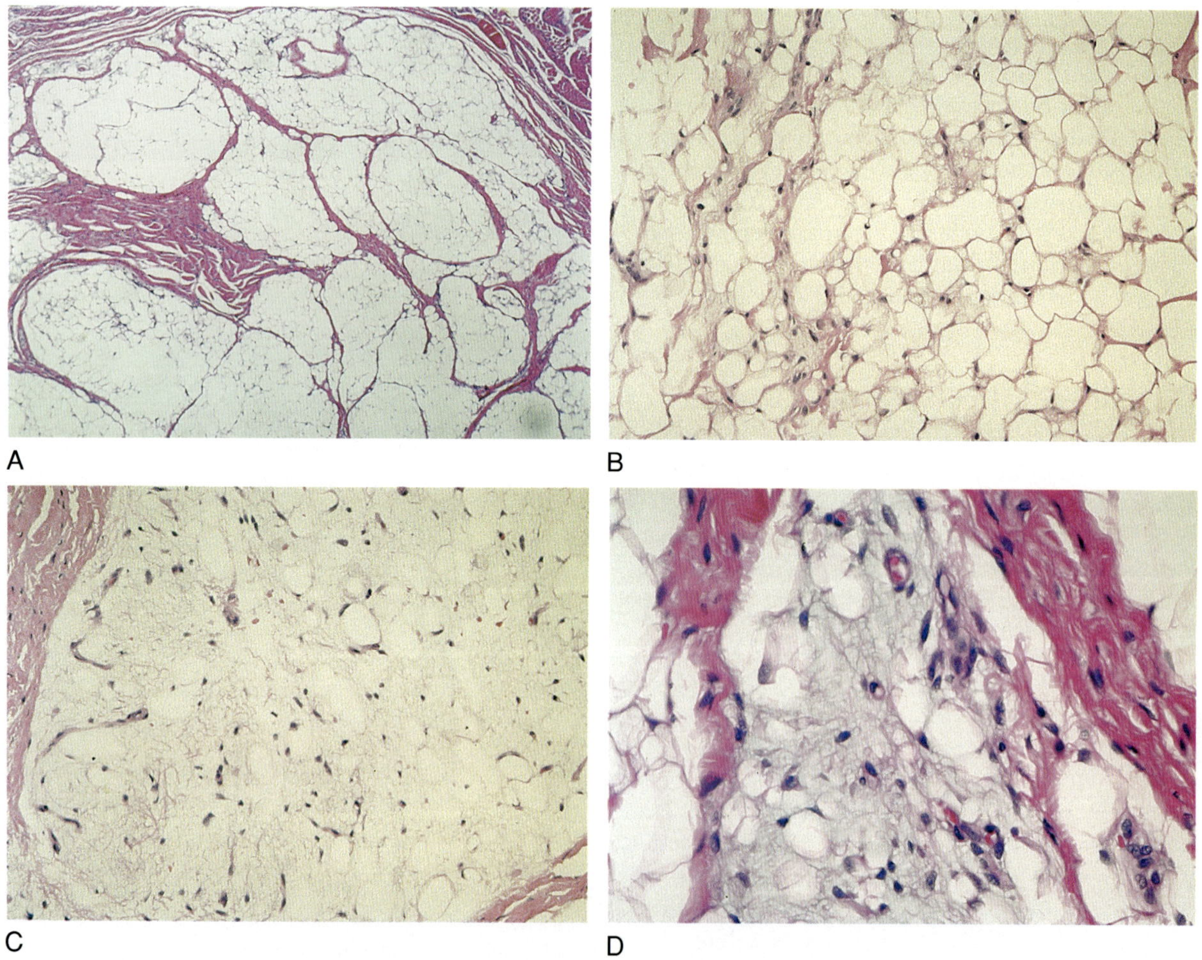

FIGURE 9.8 Lipoblastoma/lipoblastomatosis typically exhibits a lobulated pattern with fibrous bands separating nodules of mature and immature adipose tissue with lipoblasts **(A** and **B)**. Myxoid changes may result in confusion with myxoid liposarcoma **(C** and **D)**. **(A,** Low power; **B,** intermediate power; **C,** intermediate power; **D,** high power, H&E.)

Lipofibromatosis

Lipofibromatosis is a rare, recently described pediatric tumor usually seen in infants and young children. It may be present at birth.[24] Males are affected more commonly than females. The most common anatomic sites are the extremities, especially the hand, followed by the trunk and head. Morphologically, the infiltrative lesions consist of mature adipose tissue with markedly expanded and cellular fibrous tissue septa.[24] Lipofibromatosis resembles fibrous hamartoma of infancy, but the primitive myxoid component of the latter is not observed. The spindle cell fibroblastic component consists of fascicles of mostly uniform, bland spindle cells resembling infantile fibromatosis. The absence of tissue destruction and the preservation of the adipose tissue are not features of infantile fibromatosis, however. Significant nuclear atypia is absent, and mitotic activity is almost always less than 1 mitotic figure per 10 high-power fields.[24] Immunohistochemically the neoplastic cells may show focal positivity for CD99, CD34, smooth muscle actin, S-100 protein, and, infrequently, epithelial membrane antigen.[24] Local recurrence occurs in 72% of cases and is more likely to occur in males and after incomplete excision.

Angiolipoma

Clinical Features

In contrast to most adipose tissue tumors, angiolipomas are seen more frequently in adolescents and young adults. There seems to be a slight male predilection. The most common anatomic site is the forearm, followed by the trunk and upper arm.[25] Most patients present with one to multiple, small subcutaneous masses that often are described as painful. Familial forms, representing 5% of cases, have been reported.[26]

Pathologic Findings

Histology

Angiolipomas are well-circumscribed, encapsulated tumors, generally showing an admixture of mature adipocytes and aggregates of small, capillary-sized blood vessels.[25] The proportions of adipose tissue and blood vessels vary considerably from one tumor to the next, but the vascular component is usually most obvious at the periphery (subcapsular area) of the lesion. The stroma between the capillaries and blood vessels is generally hypocellular and may be focally myxoid. This lack of stromal cellularity helps distinguish angiolipomas from rare hypervascular forms of spindle cell lipoma, which have a hypercellular spindle cell stroma. The endothelial cells lining the small blood vessels reveal no significant atypia. Fibrin thrombi often are observed within these blood vessels and are a helpful diagnostic finding (Fig. 9.9).

Ancillary Studies

To date, cytogenetic analysis of angiolipomas has revealed a normal diploid karyotype in virtually all cases.[27]

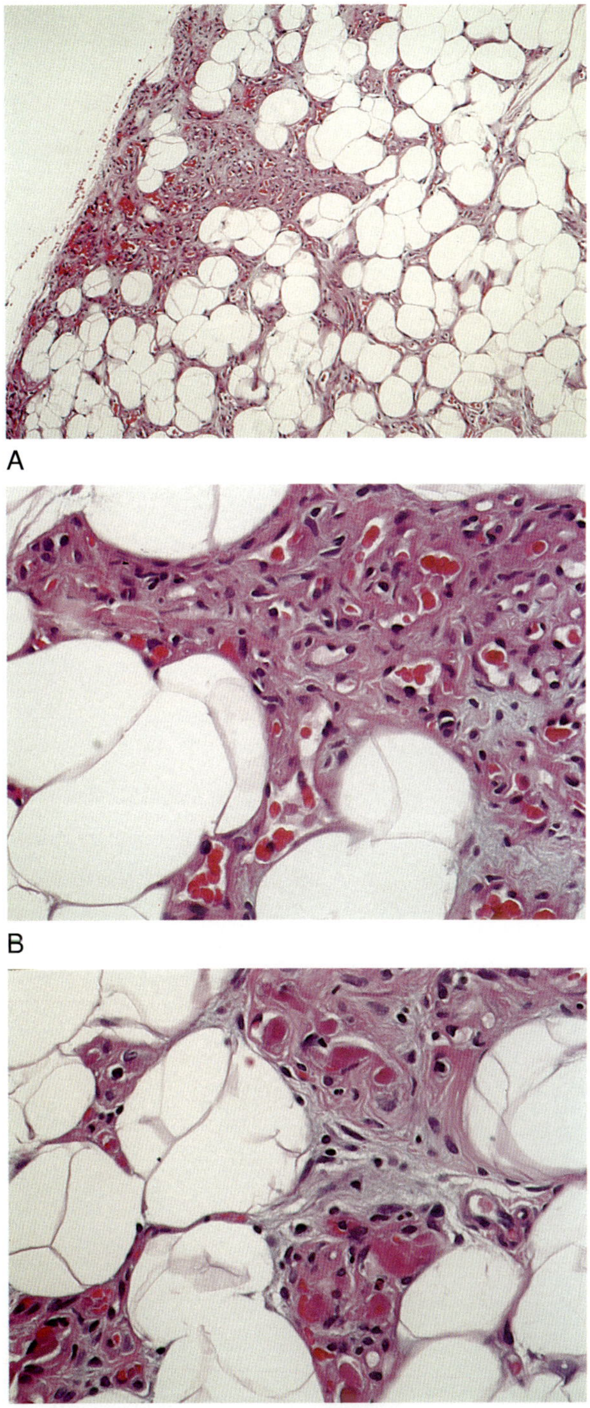

A

B

C

FIGURE 9.9 Angiolipoma is well circumscribed and consists of a mixture of mature adipose tissue and aggregates of small-caliber, benign-appearing, capillary blood vessels, often located at the periphery of the lesion **(A** and **B)**. A characteristic finding in angiolipoma is fibrin thrombi within the capillary blood vessels **(C)**. **(A,** Low power; **B,** high power; **C,** high power, H&E.)

Prognosis and Therapy

Angiolipomas are benign lesions. Local recurrence does not occur after resection.

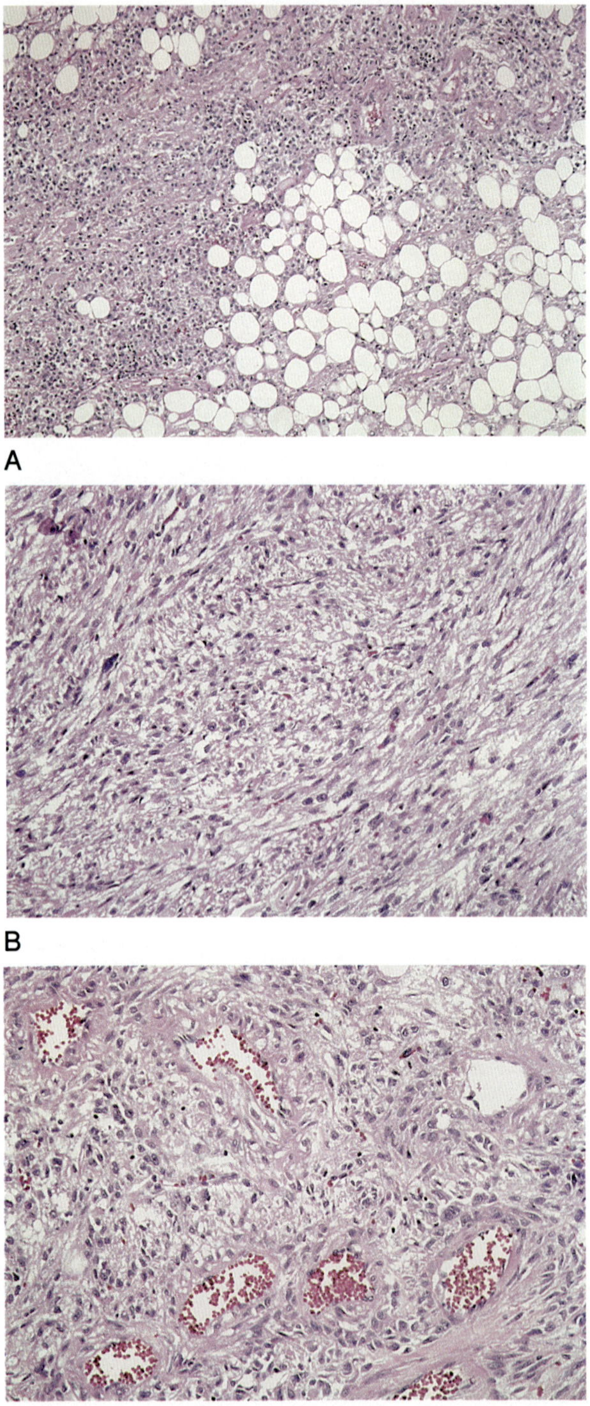

FIGURE 9.10 Angiomyolipoma, a lesion virtually exclusively seen in the kidneys, is characterized by variable mixtures of smooth muscle, fat, and thick-walled blood vessels **(A** and **B)**. In some cases, the smooth muscle component may appear more epithelioid **(C)**. **(A,** Low power; **B** and **C,** intermediate power, H&E.)

Myolipoma

Myolipoma is an extraordinarily rare, benign tumor displaying an admixture of mature adipose tissue and smooth muscle elements.[28] These tumors sometimes have been referred to as extrauterine lipoleiomyomas. Most myolipomas occur in adults and seem to be slightly more common in females. Common anatomic locations include the abdominal cavity and retroperitoneal/pelvic regions. In many cases, myolipoma is an incidental, asymptomatic finding. Occasional patients complain of localized soft tissue swelling. Morphologically, myolipomas tend to be well circumscribed and at least partially encapsulated. Although individual cases may show variable amounts of adipose tissue and smooth muscle elements, the smooth muscle component predominates in most examples.[28] Individual smooth muscle cells are arranged in short, sweeping fascicles and lack nuclear atypia. Likewise, aggregates of adipose tissue appear mature, also lacking significant atypia. Lipoblasts are never observed. As expected, the smooth muscle component shows positive immunoreactivity for smooth muscle actin and desmin. Complete surgical resection is generally curative, and local recurrence does not occur.[28]

Angiomyolipoma

Clinical Features

The diagnosis of angiomyolipoma generally refers to a specific lesion almost always arising within the parenchyma of one or both kidneys. Most patients are adults, and there is a predilection for females. Although angiomyolipoma may be an incidental, asymptomatic finding, most patients complain of abdominal pain, mass, hematuria, or fever.[29] Rare extrarenal sites of angiomyolipoma include the liver, lung, colon, heart, and mucosal surfaces of the head and neck. Most cases present as solitary, well-circumscribed masses; however, angiomyolipoma may exhibit bilateral and multiple renal masses, especially in patients with tuberous sclerosis. Radiographic imaging usually reveals a lipomatous mass admixed with variable amounts of nonlipomatous soft tissue.

Pathologic Findings

Histology

Angiomyolipoma is composed of varying amounts of three distinct soft tissue components—mature adipose tissue, thick-walled blood vessels, and fascicles or sheets of smooth muscle cells (Fig. 9.10). Rarely the last-mentioned elements may display marked nuclear pleomorphism with occasional multinucleated giant cells. Individual smooth muscle cells are usually spindle-shaped, resembling typical smooth muscle; however, more epithelioid-appearing smooth muscle cells rarely predominate, potentially confounding the diagnosis.[30]

Ancillary Studies

Ultrastructurally the smooth muscle cells show the typical features of myodifferentiation, including intermediate myofilaments, glycogen, and electron-dense, membrane-bound granules; structures resembling melanosomes or premelanosomes are observed less frequently.[31] Arguably the most distinctive features of angiomyolipoma are the immunohistochemical properties of the smooth muscle cells. In addition to smooth muscle actin and desmin, melanocytic markers, including HMB 45 and MART-1, often are expressed by the smooth muscle component (spindled and epithelioid cells) but may be focal.[29] Reported cytogenetic abnormalities in angiomyolipoma include trisomy 7; loss of heterozygosity of 3p; and, especially among cases occurring in the setting of tuberous sclerosis, loss of heterozygosity of the tuberous sclerosis complex genes, 9q34 (*TSC1*) and 16p13 (*TSC2*).[32,33]

Prognosis and Therapy

A partial nephrectomy with excision of the lesion is generally curative; complete nephrectomy may be required for larger lesions. Malignant transformation has been reported but is considered extraordinarily rare.[29] Significant nuclear pleomorphism and intravascular extension may be observed in benign forms of the disease and are not, by themselves, markers of malignancy. At present, malignancy is defined reliably only by the presence of distant metastases.

Hibernoma

Clinical Features

Despite its distinct composition of mostly brown fat, hibernomas most commonly occur in young to middle-aged adults with a slight male predominance.[34] The most common anatomic location is the thigh, followed by the trunk and upper extremity. Most tumors appear as slow-growing, painless soft tissue masses. Radiographic imaging may reveal distinct nonlipomatous septations and a signal intensity within the tumor proper intermediate between mature adipose tissue and skeletal muscle (Fig. 9.11).[35,36]

Pathologic Findings

Histology

Hibernomas show varying proportions of brown fat admixed with mature, white adipose tissue.[34,37] At low power, the lesion appears distinctly lobulated, similar to the appearance of lipoblastoma. Individual brown fat cells generally exhibit a centrally placed nucleus and a prominent nucleolus. The cytoplasm ranges from granular and eosinophilic to uniformly multivacuolated (Fig. 9.12). Nevertheless, virtually all cases of hibernoma have at least focal accumulations of mature white adipose tissue. Rare myxoid variants and spindle cell forms resembling spindle cell lipoma have been described.[34] Mitotic figures are virtually never seen; significant nuclear atypia is not a feature of hibernoma.

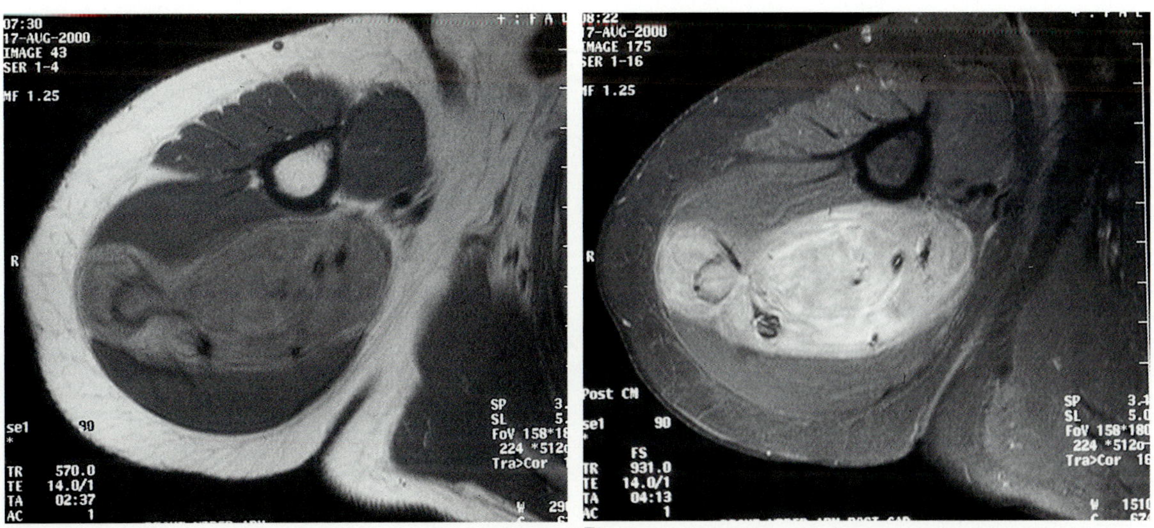

A B

FIGURE 9.11 Hibernoma. T1-weighted **(A)** and fat-suppressed T1-weighted gadolinium-enhanced **(B)** axial magnetic resonance images of the upper arm reveal a heterogeneous, enhancing mass in the triceps muscle. On the unenhanced image, the mass is of lesser signal intensity than subcutaneous fat but more intense than surrounding skeletal muscle.

Fine Needle Aspiration Biopsy

In contrast to most lipomatous lesions, the FNAB findings in hibernoma are fairly distinctive and permit an accurate diagnosis in the appropriate clinicopathologic setting. As expected, cytologic smears show aggregates of mostly brown fat with the characteristic, uniform, centrally placed nuclei and abundant granular-to-multivacuolated cytoplasm. The cytoplasmic vacuoles are generally small and uniform within an individual cell (Fig. 9.13). Significant nuclear atypia is not observed.

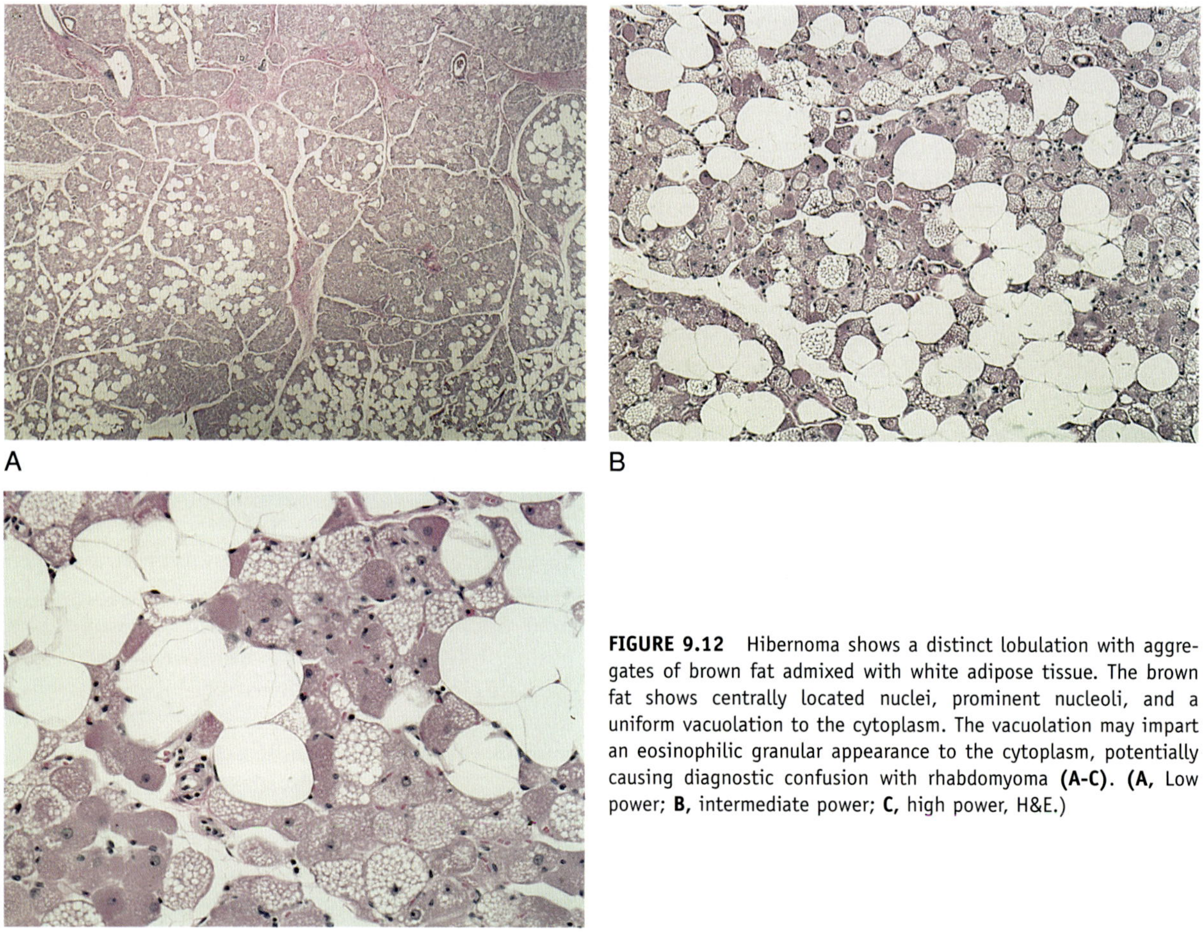

A B C

FIGURE 9.12 Hibernoma shows a distinct lobulation with aggregates of brown fat admixed with white adipose tissue. The brown fat shows centrally located nuclei, prominent nucleoli, and a uniform vacuolation to the cytoplasm. The vacuolation may impart an eosinophilic granular appearance to the cytoplasm, potentially causing diagnostic confusion with rhabdomyoma **(A-C)**. **(A,** Low power; **B,** intermediate power; **C,** high power, H&E.)

Ancillary Studies

Ultrastructural features of hibernoma include focal complex undulating plasmalemmal invaginations, multiple lipid vacuoles, and pleomorphic mitochondria.[37] Immunohistochemically, hibernomas are generally positive for S-100 protein. CD34 positivity has been observed in the spindle cell variant.[34] In most cases, cytogenetic analysis reveals structural rearrangements involving 11q13-21.[9,38]

Prognosis and Therapy

Hibernomas are benign tumors. They generally are cured completely with local but complete resection.[34]

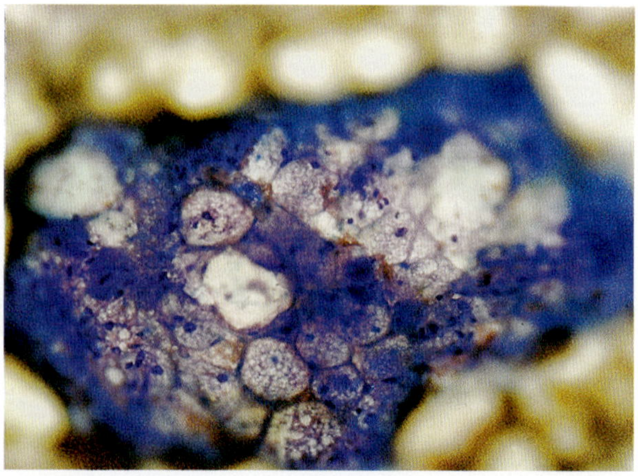

FIGURE 9.13 In contrast to most fatty tumors, fine needle aspiration biopsy of hibernoma may be diagnostic, consisting of aggregates of brown fat admixed with white adipose tissue. The brown fat consists of adipocytes with abundant multivacuolated-to-granular cytoplasm and a centrally located nucleus. (Diff-Quik.)

Chondroid Lipoma

Chondroid lipoma is a recently described but extraordinarily rare, benign lipomatous tumor.[39] Most tumors arise in adults, with a predilection for females. Common anatomic sites include the deep soft tissues of the proximal extremities and limb girdles. Most patients present with a painless soft tissue mass. Chondroid lipomas are well circumscribed and encapsulated, often exhibiting multiple lobulations. Characteristic morphologic features include the presence of univacuolated and multivacuolated lipoblasts arranged in small nests, sheets, and cords within a myxohyalinized-to-chondroid stroma.[39] Variable amounts of mature adipose tissue are admixed with lipoblasts. Individual lipoblasts appear variably vacuolated with small but uniform nuclei, ranging from round to ovoid to kidney bean–shaped (Fig. 9.14). Ultrastructurally the lipoblasts show abundant intracytoplasmic lipid, glycogen, and pinocytotic vesicles, supportive of white fat differentiation.[40] In contrast to most lipomatous tumors, chondroid lipoma typically shows weak S-100 protein positivity. Vimentin is virtually always positive. Focal cytokeratin positivity also has been reported.[39] Cytogenetic analysis has been performed on two cases, both revealing a balanced translocation, t(11;16) (q13;p12-13).[41] Chondroid lipoma is a benign lesion that, with local resection, does not recur. Metastasis has not been reported.

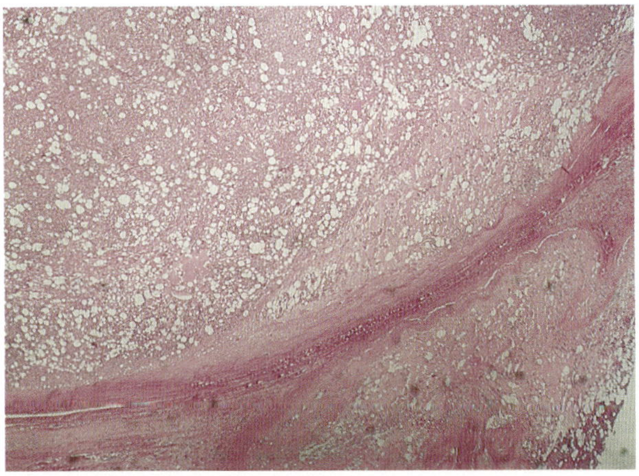

A

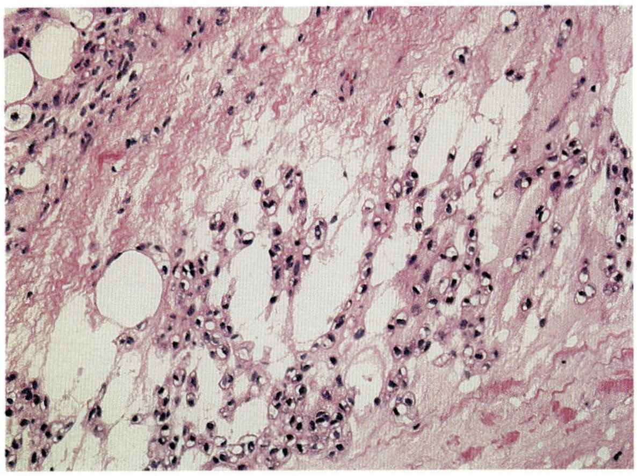

B

FIGURE 9.14 Chondroid lipoma is well circumscribed and shows mixtures of stromal cells and lipoblasts embedded within a myxohyalinized-to-chondroid stroma **(A** and **B)**. **(A,** Low power; **B,** high power, H&E.)

Spindle Cell Lipoma/Pleomorphic Lipoma

Clinical Features

Spindle cell lipoma and pleomorphic lipoma are considered to represent the end points of a spectrum of a similar entity. Spindle cell/pleomorphic lipomas typically occur in older men (>50 years old) and almost exclusively involve the shoulder, posterior neck, face, and head.[42,43] Patients typically present with complaints of a painless, mobile, superficial soft tissue mass, often of several years' duration. A familial association with multiple lesions has been reported, mostly involving men, in similar anatomic locations as the sporadic form.[44] We consider the clinical setting of spindle cell/pleomorphic lipomas to be relatively specific for this entity. Fatty tumors with similar morphology but occurring in younger age groups or different anatomic locations (e.g., lower extremities) are best considered atypical lipomas/well-differentiated liposarcomas because their biologic behavior and karyotypic abnormalities tend to support this conclusion.[45]

Pathologic Findings

Histology

Spindle cell/pleomorphic lipomas show an admixture of mature-appearing adipose tissue and a distinctive, nonlipogenic component (Fig. 9.15). The latter usually comprises

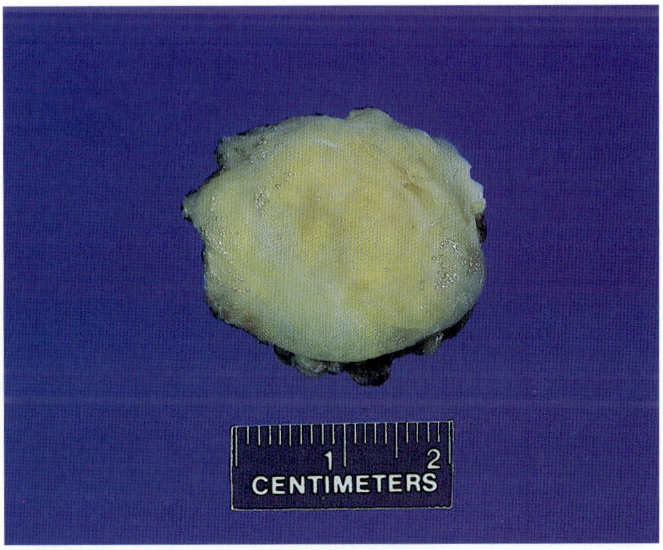

FIGURE 9.15 Spindle cell/pleomorphic lipoma with mixtures of yellow adipose tissue and white-tan fibromyxoid tissue.

bundles of collagen fibers within a variably myxoid stroma. The cells in the lipogenic areas may consist entirely of a bland, uniform-appearing spindle cell population (spindle cell lipoma) evenly distributed among the collagen bundles (Fig. 9.16).[42] At the opposite end of the spectrum, a population of atypical, multilobated-to-multinucleated giant cells with hyperchromatic nuclei (pleomorphic lipoma) may predominate (Fig. 9.17).[43] Scattered giant cells exhibit peripherally located nuclei arranged radially around the more central cytoplasm, so-called floret cells. As expected, some tumors show mixtures of spindle cell and pleomorphic lipoma. Inflammatory cells, including lymphocytes, plasma cells, and mast cells, often are seen scattered throughout the tumor. Rarely, spindle cell lipoma contains abundant vascularity and slit-like cleaves, suggesting angiosarcoma or angiolipoma (pseudoangiomatous variant) (see Fig. 9.16).

Ancillary Studies

Immunohistochemically the neoplastic cells appear diffusely and strongly positive for CD34; S-100 protein positivity is rarely seen.[46] In most cases, cytogenetic analysis reveals monosomy or partial loss of segments in chromosome 13 or 16 or both. Losses of 16q13 and 13q12 seem to be the most frequent events.[11]

Prognosis and Therapy

Spindle cell/pleomorphic lipomas are benign lesions. Surgical resection is generally curative, and local recurrence is rare.

Myelolipoma

Myelolipoma is a rare tumor, usually seen in patients older than age 40. It most commonly arises in the adrenal glands but may occur as an isolated soft tissue mass within the retroperitoneum and pelvis. Almost all extra-adrenal forms occur in females.[47,48] In contrast to extramedullary hematopoietic tumors, myelolipomas are solitary and not associated with hepatospleno-

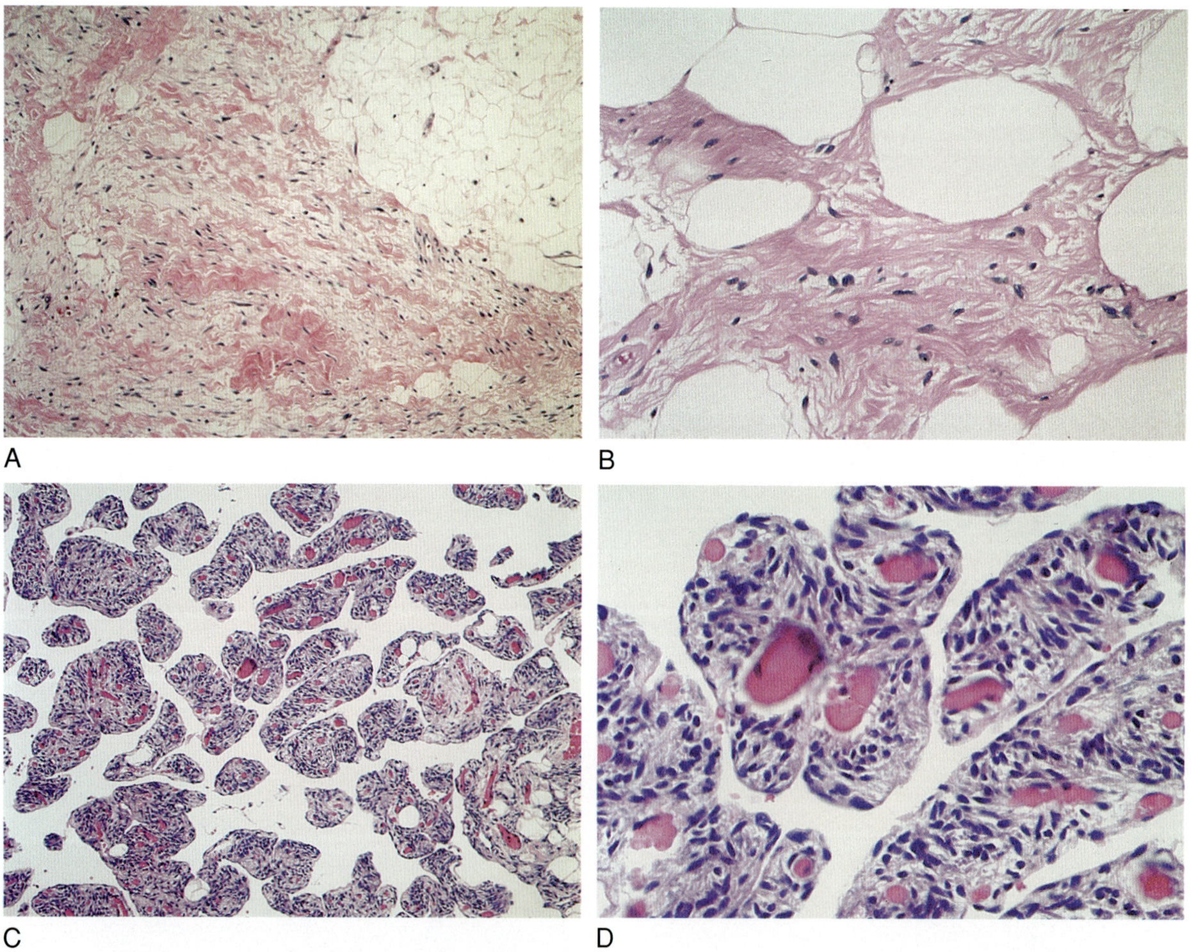

FIGURE 9.16 Spindle cell lipoma typically shows an evenly distributed, spindle cell population within a slightly fibromyxoid stroma with scattered collagen bundles. The spindle cells show uniform, ovoid, hyperchromatic nuclei **(A** and **B)**. Occasional examples may be quite vascular, exhibiting a pseudoangiomatous appearance, mimicking angiosarcoma **(C** and **D)**. **(A,** Low power; **B,** high power; **C,** low power; **D,** high power, H&E.)

megaly or an underlying hematopoietic disorder. Most patients are asymptomatic, and myelolipomas are often incidental surgical or autopsy findings. Spontaneous rupture with hemorrhage is a rare complication. Myelolipoma is typically well circumscribed and comprises varying proportions of mature adipose tissue and benign hematopoietic bone marrow elements (Fig. 9.18). It does not recur after surgical resection.

Atypical Lipoma/ Well-Differentiated Liposarcoma

The designation *atypical lipoma* is synonymous with *well-differentiated liposarcoma*, both referring to a tumor that may recur locally, but in the absence of dedifferentiation, does not metastasize. In the past, the term *atypical lipoma* has been used to delineate the superficial forms of these tumors that were believed not to dedifferentiate and only rarely locally recurred after excision. The use of this terminology has led to considerable diagnostic confusion, however. Examples of dedifferentiated liposarcoma arising from superficially located well-differentiated liposarcoma have been reported.[49,50] For these reasons, the term *atypical lipoma* should be used only if it is understood fully by the treating physician that this designation is synonymous with and may have the implications of a well-differentiated liposarcoma.

Clinical Features

Well-differentiated liposarcoma usually arises in adults older than age 40. It is virtually never seen in childhood. There is no gender predilection. Anatomic sites in decreasing order of frequency include the deep soft tissues of the extremities, especially the thigh, retroperitoneum, and paratesticular area.[51,52] Less commonly, well-differentiated liposarcoma arises within subcutaneous adipose tissue. Most patients initially present with a painless, deep-seated soft tissue mass (Fig. 9.19). Retroperitoneal lesions often are discovered incidentally.

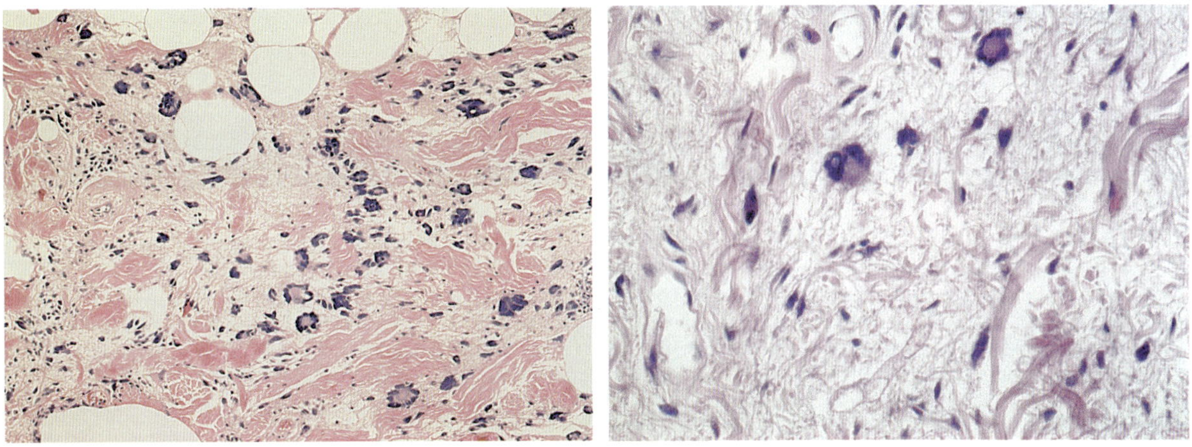

A B

FIGURE 9.17 Pleomorphic lipoma has a stromal background virtually identical to that observed with spindle cell lipoma. In pleomorphic lipoma, however, atypical, multilobated-to-multinucleated cells, often with floret-like features, predominate **(A** and **B)**. **(A,** Low power; **B,** high power, H&E.)

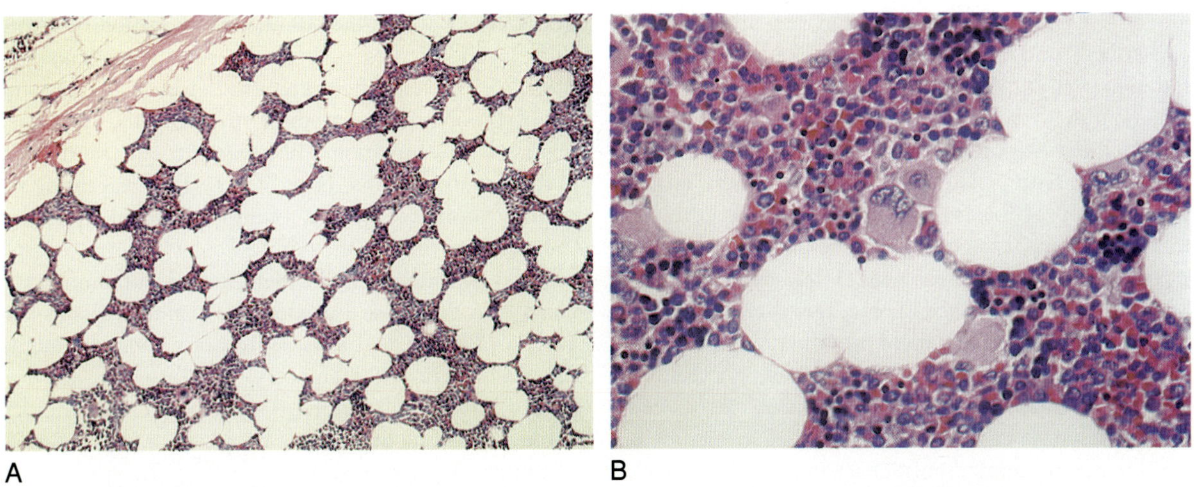

A B

FIGURE 9.18 Myelolipoma is a well-circumscribed, lipomatous lesion, consisting of hematopoietic elements indistinguishable from normal bone marrow admixed with mature adipose tissue **(A** and **B)**. **(A,** Low power; **B,** high power, H&E.)

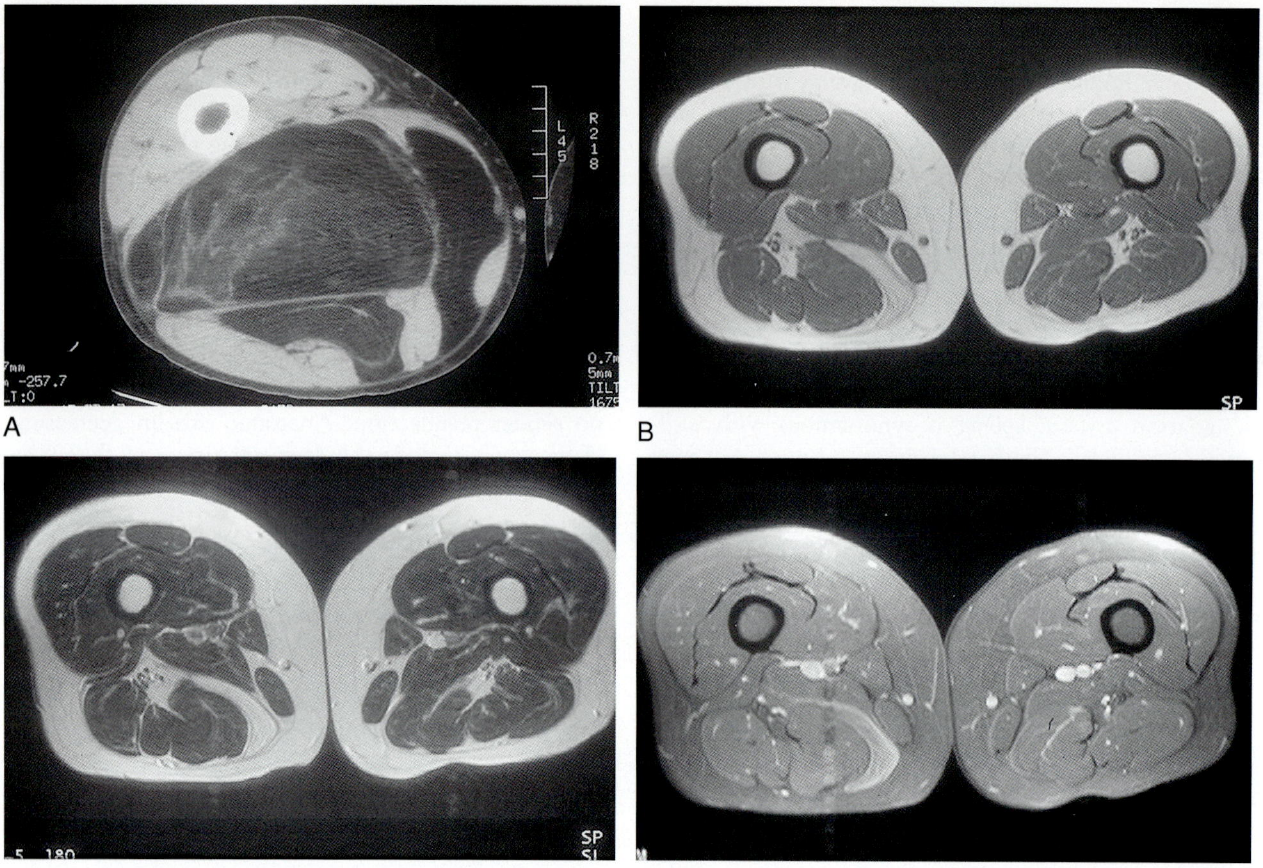

FIGURE 9.19 Atypical lipoma/well-differentiated liposarcoma. An axial computed tomographic scan of the thigh shows a large, lobulated mass in the posterior compartment of the thigh. Although most of the mass is of comparable density to nearby subcutaneous fat, the lateral aspect of the mass contains strands of soft tissue densities in excess of what would be expected for a conventional lipoma **(A)**. In another patient, T1- weighted **(B)**, T2-weighted **(C)**, and fat-suppressed T1-weighted gadolinium-enhanced **(D)** axial magnetic resonance images of the thighs show a fatty mass in the posterior compartment of the right thigh. Although most of the mass appears fatty in nature, the degree of enhancement after administration of gadolinium is more than would be expected for a simple lipoma.

Pathologic Findings

Histology

Most examples of well-differentiated liposarcoma appear large, well circumscribed, and at least partially lobulated. In the retroperitoneum, well-differentiated liposarcoma may appear multicentric. Four major subtypes of well-differentiated liposarcoma are recognized—lipoma-like, sclerosing, inflammatory, and spindle cell variants. The most common form is the lipoma-like subtype. Morphologically, well-differentiated lipoma-like liposarcoma is composed of a mature-appearing adipocyte population that in areas may closely resemble conventional lipoma. Compared with lipoma, however, the nonlipogenic fibrous tissue tends to be more prominent, and there is greater variability in size and shape of individual adipocytes. At high power, well-differentiated liposarcomas are recognized most easily by the presence of scattered atypical stromal cells with enlarged hyperchromatic, multilobated nuclei (Fig. 9.20). Multivacuolated, classic-appearing lipoblasts with centrally located, hyperchromatic, and scalloped nuclei are a helpful but less common finding (Fig. 9.21). In the presence of otherwise consistent clinicopathologic findings, classic lipoblasts are not necessary for establishing the diagnosis of well-differentiated liposarcoma. When the volume of hypocellular sclerotic fibrous tissue predominates over the adipose tissue component, the diagnosis of well-differentiated sclerosing liposarcoma is rendered. Lipoblasts and atypical stromal cells, identical to those observed in the lipoma-like variant, are found within the fibrous tissue stroma (Fig. 9.22). The sclerosing histologic pattern is observed most commonly within tumors arising in the retroperitoneum and paratesticular regions. Resembling the sclerosing variant, well-differentiated inflammatory liposarcoma also contains a predominant fibrous tissue component but, in addition, exhibits a distinctive, often abundant lymphoplasmacytic inflammatory infiltrate.[53,54] Similar to the other forms of well-differentiated liposarcoma, the diagnosis is confirmed by the presence of lipoblasts or the classic (and more common) atypical stromal cells (Fig. 9.23). The differential diagnosis of inflammatory liposarcoma includes inflammatory

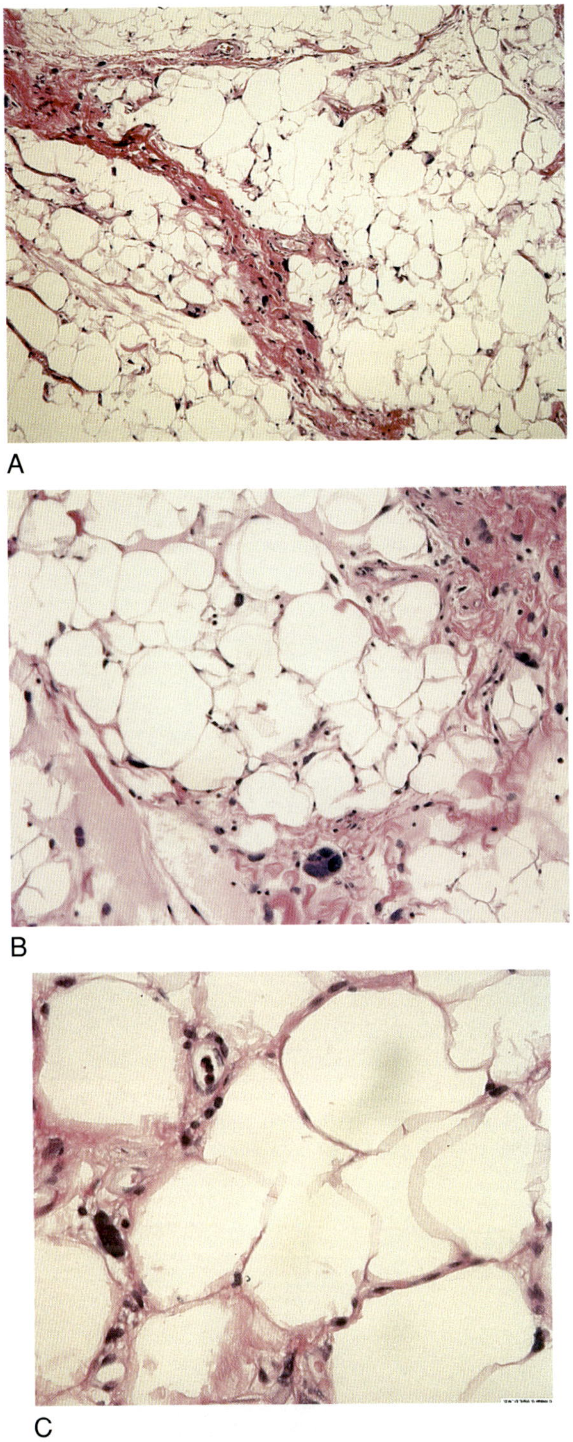

FIGURE 9.20 Well-differentiated, lipoma-like liposarcoma initially may mimic conventional lipoma. Closer inspection reveals, however, slightly more nonlipogenic fibrous tissue, adipocytes with more variable sizes and shapes, and scattered atypical stromal cells (within fibrous tissue and fat) with atypical, multilobated-to-multinucleated, enlarged and hyperchromatic nuclei **(A-C)**. (**A**, Low power; **B**, intermediate power; **C**, high power, H&E.)

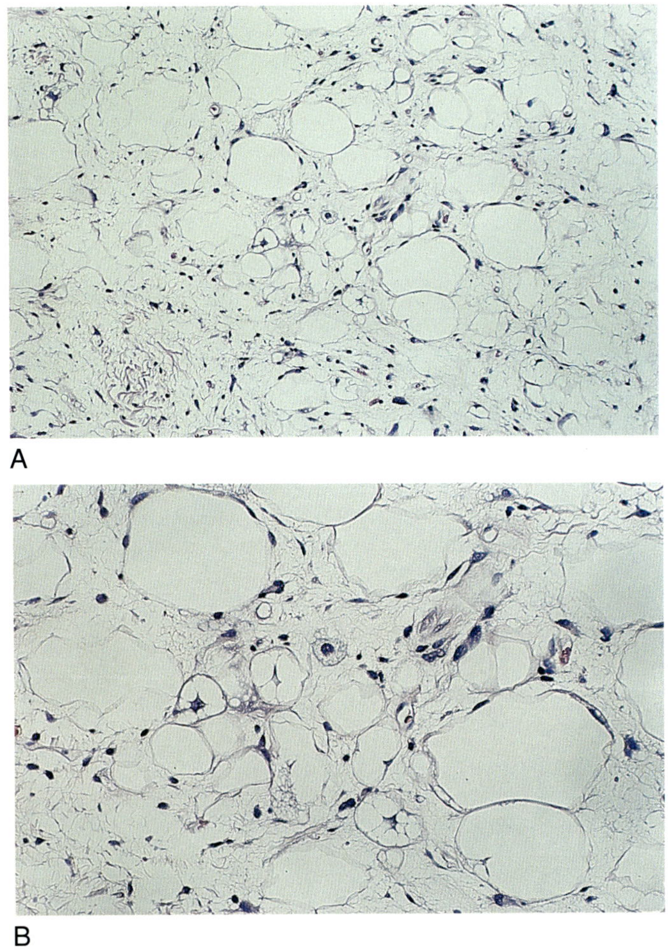

FIGURE 9.21 Well-differentiated, lipoma-like liposarcoma with a heterogeneous population of adipocytes. Compared with the atypical stromal cells, classic multivacuolated lipoblasts are observed less commonly in well-differentiated liposarcoma and are not required to establish the diagnosis **(A and B)**. (**A**, Low power; **B**, high power, H&E.)

myofibroblastic tumor and Hodgkin's disease, both of which lack the characteristic stromal cells of well-differentiated liposarcoma. In difficult cases, immunohistochemistry may be helpful to exclude Hodgkin's disease. The rarest (and most controversial) form of well-differentiated liposarcoma is the spindle cell variant.[55] Well-differentiated spindle cell liposarcoma is composed of a population of bland-appearing, spindle-shaped cells, often resembling neurofibroma. The background stroma ranges from fibrous to partially myxoid. As expected, lipoblasts or atypical stromal cells are essential for establishing the diagnosis.[55]

Fine Needle Aspiration Biopsy

As already noted, the diagnosis of atypical lipoma/well-differentiated liposarcoma is not established easily by FNAB. In most cases, cytologic smears appear variably cellular and include aggregates of bland adipose tissue (Fig. 9.24). In our experience, atypical stromal cells or lipoblasts, necessary for establishing the diagnosis, are virtually never seen (Fig. 9.25). Consequently, FNAB may rule in the diagnosis of well-differentiated liposarcoma but usually cannot completely rule out the diagnosis, especially in deep soft tissues.

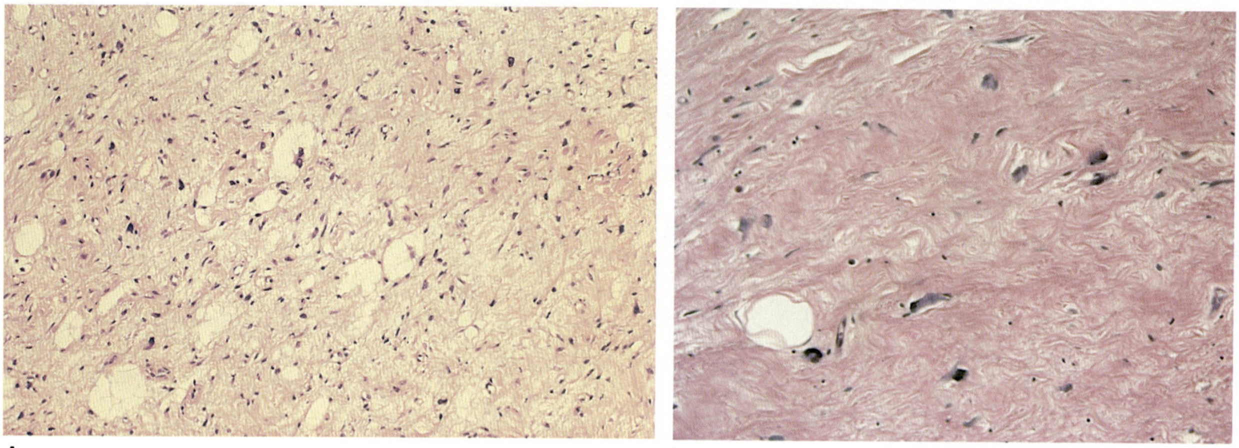

A B

FIGURE 9.22 In well-differentiated sclerosing liposarcoma, the slightly cellular to dense fibrous stroma predominates over the adipose tissue component. Atypical stromal cells, identical to the cells observed in the lipoma-like variant, are within the stroma and sometimes are accompanied by characteristic lipoblasts **(A** and **B)**. **(A,** Low power; **B,** high power, H&E.)

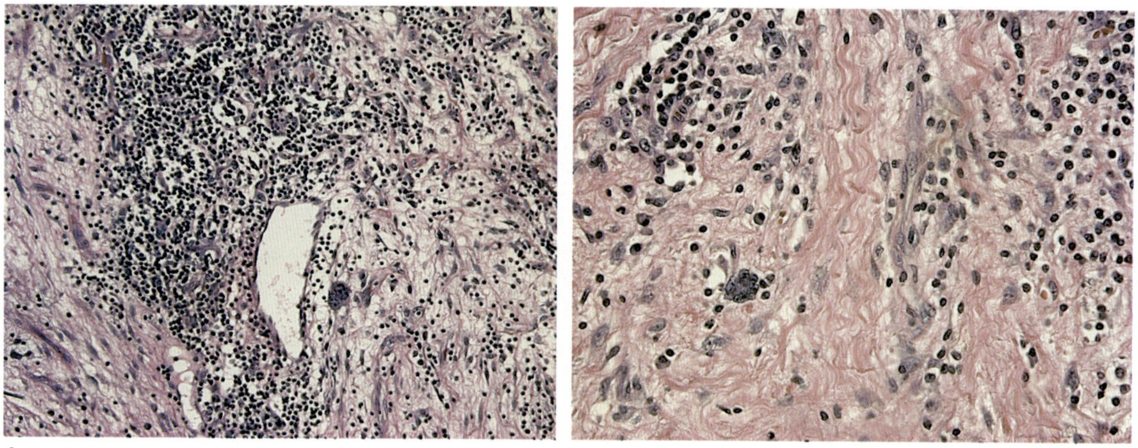

A B

FIGURE 9.23 Well-differentiated inflammatory liposarcoma resembles the sclerosing variant but has aggregates of lymphocytes and plasma cells that may mask the diagnostic atypical stromal cells **(A** and **B)**. **(A,** Low power; **B,** high power, H&E.)

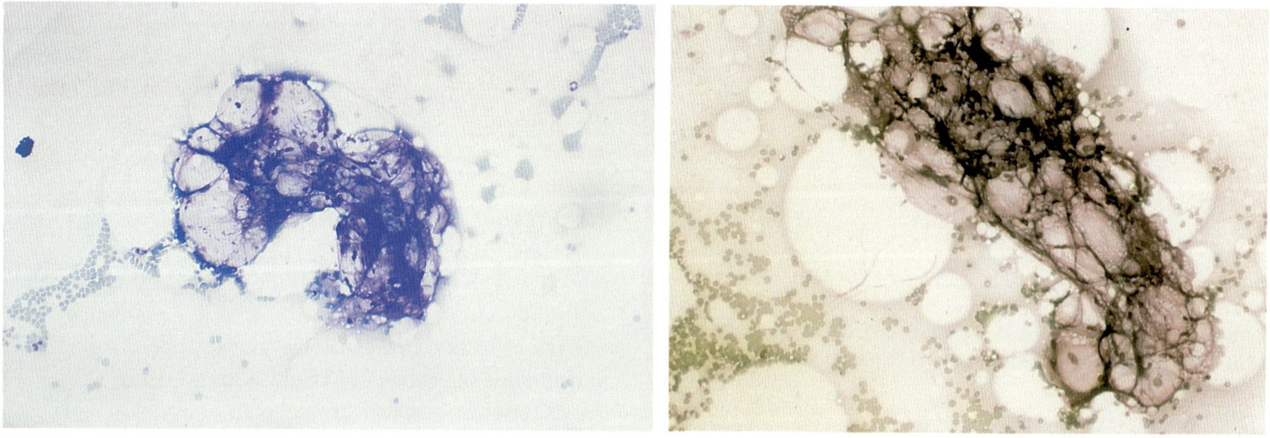

A B

FIGURE 9.24 The diagnosis of well-differentiated liposarcoma usually cannot be rendered on fine needle aspiration biopsy material alone. Most cases reveal aggregates of adipocytes indistinguishable from that observed with lipoma **(A** and **B)**. **(A,** Diff-Quik; **B,** Papanicolaou.)

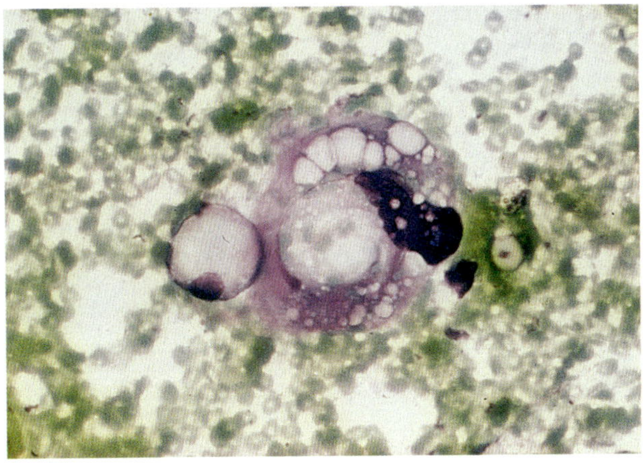

FIGURE 9.25 Rarely are the diagnostic lipoblasts or atypical stromal cells evident by fine needle aspiration biopsy. (Diff-Quik.)

Ancillary Studies

The role of immunohistochemistry in the diagnosis of well-differentiated liposarcoma is limited. As expected, S-100 protein positivity is observed in the adipocytes.

Cytogenetic analysis reveals in two thirds of cases the presence of supernumerary ring and giant marker chromosomes containing amplified sequences from 12q14-15; these abnormalities are seen more commonly in large tumors with lipoblasts and marked cytologic atypia.[56] Such cytogenetic findings have never been observed in superficial or deep lipomas.

Prognosis and Therapy

The most important prognostic factor in well-differentiated liposarcoma is anatomic location. Tumors occurring in the retroperitoneum and mediastinum are more difficult to eradicate surgically and more likely to recur locally. Superficially located lesions arising in the extremities generally do not recur after complete resection. The risk of dedifferentiation also is linked to the anatomic site. Tumors arising in the retroperitoneum are more likely to undergo dedifferentiation than are tumors occurring in the extremities. Complete resection with negative margins, when possible, is strongly recommended.[51] In the absence of dedifferentiation, metastasis does not occur. Dedifferentiated liposarcoma is discussed in greater detail in Chapter 11.

REFERENCES

1. Milgram JW: Intraosseous lipomas: A clinicopathologic study of 66 cases. Clin Orthop 1988;231:277.
2. Kenan S, Lewis MM, Abdelwahab IF, et al: Case report 652: Primary intraosseous low grade myxoid sarcoma of the scapula (myxoid liposarcoma). Skeletal Radiol 1991;20:73.
3. Torok G, Meller Y, Maor E: Primary liposarcoma of bone: Case report and review of the literature. Bull Hosp Joint Dis Orthop Inst 1983; 43:28.

Lipoma

4. Fletcher CD, Martin-Bates E: Intramuscular and intermuscular lipomas: Neglected diagnoses. Histopathology 1988;12:275.
5. Kindblom LG, Angervall L, Stener B, et al: Intermuscular and intramuscular lipomas and hibernomas: A clinical, roentgenologic, histologic, and prognostic study of 46 cases. Cancer 1974;33:754.
6. Hallel T, Lew S, Bansal M: Villous lipomatous proliferation of the synovial membrane (lipoma arborescens). J Bone Joint Surg Am 1988;70:264.
7. Miller MD, Ragsdale BD, Sweet DE: Parosteal lipomas: A new perspective. Pathology 1992;24:132.
8. Kilpatrick SE, Geisinger KR: Soft tissue sarcomas: The usefulness and limitations of fine-needle aspiration biopsy. Am J Clin Pathol 1998;110:50.
9. Kim YH, Reiner L: Ultrastructure of lipoma. Cancer 1982;50:102.
10. Oliveira AM, Nascimento AG, Lloyd RV: Leptin and leptin receptor mRNA are widely expressed in tumors of adipocytic origin. Mod Pathol 2001;14:549.
11. Fletcher CD, Akerman M, Dal Cin P, et al: Correlation between clinicopathological features and karyotype in lipomatous tumors: A report of 178 cases from the Chromosomes and Morphology (CHAMP) collaborative study group. Am J Pathol 1996;148:623.
12. Bjerregard P, Hagen K, Daugaard S, et al: Intramuscular lipoma of the lower limb: Long-term follow-up after local resection. J Bone Joint Surg Br 1989;71:812.

Lipomatosis

13. Nixon HH, Scobie WG: Congenital lipomatosis: A report of four cases. J Pediatr Surg 1971;6:742.
14. Klein FA, Smith MJ, Kasenetz I: Pelvic lipomatosis: A 35-year experience. J Urol 1988;139:998.
15. Heyns CF: Pelvic lipomatosis: A review of its diagnosis and management. J Urol 1991;146:267.
16. Cossarizza A, Mussini C, Vigano A: Mitochondria in the pathogenesis of lipodystrophy induced by anti-HIV anti-retroviral drugs: Actors or bystanders? Bioessays 2001;23:1070.

Lipoblastoma/Lipoblastomatosis

17. Collins MH, Chatten J: Lipoblastoma/lipoblastomatosis: A clinicopathologic study of 25 tumors. Am J Surg Pathol 1997;21:1131.
18. Chung EB, Enzinger FM: Benign lipoblastoma: An analysis of 35 cases. Cancer 1973;32:482.
19. Coffin CM, Williams RA: Congenital lipoblastoma of the hand. Pediatr Pathol 1992;12:856.
20. Dishop MK, O'Connor WN, Abraham S, et al: Primary cardiac lipoblastoma. Pediatr Dev Pathol 2001;4:276.
21. Matthew J, Sen S, Chandi SM, et al: Pulmonary lipoblastoma: A case report. Pediatr Surg Int 2001;17:543.
22. Bolen JW, Thorning D: Benign lipoblastoma and myxoid liposarcoma: A comparative light- and electron-microscopic study. Am J Surg Pathol 1980;4:163.
23. Mentzel T, Calonje E, Fletcher CDM. Lipoblastoma and lipoblastomatosis: A clinicopathologic study of 14 cases. Histopathology 1993;23:527.

Lipofibromatosis

24. Fetsch JF, Miettinen M, Laskin WB, et al: A clinicopathologic study of 45 pediatric soft tissue tumors with an admixture of adipose tissue and fibroblastic elements, and a proposal for classification as lipofibromatosis. Am J Surg Pathol 2000;24:1491.

Angiolipoma

25. Dixon AY, McGregor DH, Lee SH: Angiolipomas: An ultrastructural and clinicopathological study. Hum Pathol 1981;12:739.
26. Cina SJ, Radentz SS, Smialek JE: A case of familial angiolipomatosis with Lisch nodules. Arch Pathol Lab Med 1999;123:946.
27. Sciot R, Akerman M, Dal Cin P, et al: Cytogenetic analysis of subcutaneous angiolipoma: Further evidence supporting its difference from ordinary pure lipomas: A report of the CHAMP study. Am J Surg Pathol 1997;21:441.

Myolipoma

28. Meis JM, Enzinger FM: Myolipoma of soft tissue. Am J Surg Pathol 1991;15:121.

Angiomyolipoma

29. Hostis HL, Deminiere C, Ferriere JM, et al: Renal angiomyolipoma: A clinicopathologic, immunohistochemical, and follow-up study of 46 cases. Am J Surg Pathol 1999;23:1011.
30. Eble JN, Amin MB, Young RH: Epithelioid angiomyolipoma of the kidney: A report of five cases with a prominent and diagnostically confusing epithelioid smooth muscle component. Am J Surg Pathol 1997;21:1123.
31. Martigoni G, Pea M, Bonetti F, et al: Carcinomalike monotypic epithelioid angiomyolipoma in patients without evidence of tuberous sclerosis: A clinicopathologic and genetic study. Am J Surg Pathol 1998;22:663.
32. Sampson JR, Patel A, Mee AD: Multifocal renal cell carcinoma in sibs from a chromosome 9 linked (TSC1) tuberous sclerosis family. J Med Genet 1995;32:848.
33. Henske EP, Neumann HPH, Scheithauer BW, et al: Loss of heterozygosity in tuberous sclerosis (TSC2) region of chromosome band 16p13 occurs in sporadic as well as TSC-associated renal angiomyolipoma. Genes Chromosomes Cancer 1995;13:295.

Hibernoma

34. Furlong MA, Fanburg-Smith JC, Miettinen M: The morphologic spectrum of hibernoma: A clinicopathologic study of 170 cases. Am J Surg Pathol 2001;25:809.
35. Kindblom LG, Angervall L, Stener B, et al: Intermuscular and intramuscular lipomas and hibernomas: A clinical, roentgenologic, histologic, and prognostic study of 46 cases. Cancer 1974;33:754.
36. Kransdorf MJ, Moser RP Jr, Meis JM, et al: Fat-containing soft tissue masses of the extremities. Radiographics 1991;11:81.
37. Gaffney EF, Hargreaves HK, Semple E, et al: Hibernoma: Distinctive light and electron microscopic features and relationship to brown adipose tissue. Hum Pathol 1983;14:677.
38. Mertens F, Rydholm A, Brosjo H, et al: Hibernomas are characterized by rearrangements of chromosome bands 11q13-21. Int J Cancer 1994;58:503.

Chondroid Lipoma

39. Meis JM, Enzinger FM: Chondroid lipoma: A unique tumor simulating liposarcoma and myxoid chondrosarcoma. Am J Surg Pathol 1993; 17:1103.
40. Nielsen GP, O'Connell JX, Dickersin GR, et al: Chondroid lipoma, a tumor of white cells: A brief report of two cases with ultrastructural analysis. Am J Surg Pathol 1995;19:1272.
41. Kindblom LG, Meis-Kindblom JM, Mandahl N: Chondroid lipoma. In Fletcher CDM, Unni KK, Mertens F (eds): Pathology and Genetics: Tumours of Soft Tissue and Bone. World Health Organization Classification of Tumours. Lyon, France: IARC Press, 2002, p 30.

Spindle Cell/Pleomorphic Lipoma

42. Fletcher CDM, Martin-Bates E: Spindle cell lipoma: A clinicopathological study with some original observations. Histopathology 1987;11:803.
43. Shmookler BM, Enzinger FM: Pleomorphic lipoma: A benign tumor simulating liposarcoma: A clinicopathologic analysis of 48 cases. Cancer 1981;47:126.
44. Fanburg-Smith JC, Devaney KO, Miettinen M, et al: Multiple spindle cell lipomas: A report of 7 familial and 11 nonfamilial cases. Am J Surg Pathol 1998;22:40.
45. Allen PW, Strungs I, MacCormac LB: Atypical subcutaneous fatty tumors: A review of 37 referred cases. Pathology 1998;30:123.
46. Suster S, Fisher C: Immunoreactivity for the human hematopoietic progenitor cell antigen (CD34) in lipomatous tumors. Am J Surg Pathol 1997;21:195.

Myelolipoma

47. Grignon DJ, Shkrum MJ, Smout MS: Extra-adrenal myelolipoma. Arch Pathol Lab Med 1989;113:52.
48. Hunter SB, Shemankewitz EH, Patterson C, et al: Extra-adrenal myelolipoma: A report of two cases. Am J Clin Pathol 1992;97:402.

Atypical Lipoma/Well-Differentiated Liposarcoma

49. Yoshikawa H, Ueda T, Mori S, et al: Dedifferentiated liposarcoma of the subcutis. Am J Surg Pathol 1996;20:1525.
50. McCormick D, Mentzel T, Beham A, et al: Dedifferentiated liposarcoma: Clinicopathologic analysis of 32 cases suggesting a better prognostic subgroup among pleomorphic sarcomas. Am J Surg Pathol 1994;18:1213.
51. Lucas DR, Nascimento AG, Sanjay BKS, et al: Well-differentiated liposarcoma: The Mayo Clinic experience with 58 cases. Am J Clin Pathol 1994;102:677.
52. Weiss SW, Rao VK: Well-differentiated liposarcoma (atypical lipoma) of deep soft tissue of the extremities, retroperitoneum, and miscellaneous sites: A follow-up study of 92 cases with analysis of the incidence of "dedifferentiation." Am J Surg Pathol 1992;16:1051.
53. Kraus MD, Guillou L, Fletcher CDM: Well-differentiated inflammatory liposarcoma: An uncommon and easily overlooked variant of a common sarcoma. Am J Surg Pathol 1997;21:518.
54. Argani P, Facchetti F, Inghirami G, et al: Lymphocyte-rich well-differentiated liposarcoma: Report of nine cases. Am J Surg Pathol 1997;21:884.
55. Dei Tos AP, Menzel T, Newman PL, et al: Spindle cell liposarcoma, a hitherto unrecognized variant of liposarcoma: Analysis of six cases. Am J Surg Pathol 1994;18:913.
56. Rosai J, Akerman M, Dal Cin P, et al: Combined morphologic and karyotypic study of 59 atypical lipomatous tumors: Evaluation of their relationship and differential diagnosis with other adipose tumors: A report of the CHAMP study group. Am J Surg Pathol 1996;20:1182.

CHAPTER 10

Vascular Tumors of Bone and Soft Tissue

Vascular tumors of bone and soft tissue encompass lesions that are vasoformative and are composed at least partly of endothelium. These lesions are listed in Table 10.1. Probably no other category of tumors has been plagued with such a variety of confusing designations and terminologies. Hemangiomas are among the most common soft tissue lesions and constitute most vascular lesions. Among infants and children, they are the most common tumor. Controversy remains over whether some forms of hemangioma are true neoplasms, vascular malformations, or reactive processes. Although most are superficial cutaneous lesions, hemangiomas may arise in deep soft tissues, bone, or viscera. Histologic subclassification is based largely on the predominant blood vessel type (e.g., capillary, venous, arteriovenous). Except for capillary hemangioma with its tendency for spontaneous regression, classification by blood vessel type is of little prognostic relevance. It is far more important that these processes be recognized as benign and treated accordingly. Albeit extraordinarily rare, malignant transformation of hemangioma may occur and can be lethal. Fine needle aspiration biopsy (FNAB) of hemangioma generally is not useful. Cytologic smears typically are composed mostly of blood and rarely contain nonspecific blood vessels, insufficient to establish a definitive diagnosis (Fig. 10.1).

The term *hemangioendothelioma* should be used only to designate lesions with borderline-to-intermediate malignant potential. Tumors included in this category include epithelioid hemangioendothelioma, retiform hemangioendothelioma (Dabska's tumor), and kaposiform hemangioendothelioma. The criteria for rendering the diagnosis of these rare neoplasms have been well established in soft tissue types. Among primary bone tumors, only epithelioid hemangioendothelioma is recognized universally as an established entity. A group of vasoformative tumors, sometimes designated as *nonepithelioid hemangioendothelioma,* clearly exists, however, which may not have a soft tissue analogue. Whether some of these "hemangioendotheliomas" of bone are variants of hemangioma is unclear, but there is increasing evidence in support of the latter. In bone and soft tissue, high-grade vascular lesions are recognized as angiosarcomas.

Tumors of pericytes, modified smooth muscle cells functioning in thermoregulation, are far less common than

TABLE 10.1 Vascular (Endothelial) Lesions of Bone and Soft Tissue

Bone Origin	Soft Tissue Origin
Hemangioma and variants	Hemangioma and variants
Epithelioid hemangioendothelioma	Lymphangioma
Angiosarcoma	Epithelioid hemangioendothelioma
	Retiform hemangioendothelioma
	Kaposiform hemangioendothelioma
	Kaposi's sarcoma
	Angiosarcoma

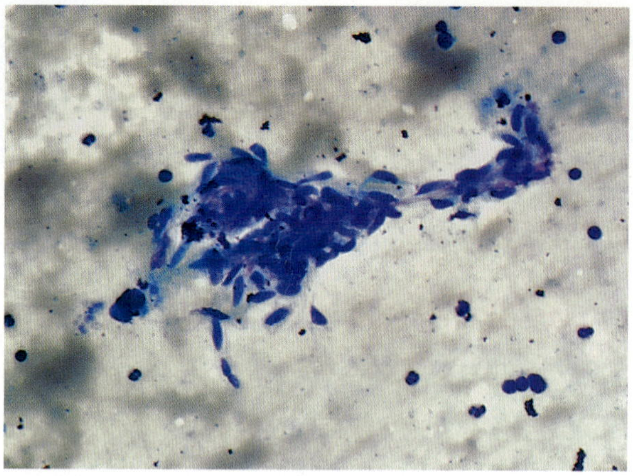

FIGURE 10.1 Fine needle aspiration biopsy of hemangioma, regardless of subtype, usually yields mostly blood and rare nonspecific vascular channels. (Diff-Quik.)

TABLE 10.2 Perivascular (Pericytic) Lesions of Bone and Soft Tissue

Glomus tumor and variants
Hemangiopericytoma*

* Currently considered to be part of a spectrum of solitary fibrous tumor.

tumors of endothelial origin. Table 10.2 lists these lesions. In the past, this category of tumors largely was dominated by the so-called hemangiopericytoma. It now is recognized that the staghorn-shaped, thin-walled blood vessels that defined hemangiopericytoma may be observed in a variety of benign and malignant lesions. Consequently, we consider the diagnosis of hemangiopericytoma to be one of exclusion. In the current World Health Organization classification, hemangiopericytomas are considered part of the spectrum of solitary fibrous tumors. The prototype pericytic tumor is the glomus tumor. Myopericytomas, also called *infantile hemangiopericytoma*, represent a spectrum of myofibroma/myofibromatosis.

Capillary (Juvenile) Hemangioma

Clinical Features

Capillary hemangiomas are the most common form of hemangioma, typically occurring during infancy and early childhood. Table 10.3 summarizes the various subtypes of hemangioma and their clinical features. Synonyms for capillary hemangioma include *cellular hemangioma*, *juvenile hemangioma*, *strawberry nevus*, and *infantile hemangioendothelioma*. Approximately 20% of cases are multiple. Females are affected slightly more often than males. The most common anatomic location is the skin and subcutaneous adipose tissue of the head and neck region. Although often considered congenital lesions, most capillary hemangiomas appear shortly after birth and continue to grow until about 1 year of age. In contrast to other forms of hemangioma, the natural history is one of initial rapid growth followed by involution often over months to years.[1,2] For this reason, recognition and distinction of capillary hemangioma from other hemangioma variants is prognostically and therapeutically important.

Pathologic Findings

Histology

Histologically, capillary hemangiomas appear distinctly lobulated with individual lobules containing centrally located, "feeder" blood vessels. The cells within the lobules are heterogeneous, composed mainly of endothelial cells with small capillary lumens and pericytes (Fig. 10.2). Fibroblasts and mast cells are scattered among these cells in lesser numbers.[1] With maturation, the vascular differentiation of the endothelial cells generally becomes more evident (cellularity decreases), as the small blood vessels progressively dilate and the endothelial cells are flattened (Fig. 10.3). Mitotic figures in the more cellular examples may be numerous but are of no prognostic significance.

TABLE 10.3 Clinical Features of Various Hemangioma Subtypes and Related Lesions

Subtype	Age	Anatomic Location	Spontaneous Regression
Capillary	Infants and children	Skin and subcutis, head and neck	Yes
Cavernous	Infants and children	Skin and subcutis, head and neck	No
Venous	Adults	Subcutis and deep tissues, extremities	No
Arteriovenous	Children and young adults	Deep soft tissues, head and neck	No
Intramuscular	Adolescents and young adults	Intramuscular, lower extremities	No
Pyogenic granuloma	All ages	Skin, fingers, head and neck, gingiva	No
Spindle cell	Adults	Skin, distal extremities	No
Epithelioid	Adults	Skin, head and neck	No
Synovial	Children and adolescents	Synovial tissues, knee	No
Bone	Adults	Axial skeleton	No

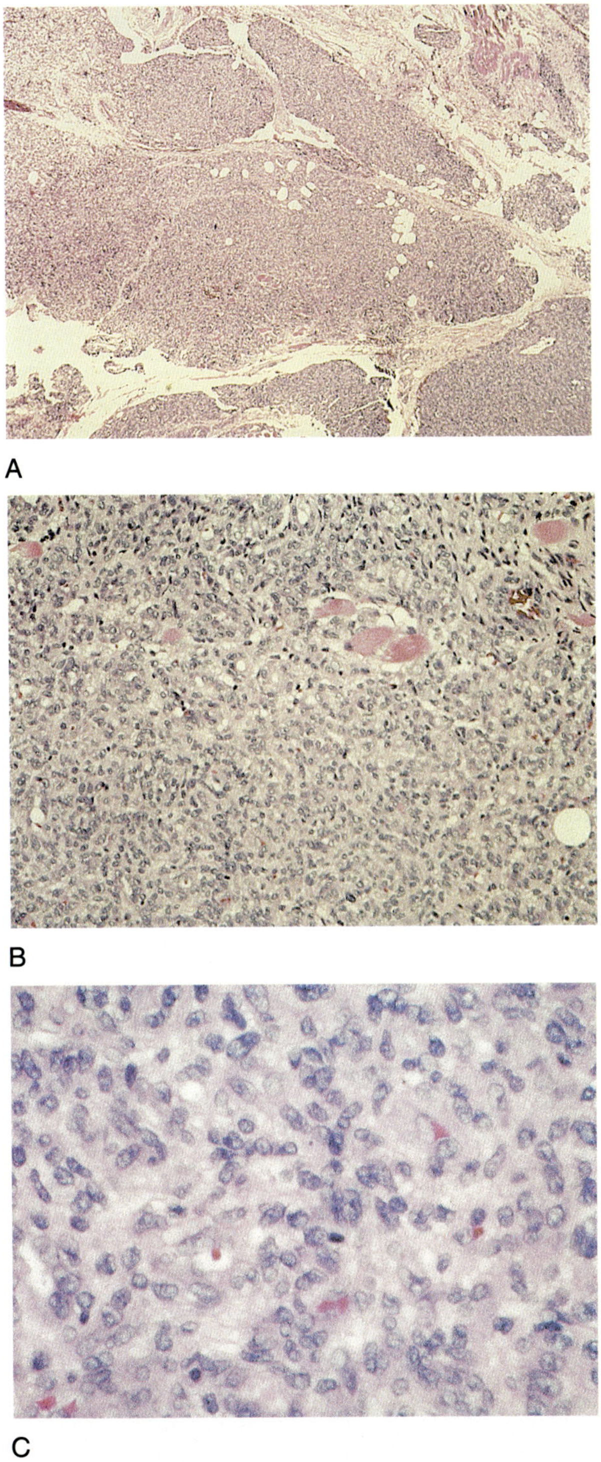

FIGURE 10.2 Capillary hemangioma has a typical lobulated appearance **(A)**. Individual lobules may appear cellular and the vascular nature less obvious **(B)**. Closer inspection reveals numerous small capillary-like blood vessels and endothelium admixed with fibroblasts and pericytes **(C)**. (**A,** low power, H&E; **B,** intermediate power, H&E; **C,** high power, H&E.)

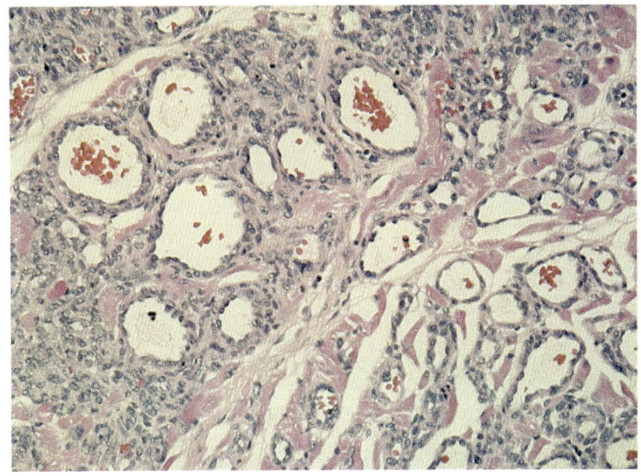

FIGURE 10.3 On maturation, the vascular differentiation of capillary hemangiomas is recognized more easily, as a result of luminal dilation. (H&E.)

Ancillary Studies

Ultrastructurally the endothelial cells appear largely immature, lacking Weibel-Palade bodies but containing peculiar crystalloid inclusions.[2] Immunohistochemistry generally is not necessary to establish a diagnosis because most cases of capillary hemangioma are diagnosed easily if close attention is paid to clinical and pathologic features. For more cellular forms of capillary hemangioma in which blood vessels appear inconspicuous, vascular endothelial markers, such as CD31, CD34, and factor 8, may be useful for highlighting the hypervascularity of the lesion. North and colleagues[3] reported the immunohistochemical presence of the erythrocyte-type glucose transporter protein, GLUT1, in virtually all cases of capillary hemangioma examined. Vascular malformations, pyogenic granulomas, and hemangioendotheliomas all were negative for GLUT1 expression. Evidence suggests that the formation of hemangiomas may be associated with somatic mutations and loss of heterozygosity on chromosome 5q.[4]

Prognosis and Therapy

Most capillary hemangiomas ultimately spontaneously regress. Consequently, the best therapeutic approach is often watchful waiting. Larger lesions compromising crucial functions (e.g., respiration) or viscera may respond to systemic steroids or interferon therapy. Surgical intervention less commonly is required.

Cavernous Hemangioma

Similar to capillary hemangiomas, cavernous hemangiomas are observed most often in the skin and subcutaneous adipose tissue of the upper body in infants and children with a slight female predominance.[5] Compared with capillary hemangiomas, cavernous hemangiomas are larger with more

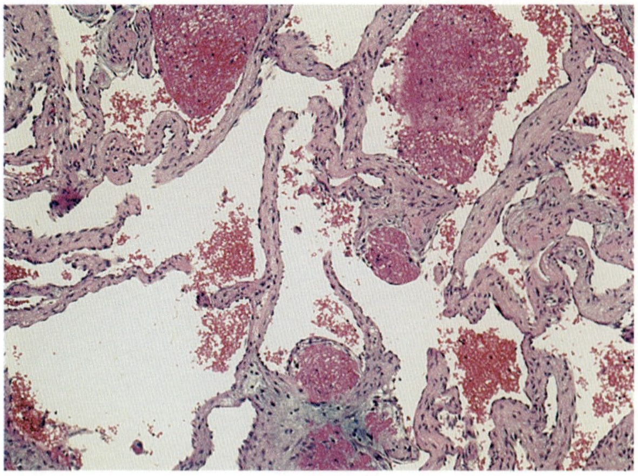

FIGURE 10.4 Cavernous hemangioma is characterized by large "cavernous" blood-filled spaces lined by thick fibrous septa and flattened banal endothelium. (H&E.)

infiltrative borders and have a tendency to involve deep soft tissue and viscera, especially the liver. Morphologically, cavernous hemangiomas consist of dilated blood-filled spaces lined by variably thickened fibrous walls and benign-appearing but flattened endothelium (Fig. 10.4). Organizing thrombi with dystrophic calcifications are frequently within the blood vessel lumina. Cavernous hemangiomas do not spontaneously regress and often require surgical resection.

Venous Hemangioma

Pure venous hemangiomas are rare and usually occur in adults. Preferred anatomic locations include the subcutaneous adipose tissue or deep soft tissues of the extremities, abdomen, or retroperitoneum. Patients often present with a history of a slowly growing tumor of long duration. Radiographic studies may reveal calcifications resulting from phleboliths.

Histologically, venous hemangiomas are composed of large thick-walled blood vessels, lacking a distinct internal elastic lamina. The lumina frequently are dilated and may contain organizing thrombi and dystrophic calcifications (Fig. 10.5). Spontaneous regression does not occur. Superficial tumors generally are cured with surgical excision; deeper lesions are more difficult to eradicate surgically and may recur locally.

Arteriovenous Hemangioma

Arteriovenous hemangioma, also called *arteriovenous malformation*, is a rare non-neoplastic disorder usually observed in children and young adults. The most common anatomic location is the head and neck region followed by the extremities. Angiography establishes the diagnosis, revealing evidence of arteriovenous shunting that rarely may be severe enough to cause heart failure. Soft tissue swelling and pain are common presenting complaints. Histologically, arteriovenous hemangiomas show an admixture of relatively large blood vessels of differing sizes and shapes frequently associated with organizing thrombosis and dystrophic calcifications. Thick-walled veins greatly outnumber the muscular-walled arteries, the latter of which may require elastic stains for confirmation (Fig. 10.6). Prognosis is related largely to the degree of involvement of the affected area. Complete excision is often difficult, and local recurrence commonly is seen.

Intramuscular Hemangioma

Intramuscular hemangioma (angioma) is observed most commonly in adolescents and young adults with most cases presenting before age 30 years.[6,7] Males and females are affected

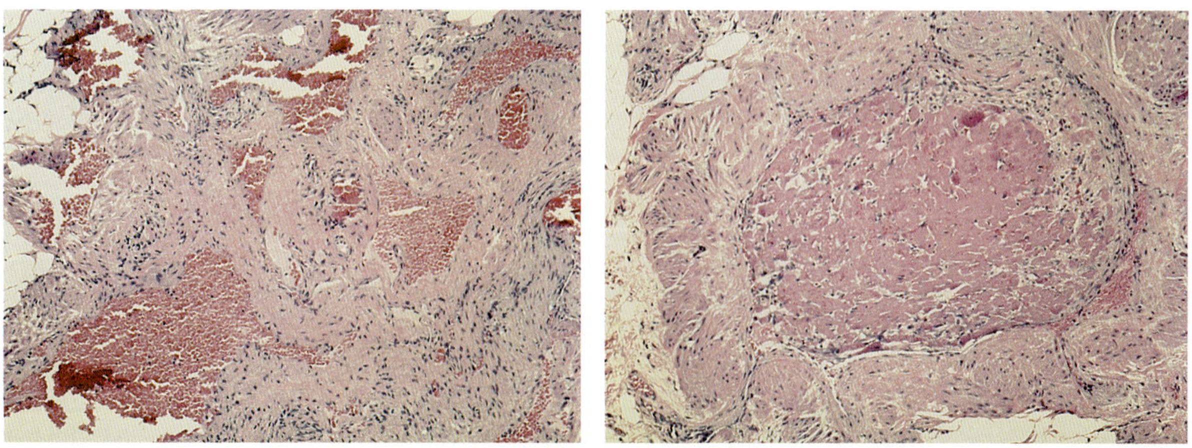

A B

FIGURE 10.5 Venous hemangioma is composed of haphazard arrangements of thick muscular-walled blood vessels **(A)**. Organizing thrombi commonly are observed within the vessel lumina **(B)**. (**A** and **B,** H&E.)

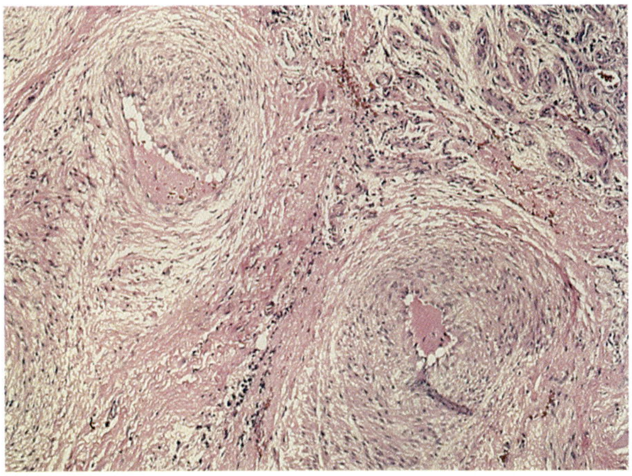

FIGURE 10.6 Arteriovenous hemangiomas can be difficult to distinguish from venous hemangiomas. In both cases, venous vessels tend to predominate, and elastic stains may be required to recognize the presence of internal elastic lamina, characteristic of muscular arteries. (H&E.)

in roughly equal numbers. The extremities, especially the lower limb, are the most common anatomic location, followed by the head and neck region and the trunk.[6] Generally, intramuscular hemangiomas present as slowly growing soft tissue masses that often are reportedly painful, especially after exertion. As with cavernous hemangiomas, radiographic evaluation may reveal calcifications resulting from phleboliths (Fig. 10.7). Variably sized blood vessels ranging from capillaries to thick-walled veins are interspersed within skeletal muscle and often admixed with adipose tissue (Fig. 10.8).[6,7] Subclassification by exclusive blood vessel type (e.g., capillary versus venous) usually is not possible because a variety of blood vessel types is observed in all cases. In many tumors, the degree of vascular involvement may be so extensive as to result in skeletal muscle atrophy in the involved areas. Wide local excision with negative margins is the recommended form of treatment. Local recurrence occurs in 50% of cases, regardless of predominant blood vessel type, and is virtually always secondary to incomplete resection.[6] Distance metastases have not been documented.

Pyogenic Granuloma (Lobular Capillary Hemangioma)

Pyogenic granulomas are exophytic capillary hemangiomas typically seen on the skin or mucosal surfaces. Pyogenic granulomas may arise at any age and show no gender predilection. The most common anatomic location is the gingiva followed by the fingers, lip, and face.[8] In one third of cases, an association with trauma is reported. The initial rapid growth phase may cause some clinical concern, but most cases stabilize and cease to grow within a few weeks of onset. At low power, pyogenic granuloma has a distinct lobulated appearance, mimicking capillary hemangioma of infancy (Fig. 10.9). Individual lobules consist of small but variably sized capillaries lined by plump but benign-appearing endothelial cells. Larger blood vessels, presumably the feeder vessels, course through the lobules (Fig. 10.10). Varying amounts of acute and chronic inflammation are seen and are more abundant if concomitant ulceration is present. In the early stages of the disease, significant mitotic activity frequently is observed within the endothelial cells and stromal fibroblasts. Most cases are cured by local excision.

Spindle Cell Hemangioma

Spindle cell hemangioma, previously called *spindle cell hemangioendothelioma*, is a rare vascular tumor usually seen in middle-aged adults. Men and women are affected equally.[9] Most arise as superficial cutaneous masses, involving the distal extremities. Rarely, spindle cell hemangiomas may arise in association with multiple enchondromas of bone (Maffucci's syndrome).[10] Although most spindle cell hemangiomas arise as solitary lesions, progression to multiple lesions within the same anatomic area is not unusual. At low power, the lesions appear to represent a combination of cavernous hemangioma and more solid-appearing Kaposi's sarcoma (Fig. 10.11). In the former, dilated, thin-walled blood vessels contain abundant hemorrhage or thrombi with dystrophic calcifications (Fig. 10.12). In the more cellular Kaposi's sarcoma–like areas, a population of rounded, epithelioid-appearing cells is admixed with a second population of uniform-appearing, spindled, fibroblast-like cells with slit-like-to-collapsed vascular spaces (Fig. 10.13). Even after wide resection, local recurrence frequently is observed. It has been suggested that these local recurrences likely represent contiguous or multifocal vascular involvement.[9] Definite distant metastasis has not been documented, however.

Epithelioid Hemangioma

Although seen at any age, most examples of epithelioid hemangioma arise within young-to-middle-aged adults. There is a roughly equal sex incidence. The most common anatomic location is the head and neck region followed by the distal extremities.[11,12] Most patients present with a localized, painless, superficial soft tissue swelling. In approximately 10% of patients, a history of prior trauma is reported.[11] Microscopically, epithelioid hemangiomas are characterized by a proliferation of small-to-medium-sized, muscular-walled blood vessels lined by a single layer of epithelioid endothelial cells. Individual endothelial cells appear large and plump with a single round-to-ovoid nucleus, inconspicuous-to-prominent nucleoli, and abundant dense-to-vacuolated cytoplasm. The background stroma contains variable numbers of lymphocytes, plasma cells, and eosinophils (Fig. 10.14). In some cases, the lymphoid proliferation may form follicles at the periphery of the lesion, mimicking a lymph node. Subcutaneous lesions often are

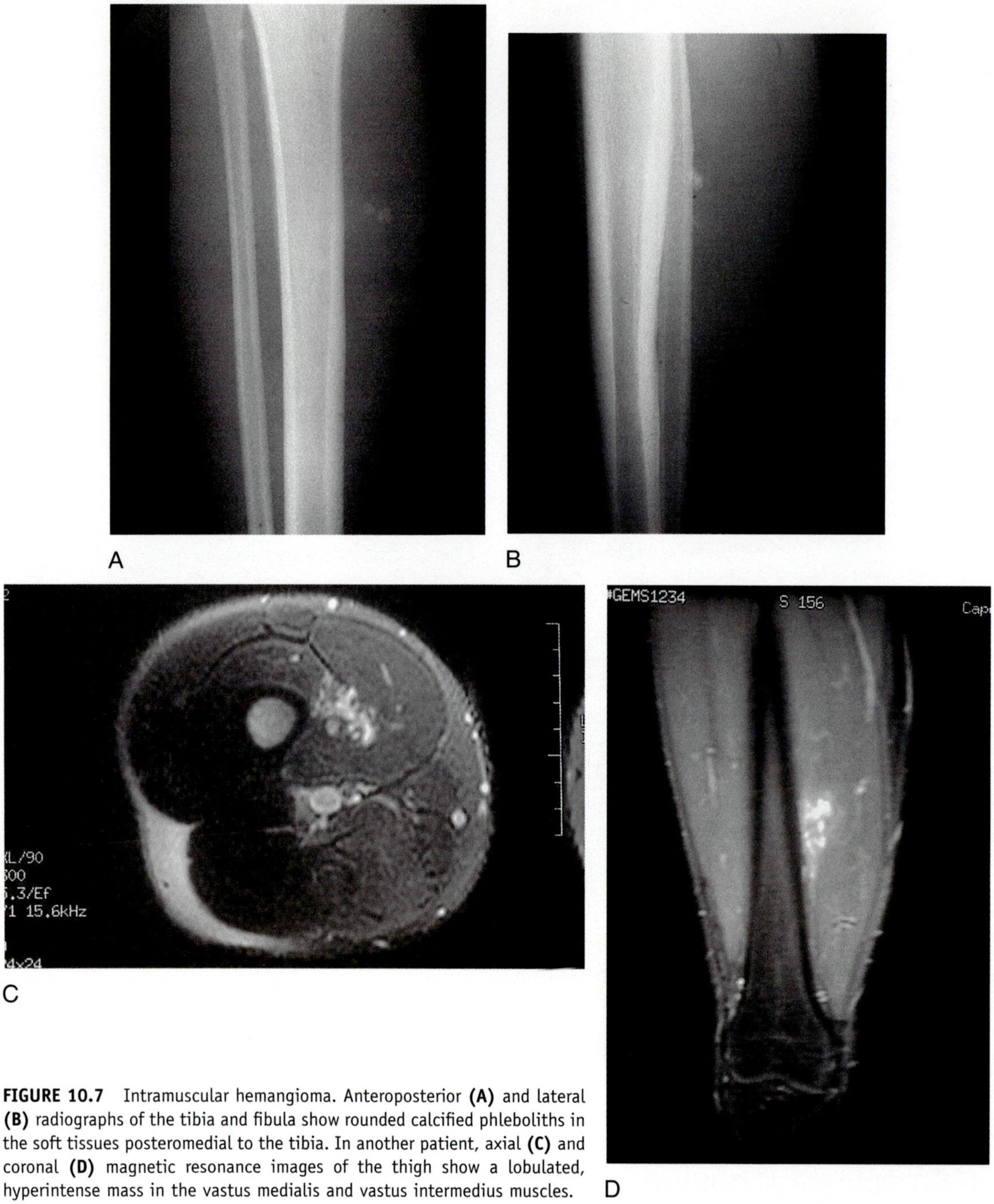

FIGURE 10.7 Intramuscular hemangioma. Anteroposterior **(A)** and lateral **(B)** radiographs of the tibia and fibula show rounded calcified phleboliths in the soft tissues posteromedial to the tibia. In another patient, axial **(C)** and coronal **(D)** magnetic resonance images of the thigh show a lobulated, hyperintense mass in the vastus medialis and vastus intermedius muscles.

organized around a centrally located larger blood vessel, usually an artery. These findings suggest that some forms of epithelioid hemangioma represent reactive processes and not true neoplasms.[11] Complete excision is the recommended therapy. Local recurrence is seen in one third of patients.[12]

Synovial Hemangioma

Synovial hemangioma essentially is a hemangioma arising from a synovial-lined surface. Synovial hemangioma is extraordinarily rare. It predominately affects children and adolescents, and there is a male predominance.[13,14] Most cases arise in the synovial tissues surrounding the knee, followed in frequency by the elbow. Clinical complaints include localized pain, soft tissue swelling, and joint effusion. On conventional radiographs, phleboliths are seen in approximately 50% of patients. Magnetic resonance imaging seems most accurate, however, revealing an intra-articular or juxta-articular soft tissue mass of intermediate signal intensity on T1-weighted images and a high signal intensity on T2-weighted images.[14] Morphologically, synovial hemangioma usually appears as a cavernous hemangioma with dilated blood vessels separated by thin-walled fibrous septa and vari-

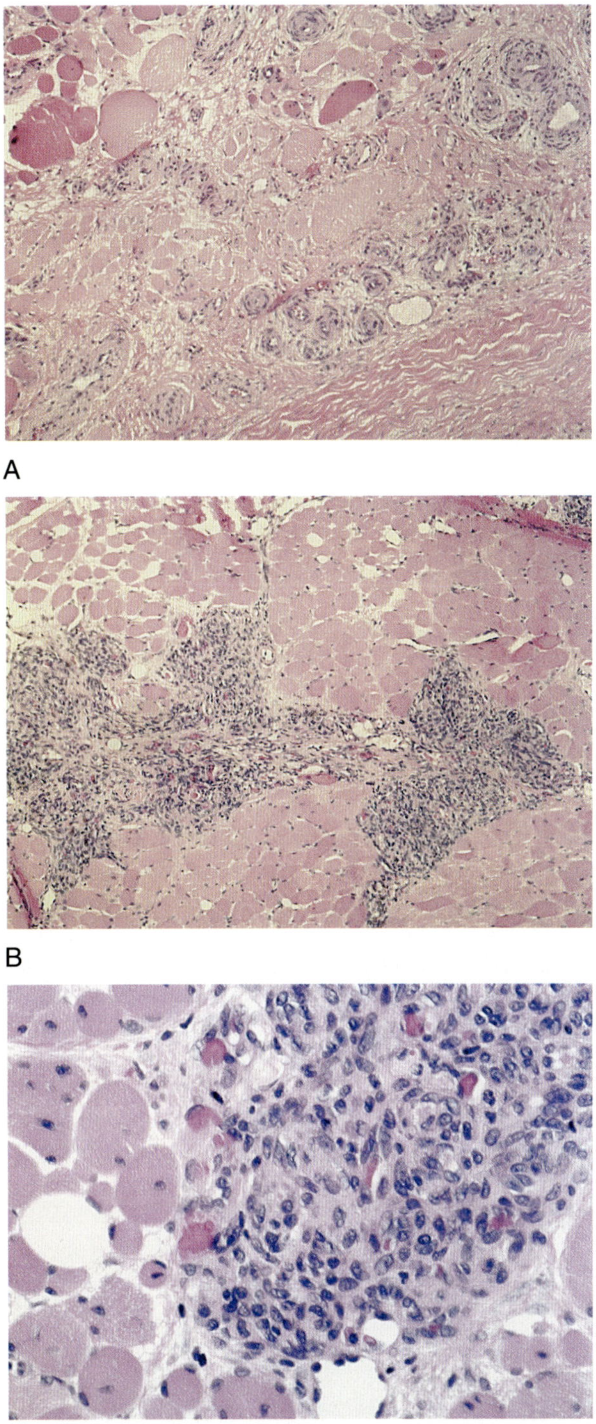

FIGURE 10.8 Intramuscular hemangiomas are vascular proliferations, ranging from dilated, thick-walled veins to inconspicuous capillaries, arising within skeletal muscle **(A-C)**. **(A** and **B,** low power, H&E; **C,** high power, H&E.)

able amounts of hemosiderin pigment deposition. Less commonly, synovial hemangioma displays a capillary or arteriovenous appearance.[13] Prognosis is related to the extent of the disease. Small pedunculated lesions are cured by simple excision; diffuse involvement of a joint may lead to persistence of the disease after incomplete surgical resection.

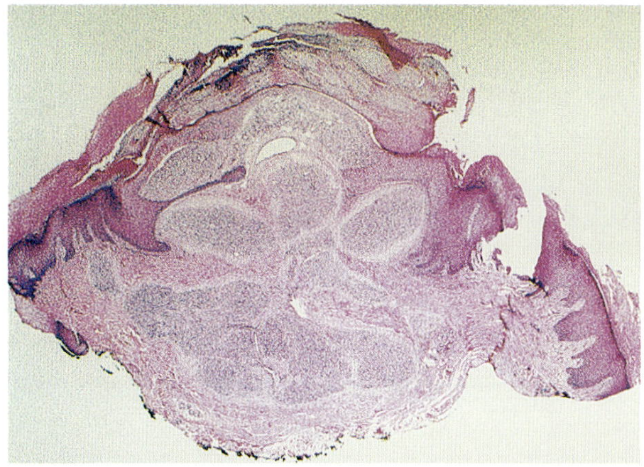

FIGURE 10.9 Low-power view of pyogenic granuloma reveals its superficial, lobulated appearance, sometimes associated with ulceration. (H&E.)

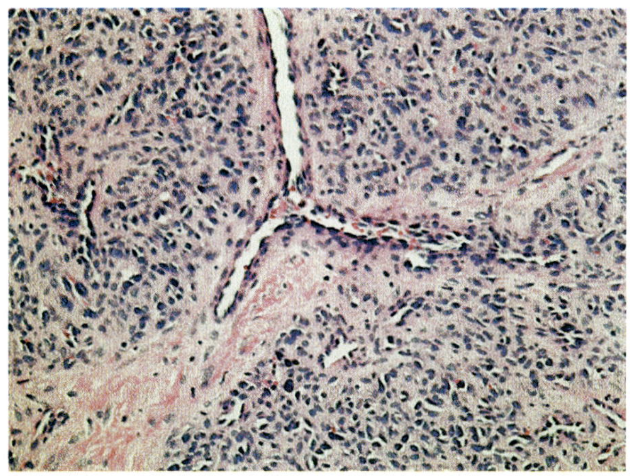

FIGURE 10.10 Pyogenic granuloma showing at least three vascular and cellular lobules being fed by a larger, central blood vessel. The composition of the individual lobules includes endothelial cells, pericytes, and fibroblasts. (H&E.)

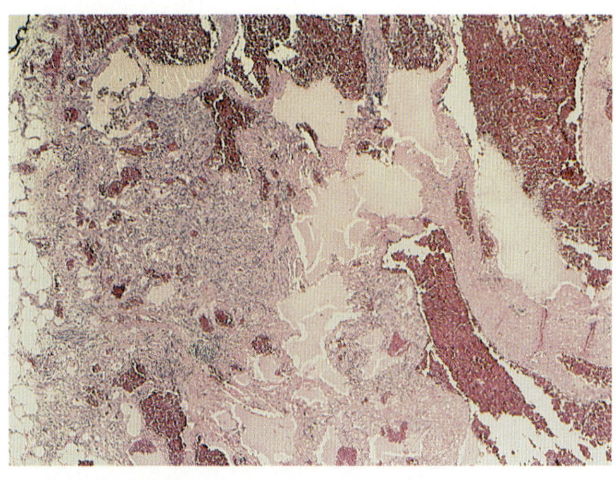

FIGURE 10.11 Spindle cell hemangioma at low power reveals a combination of dilated, blood-filled spaces alternating with more cellular, Kaposi's-like areas. (H&E.)

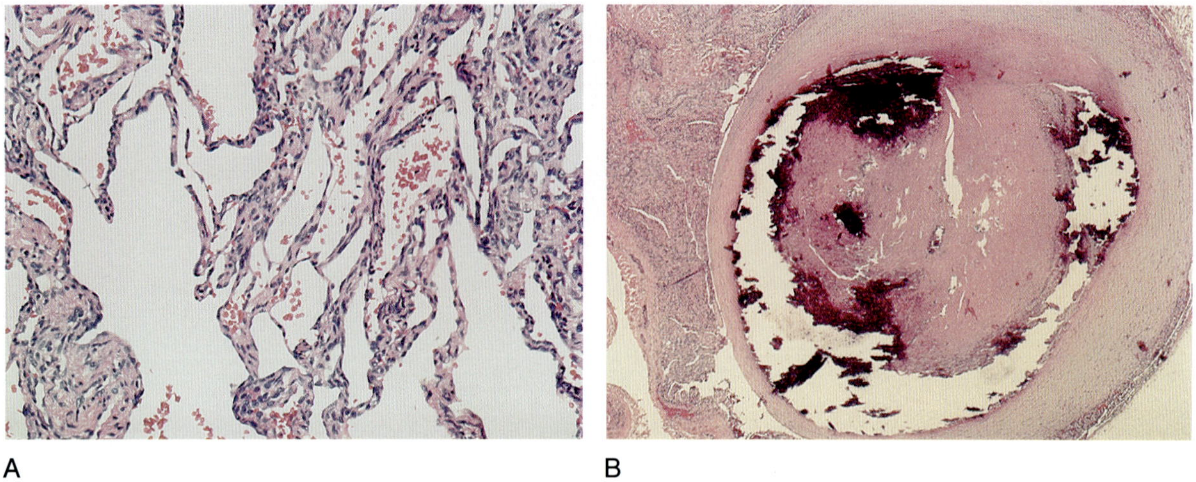

FIGURE 10.12 The cavernous hemangioma component of spindle cell hemangioma comprises dilated vascular spaces lined by variably sized fibrous septa and flattened endothelium **(A)**. Organizing thrombi with dystrophic calcifications (phleboliths) are frequent **(B)**. (**A** and **B**, H&E.)

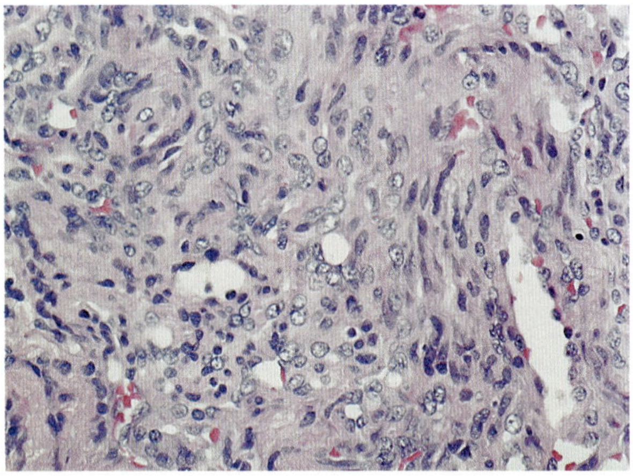

FIGURE 10.13 The Kaposi's-like areas of spindle cell hemangioma show less conspicuous vascular differentiation and a population of distinctly epithelioid cells admixed with spindled cells. (H&E.)

Hemangioma of Bone

Clinical Features

Based on autopsy studies, hemangiomas of bone are relatively common lesions, being found in approximately 10% of adults.[15] Most of these tumors are asymptomatic, however. Symptomatic lesions are observed most commonly in middle-aged and older adults. Women are affected slightly more often than men. The most common anatomic location is the vertebral body, followed by the skull and craniofacial region and the extremity long bones. Clinical symptoms depend largely on anatomic site and their relationship to adjacent structures. Many hemangiomas are incidental findings discovered during radiographic studies for evaluation of other clinical problems.[16] Involvement of the vertebral spine may

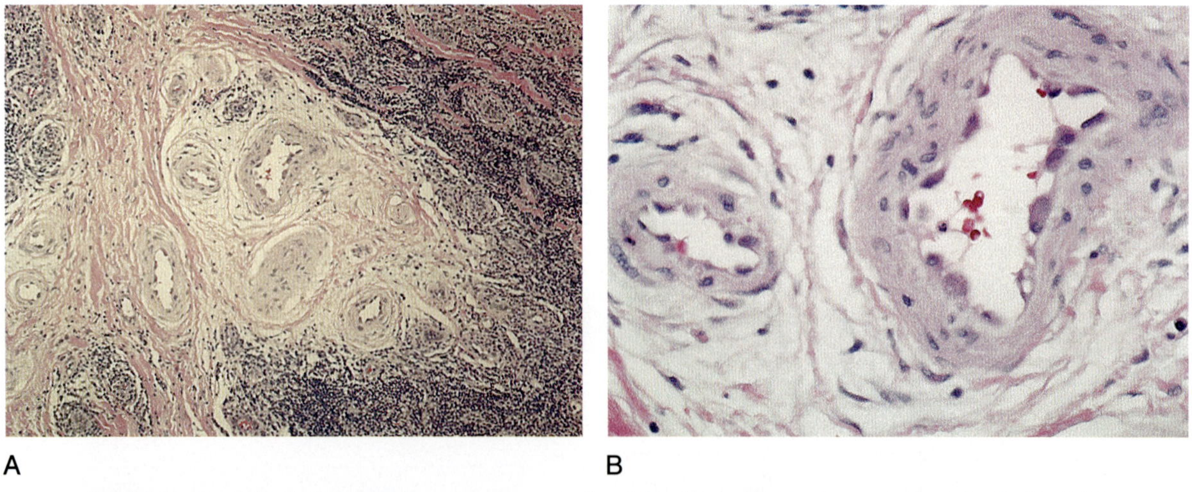

FIGURE 10.14 Epithelioid hemangioma is composed of variably thickened blood vessels lined by "epithelioid" endothelial cells that may protrude into the lumen, creating a "tombstone" appearance. The background stroma shows variable numbers of lymphocytes, plasma cells, and occasional eosinophils **(A** and **B)**. (**A,** low power, H&E; **B,** high power, H&E.)

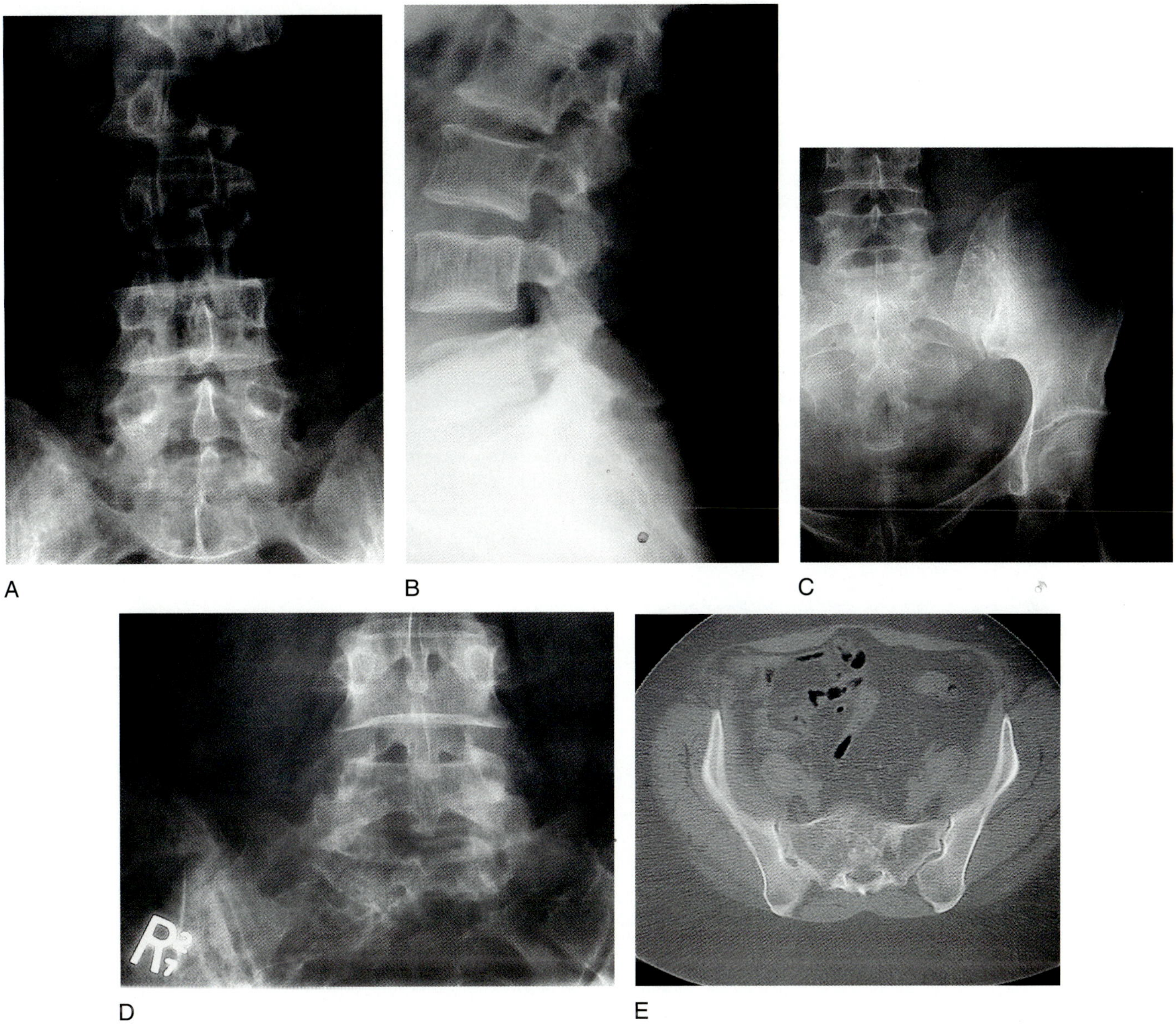

FIGURE 10.15 Intraosseous hemangioma. Anteroposterior **(A)** and lateral **(B)** radiographs of the lumbar spine reveal a lesion in L4. The vertebral body trabeculae are coarse and accompanied by surrounding lucency. In another patient, an anteroposterior radiograph of the left pelvis **(C)** shows a lytic lesion in the posterior left ilium associated with prominent remaining trabeculae. No matrix calcification is evident. An anteroposterior radiograph **(D)** and computed tomographic scan **(E)** of the sacrum shows a lytic lesion in the sacrum. Although the lesion is difficult to perceive on the radiograph, the coarsened trabeculae are obvious on the computed tomographic scan.

lead to compression fractures, resulting in cord compression and neurologic symptoms. Hemangiomas that cause expansion of the bone may manifest clinically as soft tissue swelling. Occasional patients complain of localized pain.

Radiographically, hemangiomas are lytic, well-demarcated lesions that, in the vertebral body, may exhibit vertical striations or a honeycomb appearance (Fig. 10.15). Similar features may be observed in the skull, but the tumor is usually expansile, producing a "sunburst" pattern of reactive new bone formation. In the extremities, hemangiomas may present as expansile lesions with destruction of the cortex. Multifocal lesions within the same bone or anatomic region commonly are observed, especially with the epithelioid form of hemangioma.[17,18]

Pathologic Findings

Histology

Similar to hemangiomas seen in the synovium, most hemangiomas of bone appear predominantly cavernous, consisting of thin-walled, dilated blood vessels lined by banal and flattened endothelial cells. Hemangiomas predominantly

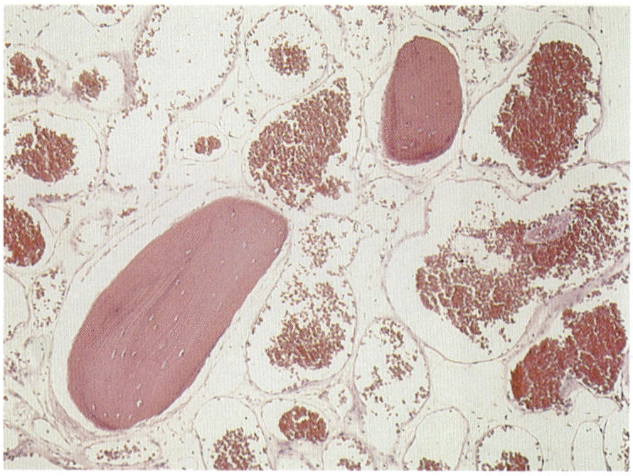

FIGURE 10.16 Hemangioma of bone usually consists of bland-appearing dilated blood vessels filled with blood and entrapping medullary bone. (H&E.)

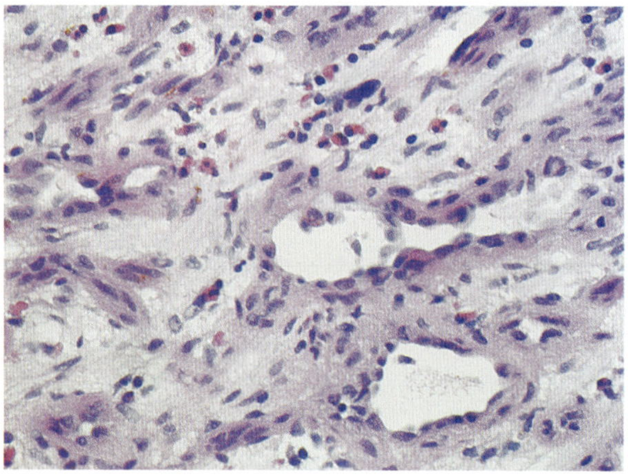

FIGURE 10.17 Epithelioid hemangioma of bone resembles its soft tissue counterpart, being composed of variably thickened blood vessels, epithelioid-appearing endothelial cells, and a background inflammatory infiltrate often containing eosinophils. (H&E.)

composed of capillary or venous components are observed less frequently. Despite being completely benign, the blood vessels appear to permeate medullary bone, surrounding and sometimes entrapping residual lamellar bone (Fig. 10.16). Rarely, reactive new bone formation with trabecular bone rimmed by prominent osteoblasts may be so prominent as to suggest initially the diagnosis of osteoblastoma.

Epithelioid hemangioma of bone is a rare form of hemangioma most commonly arising in the extremities, occasionally is multifocal, and characteristically contains variable numbers of epithelioid and spindled endothelial cells proliferating in a lobular growth pattern. The spindle cells are arranged in loose fascicles; individual cells sometimes contain primitive slit-like vacuoles and are associated with abundant extravasated red blood cells. Conversely the epithelioid endothelial cells are admixed with the more spindled cells and, in other foci, line definite vascular channels (Fig. 10.17).[17,18] Significant nuclear pleomorphism is not a feature of either cell type. Mitotic activity rarely exceeds 1 mitotic figure per 10 high-power fields. The background stroma is loose to slightly myxoid with variable numbers of inflammatory cells, including eosinophils. The chondromyxoid-to-hyalinized stroma of epithelioid hemangioendothelioma is not observed. The diagnosis of epithelioid hemangioma and its distinction from hemangioendothelioma are controversial. To date, neither locally aggressive behavior nor distant metastases have been documented among this group of tumors.[17,18]

Fine Needle Aspiration Biopsy

FNAB is rarely diagnostic for hemangiomas of bone. Because most tumors are confined to bone with little or no cortical thinning, hemangiomas are not usually amenable to FNAB analysis. Cytologic smears consist mainly of blood. We have observed one example of epithelioid hemangioma diagnosed by FNAB. The diagnosis was based almost entirely on cell block material, however, allowing assessment of the histologic features described earlier.

Ancillary Studies

Ultrastructurally the endothelial cells contain Weibel-Palade bodies. As expected, the endothelial cells exhibit immunoexpression for CD31, CD34, and factor 8. Epithelioid hemangiomas commonly are positive for cytokeratin and epithelial membrane antigen, potentially confounding the diagnosis.[18]

Prognosis and Therapy

Conservative surgical therapy generally results in a cure. Larger lesions that are inaccessible to surgical resection may be treated by radiation therapy. Rare examples of hemangiomas progressing to angiosarcoma have been described.[19]

Angiomatosis

Angiomatosis is a benign vascular hemangiomatous condition characteristically involving a large segment of the body in a contiguous fashion, including skin, soft tissues, skeletal muscle, and bone. The process may be the result of either extensive involvement of multiple tissue types vertically (e.g., skin, subcutis, skeletal muscle, bone) or diffuse involvement of the same type of tissue (e.g., multiple skeletal muscles).[20] Most cases become clinically apparent during the first 2 decades of life. Females are affected slightly more commonly than males. The most common anatomic location is the lower extremities, but the process also may be observed in the upper extremities and trunk. Clinical complaints include soft tissue swelling with or without pain of the affected

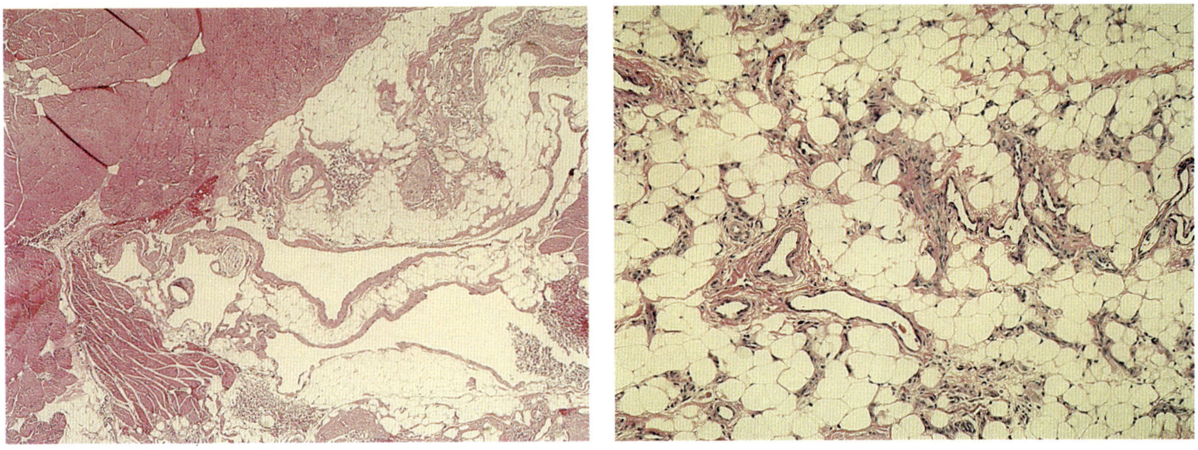

A B

FIGURE 10.18 Angiomatosis often is characterized by variably sized, ectatic vessels infiltrating subcutaneous adipose tissue and skeletal muscle (vertical extension). The endothelial cells lining these vascular spaces lack significant atypia. Clinicoradiographic correlation is needed to establish the diagnosis (**A** and **B**). (**A** and **B**, H&E.)

region; in some examples, the swelling waxes and wanes and may be worsened by physical activity. Hypertrophy or gigantism of an affected limb is seen rarely. Morphologically, variable mixtures of cavernous, venous, and capillary-type blood vessels diffusely infiltrating throughout involved soft tissues or bone characterize angiomatosis (Fig. 10.18).[20,21] Excess glomus cells sometimes are observed, in which case the process is referred to as *glomangiomatosis*. Local recurrences are seen in 90% of patients, likely resulting from the difficulties of surgical resection. Malignant transformation does not occur. For this reason, the type of surgical therapy employed should be balanced with the degree of morbidity resulting from the procedure.

Lymphangioma

Clinical Features

Lymphangiomas predominantly occur in young children and may be present at birth.[22] The most common anatomic location is the head and neck region, although involvement of the trunk or extremities is observed sometimes. Most patients complain of painless soft tissue swelling that, if palpable, is soft and fluctuant on physical examination. Rarely, lymphangioma is associated with Turner's syndrome.

Pathologic Findings

Histology

Lymphangiomas are multicystic-to-cavernous lesions consisting of large, dilated lymphatic vessels of varying sizes and shapes. The endothelial cell lining consists of bland-appearing, flattened endothelial cells. The fibrous septa separating the individual lymphatic channels are variably thickened and sometimes contain smooth muscle in their walls. Lymphoid aggregates are scattered among the dilated vessels. The luminal contents within the lymphatic vessels may be composed predominantly of proteinaceous fluid, aggregates of erythrocytes resembling hemangioma, or lymphocytes (Fig. 10.19).

Ancillary Studies

Immunohistochemistry is generally not required to establish a diagnosis. The lymphatic endothelium frequently shows expression of factor 8, CD31, and CD34, similar to that observed with vascular endothelium.[23] No reproducible cytogenetic abnormalities have been reported. Lymphangiomas of the neck sometimes are associated with Turner's syndrome, however.

Prognosis and Therapy

Surgical resection usually results in cure. Incompletely excised lesions may locally recur. Malignant transformation of lymphangioma has not been documented definitively.

Epithelioid Hemangioendothelioma

Clinical Features

Epithelioid hemangioendothelioma is a rare vascular tumor that may arise within soft tissue, bone, liver, or lung.[24–27] This discussion concentrates on the musculoskeletal forms. Within soft tissues, epithelioid hemangioendothelioma may be observed at any age; most patients are middle-aged or

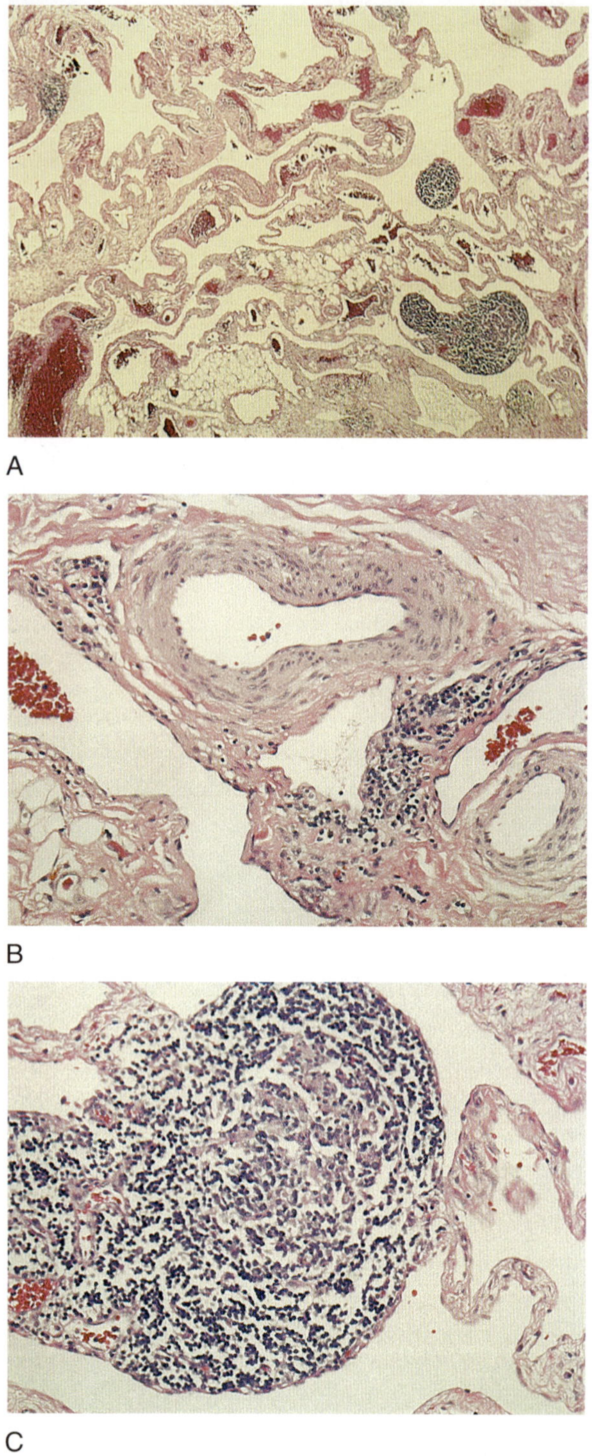

FIGURE 10.19 Lymphangiomas are composed of variably sized vascular channels that may contain blood, proteinaceous material, or lymphocytes **(A)**. The blood vessel walls range from thin strands of fibrous tissue to thick, muscular-walled forms **(B)**. Aggregates of lymphocytes typically are seen throughout the lesion, within the blood vessel lumens and on their walls **(C)**. (**A-C**, H&E.)

older adults. Children rarely are affected. There seems to be no gender bias. The extremities, especially the lower extremities, are involved most commonly followed by the head and neck and trunk regions.[24,25] Epithelioid hemangioendothelioma may arise in deep soft tissues, subcutaneous adipose tissue, or dermal sites. Among subcutaneous or deep soft tissue cases, 50% appear to originate from a blood vessel, usually a vein. Complaints of soft tissue swelling, sometimes accompanied by pain, are typical.

When epithelioid hemangioendothelioma arises in bone, there is a tendency for the disease to occur in younger patients, the peak incidence being between 10 and 40 years of age.[26] Similar to epithelioid hemangioepithelioma of soft tissues, there is no sex predilection. Most cases involve the lower extremity, especially the pelvis and femur (Fig. 10.20). Multicentric tumors involving a single bone or anatomic area are observed in 50% of patients; conversely, multicentric lesions are rare in soft tissue epithelioid hemangioendothelioma. Localized pain is the most common complaint. Radiographically, epithelioid hemangioepitheliomas are usually lytic and poorly marginated and show varying degrees of cortical expansion and destruction.[26] Periosteal reaction is rare, but surrounding sclerosis commonly is seen. Soft tissue extension is present in less than half of cases.

Pathologic Findings

Histology

With the exception of origin from a pre-existing blood vessel, the histologic features of soft tissue hemangioendothelioma are largely similar to those observed in primary bone tumors. Epithelioid endothelial cells proliferate as cords, strands, or nests of mostly round-to-cuboidal, epithelioid-appearing tumor cells containing ovoid-to-round, mostly uniform nuclei and abundant eosinophilic cytoplasm. Although easily overlooked, cytoplasmic vacuolation, which indicates primitive vascular differentiation, is present in all cases. Some of the cytoplasmic vacuoles contain a single erythrocyte (Fig. 10.21). In other cells, the cytoplasmic vacuole may be sufficiently large so as to displace the nucleus peripherally, creating a signet-ring cell appearance. The background stroma is typically loose and appears lightly basophilic myxoid to myxochondroid. Well-formed vascular channels, as observed in epithelioid hemangioma, are seen rarely and are always focal in epithelioid hemangioendothelioma. Significant nuclear pleomorphism may be present as small foci in epithelioid hemangioendothelioma, but, if prominent and seen as solid sheets, the diagnosis of epithelioid angiosarcoma more appropriately is rendered (Fig. 10.22).[25] Mitotic figures are usually less than 2 per 10 high-power fields. Metaplastic bone may be observed in soft tissue and osseous forms.

Fine Needle Aspiration Biopsy

Cytologic smears of epithelial hemangioendothelioma are generally hypercellular and composed of mostly single cells and small aggregates of ovoid to polygonal-shaped epithelioid cells. Although nuclear pleomorphism and significant atypia generally are not features of epithelioid hemangioendothe-

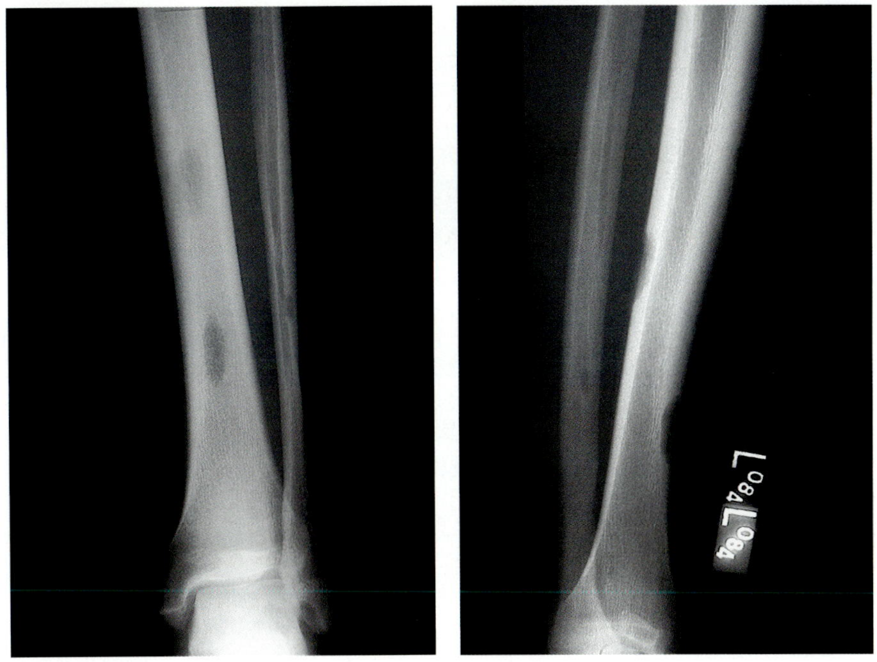

A B

FIGURE 10.20 Epithelioid hemangioendothelioma. Anteroposterior **(A)** and lateral **(B)** radiographs of the distal tibia show two well-demarcated lytic lesions in the distal tibia and one in the fibula. The areas of bone lysis are primarily cortical in location. No periosteal new bone production or matrix calcification is present.

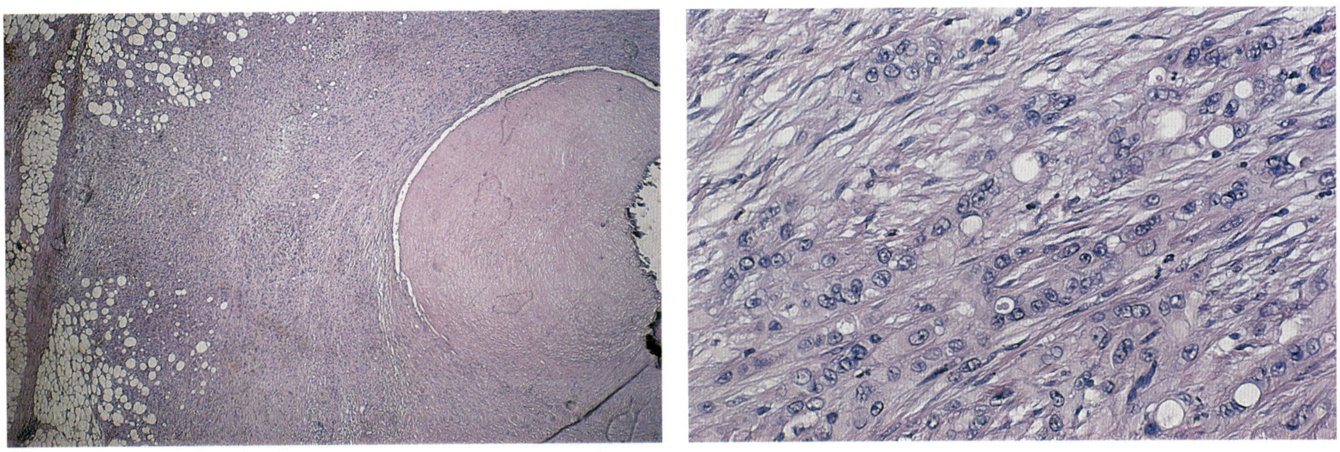

A B

FIGURE 10.21 Epithelioid hemangioendothelioma often originates from the wall of a large blood vessel **(A)**. At high power, the tumor classically is composed of infiltrating nests and single-file cords of tumor cells that may resemble a lobular carcinoma of the breast. The background stroma appears slightly myxoid. Individual cells exhibit cytoplasmic vacuoles sometimes containing erythrocytes **(B)**. (**A** and **B**, H&E.)

lioma, the nuclei show significant variability, ranging from ovoid and reniform to round and polylobated, surrounded by an abundant amount of dense cytoplasm. Binucleated epithelioid cells are seen frequently (Fig. 10.23).[28] Rarely the neoplastic cells contain a single, sharply demarcated intracytoplasmic vacuole, representing primitive vascular differentiation (Fig. 10.24). Nuclear cytoplasmic pseudoinclusions also are observed rarely (Fig. 10.25).[28] In Romanowsky preparations, the myxohyalinized-to-myxochondroid stroma appears as metachromatic stromal fragments. Because of significant morphologic overlap with epithelioid sarcoma and metastatic carcinoma, establishing a diagnosis of epithelioid hemangioendothelioma by FNAB requires ancillary studies, principally immunohistochemistry.

Ancillary Studies

Ultrastructurally the neoplastic cells are surrounded by a variably thickened basal lamina with numerous pinocytotic vesicles and scattered Weibel-Palade bodies. Small microvilli or cytoplasmic flaps, mimicking the luminal surface of normal endothelium, line the intracytoplasmic vacuoles.[24]

The neoplastic cells of epithelioid hemangioendothelioma generally express CD31, CD34, and factor 8. At least focal cytokeratin positivity may be observed in 20% to 30% of cases.[25,26] Almost 50% of cases show focal immunoexpression of α smooth muscle actin.[25] S-100 protein and desmin are uniformly negative. Although data are limited to two cases, cytogenetic analysis has revealed a unique chromosomal

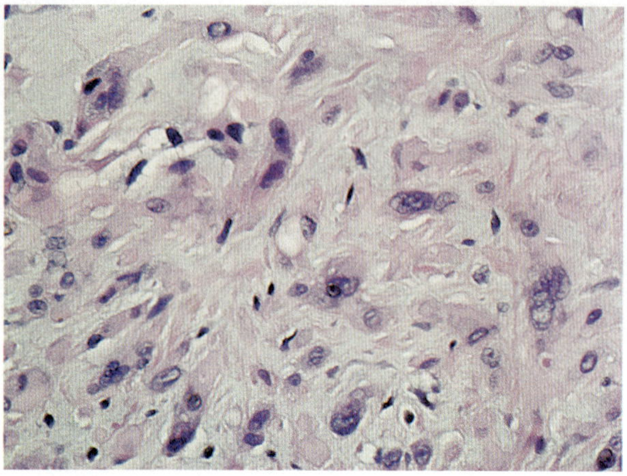

FIGURE 10.22 Less frequently, epithelioid hemangioendothelioma may show focal areas of atypia. (H&E.)

translocation, t(1;3)(p36.3;q25), that may be specific for epithelioid hemangioendothelioma.[29]

Prognosis and Therapy

The prognosis of epithelioid hemangioendothelioma should be considered intermediate (but definitely malignant) between that of hemangiomas and angiosarcoma. There is no clear association, however, between histologic features and clinical outcome. In patients with bone lesions, concomitant involvement of visceral organs is a poor prognostic sign.[26] Local recurrence occurs in approximately 10% to 15% of patients; distant metastases have been reported in approximately 20% to 25% of patients.[24,25] Death occurs in 15% to 20% of patients, regardless of anatomic site (e.g., bone versus

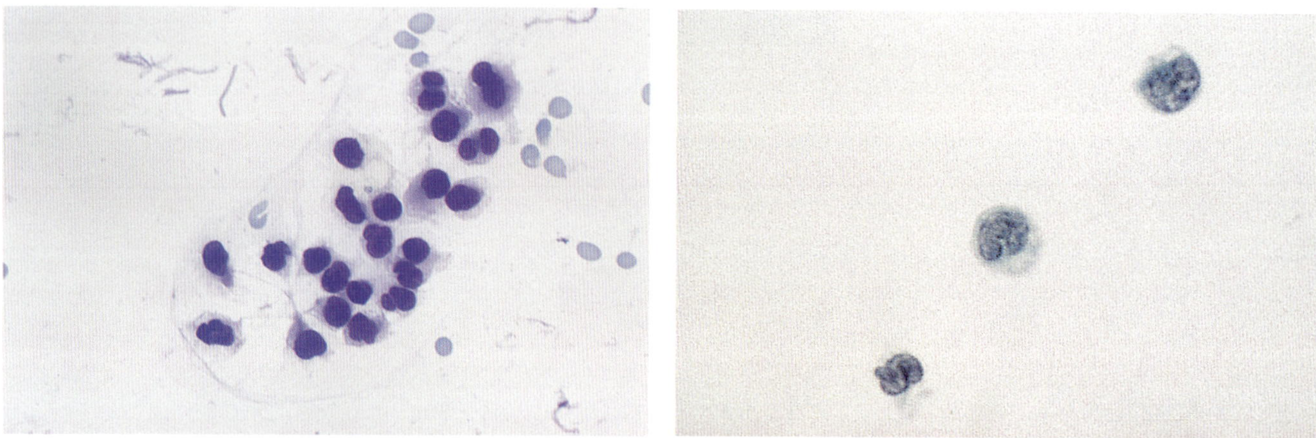

A B

FIGURE 10.23 Fine needle aspiration biopsy of epithelioid hemangioendothelioma typically yields hypercellular smears composed of discohesive cells. Although the neoplastic cells do not show marked nuclear pleomorphism, individual cells exhibit significant nuclear variation, ranging from ovoid and reniform to lobulated and binucleated forms (**A** and **B**). (**A,** Diff-Quik; **B,** Papanicolaou.)

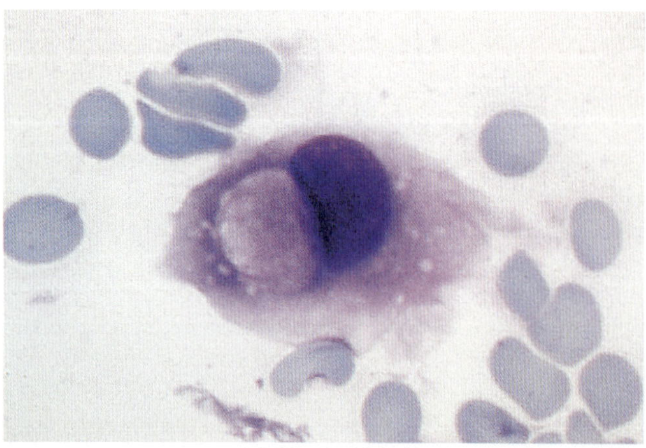

FIGURE 10.24 Primitive vascular differentiation in the form of a single large intracytoplasmic vacuole is observed rarely in cytologic smears of epithelioid hemangioendothelioma. (Diff-Quik.)

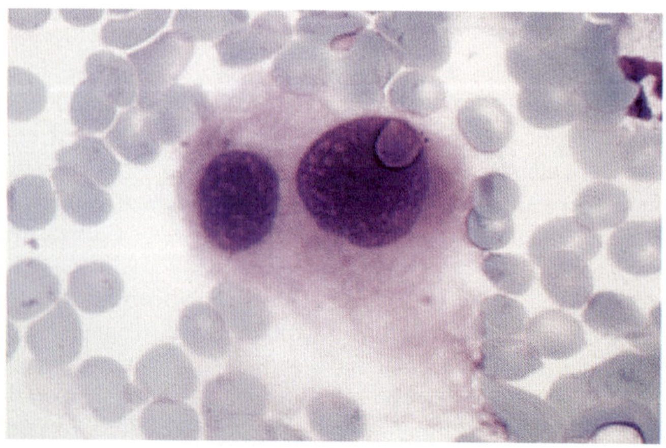

FIGURE 10.25 Intranuclear cytoplasmic pseudoinclusions are seen rarely in epithelioid hemangioendothelioma. (Diff-Quik.)

soft tissue).[24–26] Wide surgical resection is the therapy of choice. Radiation therapy may be used for surgically inaccessible lesions or multicentric tumors. The role of chemotherapy is unclear.

Retiform Hemangioendothelioma

Retiform hemangioendothelioma, also called *hobnail hemangioendothelioma,* is a rare low-grade vascular neoplasm. We believe that papillary intralymphatic angioendothelioma (Dabska's tumor) and retiform hemangioendothelioma are a spectrum of a similar entity. Retiform hemangioendothelioma occurs predominantly in children and young adults. The superficial soft tissues of the distal extremities, especially the lower limb, are affected most frequently. Clinically, patients present with slow-growing, exophytic or plaque-like cutaneous or subcutaneous soft tissue lesions.[30] Cardinal histologic features include arborizing vascular channels, resembling the rete testis, lined by a mostly uniform-appearing population of endothelial cells with protuberant nuclei, imparting a "hobnail" appearance. Individual endothelial cells have high nuclear-to-cytoplasmic ratios with scanty cytoplasm. Immediately surrounding the arborizing blood vessels, the stroma appears fibrotic and may contain a prominent lymphoid infiltrate (Fig. 10.26). Less frequently, retiform hemangioendothelioma displays prominent intraluminal papillae with hyalinized cores, identical to that described in papillary intralymphatic angioendothelioma (Fig. 10.27).[30] The endothelial cells express the usual vascular markers, including CD31, CD34, and factor 8. Wide surgical resection is the therapy of choice. Less than complete excision leads to local recurrence in most cases. Although metastasis to a regional lymph node has been described in a single case, distant metastases have not been reported, and no patients have died of the disease.[30]

Kaposiform Hemangioendothelioma

Kaposiform hemangioendothelioma is a rare low-grade malignant vascular neoplasm closely resembling Kaposi's sarcoma.[31] Most examples occur in infancy and childhood; adults are affected rarely.[32] Although a variety of anatomic locations have been reported, the skin and the retroperitoneum are the most common anatomic sites. Clinical symptoms relate to the anatomic location of origin. Tumors arising in the retroperitoneum may be associated with mass effect, ascites, or jaundice. Cutaneous lesions produce ill-defined plaques. Histologically, kaposiform hemangioendothelioma shows a distinct lobular or nodular architecture of densely packed, spindle-shaped tumor cells, many of which contain slit-like vascular lumina. Nuclear atypia is minimal. Mitotic activity tends to be rare. Intermingled with the spindle cells are numerous capillaries, often containing fibrin thrombi.[32]

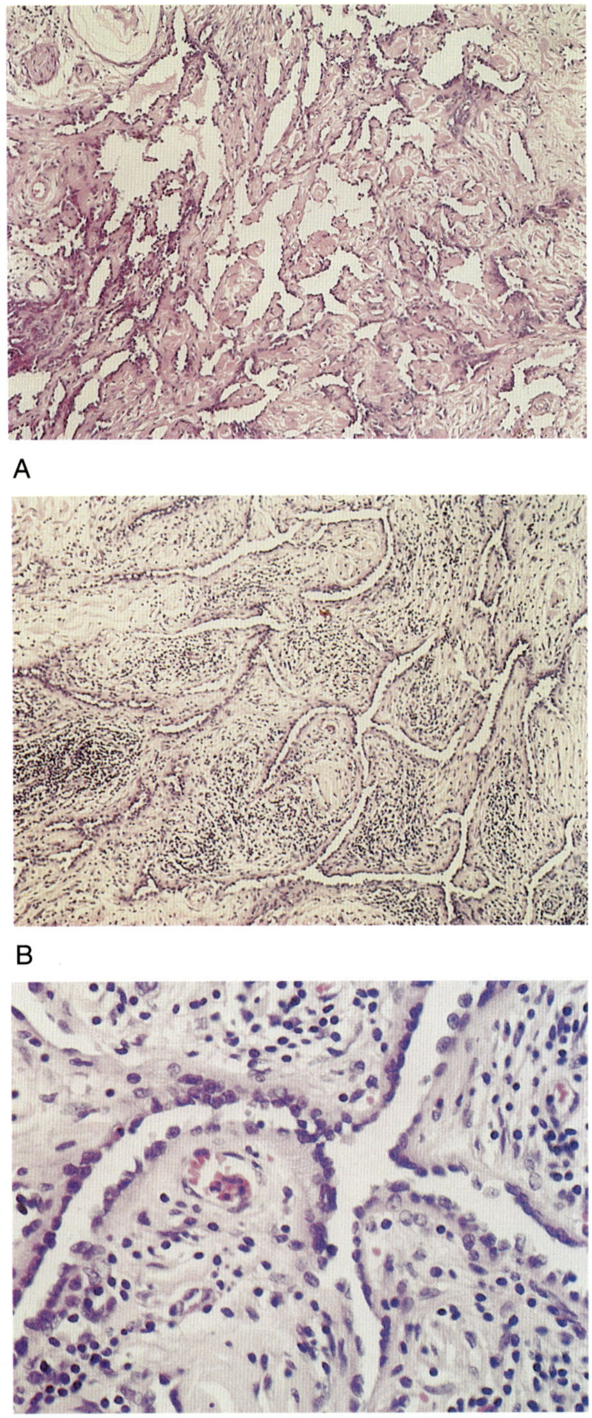

A

B

C

FIGURE 10.26 Retiform hemangioendothelioma is a rare neoplasm of superficial soft tissues characterized by an arborizing vascular proliferation resembling the rete testis. A uniform population of "hobnail" endothelial cells with high nuclear-to-cytoplasmic ratios lines these blood vessels. The stroma immediately surrounding the blood vessels often contains a lymphocytic infiltrate **(A-C)**. (**A** and **B**, low power, H&E; **C**, high power, H&E.)

Immunohistochemically the tumor cells are usually negative for factor 8 and show only focal positivity for CD34 and CD31. Overall, the prognosis depends on the extent of the disease and the anatomic site. Large intra-abdominal tumors arising in infancy and complicated by Kasabach-Merritt

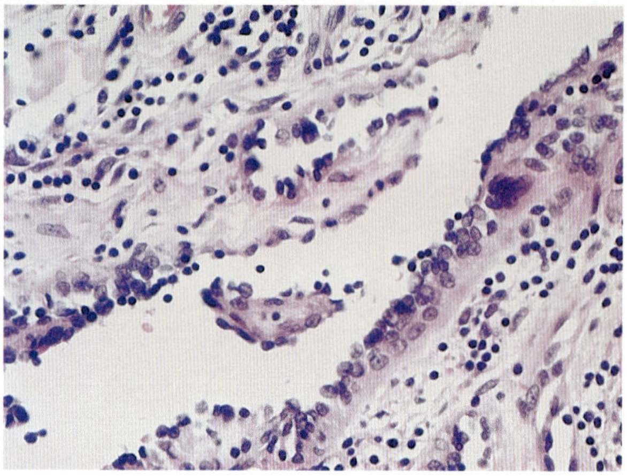

FIGURE 10.27 Retiform hemangioendothelioma may exhibit intravascular papillary tufts, evidence of a close relationship or spectrum with Dabska's tumor. (H&E.)

syndrome have a poor prognosis. Superficially located lesions are usually curable by complete resection. Kaposiform hemangioendothelioma does not spontaneously regress. Distant metastases do not occur.[31]

Kaposi's Sarcoma

Clinical Features

Kaposi's sarcoma is a locally aggressive vascular neoplasm that exists as four different clinical forms—classic indolent, African endemic, iatrogenic, and acquired immunodeficiency syndrome (AIDS)–associated types.[33–35] In most cases, the skin is involved, but lymph nodes, mucosal membranes, or visceral organs may be affected during the course of the disease. Involvement of viscera may be asymptomatic.

The classic indolent type of Kaposi's sarcoma is rare but especially prevalent among Ashkenazi Jews and patients of Mediterranean descent, affecting men more often than women. Most of these patients are older than age 50 at diagnosis.[35] The disease is characterized by the presence of red-purple plaques, macules, or nodules that have a predilection for the lower extremities. In one third of patients, a second malignancy, usually lymphoma, complicates the clinical picture.

In contrast to the classic subtype, the endemic form of Kaposi's sarcoma is relatively common in blacks from equatorial Africa. Affected individuals tend to be younger, and the disease is more aggressive. In younger children, lymph node involvement is frequently extensive and unassociated with cutaneous lesions. This disease is often rapidly fatal.

Iatrogenic Kaposi's sarcoma is also more common than the classic form. It may occur a few months to years after solid organ transplantation or intense immunosuppressive therapy. Cessation of immunosuppressive therapy sometimes results in resolution of the lesions.[33]

AIDS-related Kaposi's sarcoma is one of the most aggressive forms of the disease, predominantly affecting young, homosexual men. The skin lesions may be widely disseminated but tend to involve the face, genitalia, and lower extremities. Extensive involvement of lymph nodes, viscera, and mucous membranes, particularly in the gastrointestinal tract, is observed frequently.[34]

Pathologic Findings

Histology

Regardless of clinical subtype, the morphologic features of Kaposi's sarcoma are similar. In the early patch stage, increased, irregular, and thin-walled vascular spaces appear to dissect through the dermis with a predilection toward preexisting vascular spaces and adnexal structures. Individual endothelial cells show little or no atypia. The background stroma shows variable numbers of lymphocytes, plasma cells, and hemosiderin pigment deposition (Fig. 10.28). In the plague stage of Kaposi's sarcoma, all of the aforementioned features become more pronounced with involvement of the entire dermis and upper subcutaneous adipose tissue. The vascular proliferation is more prominent, and increasing numbers of inflammatory cells are observed. Eosinophilic hyaline globules may be prominent. The nodular stage is characterized by solid-appearing nodules of uniform spindled cells arranged in interweaving fascicles and displaying slit-like clefts containing red blood cells.[34] Intracellular and extracellular hyaline globules are observed (Fig. 10.29). Ectatic vascular spaces often are seen peripherally.

Fine Needle Aspiration Biopsy

FNAB of Kapsosi's sarcoma usually yields loosely cohesive clusters of bland-appearing spindled cells.[36] Individual cells have elongated nuclei, inconspicuous nucleoli, and ill-defined cytoplasmic borders. Hemosiderin pigment deposition may be observed. Variable numbers of plasma cells and lymphocytes are within the background. Overall the cytologic features are nonspecific and bear a strong resemblance to granulation tissue. Ancillary studies are required for definitive diagnosis.

Ancillary Studies

The vascular spaces show positivity for the typical vascular markers, including CD31, CD34, and factor 8. FLI-1, a nuclear transcription factor, also is expressed in most cases.[37] The spindle cells show diffuse positivity for CD34 but are negative for factor 8. No reproducible cytogenetic abnormalities have been discovered in Kaposi's sarcoma. The causative agent, present in all forms of the disease, is human herpesvirus 8.[38]

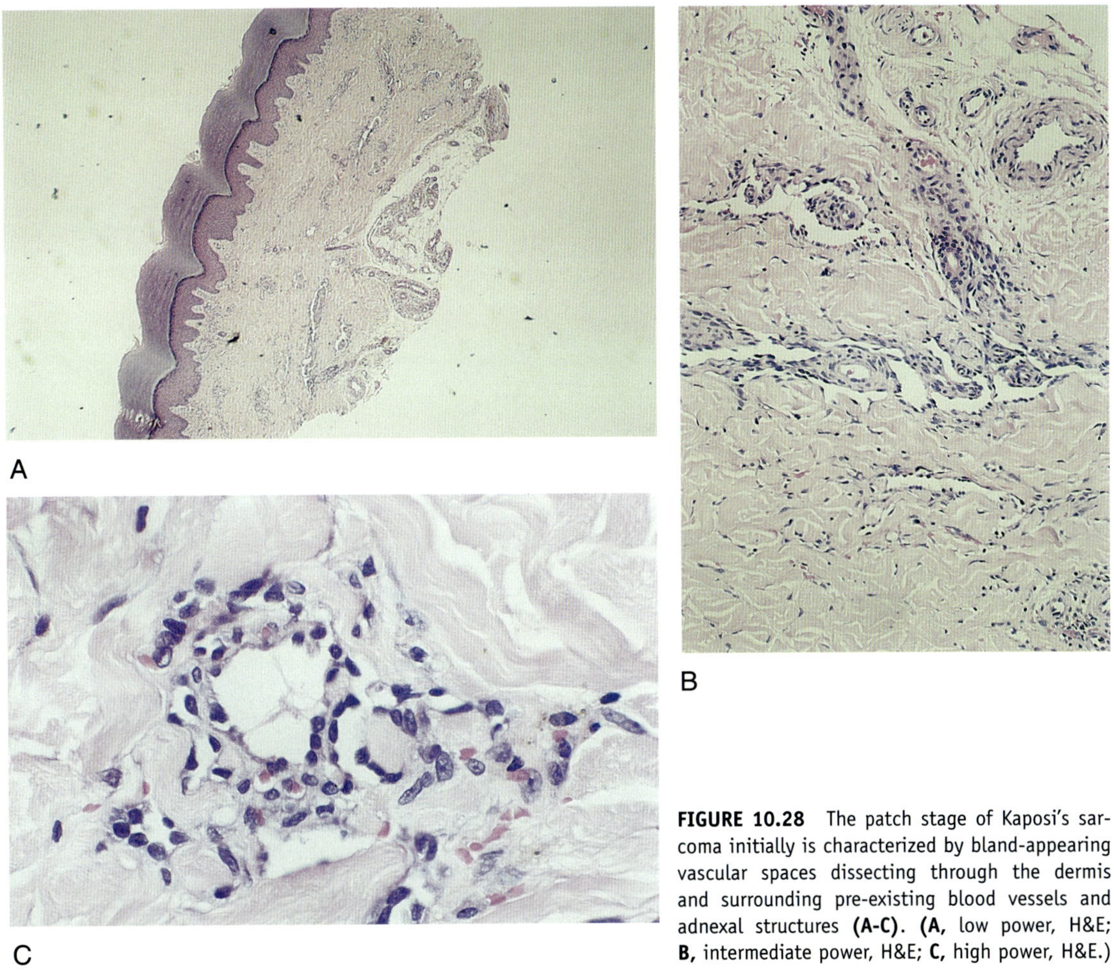

FIGURE 10.28 The patch stage of Kaposi's sarcoma initially is characterized by bland-appearing vascular spaces dissecting through the dermis and surrounding pre-existing blood vessels and adnexal structures **(A-C)**. (**A,** low power, H&E; **B,** intermediate power, H&E; **C,** high power, H&E.)

Prognosis and Therapy

As mentioned previously, the prognosis largely depends on the type of Kaposi's sarcoma and the extent of disease. Widespread visceral involvement is generally a poor prognostic sign. Among cases of classic Kaposi's sarcoma, older age (>50 years old) and immunosuppression are associated with poor clinical outcome.[35] Local excision, radiation therapy, and chemotherapy all may be employed depending on the extent of the disease.

Angiosarcoma

Clinical Features

In contrast to most sarcomas, angiosarcomas most often arise in the skin with a predilection for the head and neck region. Other common sites include the breast, liver, spleen, and bone.[39–41] Angiosarcoma arising in the deep soft tissue or the retroperitoneum is a relatively rare event. In contrast to the cutaneous form, angiosarcomas of soft tissues are observed most frequently in the extremities, especially the thigh, followed by the trunk and head and neck. Within the skeleton, angiosarcomas show a wide distribution; the extremity long bones and the spine are probably the most common skeletal locations. Among all musculoskeletal forms, 22% of skeletal and 6% of deep soft tissue tumors are multicentric, generally within the same bone, extremity, or anatomic location.[39,40] Angiosarcomas occurring in skin or soft tissue typically involve elderly patients but may be seen over a wide age distribution. Males are affected slightly more often than females. Skeletal angiosarcomas show no obvious peak age range or gender bias. Soft tissue swelling, sometimes associated with pain, is reported by most patients with angiosarcoma of soft tissue, whereas patients with skeletal forms virtually always have localized pain with or without a concomitant soft tissue mass.

Radiographically, angiosarcomas within the skeleton are generally purely lytic lesions with poor margination. Extension into soft tissues is observed with higher grade tumors. Angiosarcomas may arise as a complication of radiation therapy or severe lymphedema of the extremities, observed frequently in the past after radical mastectomies.[41]

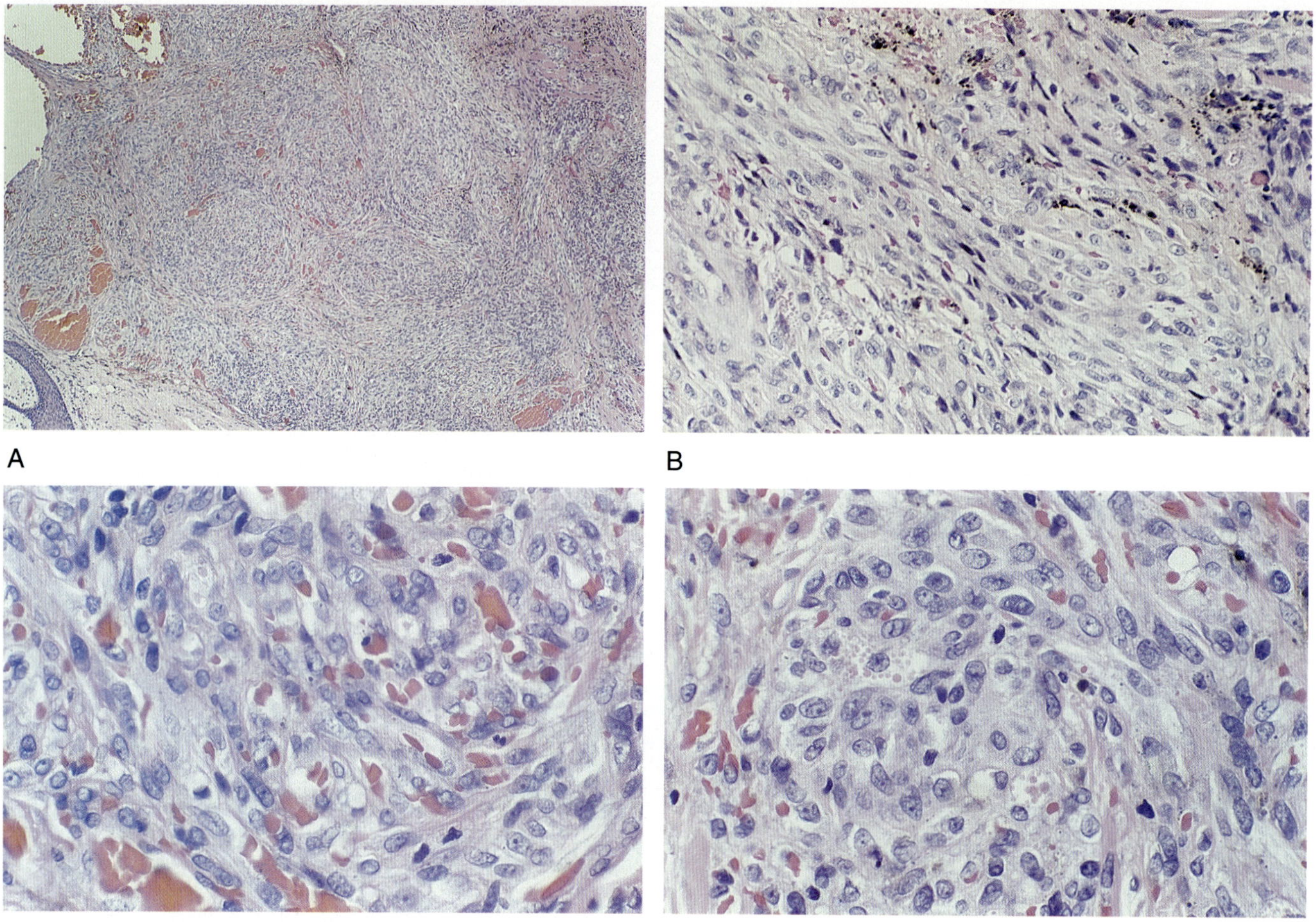

A B C D

FIGURE 10.29 The nodular stage of Kaposi's sarcoma exhibits a solid proliferation of uniform-appearing spindled cells arranged in nests and fascicles and containing slit-like vascular spaces **(A-C)**. Extraintracellular and intracellular hyaline globules are frequently present **(D)**. **(A,** low power, H&E; **B,** intermediate power, H&E; **C,** high power, H&E; **D,** high power, H&E.)

Pathologic Findings

Histology

Regardless of anatomic site, angiosarcoma shows considerable morphologic variability, ranging from well-differentiated tumors forming obvious vascular channels to poorly differentiated epithelioid lesions resembling carcinoma. Most angiosarcomas are high-grade neoplasms. Among cutaneous lesions, angiosarcomas typically show intersecting and gaping vascular channels dissecting dermal collagen, freely communicating with one another, and surrounding pre-existing adnexal structures. Nuclear atypia is minimal to moderate in the endothelial cells (Fig. 10.30). Conversely, angiosarcomas of deep soft tissue are more often epithelioid, arranged in nests, sheets, papillae, or gaping, irregular vascular structures (Figs. 10.31 and 10.32).[39] Abundant reactive-appearing bone rimmed by osteoblasts, most often at the outer edges of the tumor, may confound the diagnosis of skeletal angiosarcoma. Hemorrhage is a consistent feature in all angiosarcomas and may be so extensive as to suggest hematoma.

Fine Needle Aspiration Biopsy

The cytologic features of angiosarcoma are nonspecific, but most tumors appear obviously malignant with moderate-to-marked nuclear pleomorphism.[42,43] Individual cells are seen singly and in solitary clusters, ranging from predominantly spindled to epithelioid. Nuclei are round to ovoid with scant-to-moderate amounts of dense-to-vacuolated cytoplasm; nucleoli are often prominent. Definite vascular differentiation is not usually evident. Inflammatory cells, primarily neutrophils, may dominate the background. A helpful diagnostic clue is the presence of intracytoplasmic hemosiderin deposits or red blood cells.[43] Nevertheless, definitive diagnosis virtually always requires ancillary studies.

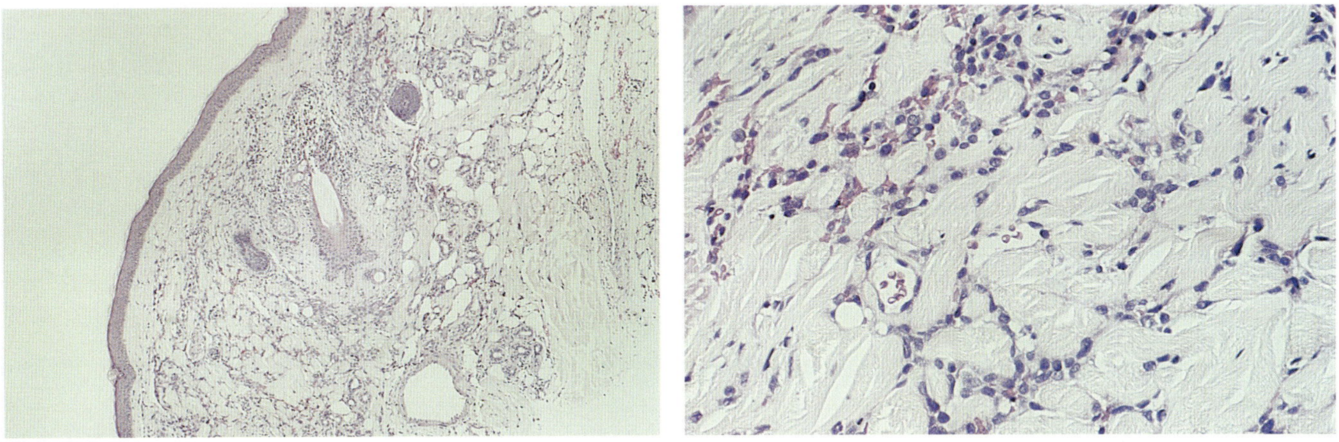

A B

FIGURE 10.30 Intersecting and anastomosing vascular channels characterize cutaneous angiosarcoma. The neoplastic endothelial cells have high nuclear-to-cytoplasmic ratios, appear hyperchromatic, and show mild-to-moderate nuclear pleomorphism **(A** and **B)**. **(A,** low power, H&E; **B,** high power, H&E.)

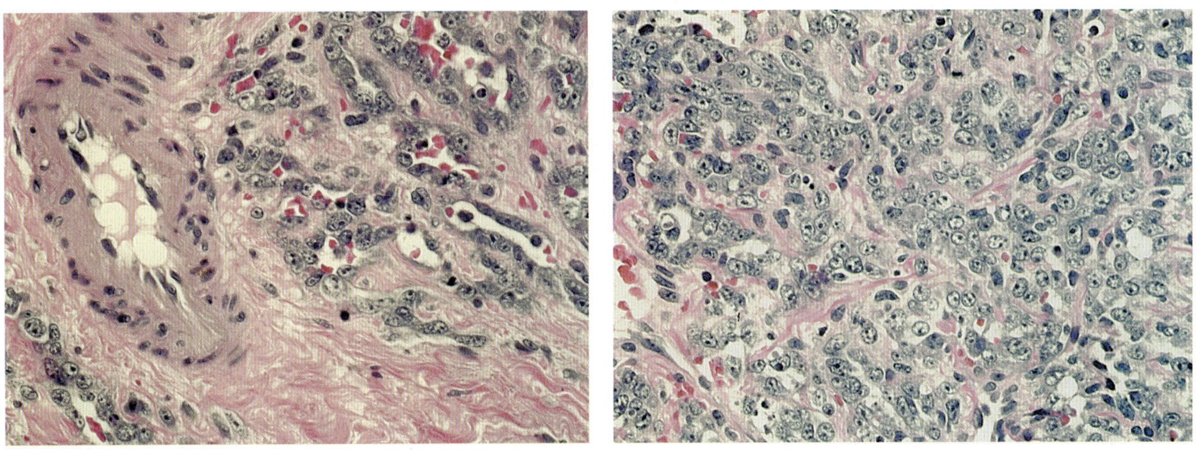

A B

FIGURE 10.31 When angiosarcoma arises in deep soft tissues, the neoplastic cells generally appear more epithelioid and are arranged in nests and gaping vascular channels **(A** and **B)**. (**A** and **B,** H&E.)

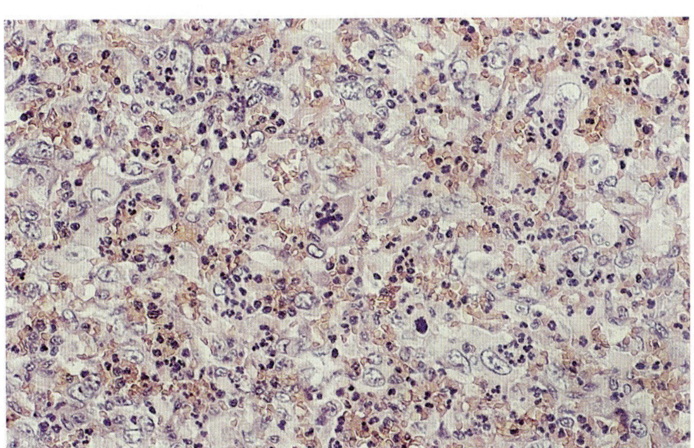

FIGURE 10.32 Poorly differentiated epithelioid angiosarcoma with abundant stromal hemorrhage but lacking obvious vascular differentiation. These cases require ancillary studies for definitive diagnosis. (H&E.)

Ancillary Studies

Ultrastructurally the malignant endothelial cells rarely show the characteristic Weibel-Palade bodies. Abundant intermediate filaments and surface pinocytotic vesicles are characteristic.

Virtually all angiosarcomas show positivity for vimentin and at least one vascular marker, CD31, CD34, or factor 8. Up to 35% of cases, especially more epithelioid forms, are positive for cytokeratin. A pericytic component, when present, expresses smooth muscle actin. Epithelial membrane antigen, S-100 protein, and HMB 45 are uniformly negative.[39] A subset of angiosarcomas shows CD117 (*c-kit*) immunoexpression but is not associated with mutations of the tyrosine kinase domains of the *c-kit* gene.[44]

No reproducible cytogenetic abnormalities have been identified in angiosarcoma. Most studies have revealed nonspecific complex karyotypes.[45,46]

Prognosis and Therapy

Angiosarcomas are typically high-grade lesions that behave in an aggressive manner. Adverse prognostic indicators include older age, large tumor size, and localization in the retroperitoneum.[39] Local recurrences occur in 20% to 60% of patients; distant metastases, mostly to the lung, liver, lymph nodes, and bone, are observed in 40% to 50% of cases. Studies with prolonged follow-ups have shown 50% to 60% of patients die of the disease.[39,40] Wide surgical resection combined with radiation therapy offers the best chance for local control.[40] The role of chemotherapy is unclear; most studies have not shown a definite survival benefit.[47]

Glomus Tumor

Clinical Features

Glomus tumors are relatively rare lesions, occurring most commonly in the skin and superficial soft tissues of the distal extremities, especially the subungual region.[48,49] Up to 10% of patients may have multiple lesions. Rare anatomic sites include bone, particularly phalanges; stomach; mediastinum; and lung.[50,51] The peak incidence is the third to fifth decades of life. In the subungual region, glomus tumors are observed more frequently in women; elsewhere, there is no gender bias.[49] Superficial lesions usually appear as small, red-purple to blue nodules, often associated with pain that is sharp, paroxysmal, or radiating in nature. Deeply seated tumors may be asymptomatic. Malignant lesions are more likely to be larger (>2 cm) and localized in deep soft tissues.[49]

Tumors in soft tissues may erode the underlying bone. Radiographically, intraosseous lesions are generally lytic and well marginated and may show a marginal sclerotic rim (Fig. 10.33).[50]

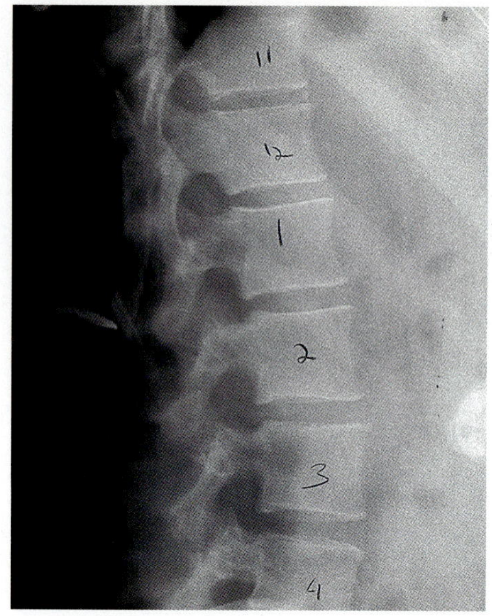

FIGURE 10.33 Glomus tumor. A lateral radiograph of the spine reveals a lytic lesion in the L1 pedicle. The lesion is sharply defined.

Pathologic Findings

Histology

Classic glomus tumors are composed of solid sheets and cords of uniform-appearing rounded cells, often forming collars around scattered capillary-sized blood vessels. Individual nuclei are regular, round to ovoid, centrally placed, with small nucleoli and abundant dense-to-eosinophilic cytoplasm. Mitotic figures rarely are seen. The background stroma often shows hyalinization and myxoid changes (Fig. 10.34). Glomangiomas essentially are a combination of cavernous hemangioma and glomus tumor (Fig. 10.35). Glomangiomyomas, the least common form of glomus tumor, are characterized by the presence of transitional areas of smooth muscle differentiation.

Folpe and colleagues[49] provided clinical and pathologic criteria for defining malignancy in glomus tumors (Table 10.4). The diagnosis of malignant glomus tumor should be rendered only for tumors that are deeply seated and large (>2 cm), contain atypical mitotic figures, or show moderate-to-marked nuclear atypia with any level of mitotic activity. The malignant component may resemble leiomyosarcoma or be composed of sheets of obviously malignant round tumor cells. The authors also defined *glomus tumor of uncertain malignant potential* as having at least one of the aforementioned atypical features (not including nuclear atypia) but not completely fulfilling the criteria for malignancy.[49] *Symplastic glomus tumor* is an otherwise typical glomus tumor with prominent nuclear atypia but no other malignant features.

Fine Needle Aspiration Biopsy

FNAB of glomus tumor has been reported only rarely.[52] Cytologic smears are cellular and composed of clusters of uniform, round-to-ovoid tumor cells, often admixed with metachromatic stromal material. Individual nuclei are round to ovoid with variable amounts of dense cytoplasm. In the appropriate clinical context, a diagnosis can be rendered by FNAB.[52]

Ancillary Studies

Ultrastructurally, glomus tumors show features of pericytes, including prominent external lamina; intracytoplasmic thin filaments; and short, interdigitating cell processes.[53] All glomus tumors show immunoexpression of vimentin and smooth muscle actin. Most also appear positive for caldesmon. Less frequently, positivity for desmin and CD34 is

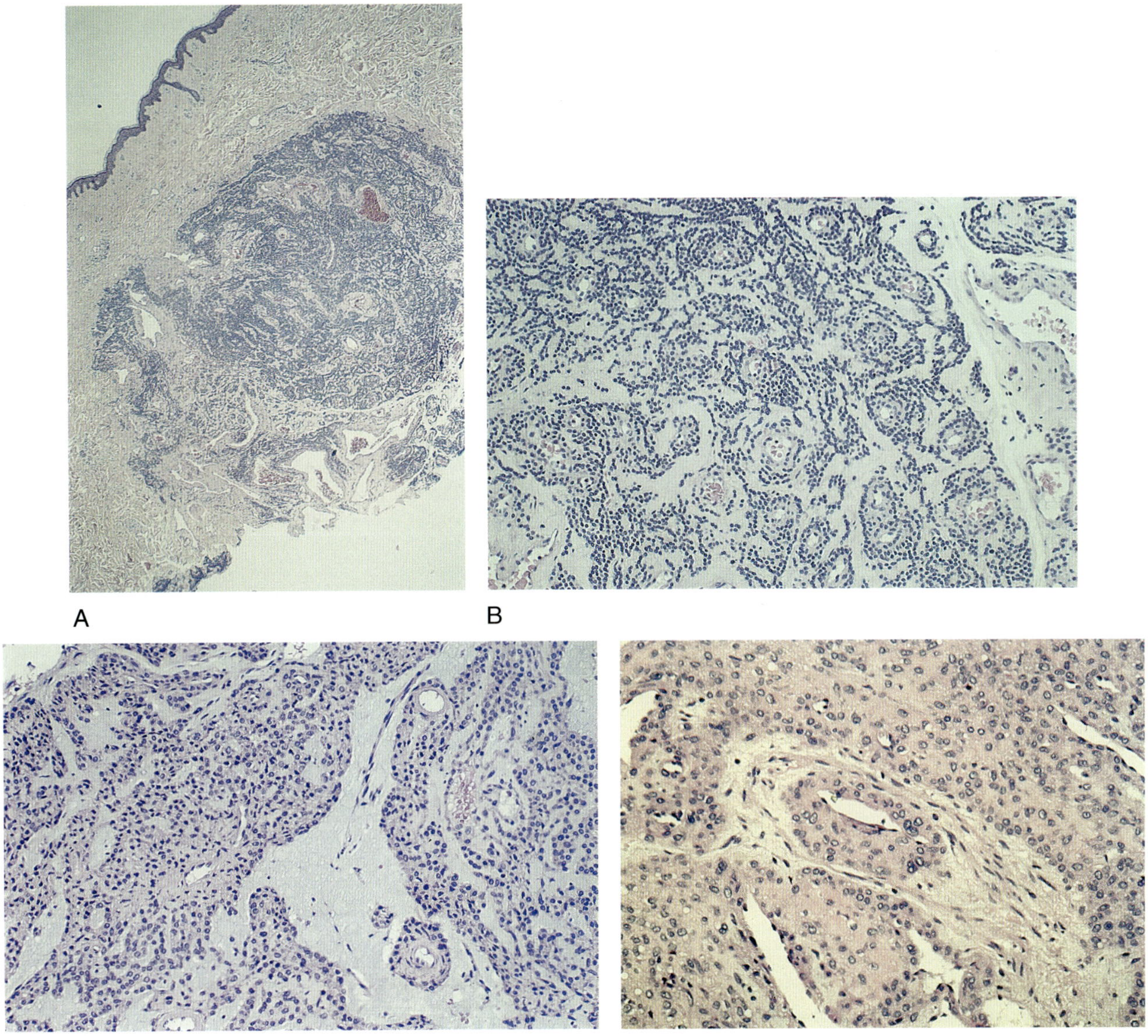

A B C D

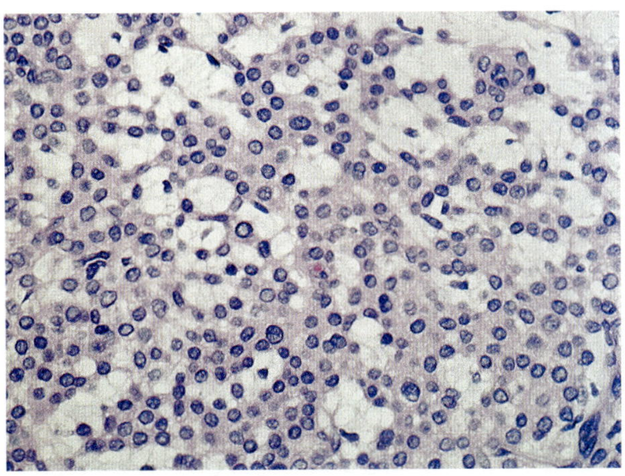

E

FIGURE 10.34 Glomus tumors usually are superficially located and well-circumscribed lesions, most often involving the distal extremities **(A)**. The neoplastic cells are arranged in nests, sheets, and cords, often forming collars around small blood vessels. The background stroma appears myxoid. Cytologically, individual cells typically appear remarkably uniform with round-to-ovoid nuclei and scant-to-abundant eosinophilic cytoplasm **(B-E)**. **(A,** H&E; **B** and **C,** low power, H&E; **D,** intermediate power, H&E; **E,** high power, H&E.)

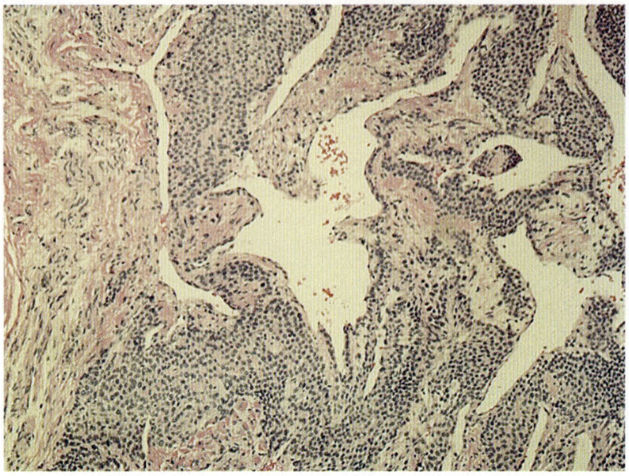

FIGURE 10.35 Glomangiomas are glomus tumors associated with dilated, cavernous blood vessels. The diagnosis may be missed if a closer inspection of the glomus cells immediately surrounding the blood vessels is not done. (H&E.)

TABLE 10.4 Criteria for Malignancy (and Atypical Features) in Glomus Tumors

Malignant Glomus Tumor	Glomus Tumor of Uncertain Malignant Potential
>2 cm and deep	>2 cm *only*
or	*or*
Atypical mitotic figures	Deep location *only*
or	*or*
Moderate to high nuclear grade and ≥5 mitoses/50 HPF	Superficial location and ≥5 mitoses/50 HPF
Symplastic Glomus Tumor	
Only high nuclear grade	

HPF, high-power fields.
Based on the results of Folpe AL, Fanburg-Smith JC, Miettinen M, et al: Atypical and malignant glomus tumors: Analysis of 52 cases, with a proposal for the reclassification of glomus tumors. Am J Surg Pathol 2001;25:1.

observed. The neoplastic cells appear uniformly negative for S-100 protein and cytokeratin.[49]

No reproducible cytogenetic abnormality has been discovered for glomus tumors. An autosomal dominant inheritance pattern with a link to chromosome 1p has been reported for multiple familial examples.[54] An association with neurofibromatosis 1 also has been documented.[55]

Prognosis and Therapy

Glomus tumors usually are cured by simple excision or, for bone lesions, curettage. Local recurrence rarely is seen. Using the definition provided by Folpe and colleagues,[49] lesions fulfilling the criteria for malignancy develop metastases in approximately 38% of patients. In Folpe and colleagues'[49] series, metastatic disease was not observed in symplastic glomus tumors or glomus tumors of uncertain malignant potential.

REFERENCES

Hemangioma and Variants

1. Gonzalez-Crussi F, Reyes-Mugica M: Cellular hemangiomas ("hemangioendotheliomas") in infants: Light microscopic, immunohistochemical, and ultrastructural observations. Am J Surg Pathol 1991;15:769.
2. Pysyk KA, Grabb WC, Cherry GW: Cellular hemangiomas: Light and electron microscopic studies of two cases. Virchows Arch A Pathol Anat Histol 1982;396:103.
3. North PE, Waner M, Mizeracki A, et al: GLUT1: A newly discovered immunohistochemical marker for juvenile hemangioendotheliomas. Hum Pathol 2000;31:11.
4. Berg JN, Walter JW, Thisanagayam U, et al: Evidence of loss of heterozygosity of 5q in sporadic haemangiomas: Are somatic mutations involved in haemangioma formation? J Clin Pathol 2001;54:249.
5. Weiss SW, Goldblum JR: Benign tumors and tumor-like lesions of blood vessels. In Enzinger and Weiss's Soft Tissue Tumors, 4th ed. St. Louis: Mosby, 2001, pp 839-890.
6. Beham A, Fletcher CDM: Intramuscular angioma: A clinicopathologic analysis of 74 cases. Histopathology 1991;18:53.
7. Allen PW, Enzinger FM: Hemangioma of skeletal muscle: An analysis of 89 cases. Cancer 1972;29:8.
8. Kerr DA: Granuloma pyogenicum. Oral Surg Oral Med Oral Pathol 1951;4:158.
9. Perkins P, Weiss SW: Spindle cell hemangioendothelioma: An analysis of 78 cases with reassessment of its pathogenesis and biologic behavior. Am J Surg Pathol 1996;20:1196.
10. Fanburg JC, Meis-Kindblom JM, Rosenberg AE: Multiple enchondromas associated with spindle-cell hemangioendotheliomas: An overlooked variant of Maffucci's syndrome. Am J Surg Pathol 1995;19:1029.
11. Fetsch JF, Weiss SW: Observations concerning the pathogenesis of epithelioid hemangiomas (angiolymphoid hyperplasia). Mod Pathol 1991;4:449.
12. Olsen TG, Helwig EB: Angiolymphoid hyperplasia with eosinophilia: A clinicopathologic study of 116 patients. J Am Acad Dermatol 1985;12:781.
13. Devaney K, Vinh TN, Sweet DE: Synovial hemangiomas: A report of 20 cases with differential diagnostic considerations. Hum Pathol 1993;24:737.
14. Greenspan A, Azouz EM, Matthews J, et al: Synovial hemangiomas: Imaging features in eight histologically proven cases, review of the literature, and differential diagnosis. Skeletal Radiol 1995;24:583.
15. Adler CP: Hemangioma of the bone. In Bone Diseases. Springer, Berlin, 2000, pp 370-375.
16. Kaleem Z, Kyriakos M, Totty WG: Solitary skeletal hemangiomas of the extremities. Skeletal Radiol 2000;29:502.
17. Keel SB, Rosenberg AE: Hemorrhagic epithelioid and spindle cell hemangioma: A newly recognized, unique vascular tumor of bone. Cancer 1999;85:1966.
18. O'Connell JX, Kattapuram SV, Mankin HJ, et al: Epithelioid hemangioma of bone: A tumor often mistaken for low-grade angiosarcoma or malignant hemangioendothelioma. Am J Surg Pathol 1993;17:610.
19. Esparza J, Castro S, Portillo JM, et al: Vertebral hemangiomas: Spinal angiography and preoperative embolization. Surg Neurol 1978;10:171.
20. Rao VK, Weiss SW: Angiomatosis of soft tissue: An analysis of the histologic features and clinical outcome in 51 cases. Am J Surg Pathol 1992;16:764.
21. Devaney K, Vinh TN, Sweet DE: Skeletal-extraskeletal angiomatosis: A clinicopathologic study of fourteen patients and nosologic considerations. J Bone Joint Surg Am 1994;76:878.

22. Alqahtani A, Nguyen LT, Flageole H, et al: 25 years' experience with lymphangiomas in children. J Pediatr Surg 1999;34:1164.
23. Folpe AL, Veikkola T, Valtola R, et al: Vascular endothelial growth factor receptor-3 (VEGFR-3): A marker of vascular tumors with presumed lymphatic differentiation, including Kaposi's sarcoma, kaposiform and Dabska-type hemangioendotheliomas, and a subset of angiosarcomas. Mod Pathol 2000;13:180.

Epithelioid Hemangioendothelioma

24. Weiss SW, Enzinger FM: Epithelioid hemangioendothelioma: A vascular tumor often mistaken for a carcinoma. Cancer 1982;50:970.
25. Mentzel T, Beham A, Calonje E, et al: Epithelioid hemangioendothelioma of skin and soft tissues: Clinicopathologic and immunohistochemical study of 30 cases. Am J Surg Pathol 1997;21:363.
26. Kleer CG, Unni KK, McLeod RA: Epithelioid hemangioendothelioma of bone. Am J Surg Pathol 1996;20:1301.
27. Makhlouf HR, Ishak KG, Goodman ZD: Epithelioid hemangioendothelioma of the liver: A clinicopathologic study of 137 cases. Cancer 1999;85:562.
28. Kilpatrick SE, Koplyay PD, Ward WG, et al: Epithelioid hemangioendothelioma of bone and soft tissue: A fine-needle aspiration biopsy study with histologic and immunohistochemical confirmation. Diagn Cytopathol 1998;19:38.
29. Mendlick MR, Nelson M, Pickering D, et al: Translocation t(1;3)(p36.3;q25) is a nonrandom aberration in epithelioid hemangioendothelioma. Am J Surg Pathol 2001;25:684.

Rare Forms of Hemangioendothelioma

30. Calonje E, Fletcher CDM, Wilson-Jones E, et al: Retiform hemangioendothelioma: A distinctive form of low-grade angiosarcoma delineated in a series of 15 cases. Am J Surg Pathol 1994;18:115.
31. Mac-Moune F, Fai To K, Choi PC, et al: Kaposiform hemangioendothelioma: Five patients with cutaneous lesions and long follow-up. Mod Pathol 2001;14:1087.
32. Mentzel T, Mazzoleni G, Dei Tos AP, et al: Kaposiform hemangioendothelioma in adults: Clinicopathologic and immunohistochemical analysis of three cases. Am J Clin Pathol 1997;108:450.

Kaposi's Sarcoma

33. Trattner A, Hodak E, David M, et al: The appearance of Kaposi sarcoma during corticosteroid therapy. Cancer 1993;72:1779.
34. Gottlieb GJ, Ackerman AB: Kaposi's sarcoma: An extensively disseminated form in young homosexual men. Hum Pathol 1982;13:882.
35. Brenner B, Weissman-Brenner A, Rakowsky E, et al: Classical Kaposi sarcoma: Prognostic factor analysis of 248 patients. Cancer 2002;95:1982.
36. Layfield LJ, Glasgow BJ: Aspiration biopsy cytology of primary cutaneous tumors. Acta Cytol 1993;37:679.
37. Folpe AL, Chand EM, Goldblum JR, et al: Expression of Fli-1, a nuclear transcription factor, distinguishes vascular neoplasms from potential mimics. Am J Surg Pathol 2001;25:1061.
38. Chang Y, Cesarman E, Pessin MS, et al: Identification of herpesvirus-like DNA sequences in AIDS-associated Kaposi's sarcoma. Science 1994;266:1865.

Angiosarcoma

39. Meis-Kindblom JM, Kindblom LG: Angiosarcoma of soft tissue: A study of 80 cases. Am J Surg Pathol 1998;22:683.
40. Wold LE, Unni KK, Beabout JW, et al: Hemangioendothelial sarcoma of bone. Am J Surg Pathol 1982;6:59.
41. Mark RJ, Poen JC, Tran LM, et al: Angiosarcoma: A report of 67 patients. Cancer 1996;77:2400.
42. Boucher LD, Swanson PE, Stanley MW, et al: Cytology of angiosarcoma: Findings in fourteen fine-needle aspiration biopsy specimens and one pleural fluid specimen. Am J Clin Pathol 2000;114:210.
43. Liu K, Layfield LJ: Cytomorphologic features of angiosarcoma on fine needle aspiration biopsy. Acta Cytol 1999;43:407.
44. Miettinen M, Sarlomo-Rikala M, Lasota J: KIT expression in angiosarcomas and fetal endothelial cells: Lack of mutations of exon 11 and exon 17 of C-kit. Mod Pathol 2000;13:536.
45. Gil-Benso R, Lopez-Gines C, Soriano P, et al: Cytogenetic study of angiosarcoma of the breast. Genes Chromosomes Cancer 1994;10:210.
46. Schuborg C, Mertens F, Rydholm A, et al: Cytogenetic analysis of four angiosarcomas from deep and superficial soft tissue. Cancer Genet Cytogenet 1998;100:52.
47. Elias AD, Antman KH: Adjuvant chemotherapy for soft tissue sarcomas: An approach in search of an effective regimen. Semin Oncol 1989;16:305.

Glomus Tumor

48. Van Geertruyden J, Lorea P, Goldschmidt D, et al: Glomus tumours of the hand: A retrospective study of 51 cases. J Hand Surg Br 1996;21:257.
49. Folpe AL, Fanburg-Smith JC, Miettinen M, et al: Atypical and malignant glomus tumors: Analysis of 52 cases, with a proposal for the reclassification of glomus tumors. Am J Surg Pathol 2001;25:1.
50. Robinson JC, Kilpatrick SE, Kelly DL Jr: Introsseous glomus tumor of the spine: Case report and review of the literature. J Neurosurg 1996;85:344.
51. Gaertner EM, Steinberg DM, Huber M, et al: Pulmonary and mediastinal glomus tumors: Report of five cases including a pulmonary glomangiosarcoma: A clinicopathologic study with literature review. Am J Surg Pathol 2000;24:1105.
52. Handa U, Palta A, Mohan H, et al: Aspiration cytology of glomus tumor: A case report. Acta Cytol 2001;45:1073.
53. Miettinen M, Lehto VP, Virtanen I: Glomus tumor cells: Evaluation of smooth muscle and endothelial cell properties. Virchows Arch B Cell Pathol Incl Mol Pathol 1983;43:139.
54. Boon LM, Brouillard P, Irrthum A, et al: A gene for inherited cutaneous venous anomalies ("glomangiomas") localizes to chromosome 1p21–22. Am J Hum Genet 1999;65:125.
55. Kim YC: An additional case of solitary subungual glomus tumor associated with neurofibromatosis 1. J Dermatol 2000;27:418.

CHAPTER 11

Pleomorphic Cell Tumors of Bone and Soft Tissue

With the exception of the extraordinarily rare pleomorphic hyalinizing angiectatic tumor of soft parts, we consider the pleomorphic cell tumor group to consist almost entirely of pleomorphic sarcomas. Simply, a *pleomorphic sarcoma* is a tumor showing marked nuclear pleomorphism, usually containing tumor giant cells, and arising in adults (Figure 11.1). Consequently, pleomorphic sarcomas are virtually always high-grade lesions. A variety of tumors occasionally may exhibit significant nuclear pleomorphism; however, some sarcomas, by definition, consistently comprise diagnostic pleomorphic tumor cells. The latter are summarized in Table 11.1. Pleomorphic sarcomas may arise as a result of dedifferentiation of a low-grade malignancy, most commonly observed in well-differentiated liposarcoma and skeletal chondrosarcoma. Most examples of skeletal and extraskeletal osteosarcomas also include a pleomorphic tumor cell population (Table 11.2). In certain instances, especially among tumors arising in visceral organs, the diagnosis of sarcomatoid carcinoma also must be considered in the differential diagnosis of pleomorphic sarcoma. Other potential mimics of pleomorphic sarcoma include malignant melanoma and anaplastic lymphoma.

Despite varying clinicopathologic features among pleomorphic sarcomas, "it is difficult to make a strong case that the various pleomorphic sarcomas are behaviorally significantly different from one another."[1] At present, all adult, high-grade pleomorphic sarcomas are treated similarly, usually by complete surgical excision accompanied by radiation therapy or chemotherapy or both. Consequently, among the pleomorphic sarcoma group, histologic subtyping is usually not essential for adequate therapy. With the exception of dedifferentiated liposarcoma, cytogenetic analysis has not revealed any specific chromosomal abnormalities in any of the pleomorphic sarcomas. All are

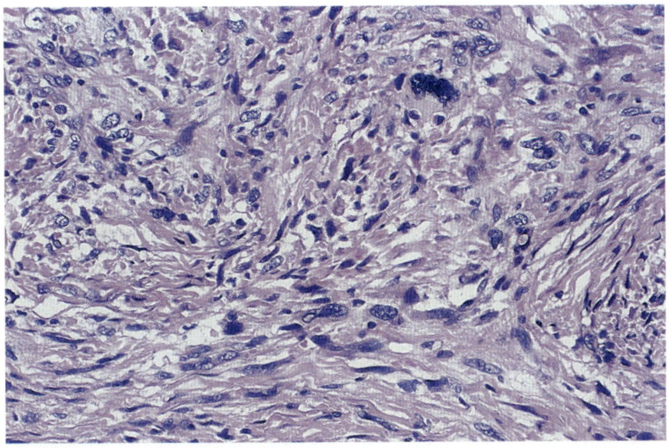

FIGURE 11.1 Pleomorphic sarcoma with spindled anaplastic tumor cells arranged in fascicles and storiform patterns within a variably collagenous background. These findings are nonspecific and may be observed within any of the pleomorphic sarcoma subtypes. (H&E.)

TABLE 11.1 Bone and Soft Tissue Tumors Primarily Occurring in Adults in Which Pleomorphic Tumor Cells Are Definitionally Part of the Lesion

Bone Origin	Soft Tissue Origin
MFH*	MFH*
Pleomorphic leiomyosarcoma	Pleomorphic leiomyosarcoma
	Pleomorphic liposarcoma
	Pleomorphic rhabdomyosarcoma
	Myxofibrosarcoma (myxoid MFH)
	Malignant mesenchymoma
	Pleomorphic hyalinizing angiectatic tumor of soft parts

*Includes the following MFH subtypes: pleomorphic/storiform, giant cell, and inflammatory.

MFH, malignant fibrous histiocytoma.

TABLE 11.2 Bone and Soft Tissue Tumors That Frequently Contain Pleomorphic Tumor Cells

Bone	Soft Tissue
Dedifferentiated chondrosarcoma	Dedifferentiated liposarcoma
Osteosarcoma	Osteosarcoma
Angiosarcoma	Angiosarcoma
	Malignant peripheral nerve sheath tumor

generally aneuploid and show a variety of complex chromosomal aberrations.

Nevertheless, it is unwise to conclude that histologic subtyping of pleomorphic sarcomas is not useful. In the past, an absence of uniform diagnostic guidelines for the various pleomorphic sarcoma subtypes made comparison among these subgroups difficult and inconsistent. More recent studies have begun to provide more reproducible criteria for the histologic subtyping of pleomorphic sarcomas.[2] Figure 11.2 illustrates application of these criteria in the work-up of a pleomorphic sarcoma. Limited early data suggest that prognostic subgroups exist among the pleomorphic sarcomas. The metastatic rate of dedifferentiated liposarcoma ranges from 15% to 20%; high-grade myxofibrosarcoma is associated with higher metastatic rates of 30% to 35%.[3] Pleomorphic rhabdomyosarcoma may produce metastases in 70% of cases. Most importantly, the separation of pleomorphic sarcoma from malignant melanoma, sarcomatoid carcinoma, or anaplastic lymphoma is essential for appropriate therapy. At some institutions, extraskeletal osteosarcoma is treated with osteosarcoma protocols, similar to those used in children.

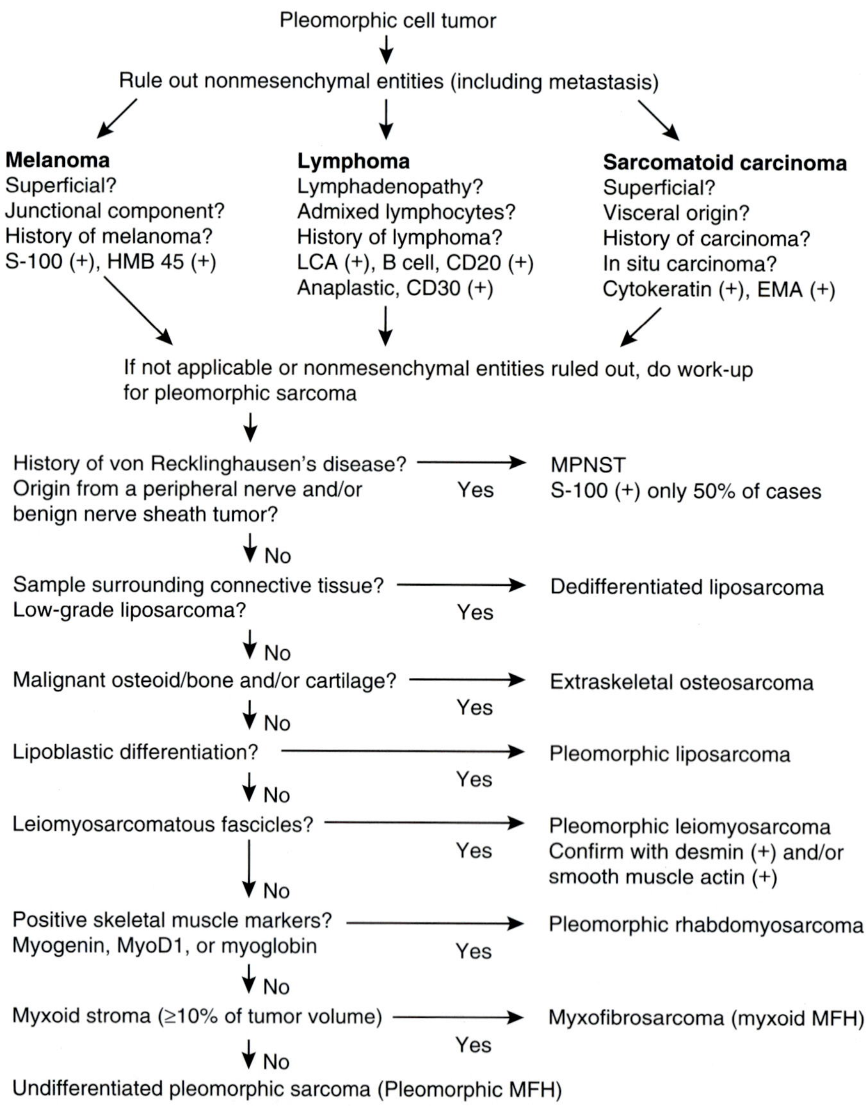

FIGURE 11.2 Work-up of an adult pleomorphic cell tumor of soft tissues. MFH, malignant fibrous histiocytoma; MPNST, malignant peripheral nerve sheath tumor.

Pleomorphic Malignant Fibrous Histiocytoma (Undifferentiated High-Grade Pleomorphic Sarcoma)

Pleomorphic malignant fibrous histiocytoma is best considered a diagnosis of exclusion reserved for pleomorphic sarcomas lacking an obvious line of differentiation (e.g., lipoblastic, smooth muscle, striated muscle, or bone/cartilage production). In the past, pleomorphic malignant fibrous histiocytoma has been considered the most common form of adult sarcoma. With the development of more reproducible diagnostic criteria for other pleomorphic sarcoma subtypes and improved immunohistochemical techniques, the incidence of malignant fibrous histiocytoma has decreased considerably.

Clinical Features

Pleomorphic malignant fibrous histiocytoma is observed most commonly in patients older than age 50. Rarely, similar tumors have been described in adolescents and young adults. Males are affected more commonly than females. Most cases arise in the deep soft tissues, and the lower extremity is the most common anatomic site.[4] Patients often report the presence of a large soft tissue mass, sometimes associated with pain (Fig. 11.3). Rare examples may arise at the site of prior radiation therapy.[5]

Pleomorphic malignant fibrous histiocytoma rarely arises within bones, most commonly the long bones of the

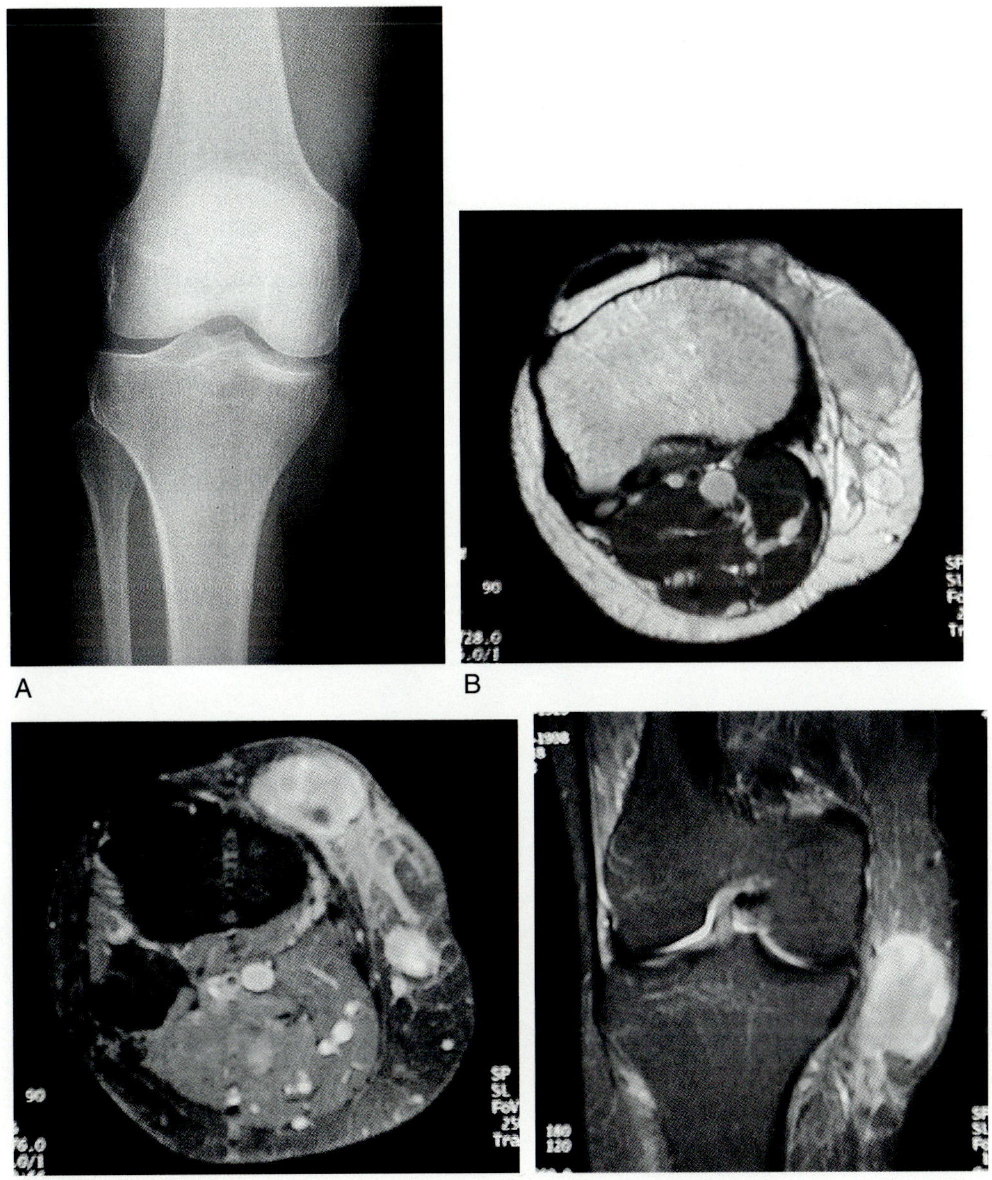

A B C D

FIGURE 11.3 Pleomorphic malignant fibrous histiocytoma. An anteroposterior radiograph of the knee shows a soft tissue mass medially just distal to the tibial plateau. No soft tissue calcification or underlying bone erosion is apparent **(A)**. Proton density axial **(B)**, fat-suppressed T1-weighted gadolinium-enhanced **(C)**, and coronal short tau inversion recovery (STIR) **(D)** magnetic resonance images reveal a large, densely but heterogeneously enhancing lesion adjacent to the proximal tibia. A smaller nodule of tumor is seen posterior to the large mass. Although the size, heterogeneity, and irregular enhancement of the lesion are typical magnetic resonance imaging findings associated with a high-grade soft tissue sarcoma, they are not specific for any particular histologic diagnosis and could be produced by any of the lesions discussed in this chapter.

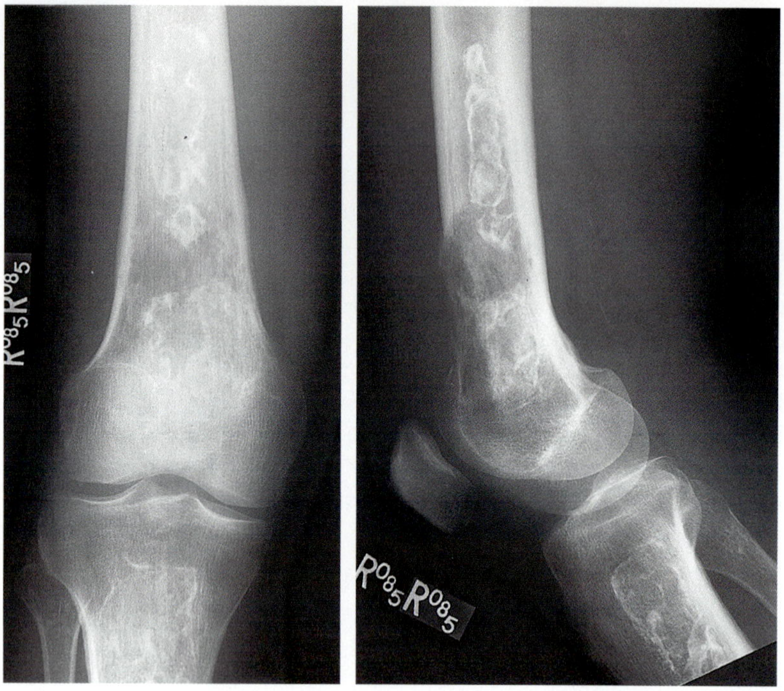

A B

FIGURE 11.4 Pleomorphic malignant fibrous histiocytoma of bone. Anteroposterior **(A)** and lateral **(B)** radiographs of the knee show serpentine calcifications in the medullary canals of the distal femur and proximal tibia, typical in appearance for bone infarction. The lateral view shows, however, a focal destructive bone lesion proximal to the patella with destruction of the anterior femoral cortex.

lower extremities, especially the femur and tibia.[6] Most patients are older than age 40. Pain with or without a soft tissue mass is the most common reported complaint. Radiographically, most tumors are lytic, are metaphyseal centered, and have a permeative destructive pattern with ill-defined margins (Fig. 11.4). Soft tissue extension frequently is seen. Of osseous cases of malignant fibrous histiocytoma, 22% develop secondary to a pre-existing bone condition (e.g., Paget's disease, bone infarct, fibrous dysplasia) or at the site of previous radiation therapy for a nonmesenchymal tumor.[6]

Pathologic Findings

Histology

Pleomorphic malignant fibrous histiocytoma exhibits a population of markedly atypical, polygonal to spindle-shaped tumor cells with multilobated-to-multiple nuclei, admixed with a population of spindle cells arranged in short fascicles and storiform patterns. The background stroma is variably fibrous (Fig. 11.5). The so-called inflammatory malignant fibrous histiocytoma is a form of pleomorphic

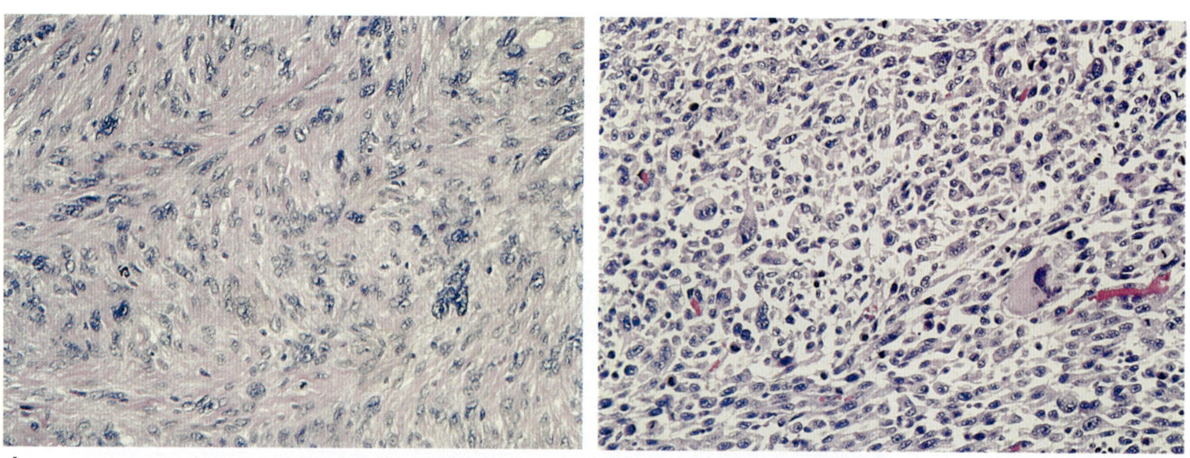

A B

FIGURE 11.5 Pleomorphic malignant fibrous histiocytoma with the characteristic (but nonspecific) anaplastic spindle cells and tumor giant cells arranged in fascicles, vague storiform patterns, and sheets within a variably collagenous background **(A** and **B)**. **(A** and **B**, H&E.)

malignant fibrous histiocytoma in which the background stroma is dominated by inflammatory cells, principally foamy histiocytes (Fig. 11.6). All of these findings are relatively nonspecific, however, and may be seen in virtually any of the pleomorphic sarcoma subtypes. It is essential that complete and thorough sampling (at least one section per 1 cm of tumor) be performed to exclude a specific differential diagnosis (see Fig. 11.2). The presence of malignant osteoid/bone confirms the diagnosis of extraskeletal osteosarcoma. The finding of lipoblasts supports the diagnosis of pleomorphic liposarcoma. Individual anaplastic tumor cells with abundant eosinophilic cytoplasm suggest the possibilities of pleomorphic leiomyosarcoma, pleomorphic rhabdomyosarcoma, sarcomatoid carcinoma, and malignant melanoma. Correlation with clinical history and judicious use of immunohistochemical stains help in the subclassification of these lesions.

Fine Needle Aspiration Biopsy

Fine needle aspiration biopsy (FNAB) yields slightly to moderately cellular smears. The tumor cells are dispersed individually or arranged in small clusters. Significant nuclear pleomorphism is present with neighboring cells appearing several times larger than one another. The cytomorphology may be variable, ranging from spindle to epithelioid-appearing forms with one or more nuclei; prominent nucleoli; and scant-to-abundant, clear-to-dense cytoplasm (Fig. 11.7). Similar to the histologic findings, the cytologic features are completely nonspecific. In the absence of specific clinicopathologic features, we render the diagnosis of "pleomorphic sarcoma, not otherwise specified" and reserve histologic subtyping for examination of the resected specimen.

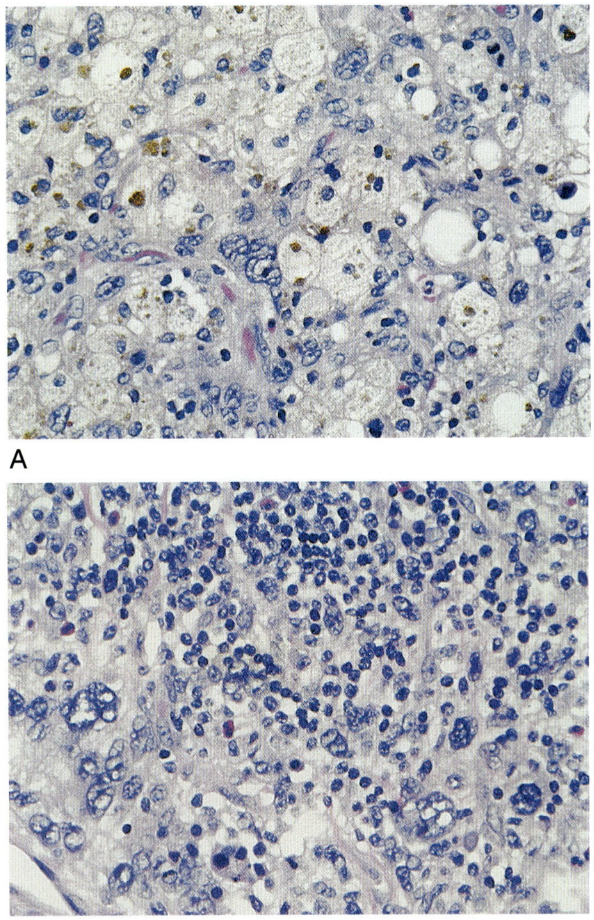

A

B

FIGURE 11.6 So-called inflammatory malignant fibrous histiocytoma with anaplastic tumor cells scattered among numerous foamy and pigmented histiocytes **(A)**. In some cases, other inflammatory cells, such as lymphocytes, eosinophils, or neutrophils, may be present in numbers sufficient to confound the diagnosis of malignancy **(B)**.

Ancillary Studies

Ultrastructural examination of pleomorphic malignant fibrous histiocytoma has revealed variable results, probably because of differing criteria for establishing the diagnosis. Most tumor cells show features suggestive of fibroblastic/myofibroblastic differentiation, including prominent endoplasmic reticulum, abundant intermediate filaments, and occasional lysosomes.[7]

The immunohistochemical features of pleomorphic malignant fibrous histiocytoma are largely nonspecific. As expected, virtually all cases show diffuse and strong immunoexpression with vimentin. Markers of histiocytic differentiation generally are not expressed by the tumor cells of malignant fibrous histiocytoma.[8] Focal smooth muscle actin or desmin positivity is also frequently observed, reflecting myofibroblastic differentiation.[9,10] Diffuse and strong immunoreactivity for these markers should suggest the diagnosis of pleomorphic leiomyosarcoma. Although focal keratin positivity has been described in pleomorphic malignant fibrous histiocytoma, its presence in similar-appearing tumors arising in visceral organs almost assuredly indicates sarcomatoid carcinoma. Similarly, strong and diffuse immunopositivity for S-100 protein should be considered melanoma until proved otherwise.

No reproducible chromosomal abnormalities specific for the diagnosis of pleomorphic malignant fibrous histiocytoma have been discovered. Most examples reveal highly complex karyotypes with numerous chromosomal abnormalities.[11]

Prognosis and Therapy

Pleomorphic malignant fibrous histiocytomas are high-grade, aggressive lesions with reported 5-year survival rates of 50% to 60%.[3] Adverse prognostic factors include large tumor size, incomplete resection, deep (below the superficial fascia) location, and metastasis at diagnosis. For primary skeletal malignant fibrous histiocytoma, the most important prognostic factors seem to be adequacy of surgical resection.[6] The overall survival rate for skeletal malignant fibrous histiocytoma is

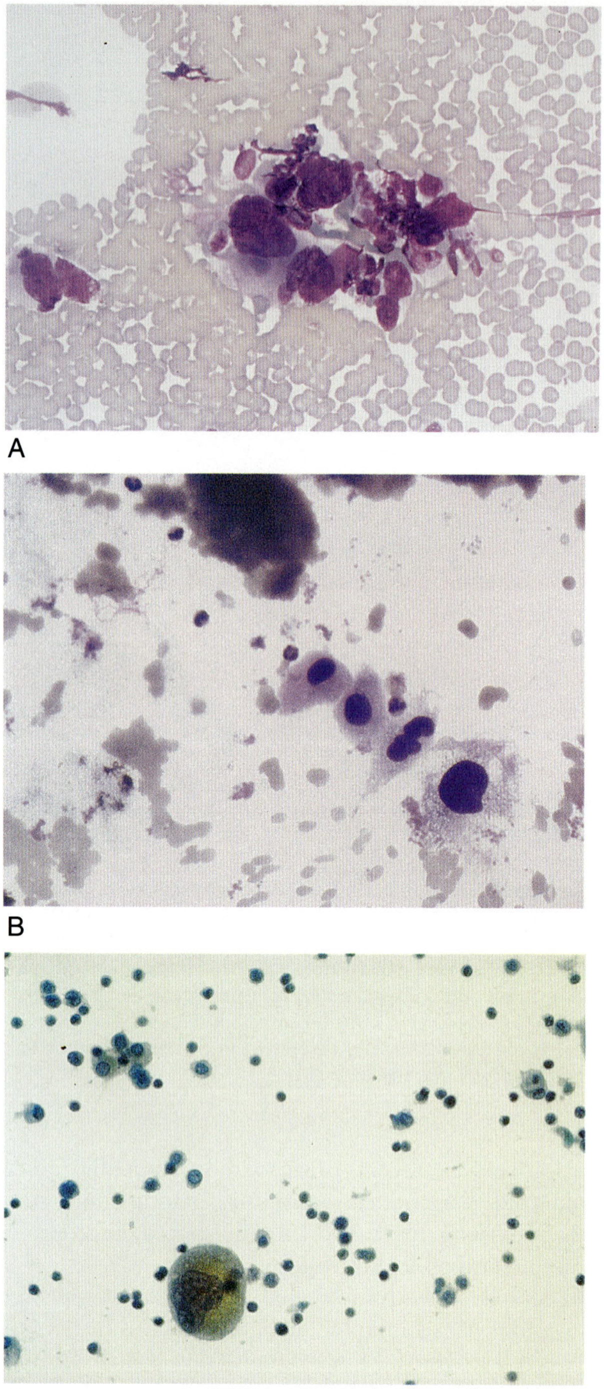
A
B
C

FIGURE 11.7 Fine needle aspiration biopsy specimens of malignant fibrous histiocytoma are nonspecific and generally comprise mostly individually dispersed and clusters of markedly atypical, spindled to polygonal-shaped tumor cells. Occasional multinucleated tumor giant cells also are observed **(A-C)**. (**A** and **B,** Diff-Quik; **C,** Papanicolaou.)

similar to that observed with osteosarcoma.[6] In some institutions, osseous malignant fibrous histiocytoma is treated with preoperative chemotherapy, and reported response rates (percentage of postchemotherapy necrosis) have been similar to osteosarcoma.[12]

Pleomorphic Liposarcoma

Clinical Features

Pleomorphic liposarcoma is a rare subtype of liposarcoma, representing approximately 5% of all liposarcoma cases. Most tumors arise in elderly (>60 years) patients and most commonly occur in the deep soft tissues of the lower extremities and the retroperitoneum.[13,14] Rare sites of tumor involvement include the mediastinum and paratesticular region. Most patients present with pain and soft tissue swelling.

Pathologic Findings

Histology

In most cases, pleomorphic liposarcoma closely resembles pleomorphic malignant fibrous histiocytoma, dominated by the presence of pleomorphic spindle-shaped tumor cells and anaplastic tumor giant cells, arranged in short fascicles and storiform growth patterns (Fig. 11.8). The diagnosis rests on the finding of lipoblastic differentiation that may be focal, requiring extensive sampling to exclude the diagnosis completely.[14] Less commonly, pleomorphic liposarcoma has a predominance of epithelioid cells with mostly round nuclei, inconspicuous-to-prominent nucleoli, and abundant cytoplasm, ranging from eosinophilic to markedly vacuolated (Fig. 11.9).[15] The epithelioid tumor cells may be arranged in solid, cohesive clusters and sheets. A characteristic feature of the epithelioid and malignant fibrous histiocytoma-like forms is the presence of pleomorphic and multiloculated lipoblasts containing bizarre-shaped, hyperchromatic, and scalloped nuclei. Intracellular and extracellular eosinophilic droplets, possibly lysosomal bodies, frequently are observed in the lipoblastic areas (Fig. 11.10). The degree of necrosis is variable but may be extensive. Likewise, mitotic activity is variable; however, the mitotic rate seems to be higher in the epithelioid form.

Fine Needle Aspiration Biopsy

FNAB of pleomorphic liposarcoma is usually not diagnostic. The cellular cytologic smears consist mainly of tumor cells closely resembling malignant fibrous histiocytoma (pleomorphic sarcoma, not otherwise specified) (Fig. 11.11). In rare instances, lipoblastic differentiation is observed, permitting the diagnosis of pleomorphic liposarcoma (Fig. 11.12).

Ancillary Studies

Ultrastructurally the neoplastic cells of pleomorphic liposarcoma show features of lipoblastic differentiation with abundant lipid droplets, numerous organelles, and a surrounding plasma cell membrane.[16] Despite definite lipoblastic differen-

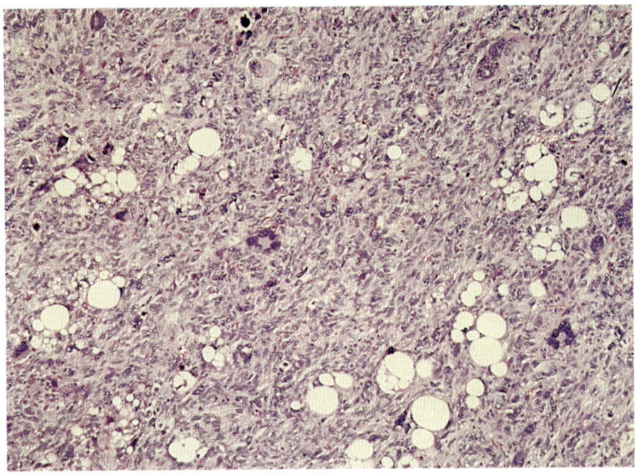
A

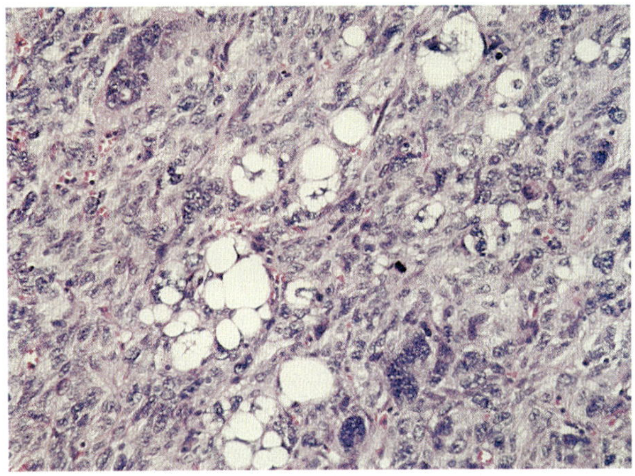
B

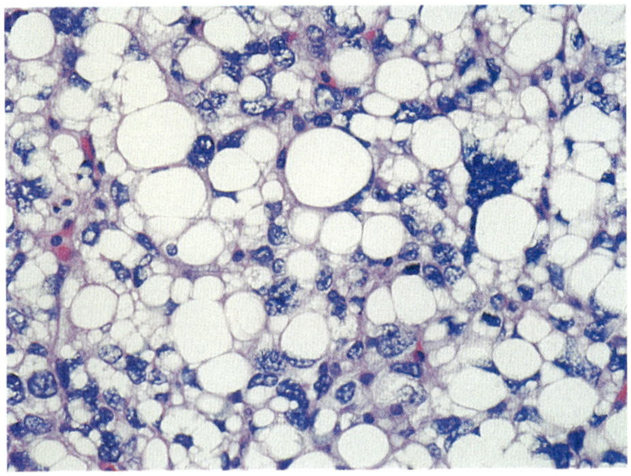
C

FIGURE 11.8 Pleomorphic liposarcoma, malignant fibrous histiocytoma type. Most of the tumor resembles pleomorphic malignant fibrous histiocytoma; however, focal aggregates of lipoblasts are diagnostic of pleomorphic liposarcoma **(A** and **B)**. At high power, the classic lipoblasts show atypical and bizarre-shaped nuclei that appear scalloped by their multivacuolated, lipid-laden cytoplasm **(C)**. **(A,** Low power, H&E; **B,** intermediate power, H&E; **C,** high power, H&E.)

tiation, only about 50% of cases show focal expression of S-100 protein. Potentially confounding the diagnosis, the epithelioid variant of pleomorphic liposarcoma may show cytokeratin or epithelial membrane positivity in approximately 40% of cases.[15,17] In the nonlipogenic areas, focal immunoreactivity for CD68, smooth muscle actin, desmin, and CD34 may be observed.[17]

To date, only 11 pleomorphic liposarcomas have documented karyotypic data. Similar to other adult pleomorphic sarcomas, all showed complex karyotypes and rearrangements.

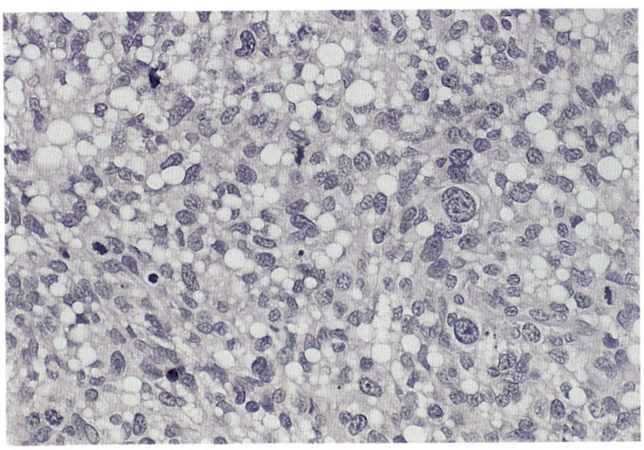

FIGURE 11.9 Pleomorphic liposarcoma, epithelioid subtype, is composed of a population of pleomorphic lipoblasts with round, epithelioid features, resembling carcinoma. (H&E.)

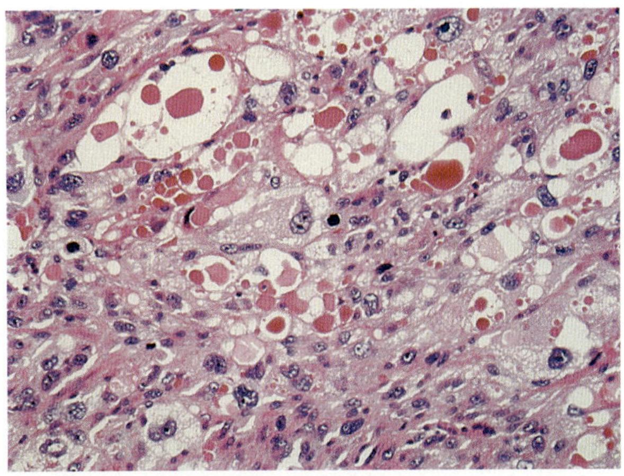

FIGURE 11.10 In the lipoblastic areas of pleomorphic liposarcoma, intracellular and extracellular eosinophilic droplets, possibly lysosomal bodies, sometimes are observed. (H&E.)

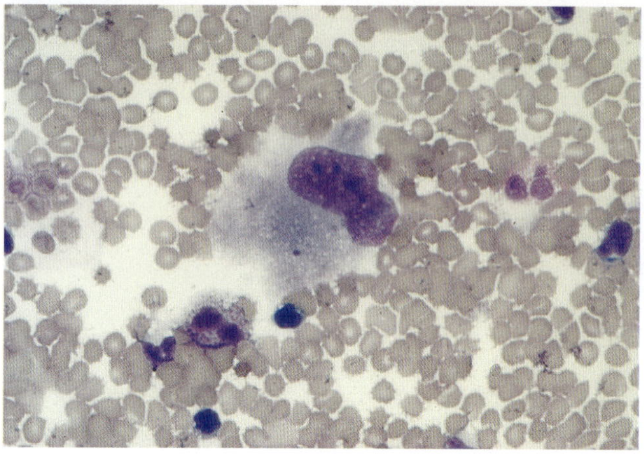

FIGURE 11.11 Fine needle aspiration biopsy of pleomorphic liposarcoma is usually nondiagnostic. Cytologic smears appear similar to malignant fibrous histiocytoma with pleomorphic tumor cells accompanied by scattered binucleated-to-multinucleated tumor giant cells. (Diff-Quik.)

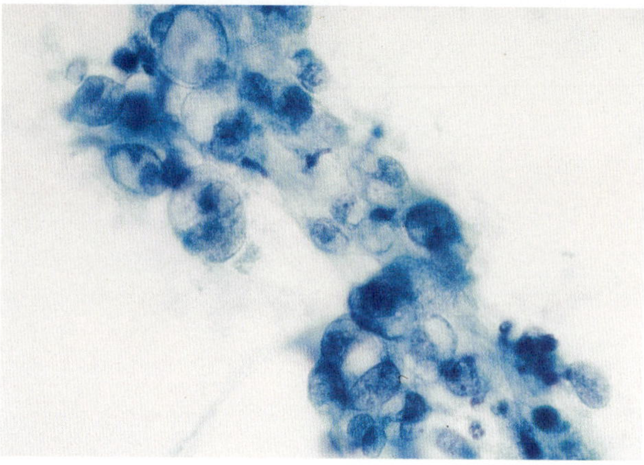

FIGURE 11.12 Rarely, fine needle aspiration biopsy reveals aggregates of diagnostic univacuolated-to-multivacuolated lipoblasts. (Papanicolaou.)

No specific or reproducible chromosomal abnormality has been reported.[18]

Prognosis and Therapy

The overall prognosis for pleomorphic liposarcoma is poor. The 5-year overall survival rate ranges from 40% to 60%; 50% of patients develop distant metastases, usually involving the lung.[13,17] Adverse prognostic factors include large tumor size (>5 cm), truncal location, deep position, vascular invasion, and incomplete tumor excision.[17] Histologic grade does not affect patient outcome. Recommended therapy includes wide or radical surgical resection accompanied by radiation therapy or chemotherapy or both.

Dedifferentiated Liposarcoma

Dedifferentiated liposarcoma is defined by the presence of a usually high-grade, nonliposarcomatous sarcoma arising concurrently (and adjacent to) a well-differentiated liposarcoma (primary) or occurring at the anatomic site of a previously resected well-differentiated liposarcoma (secondary). The incidence of dedifferentiation of a low-grade liposarcoma is difficult to determine but probably ranges from 5% to 10%, with liposarcomas located in the retroperitoneum representing the high end of this range.

Clinical Features

Dedifferentiated liposarcoma typically occurs in adult patients, almost always older than age 50. Men and women are affected roughly equally. The most common anatomic location is the retroperitoneum followed by the deep soft tissues of the extremities, spermatic cord/scrotum, and trunk.[19,20] Dedifferentiated liposarcoma rarely has been reported arising in subcutaneous adipose tissue.[21] Most patients present with painless soft tissue swelling, often of long duration. Radiographic examination may reveal the presence of the low-grade (fatty) and high-grade (nonfatty) components; however, this is not often readily appreciated.

Pathologic Findings

Histology

Dedifferentiated liposarcoma is characterized by the presence of well-differentiated liposarcoma usually sharply juxtaposed to a nonlipogenic sarcoma that is most often high grade (Fig. 11.13).[19,20] In some cases, the transition between the lower and higher grade components may be gradual and intermingled. Also, the volume of the dedifferentiated component is variable, ranging from microscopic foci to extraordinarily large (>10 cm) tumors. The dedifferentiated component is usually high grade, resembling pleomorphic malignant fibrous histiocytoma with fascicles of spindled tumor cells admixed with multinucleated tumor giant cells (Fig. 11.14). Less commonly, the dedifferentiated component is less cellular, however, and of a lower grade (Fig. 11.15).[19] Heterologous components involve the dedifferentiated component in 5% to 10% of cases. This component may include osteosarcomatous, chondrosarcomatous, angiosarcomatous, rhabdomyosarcomatous, and leiomyosarcomatous elements (Fig. 11.16).[22] Rare examples of dedifferentiated liposarcoma exhibit a neural-like whorling pattern, resembling neural tumors or meningiomas.[23] Because the diagnosis of dedifferentiated liposarcoma requires establishing the presence of the low-grade liposarcoma component, sampling of the adjacent connective tissue at the tumor–soft tissue interface should be standard pathology grossing practice.

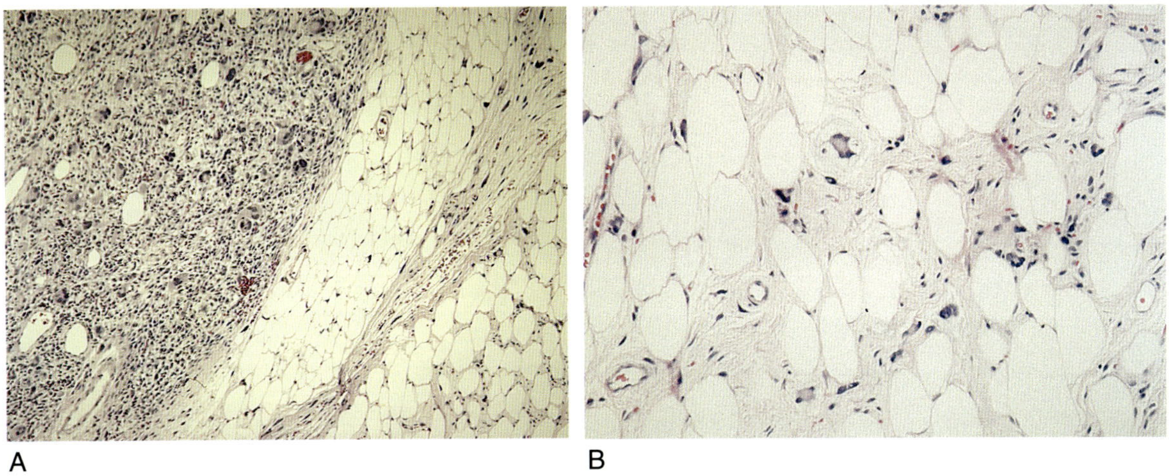

FIGURE 11.13 Dedifferentiated liposarcoma showing the classic sharp juxtaposed border between the well-differentiated liposarcoma component and the high-grade nonlipogenic component **(A)**. The low-grade component shows the classic features of atypical lipoma/well-differentiated liposarcoma with scattered, atypical stromal cells and lipoblasts **(B)**. (**A** and **B**, H&E.)

Fine Needle Aspiration Biopsy

Our experience with the cytologic findings of dedifferentiated liposarcoma is limited. As with other dedifferentiated sarcomas (e.g., dedifferentiated chondrosarcoma), however, FNAB usually samples only the high-grade dedifferentiated component. In these cases, the diagnosis of pleomorphic sarcoma, not otherwise specified, is sufficient for initiation of therapy. Unless a prior history of low-grade liposarcoma has been established at the anatomic site, the diagnosis of dedifferentiated liposarcoma usually cannot be rendered by cytologic examination alone.

Ancillary Studies

Immunohistochemistry is not useful in the diagnosis of dedifferentiated liposarcoma. Although smooth muscle actin and desmin may decorate the nonlipogenic component, the histologic presence of the low-grade component establishes the diagnosis.

Ring or giant marker chromosomes usually derived from 12q13-15 characterize well-differentiated and dedifferentiated liposarcomas.[20] Additional chromosomal aberrations often are detected in the dedifferentiated forms.

Prognosis and Therapy

Local recurrence of dedifferentiated liposarcoma occurs in approximately 40% of patients. Between 10% and 20% of patients develop distant metastasis, most commonly involving the lungs. Mortality rates range from 20% to 30%, significantly lower than rates observed with other adult pleomorphic sarcomas.[19,20] The most important prognostic factor seems to be anatomic location, with tumors located in the retroperitoneum exhibiting more aggressive behavior than tumors located in the extremities.[19] Neither the percentage of the dedifferentiated component nor its grade accurately predicts clinical outcome. Therapy is similar to other adult pleomorphic sarcomas.

Dedifferentiated Chondrosarcoma

Dedifferentiated chondrosarcoma is defined by the presence of a high-grade, nonchondrosarcomatous sarcoma sharply juxtaposed to a low-grade chondrosarcoma. Most examples arise from intramedullary, so-called central chondrosarcomas. Rarely, dedifferentiated chondrosarcoma also may arise from a pre-existing osteochondroma (peripheral chondrosarcomas).

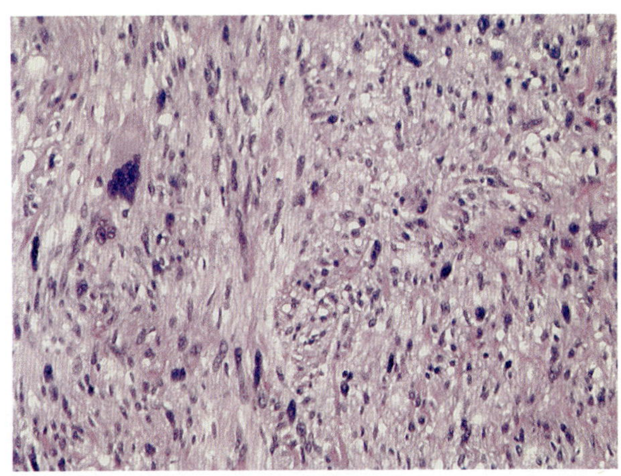

FIGURE 11.14 In most cases, the dedifferentiated component of dedifferentiated liposarcoma is indistinguishable from pleomorphic malignant fibrous histiocytoma. (H&E.)

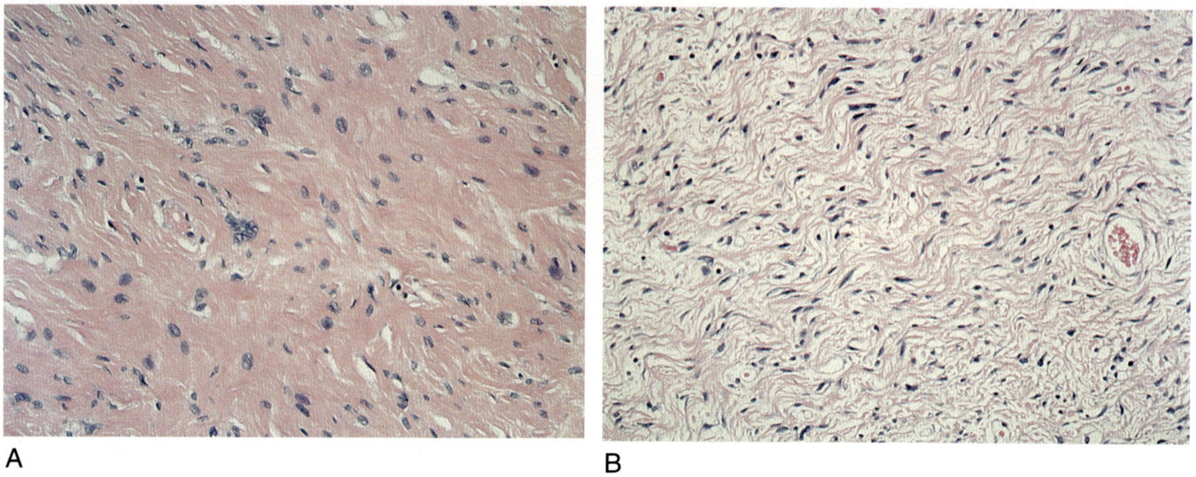

FIGURE 11.15 Less commonly, the dedifferentiated component may be less cellular and more collagenous **(A)**. Other lower grade examples may show features suggestive of nerve sheath differentiation **(B)**. (**A** and **B**, H&E.)

Clinical Features

Dedifferentiated chondrosarcoma represents approximately 10% of reported cases of chondrosarcomas. Most patients are older than age 50 at diagnosis. Common anatomic sites include the pelvic bones, femur, and humerus. The most common presentation is pain often associated with a soft tissue mass.[24,25]

Radiographically the low-grade cartilaginous component shows the typical mineralization of a cartilage tumor, whereas the dedifferentiated portion appears ill defined, permeative, and lytic and is associated with extraosseous extension. In many cases, the dedifferentiated component completely dwarfs the smaller, low-grade cartilaginous portion (Fig. 11.17).

Pathologic Findings

Histology

In resected specimens, the diagnosis of dedifferentiated chondrosarcoma is relatively straightforward if the low-grade cartilaginous component is recognized as malignant. The histologic hallmark is the finding of low-grade chondrosarcoma sharply juxtaposed to a high-grade, often spindle cell sarcoma, giving the appearance of two separate neoplasms (Fig. 11.18). Similar to dedifferentiated liposarcoma, focal areas may show a more gradual transition between the two components (Fig. 11.19). Histologically the high-grade portion most frequently masquerades as a nonmatrix-producing, spindle cell pleomorphic sarcoma. Most of these cases morphologically resemble malignant fibrous histiocytoma.[24,25] Additional reports of osteosarcoma and malignant mesenchymoma with rhabdomyosarcomatous components have been documented (Fig. 11.20).[25,26]

Fine Needle Aspiration Biopsy

Pathologists and clinicians should be aware that the diagnosis of dedifferentiated chondrosarcoma may be missed in FNAB and core needle biopsy specimens. In most cases, these biopsy specimens yield only the high-grade pleomorphic sarcoma component, indistinguishable from other pleomorphic sarcomas (Fig. 11.21).[27] Clinical and radiographic correlation is essential to establishing the diagnosis of dedifferentiated chondrosarcoma.

Ancillary Studies

Immunohistochemistry is not generally helpful for the diagnosis of dedifferentiated chondrosarcoma. Cytogenetic analysis has revealed no reproducible, specific chromosomal

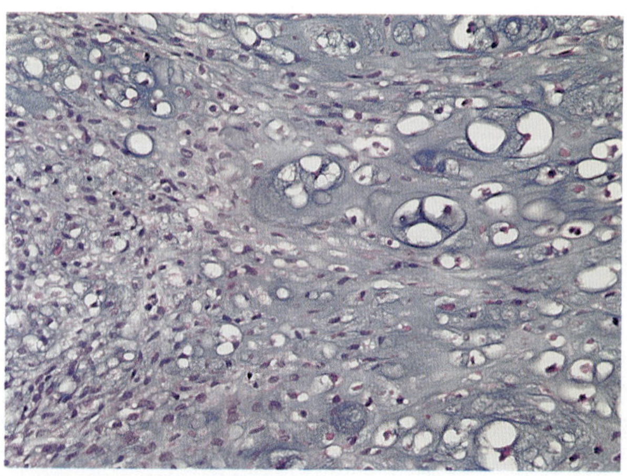

FIGURE 11.16 Dedifferentiated liposarcoma with heterologous differentiation (cartilaginous component). (H&E.)

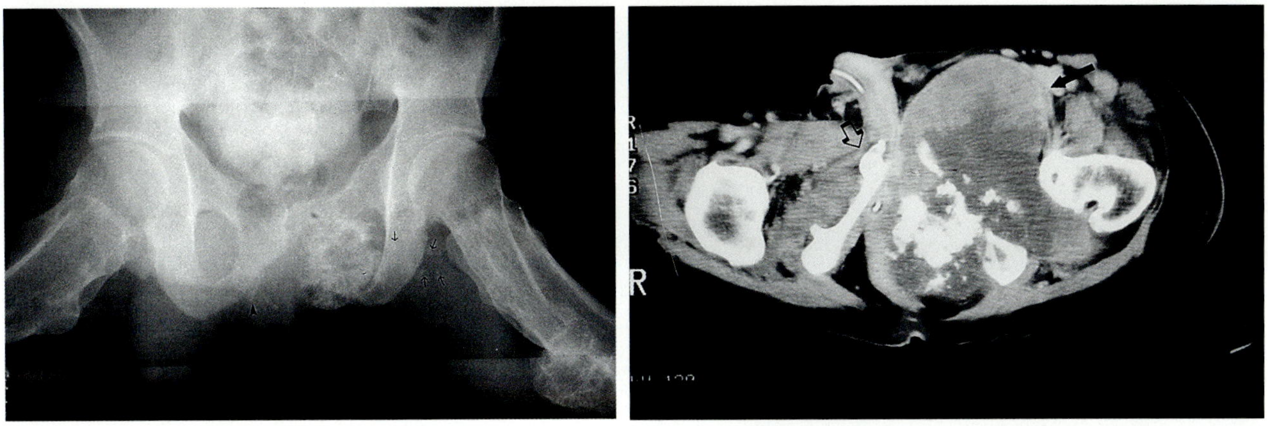

A B

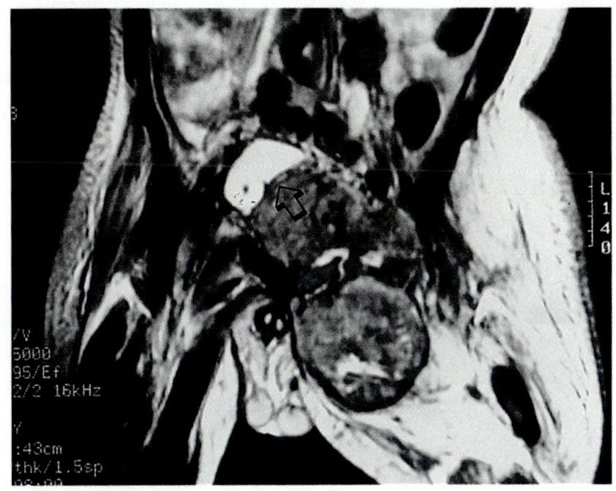

C

FIGURE 11.17 Dedifferentiated chondrosarcoma arising in a patient with multiple osteochondromatosis. An anteroposterior radiograph of the pelvis shows multiple osteochondromas *(arrowheads)*. A large soft tissue mass is accompanied by multiple irregular, chondroid calcifications at the left pubic ramus *(arrows)* **(A)**. An axial computed tomographic scan shows the extension of soft tissue mass anterior *(dark arrow)* and posterior to the left pubic rami. The neurovascular structures are displaced by the mass. The mass is markedly heterogeneous, probably reflecting necrosis within the mass. Calcifications are seen throughout much of the mass. Note the osteochondroma *(open arrow)* arising from the right pubic ramus **(B)**. A T1-weighted coronal magnetic resonance image shows the large, heterogeneous mass. Areas of decreased (black) signal intensity in the lesion reflect the calcifications evident on the radiograph and computed tomographic scan. The bladder is displaced by the intrapelvic extent of the mass *(arrow)* **(C)**.

aberrations in dedifferentiated chondrosarcoma. A variety of structural and numerical aberrations have been reported.[28]

Prognosis and Therapy

The prognosis of patients with dedifferentiated chondrosarcoma is uniformly poor, regardless of the form of therapy employed. Most patients die of distant metastases within 1 year after the initial diagnosis.

Pleomorphic Rhabdomyosarcoma

Clinical Features

In contrast to most other subtypes of rhabdomyosarcoma that predominately occur in children, pleomorphic rhabdomyosarcoma is seen almost exclusively in adults. Men are affected more commonly than women, and most cases arise in elderly (>50 years old) patients. Most patients present with a rapidly growing soft tissue mass.[29,30]

Pathologic Findings

Histology

Pleomorphic rhabdomyosarcoma usually comprises spindle-shaped to round and polygonal-shaped tumor cells arranged in sheets and vague fascicles. Additionally, numerous polygonal-shaped tumor cells with multilobated, hyperchromatic nuclei and abundant eosinophilic cytoplasm are typical (Fig. 11.22). Furlong and colleagues[30] classified pleomorphic rhabdomyosarcoma into various subtypes based on the predominant cytomorphology—classic (pleomorphic rhabdomyoblasts arranged in sheets), round cell, and spindle cell subtypes (Fig. 11.23).[30] Regardless of subtype, identifiable cross striations in eosinophilic tumor cells are extraordinarily rare. Establishing the diagnosis of pleomorphic rhabdomyosarcoma generally requires immunohistochemical evidence of skeletal muscle differentiation.[30]

Fine Needle Aspiration Biopsy

FNAB of pleomorphic rhabdomyosarcoma yields moderately highly cellular smears with anaplastic tumor cells and multinucleated tumor giant cells, indistinguishable from cells

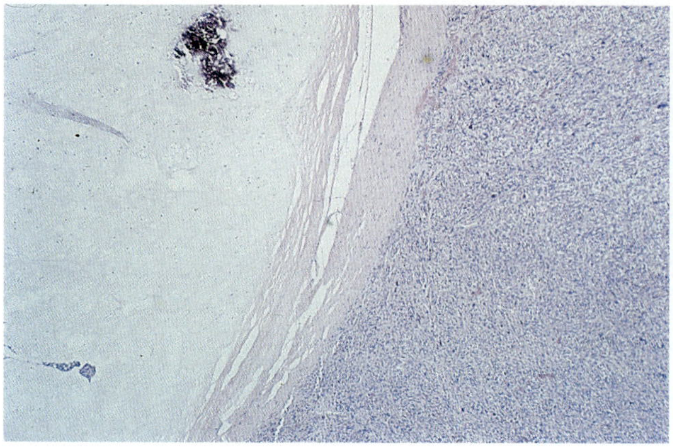

A

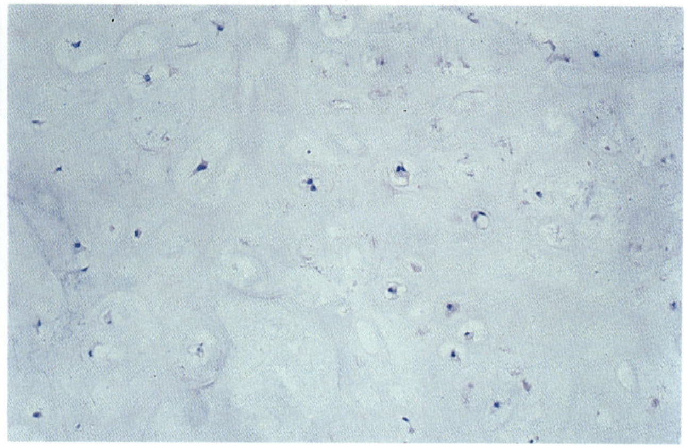

B

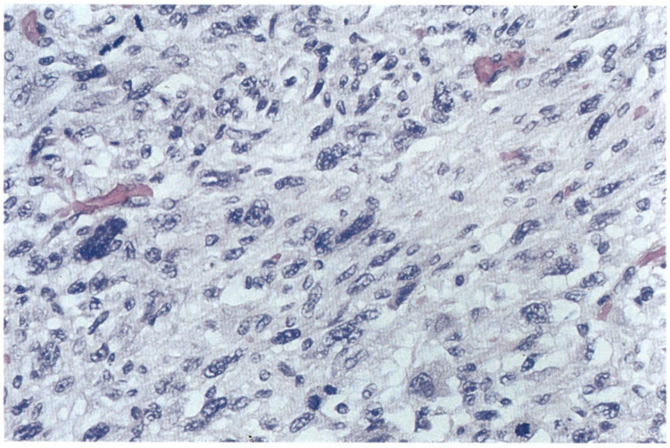

C

FIGURE 11.18 Dedifferentiated chondrosarcoma characterized by sharp juxtaposition of the low-grade cartilaginous component and the noncartilaginous, high-grade spindle cell component **(A)**. The cartilaginous component has the typical bland features of low-grade chondrosarcoma **(B)**, whereas the high-grade, spindle cell portion is virtually indistinguishable from malignant fibrous histiocytoma **(C)**. **(A-C,** H&E.)

observed with other pleomorphic sarcomas. As with tissue biopsies, ancillary studies are required for definitive diagnosis.

Ancillary Studies

Ultrastructural examination of pleomorphic rhabdomyosarcoma reveals prevalent sarcomere formation with Z-band material and thick myosin and thin actin filaments.[30] In the absence of ultrastructural evidence of myogenic differentiation, establishing a diagnosis of adult pleomorphic rhabdomyosarcoma requires immunopositivity for at least one specific skeletal muscle marker (e.g., myogenin, MyoD1, or myoglobin).[30,31] Desmin and, less frequently, actin are usually diffusely positive but, by themselves, are not considered specific enough to establish a diagnosis of pleomorphic rhabdomyosarcoma.

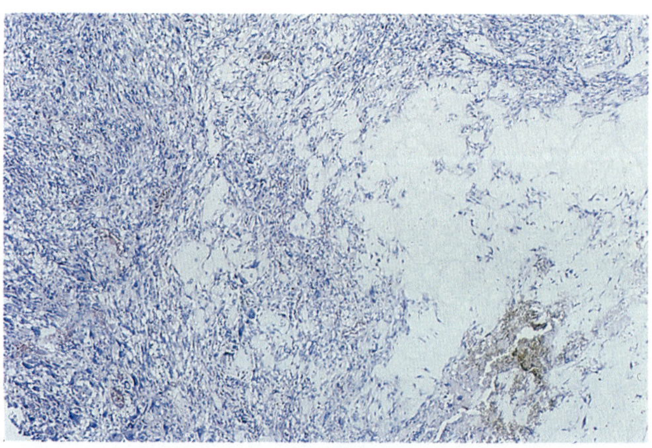

FIGURE 11.19 Dedifferentiated chondrosarcoma revealing a more gradual, intermingled transition between the low-grade chondrosarcoma and the higher grade, dedifferentiated component. (H&E.)

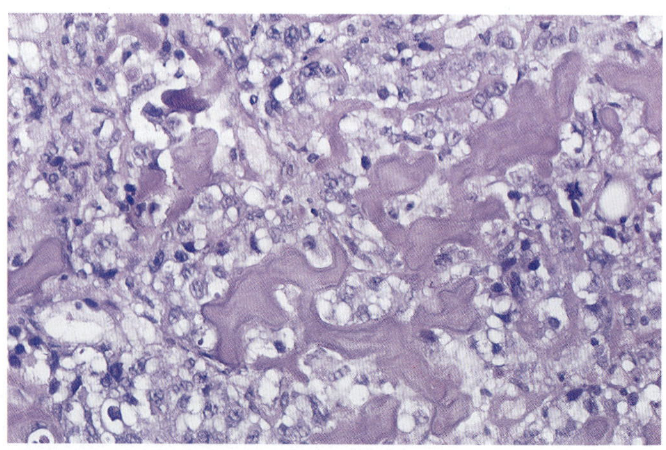

FIGURE 11.20 Less commonly, dedifferentiated chondrosarcoma may exhibit heterologous differentiation, including osteosarcoma. (H&E.)

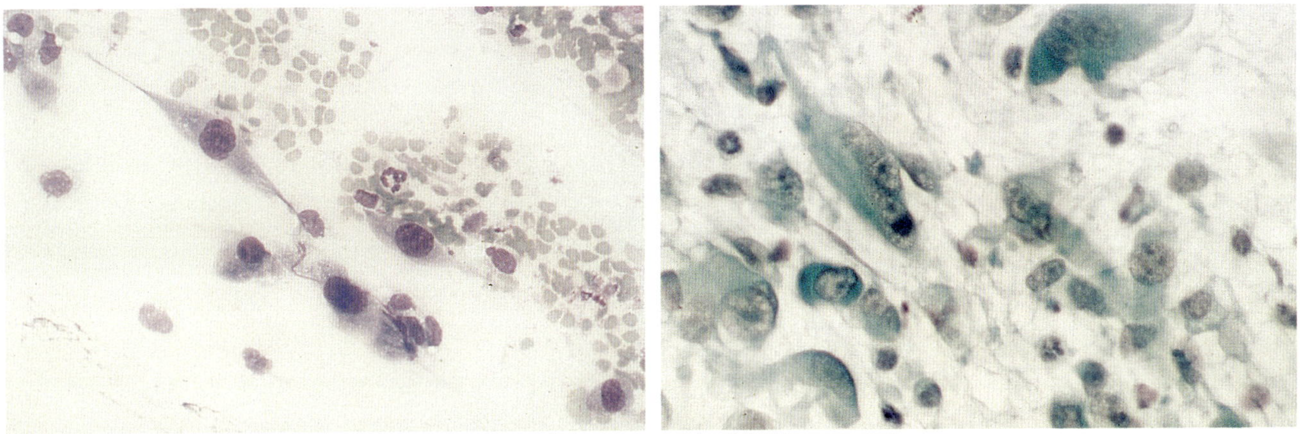

A B

FIGURE 11.21 Fine needle aspiration biopsy specimen from dedifferentiated chondrosarcoma usually reveals non-specific features of high-grade, pleomorphic sarcoma. The low-grade cartilaginous component is generally not sampled **(A** and **B)**. **(A,** Diff-Quik; **B,** Papanicolaou.)

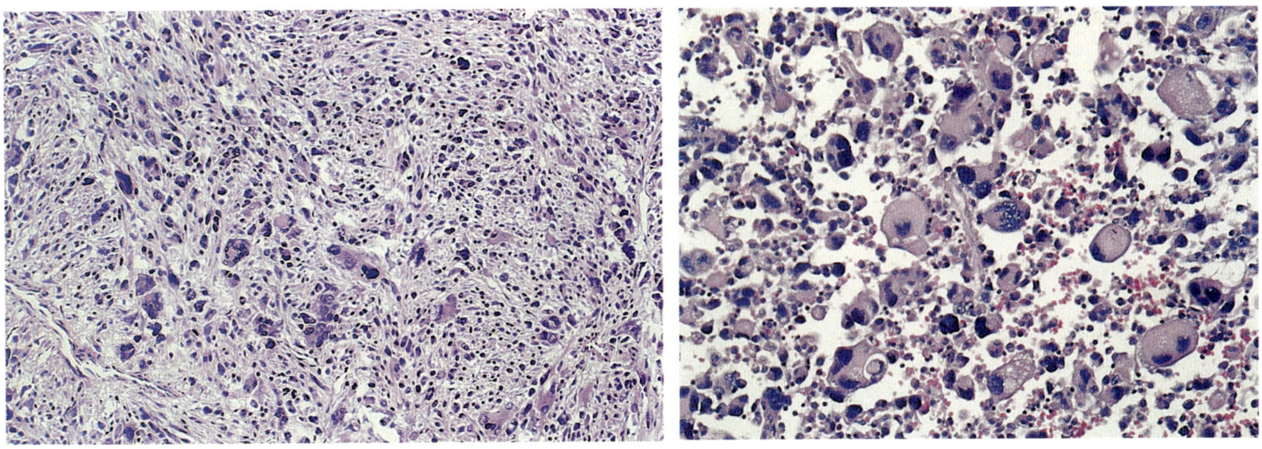

A B

FIGURE 11.22 Pleomorphic rhabdomyosarcoma with characteristic pleomorphic rhabdomyoblasts with one or more nuclei and abundant eosinophilic cytoplasm, accompanied by a population of smaller, round-to-ovoid tumor cells **(A** and **B)**. **(A,** Low power; **B,** high power, H&E.)

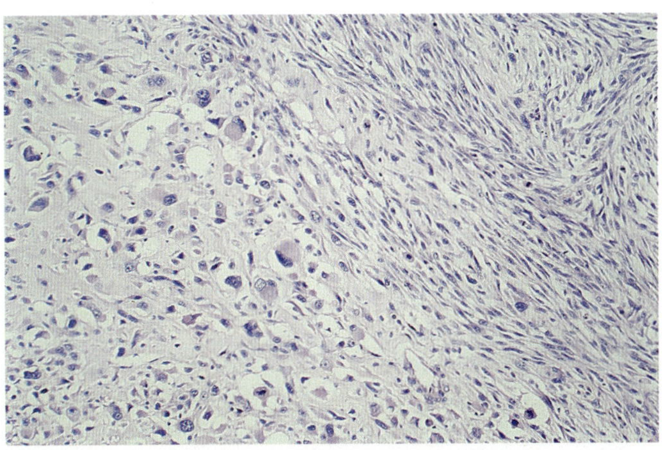

FIGURE 11.23 Pleomorphic rhabdomyosarcoma with fascicular areas and spindled cells juxtaposed to the more characteristic rhabdomyoblasts (H&E).

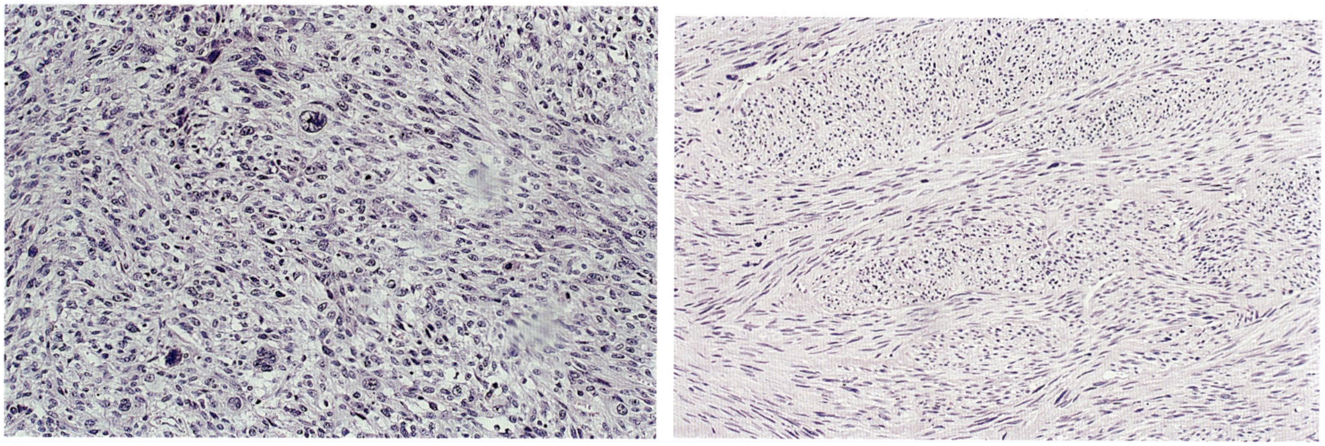

A B

FIGURE 11.24 Pleomorphic leiomyosarcoma with a mixture of anaplastic tumor cells and spindled cells, resembling malignant fibrous histiocytoma **(A)**. Establishing the diagnosis of pleomorphic leiomyosarcoma requires the presence (at least focally) of the typical intersecting-perpendicular leiomyosarcomatous fascicles and positivity for at least one smooth muscle marker (desmin, actin, smooth muscle actin) **(B)**. (H&E.)

Of six adult pleomorphic rhabdomyosarcomas that have been examined by cytogenetic analysis, all have shown complex karyotypes with numerous chromosomal aberrations.[11] No reproducible chromosomal aberrations exist, permitting the specific diagnosis of adult pleomorphic rhabdomyosarcoma by cytogenetic analysis alone.

Prognosis and Therapy

Among adult pleomorphic sarcomas, pleomorphic rhabdomyosarcoma is associated with the most aggressive clinical behavior and poorest survival rate. Of patients, 70% die of the disease; 40% to 50% develop metastases, often within 1 year of initial diagnosis.[29,30] Therapy is similar to that of other adult pleomorphic sarcomas.

Pleomorphic Leiomyosarcoma

Rarely, leiomyosarcoma may exhibit significant nuclear pleomorphism, resembling that observed in malignant fibrous histiocytoma. A more detailed discussion of leiomyosarcoma is presented in Chapter 6. In this chapter, we focus on the pleomorphic variant of leiomyosarcoma. Pleomorphic leiomyosarcoma usually arises in elderly patients (>50 years old). Males and females are affected equally.[32] The most common anatomic sites in decreasing order of frequency are the extremities, retroperitoneum and pelvis, and trunk. In bone, leiomyosarcoma most commonly involves the long bones of the extremities, especially those around the knee.[33] Differentiating pleomorphic leiomyosarcoma from other adult pleomorphic sarcomas requires the presence, at least focally, of a leiomyosarcoma fascicular pattern (e.g., intersecting perpendicular fascicles of spindled tumor cells with elongated nuclei and abundant eosinophilic cytoplasm) (Fig. 11.24).[32] Immunohistochemical evidence of myogenic differentiation should be confirmed with at least one smooth muscle marker (desmin, muscle-specific actin, or smooth muscle actin) in the fascicular areas. FNAB specimens appear indistinguishable from specimens of other adult pleomorphic sarcomas, requiring ancillary studies for definitive diagnosis (Fig. 11.25). Similar to pleomorphic rhabdomyosarcoma, limited data on pleomorphic leiomyosarcoma suggest more aggressive behavior. In one series, 15 of 23 patients (65.2%) died of metastatic disease.[32]

Malignant Mesenchymoma

The designation *malignant mesenchymoma* generally has been applied to sarcomas exhibiting two or more lines of specific differentiation.[34,35] Such differentiation includes lipoblastic,

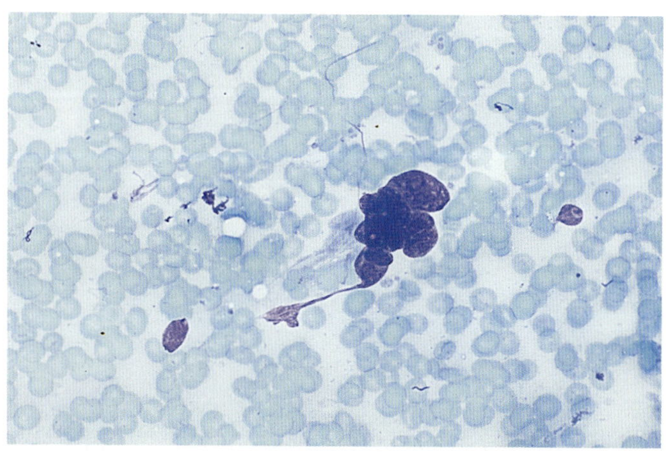

FIGURE 11.25 Fine needle aspiration biopsy specimen of pleomorphic leiomyosarcoma with a nonspecific, anaplastic tumor giant cell. (Diff-Quik.)

osteosarcomatous/chrondrosarcomatous, rhabdomyosarcomatous, or leiomyosarcomatous areas (Fig. 11.26). It has become increasingly clear, however, that the designation of malignant mesenchymoma encompasses a variety of other neoplasms that may exhibit heterologous differentiation, including malignant peripheral nerve sheath tumor, rhabdomyosarcoma, well-differentiated liposarcoma, and dedifferentiated liposarcoma. In our experience, the diagnosis of malignant mesenchymoma is extraordinarily rare and generally is applied to a subgroup of high-grade adult pleomorphic sarcomas exhibiting two or more lines of specialized differentiation. Most reported examples arise in adults and predominately occur in the deep soft tissues of the thigh and retroperitoneum.[34,35] Rare examples also have been described in bone.[36] Reports regarding prognosis have been conflicting, although it generally has been regarded as a high-grade neoplasm. Newman and Fletcher[34] analyzed nine cases of malignant mesenchymoma and found that the biologic behavior was "not as aggressive as the histology would imply." Brady and colleagues[35] evaluated eight patients with malignant mesenchymoma; six died of tumor, and two were alive with evidence of residual disease. In neither of these studies did microscopic appearance correlate with clinical behavior, albeit absolute numbers of patients were small.

Pleomorphic Hyalinizing Angiectatic Tumor of Soft Parts

Pleomorphic hyalinizing angiectatic tumor of soft parts is a more recently described but extraordinarily rare entity. Most of the reported examples have arisen in adults, and there is no gender bias. More than 50% of cases involve the subcutaneous adipose tissue of the lower extremity.[37] Patients typically report the presence of a painless, slow-growing soft tissue mass. Morphologically, pleomorphic hyalinizing angiectatic tumor of soft parts is infiltrative and characterized by thin-walled, hyalinized ectatic blood vessels within a background of spindled tumor cells. The surrounding stroma appears partially myxoid to hyalinized. Individual tumor cells are spindled with ovoid-to-spindled, pleomorphic nuclei and often contain intranuclear cytoplasmic inclusions (Fig. 11.27).[37] Despite the presence of nuclear pleomorphism, mitotic activity is generally significantly less than 1 mitotic figure per 10 high-power fields. Immunohistochemical expression of CD34 and vimentin often is observed, but the tumor cells are uniformly negative for S-100 protein, helping to distinguish it from schwannoma. Pleomorphic hyalinizing angiectatic tumor of soft parts should be considered a borderline to low-grade malignancy.

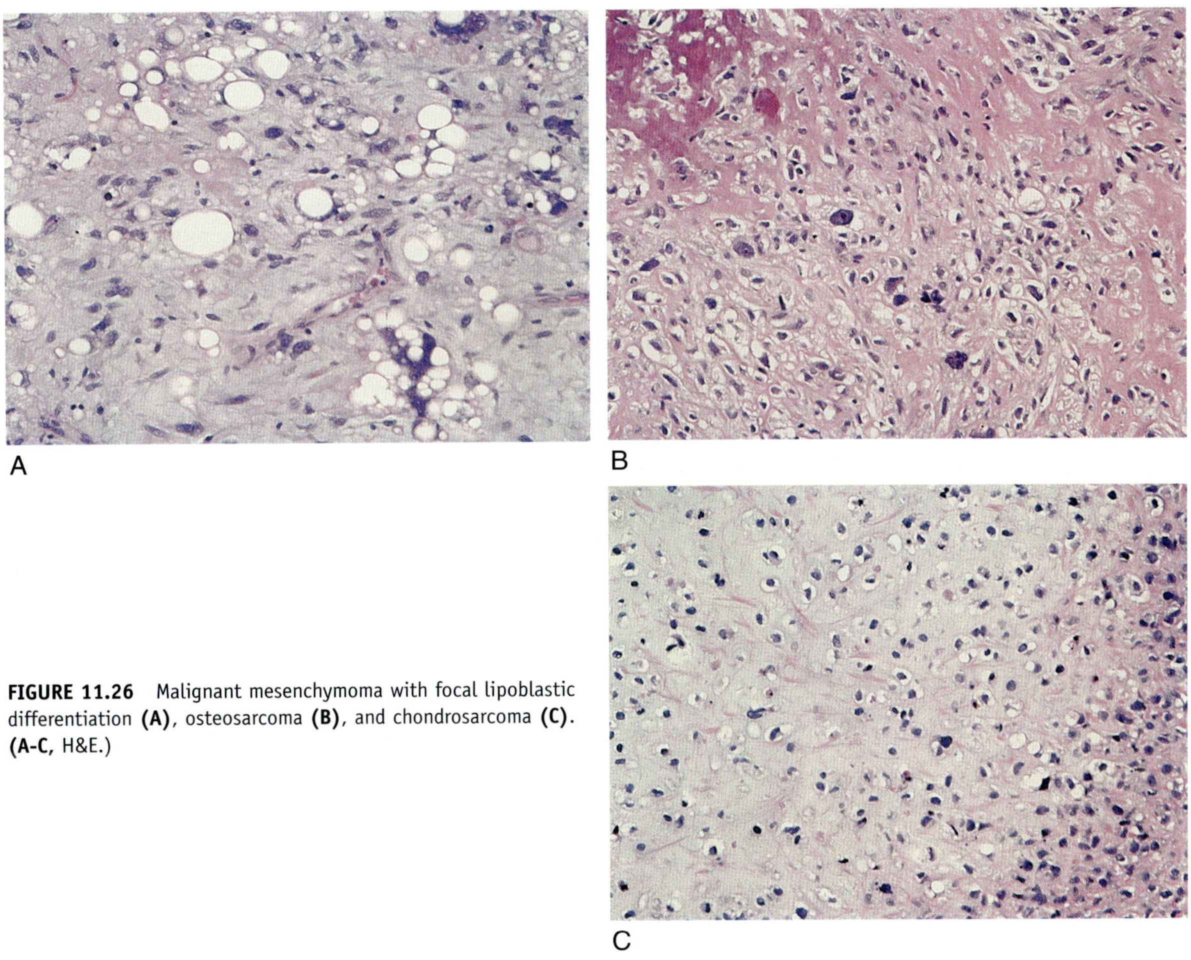

FIGURE 11.26 Malignant mesenchymoma with focal lipoblastic differentiation **(A)**, osteosarcoma **(B)**, and chondrosarcoma **(C)**. **(A-C,** H&E.)

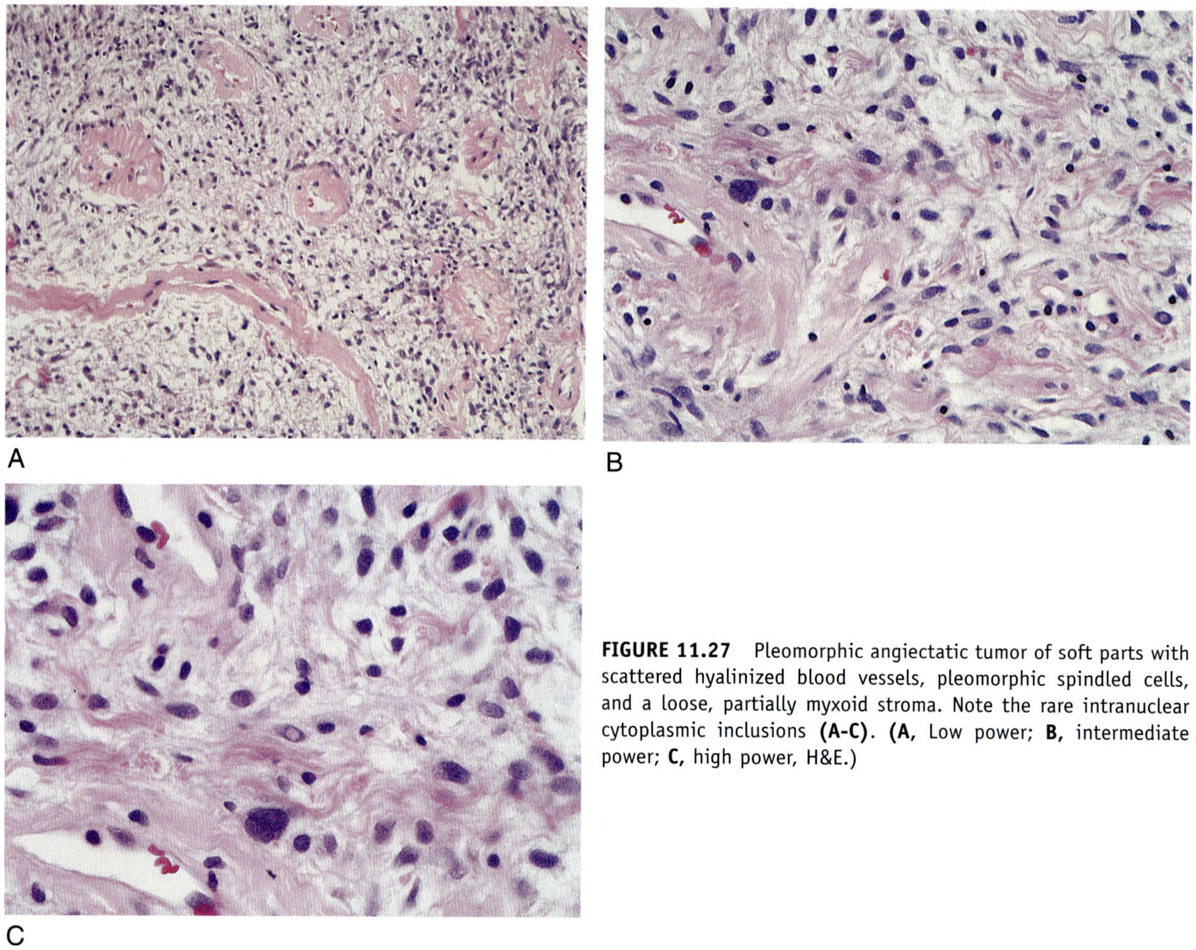

FIGURE 11.27 Pleomorphic angiectatic tumor of soft parts with scattered hyalinized blood vessels, pleomorphic spindled cells, and a loose, partially myxoid stroma. Note the rare intranuclear cytoplasmic inclusions **(A-C)**. (**A,** Low power; **B,** intermediate power; **C,** high power, H&E.)

Local recurrence occurs in 50% of cases, but distant metastasis has never been documented.[37]

REFERENCES

Malignant Fibrous Histiocytoma

1. Weiss SW: 44th Maude Abbott Lecture: Soft tissue sarcomas: Lessons from the past, challenges for the future. Mod Pathol 2002;15:77.
2. Fletcher CDM: Pleomorphic malignant fibrous histiocytoma: Fact or fiction? A critical appraisal based on 159 tumors diagnosed as pleomorphic sarcoma. Am J Surg Pathol 1992;16:213.
3. Fletcher CDM, van den Berg E, Molenaar WM: Pleomorphic malignant fibrous histiocytoma/undifferentiated high grade pleomorphic sarcoma. In Fletcher CDM, Unni KK, Mertens F (eds): Pathology and Genetics: Tumours of Soft Tissue and Bone. World Health Organization Classification of Tumours. Lyon, France: IARC Press, 2002, pp 120–122.
4. Weiss SW: Malignant fibrous histiocytoma: A reaffirmation. Am J Surg Pathol 1982;6:773.
5. Laskin WB, Silverman TA, Enzinger FM: Postradiation soft tissue sarcomas: An analysis of 53 cases. Cancer 1988;62:2330.
6. Nishida J, Sim FH, Wenger DE, et al: Malignant fibrous histiocytoma of bone: A clinicopathologic study of 81 patients. Cancer 1997;79:482.
7. Erlandson RA, Woodruff JM: Role of electron microscope in the evaluation of soft tissue neoplasms with emphasis on spindle cell and pleomorphic tumors. Hum Pathol 1998;29:1372.
8. Wood GS, Beckstead JH, Turner RR, et al: Malignant fibrous histiocytoma tumor cells resemble fibroblasts. Am J Surg Pathol 1986;10:323.
9. Hirose T, Kudo E, Hasegawa T, et al: Expression of intermediate filaments in malignant fibrous histiocytomas. Hum Pathol 1989;20:871.
10. Lawson CW, Fisher C, Gatter KC: An immunohistochemical study of differentiation in malignant fibrous histiocytoma. Histopathology 1987;11:375.
11. Mertens F, Fletcher CDM, Dal Cin P, et al: Cytogenetic analysis of 46 pleomorphic soft tissue sarcomas and correlation with morphologic and clinical features: A report of the CHAMP group. Genes Chromosomes Cancer 1998;22:16.
12. Urban C, Rosen G, Huvos AG, et al: Chemotherapy of malignant fibrous histiocytoma of bone: A report of five cases. Cancer 1983;51:795.

Pleomorphic Liposarcoma

13. Oliveria AM, Nascimento AG: Pleomorphic liposarcoma. Semin Diagn Pathol 2001;18:274.
14. Downes KA, Goldblum JR, Montgomery EA: Pleomorphic liposarcoma: A clinicopathologic analysis of 19 cases. Mod Pathol 2001;14:179.
15. Miettinen M, Enzinger FM: Epithelioid variant of pleomorphic liposarcoma: A study of 12 cases of a distinctive variant of high-grade liposarcoma. Mod Pathol 1999;12:722.
16. Weiss LM, Warhol MJ: Ultrastructural distinctions between adult pleomorphic rhabdomyosarcomas, pleomorphic liposarcomas, and pleomorphic malignant fibrous histiocytomas. Hum Pathol 1984;15:1025.
17. Gebhard S, Coindre JM, Michels JJ, et al: Pleomorphic liposarcoma: Clinicopathologic and immunohistochemical study of 63 cases: A study of the French Sarcoma Group. Am J Surg Pathol 2002;26:601.
18. Sreekantaiah C, Karakousis CP, Leong SP, et al: Cytogenetic findings in liposarcoma correlate with histopathologic subtypes. Cancer 1992;69:2484.

Dedifferentiated Liposarcoma

19. Henricks WH, Chu YC, Goldblum JR, et al: Dedifferentiated liposarcoma: A clinicopathologic analysis of 155 cases with a proposal for an expanded definition of dedifferentiation. Am J Surg Pathol 1997;21:271.
20. Nascimento AG: Dedifferentiated liposarcoma. Semin Diagn Pathol 2001;18:263.
21. McCormick D, Mentzel T, Beham A, et al: Dedifferentiated liposarcoma: Clinicopathologic analysis of 32 cases suggesting a better prognostic subgroup among pleomorphic sarcomas. Am J Surg Pathol 1994;18:1213.
22. Evans HL, Khurana KK, Kemp BL, et al: Heterologous elements in the dedifferentiated component of dedifferentiated liposarcoma. Am J Surg Pathol 1994;18:1150.
23. Nascimento AG, Kurtin PJ, Guillou L, et al: Dedifferentiated liposarcoma: A report of nine cases with a peculiar neurallike whorling pattern associated with metaplastic bone formation. Am J Surg Pathol 1998;22:945.

Dedifferentiated Chondrosarcoma

24. Dahlin DC, Beabout JW: Dedifferentiation of low-grade chondrosarcomas. Cancer 1971;28:461.
25. Johnson S, Tetu B, Ayala AG, et al: Chondrosarcoma with additional mesenchymal component (dedifferentiated chondrosarcoma): A clinicopathologic study of 26 cases. Cancer 1986;58:278.
26. Reith JD, Bauer TW, Fischler DF, et al: Dedifferentiated chondrosarcoma with rhabdomyosarcomatous differentiation. Am J Surg Pathol 1996;20:293.
27. Kilpatrick SE, Pike EJ, Ward WG, et al: Dedifferentiated chondrosarcoma in patients with multiple osteochondromatosis: Report of a case and review of the literature. Skeletal Radiol 1997;26:370.
28. O'Malley DP, Opheim KE, Barry TS, et al: Chromosomal changes in dedifferentiated chondrosarcoma: A case report and review of the literature. Cancer Genet Cytogenet 2001;124:105.

Pleomorphic Rhabdomyosarcoma

29. Gaffney EF, Dervan PA, Fletcher CDM: Pleomorphic rhabdomyosarcoma in adulthood: Analysis of 11 cases with definition of diagnostic criteria. Am J Surg Pathol 1993;17:601.
30. Furlong MA, Mentzel T, Fanburg-Smith JC: Pleomorphic rhabdomyosarcoma in adults: A clinicopathologic study of 38 cases with emphasis on morphologic variants and recent skeletal muscle-markers. Mod Pathol 2001;14:595.
31. Wesche WA, Fletcher CDM, Dias P, et al: Immunohistochemistry of MyoD1 in adult pleomorphic soft tissue sarcomas. Am J Surg Pathol 1995;19:261.

Pleomorphic Leiomyosarcoma

32. Oda Y, Miyajima K, Kawaguchi K, et al: Pleomorphic leiomyosarcoma: Clinicopathologic and immunohistochemical study with special emphasis on its distinction from ordinary leiomyosarcoma and malignant fibrous histiocytoma. Am J Surg Pathol 2001;25:1030.
33. Antonescu CR, Erlandson RA, Huvos AG: Primary leiomyosarcoma of bone: A clinicopathologic, immunohistochemical, and ultrastructural study of 33 patients and a literature review. Am J Surg Pathol 1997;21:1281.

Malignant Mesenchymoma

34. Newman PL, Fletcher CDM: Malignant mesenchymoma: Clinicopathologic analysis of a series with evidence of low-grade behavior. Am J Surg Pathol 1991;15:607.
35. Brady MS, Perino G, Tallini G, et al: Malignant mesenchymoma. Cancer 1996;77:467.
36. Van Dorpe J, Sciot R, Samson I, et al: Primary osteorhabdomyosarcoma (malignant mesenchymoma) of bone: A case report and review of the literature. Mod Pathol 1997;10:1047.

Pleomorphic Hyalinizing Angiectatic Tumor of Soft Parts

37. Smith ME, Fisher C, Weiss SW: Pleomorphic hyalinizing angiectatic tumor of soft parts: A low-grade neoplasm resembling neurilemoma. Am J Surg Pathol 1996;20:21.

CHAPTER 12

Osseous Tumors of Bone and Soft Tissue

Osseous tumors, as pertain to this chapter, concern chiefly solid lesions that contain (or produce) osteoid or bone or both as part of their stroma. Table 12.1 lists tumors generally associated with bone production. Ossifying fibromyxoid tumor perhaps is best considered in the differential diagnosis of myxoid lesions. Bone cysts are discussed in Chapter 14. Metaplastic bone may occur in a variety of generally non–bone-forming tumors. Table 12.2 summarizes soft tissue neoplasms most frequently associated with metaplastic ossification. Most of the tumors discussed in this chapter are not evaluable by fine needle aspiration biopsy (FNAB) because of excessive ossification. The exception to the rule is high-grade osteosarcoma, in which FNAB is not only possible, but also a highly accurate technique for establishing the diagnosis.

TABLE 12.1 Osteoid and Bone-Forming Tumors of Skeletal and Extraskeletal Tissues

Bone Origin	Soft Tissue Origin
Bone island	Myositis ossificans and variants
Osteoma	Ossifying fibromyxoid tumor
Osteoid osteoma	Osteosarcoma
Osteoblastoma	
Osteosarcoma	
Fibrous dysplasia	
Osteofibrous dysplasia (ossifying fibroma)	
Simple and aneurysmal bone cysts	
Hamartoma of the chest wall	

Myositis Ossificans

Strictly defined, myositis ossificans is a localized, self-limited, typically ossifying process that often occurs in response to soft tissue trauma. Nevertheless, the designation *myositis ossificans* is a misnomer because it is not always confined to the musculature, it lacks significant ossification in its early formative stages, and it is virtually never associated with significant inflammation.[1,2] Morphologically similar-appearing lesions also may occur within the skin, subcutaneous fat, tendons, nail bed, and periosteum (juxtacortical), encompassing a variety of seemingly distinct diagnostic entities, including osteoma cutis, florid reactive periostitis (fibro-osseous pseudotumor of the digits), bizarre parosteal osteochondromatous proliferation, and Dupuytren's subungual exostosis (Table 12.3). This vast plethora of terms describing what histologically represents closely related entities may cause considerable diagnostic confusion, not only for the pathologist, but also for the surgeon faced with the dilemma of appropriate therapy and clinical management.

TABLE 12.2 Soft Tissue Lesions Often Associated with Metaplastic Ossification

Ossifying fibromyxoid tumor
Mixed tumor/myoepithelioma
Malignant peripheral nerve sheath tumor
Synovial sarcoma
Mesenchymal chondrosarcoma
Dedifferentiated liposarcoma
Malignant mesenchymoma

Classic Myositis Ossificans

Clinical Features

Myositis ossificans generally affects young, often athletic adults, aged 20 to 30 years.[1] Most patients complain of a rapidly growing, tender, intramuscular soft tissue mass. A history of antecedent trauma to the affected region frequently is reported. The extremities are the most commonly affected sites, specifically the quadriceps, gluteus, and brachialis muscles.[1] Rarely, myositis ossificans may be a component of a rare genetic disorder, fibrodysplasia ossificans progressiva, in which multifocal heterotopic ossification leads to severe joint morbidity and death.

Radiologically, myositis ossificans usually manifests as a localized but diffusely calcified soft tissue mass (Fig. 12.1). The zonal phenomenon may be evident, exemplified by a distinctly more radiodense periphery contrasting with a radiolucent center (Fig. 12.2).[3,4] Less commonly, myositis ossificans may undergo cystic degeneration centrally, leaving behind only a peripheral rim of ossification. Older examples (>6 weeks' duration) may lack this distinct zoning pattern, displaying instead uniform and diffuse ossification.[5] In contrast, the early phases (<3 weeks' duration) of myositis ossificans may lack detectable ossification, exhibiting only a soft tissue density. When myositis ossificans evolves from periosteum (periostitis ossificans), longitudinal periosteal lamellations mimicking Ewing's sarcoma may occur; conversely, these changes may mimic florid reactive periostitis (Fig. 12.3).[6] Despite advances in technology, plain film radiographic interpretation remains the gold standard for analysis of orthopedic lesions. Myositis ossificans may appear aggressive on magnetic resonance imaging, causing diagnostic confusion with soft tissue sarcoma, especially if conventional radiographs are unavailable (Fig. 12.4).

TABLE 12.3 Myositis Ossificans and Variants

Classic myositis ossificans
Florid reactive periostitis (fibro-osseous pseudotumor of the digits)
Bizarre parosteal osteochondromatous proliferation (Nora's lesion)
Dupuytren's subungual exostosis
Osteoma cutis

Pathologic Findings

Histology

As with the radiologic findings, the pathologic features observed in myositis ossificans depend on the stage at which it is diagnosed. More classic examples of myositis ossificans are well circumscribed and characterized by a distinct zoning pattern (Figs. 12.5 and 12.6). The central portion of the tumefaction is composed of a loose "tissue culture" proliferation of immature but uniform-appearing fibroblasts closely resembling those observed in nodular fasciitis. Increased mitotic activity may be alarmingly evident. Inflammatory elements,

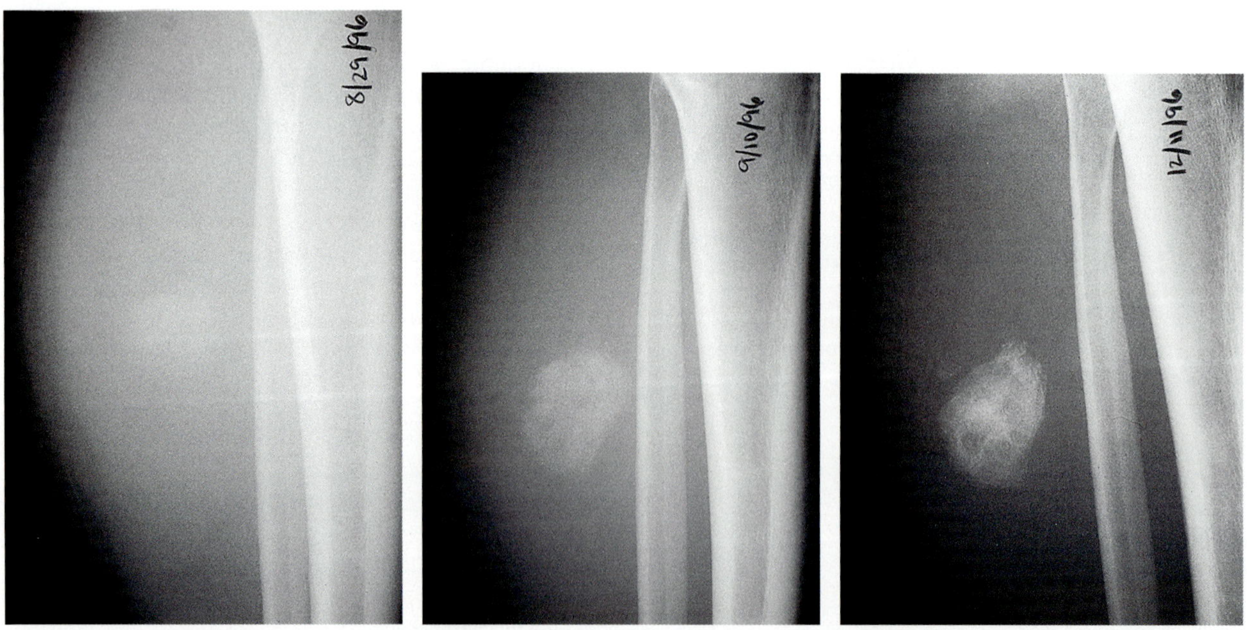

A B C

FIGURE 12.1 Myositis ossificans. A lateral radiograph 10 days after trauma shows a faintly calcified soft tissue mass posterior to the tibia **(A)**. A film 4 weeks later shows the mass is more densely calcified **(B)**. Another lateral film 2 weeks later shows progressive calcification of the mass with a developing peripheral rim of ossification **(C)**.

especially lymphocytes and histiocytes, are scattered among the fibroblasts, but neutrophils are rarely prominent. Variable amounts of benign-appearing, osteoclast-type giant cells also may be seen.[7] At the periphery, osteoid appears to emanate from the nodular fasciitis-like stroma, gradually calcifying and evolving to more mature woven or lamellar bone. Islands of immature-to-mature cartilage sometimes may predominate (Fig. 12.7), sometimes preceding bone formation and providing a template for its production.[1,6] In some examples of myositis ossificans, the central portion of the lesion may undergo cystic degeneration, leaving behind a fluid-filled space and a peripheral rim of ossification (Fig. 12.8). Such cases may represent examples of so-called primary aneurysmal bone cysts of soft tissues.[8,9] Older lesions often show complete ossification consisting of mature lamellar bone admixed with normal fat or bone marrow elements (Fig. 12.9). If juxtacortical, the latter may be difficult to distinguish from a parosteal osteoma. Some cases of myositis ossificans may lack the

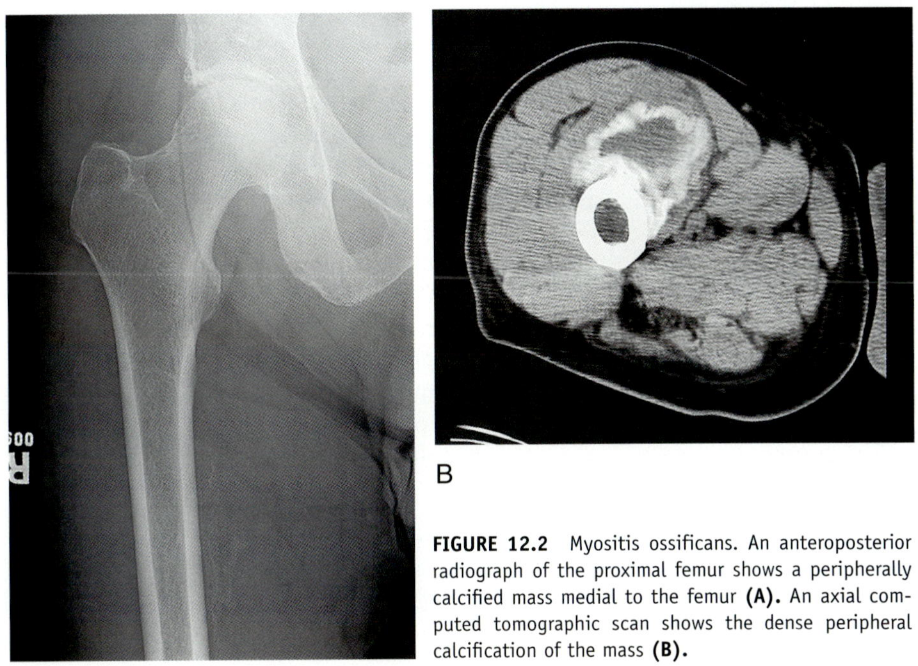

A B

FIGURE 12.2 Myositis ossificans. An anteroposterior radiograph of the proximal femur shows a peripherally calcified mass medial to the femur **(A)**. An axial computed tomographic scan shows the dense peripheral calcification of the mass **(B)**.

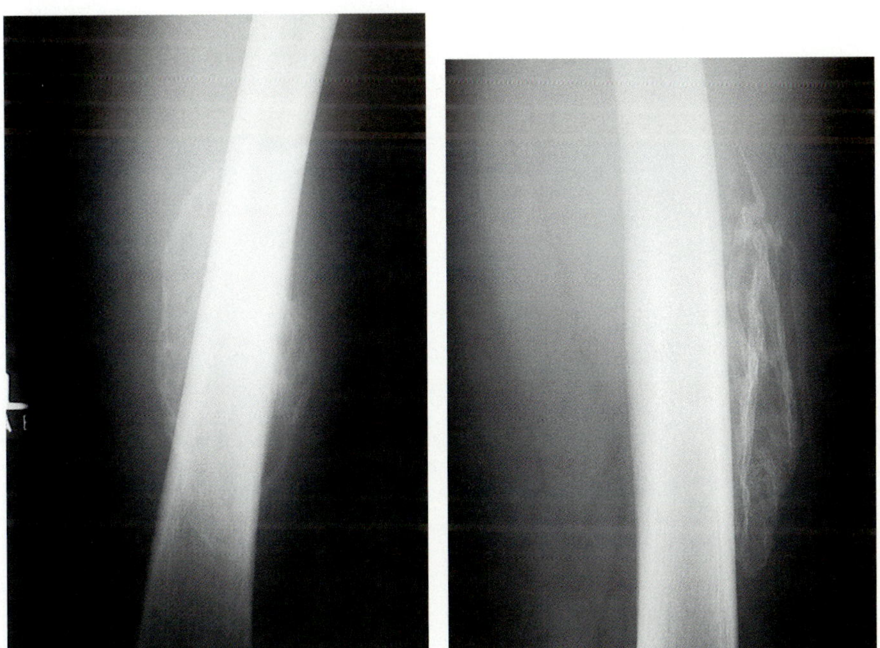

A B

FIGURE 12.3 Periostitis ossificans. Anteroposterior **(A)** and lateral **(B)** radiographs of the femur show a mass of mature periosteal new bone production abutting the shaft of the femur. The underlying femoral cortex is intact.

distinctive and pathognomonic zonation pattern of classic myositis ossificans (Fig. 12.10). Such examples appear more commonly in tumors originating in subcutaneous fat and may exhibit multiple "zonation" centers of ossification.[1] The differential diagnosis includes nodular fasciitis, proliferative fasciitis, and proliferative myositis, all of which rarely may show foci of metaplastic osteoid bone.[1,10,11] Nevertheless, the amount of metaplastic bone observed in these proliferations is never enough to cause diagnostic confusion with myositis ossificans.

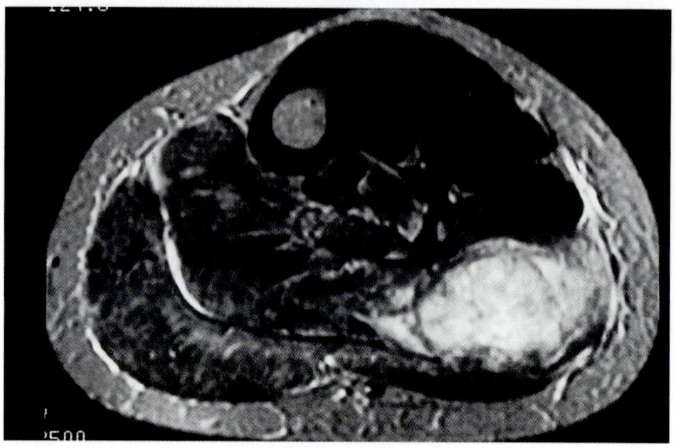

FIGURE 12.4 Myositis ossificans. An axial magnetic resonance image reveals a heterogeneous mass lateral to the midfibula. Although the peripheral rim of decreased signal intensity suggests calcification, the magnetic resonance imaging appearances are not specific and could represent a soft tissue sarcoma.

Fine Needle Aspiration Biopsy

As mentioned, FNAB is usually not successful in establishing the diagnosis of myositis ossificans because of extensive ossification. Consequently, smears generally consist of sparse to no material and are regarded as unsatisfactory. In the earlier, less ossified stages of myositis ossificans, cytologic preparations closely resemble that observed in nodular or proliferative fasciitis, appearing cellular and composed of reactive-appearing fibroblasts arranged singly and as small clusters. In Diff-Quik preparations, metachromatic stromal material consistent with osteoid/bone is variably present. Correlation with radiologic findings permits an accurate diagnosis. It has been our practice to recommend following these patients with serial radiographs to confirm subsequent maturation. If the latter does not occur, open incisional biopsy is indicated.

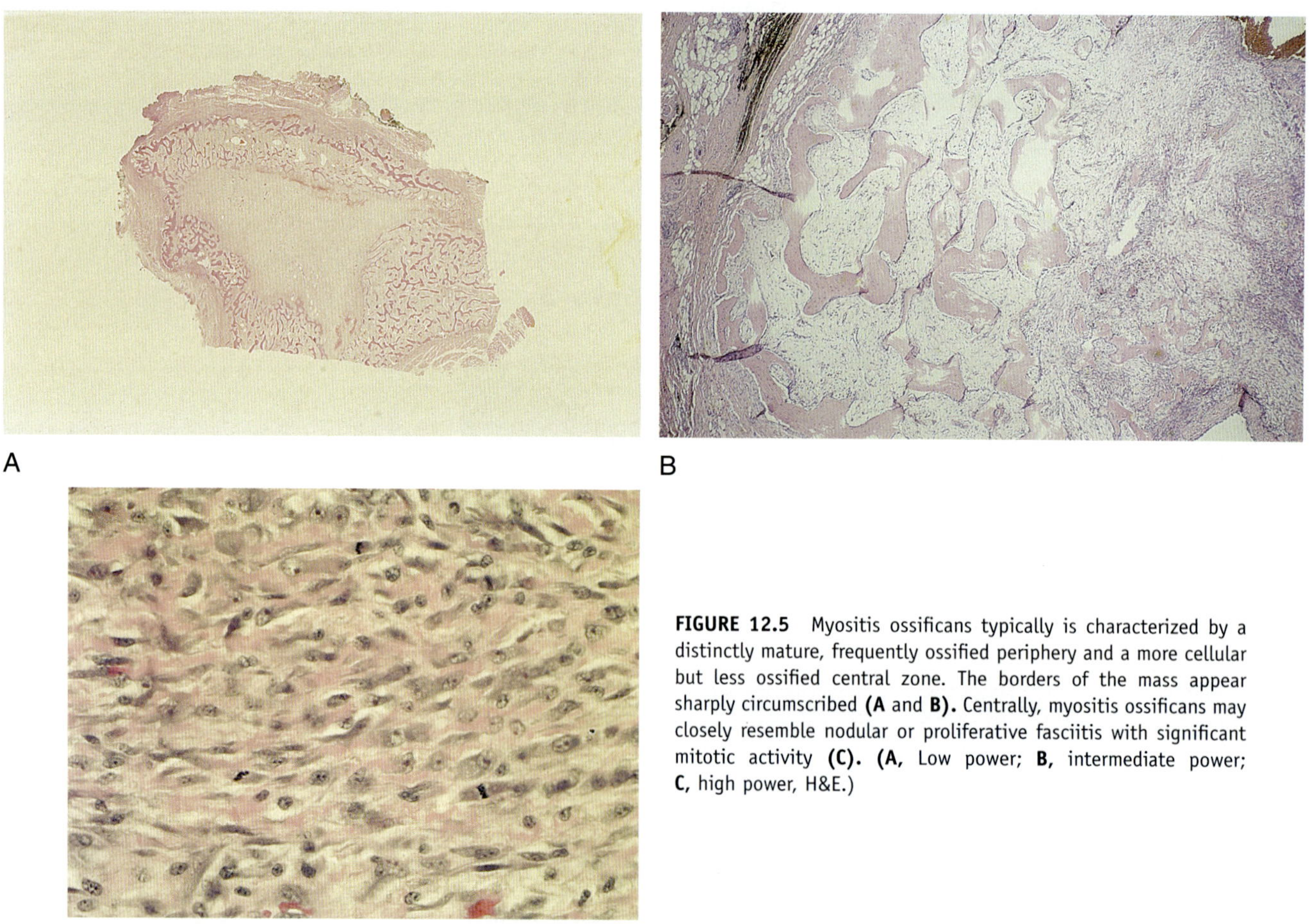

A

B

C

FIGURE 12.5 Myositis ossificans typically is characterized by a distinctly mature, frequently ossified periphery and a more cellular but less ossified central zone. The borders of the mass appear sharply circumscribed **(A** and **B)**. Centrally, myositis ossificans may closely resemble nodular or proliferative fasciitis with significant mitotic activity **(C)**. **(A,** Low power; **B,** intermediate power; **C,** high power, H&E.)

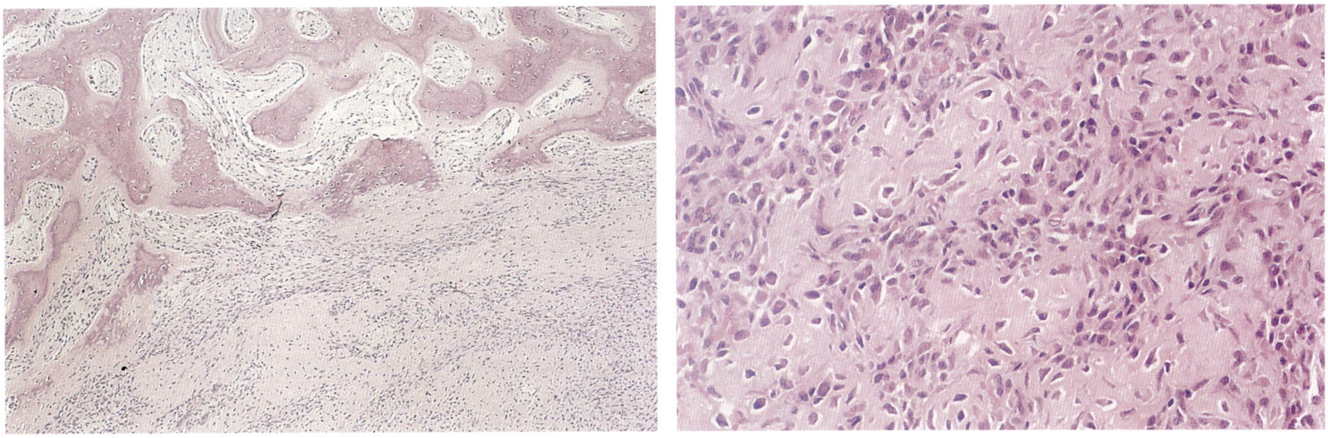

A B

FIGURE 12.6 Myositis ossificans with a peripheral zone of woven bone deposition and a more central, noncalcified region of osteoid deposition **(A).** At high power, the more central zone of osteoid deposition appears to comprise proliferating fibroblasts and osteoblasts **(B).** **(A** and **B,** H&E.)

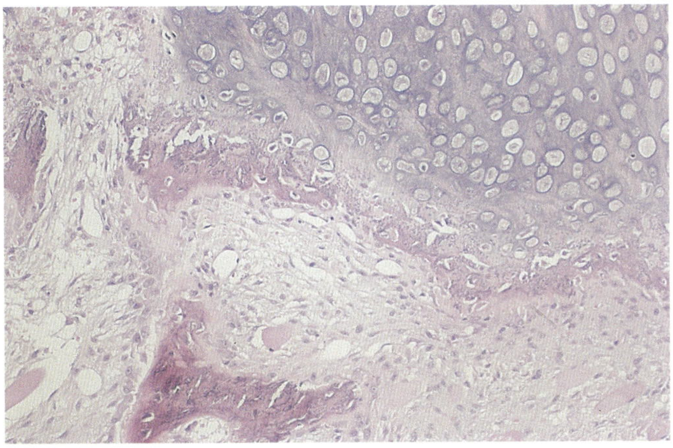

FIGURE 12.7 Mature hyaline cartilage is occasionally identified in myositis ossificans. (H&E.)

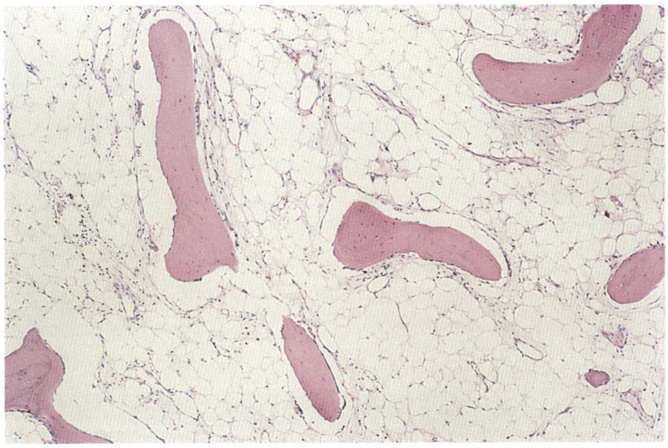

FIGURE 12.9 Older examples of myositis ossificans may become completely ossified with mature lamellar bone and intervening marrow elements and fat. (H&E.)

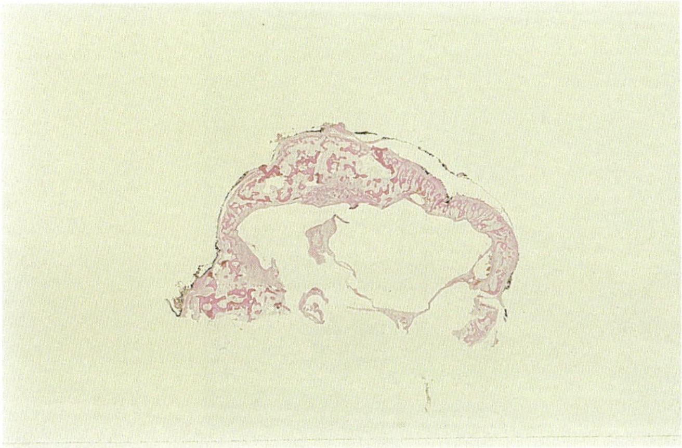

FIGURE 12.8 Rarely the central portions of myositis ossificans may undergo cystic degeneration, mimicking an aneurysmal bone cyst. (H&E.)

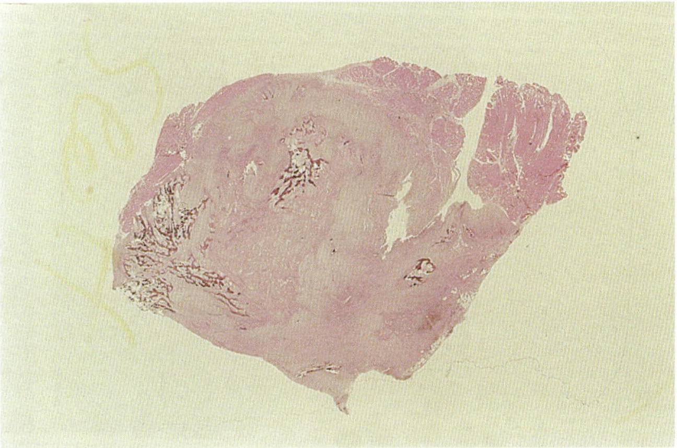

FIGURE 12.10 Myositis ossificans with an incomplete rim of ossification. (H&E.)

Prognosis and Therapy

Myositis ossificans is a benign and self-limited lesion. When the diagnosis is established, the overall prognosis is excellent, and patients generally require no further therapy. In some patients, myositis ossificans may be removed for cosmetic reasons or to alleviate patient anxiety. Biopsies performed during the early, active growth phase of the lesion may leave behind residual tumor that continues to grow. It is best to consider this phenomenon as "persistence" of myositis ossificans and not evidence of "local recurrence." These patients should be followed by serial radiographs to confirm maturation of the lesion and ultimate cessation of growth. We have never observed a convincing example of malignant transformation of myositis ossificans.

Florid Reactive Periostitis (Fibro-osseous Pseudotumor of the Digits)

Although florid reactive periostitis may occur at any age, most affected patients are young adults, usually between 20 and 30 years old. There seems to be a slight female predominance.[12,13] Many patients have a history of trauma. The most common clinical complaint is painful soft tissue swelling. Characteristic radiographic features include significant soft tissue swelling, juxtacortical calcifications, and often a periosteal reaction, which may be mature or laminated (Fig. 12.11). The underlying bony cortex is always intact.[13,14] The distal upper extremities are affected far more commonly than the distal lower extremities. The most commonly involved underlying bones are the proximal phalanges, closely followed by the distal and middle phalanges. Metacarpal and metatarsal involvement also has been documented.

Florid reactive periostitis is characterized by a proliferation of haphazardly arranged reactive-appearing osteoid/bone within a proliferating but benign-appearing fibrous stroma.[12,13] Mitotic figures frequently are seen within the stromal cells, but atypical forms are never encountered (Fig. 12.12). Immature-to-mature–appearing hyaline cartilage rarely may be evident. Rare examples of florid reactive periostitis may show evidence of "zonation," in which focal areas display immature, uncalcified osteoid centrally blending imperceptibly with more mature-appearing lamellar bone peripherally.[13] Surgical excision is also the therapy of choice for florid reactive periostitis. Local recurrence rarely occurs.

Bizarre Parosteal Osteochondromatous Proliferation (Nora's Lesion)

Most cases of bizarre parosteal osteochondromatous proliferation occur in young adults 25 to 35 years old.[15] There seems to be a slight female predominance. Symptoms, usually

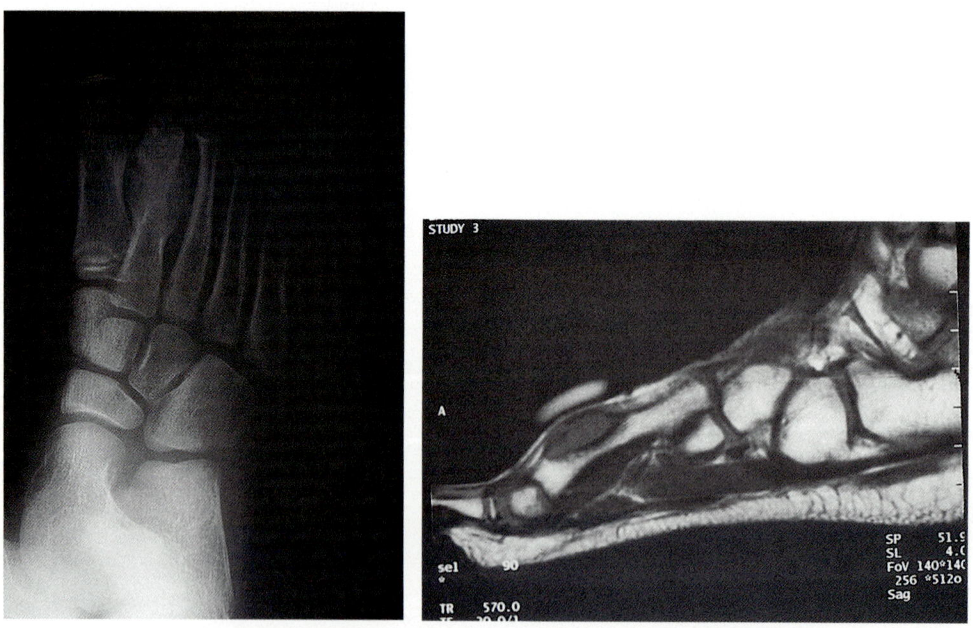

A B

FIGURE 12.11 Florid reactive periostitis. An oblique radiograph of the foot shows a circumferential mass of mature periosteal new bone production, encircling the distal second metatarsal **(A)**. A sagittal magnetic resonance image shows the mass along the dorsal surface of the second metatarsal, centered at the cortex **(B)**.

related to the tumefactions, include soft tissue swelling and limitation of movement. In contrast to florid reactive periostitis, pain is not universally present, and patients less commonly report a prior history of trauma.[15,16] Radiographically, bizarre parosteal osteochondromatous proliferations are sessile-to-pedunculated, osteochondroma-like masses that arise directly from the cortical surface of the underlying bone without significant alteration of the cortex.[15,17] In contrast to osteochondroma, bizarre parosteal osteochondromatous proliferation shows no medullary continuity at its base with the parent bone (Fig. 12.13). Most cases involve the small tubular bones of the hands and feet, especially the proximal and middle phalanges of the hands. Less commonly, the long bones of the upper and lower extremities are involved (Fig. 12.14).[17]

Pathologic examination reveals an alarmingly hypercellular cartilaginous cap, which often contains atypical chondrocytes and binucleated forms. The underlying bony trabeculae arising from enchondral ossification are mostly mature lamellar bone and tend to have a characteristic deep "blue" basophilia, which persists beyond the immediate zone of enchondral ossification.[15,17] The osteochondral junction tends to be less uniform and consistent than that observed in osteochondroma. The intertrabecular spaces exhibit a uniform and loose-appearing fibroblastic proliferation (Fig. 12.15). Although mitotic activity may be prominent, atypical mitotic figures are absent.

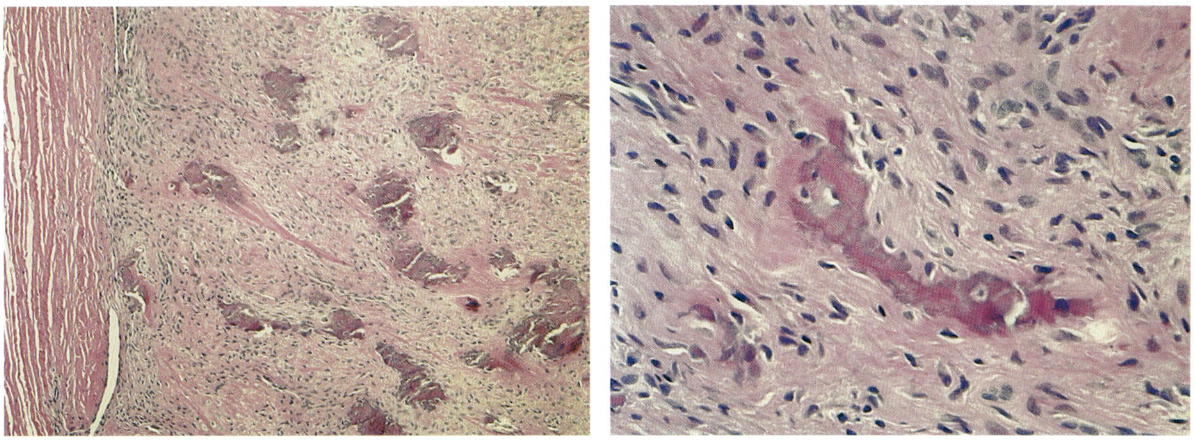

FIGURE 12.12 Florid reactive periostitis appears sharply circumscribed from the adjacent soft tissues **(A)**. At high power, spicules of woven bone are admixed with a bland-appearing fibrous stroma **(B)**. (**A,** Low power; **B,** high power, H&E.)

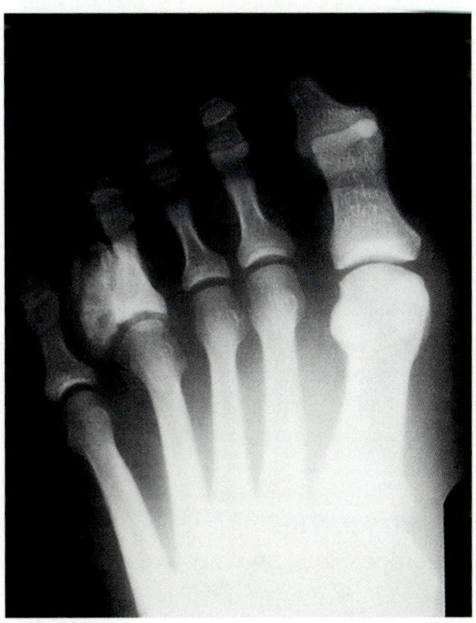

FIGURE 12.13 Bizarre parosteal osteochondromatous proliferation. An anteroposterior view of the forefoot shows a dense, peripherally calcified mass lateral to the proximal phalanx of the fourth toe.

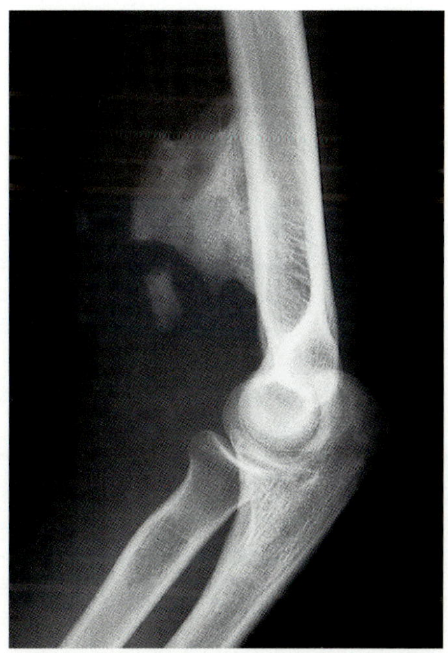

FIGURE 12.14 Bizarre parosteal osteochondromatous proliferation. A lateral radiograph of the elbow reveals a densely calcified excrescence arising from the distal humerus. The subjacent cortex is intact, and there is no medullary invasion.

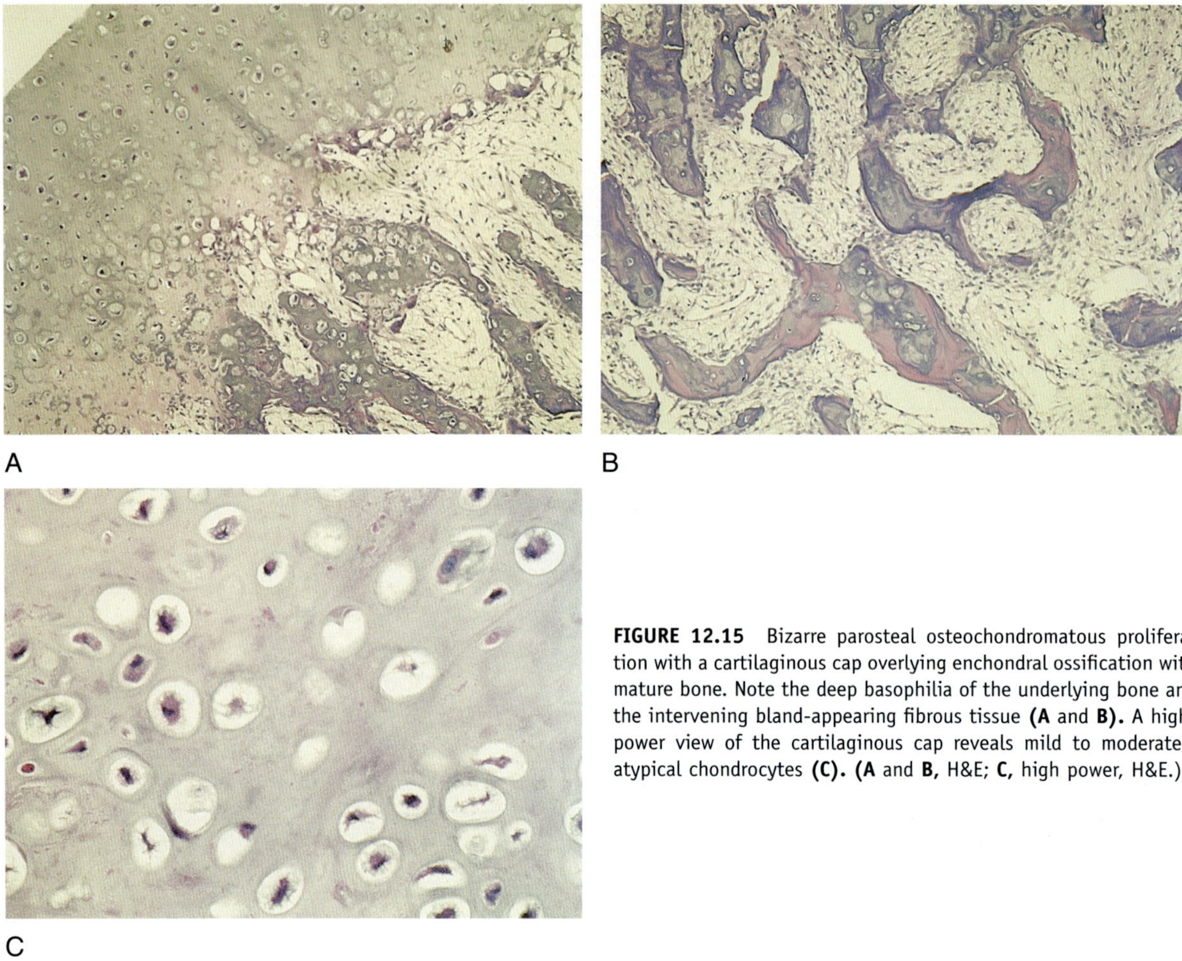

FIGURE 12.15 Bizarre parosteal osteochondromatous proliferation with a cartilaginous cap overlying enchondral ossification with mature bone. Note the deep basophilia of the underlying bone and the intervening bland-appearing fibrous tissue **(A** and **B)**. A high-power view of the cartilaginous cap reveals mild to moderately atypical chondrocytes **(C)**. **(A** and **B,** H&E; **C,** high power, H&E.)

Therapy generally consists of surgical excision. Approximately 50% may recur locally, and multiple recurrences are commonly observed.

Dupuytren's Subungual Exostosis

Dupuytren's subungual exostosis may occur at any age but is observed most commonly in patients 15 to 25 years old.[18] Males and females seem affected equally. The most common presenting complaint is a painful subungual mass, usually located dorsomedially and often associated with elevation and ultimately ulceration of the nail plate and bed. A few patients report a history of antecedent trauma. Radiographically, Dupuytren's subungual exostosis shows a soft tissue mass adjacent to but without medullary continuity to the underlying bone.[18] A periosteal reaction is typically absent (Fig. 12.16). Dupuytren's subungual exostosis involves the dorsal and dorsal-medial distal phalanges, especially the dorsal-medial aspect of the great toe in 75% of cases.

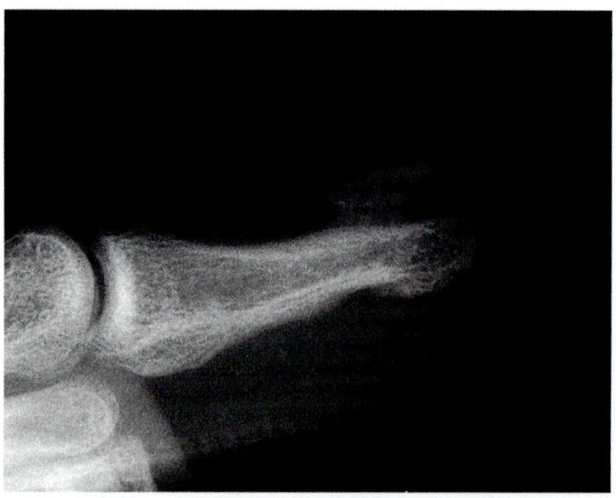

FIGURE 12.16 Dupuytren's subungual exostosis. A lateral radiograph of the great toe shows a well-defined exostosis arising from the dorsal surface of the distal phalanx and extending toward the nail bed. The excrescence arises from the cortex, but the cortex is intact.

Overall the pathologic findings of Dupuytren's subungual exostosis show a striking resemblance to findings of bizarre parosteal osteochondromatous proliferation. A proliferating fibrocartilage–to–hyaline cartilage cap blends imperceptibly with the nail bed, surrounding a haphazard arrangement of mostly mature-appearing, woven-to-lamellar bone arising partially as a result of enchondral ossification (Fig. 12.17). Within the intertrabecular spaces is proliferating fibrous tissue composed of plump, reactive-appearing fibroblasts.[18,19] As in bizarre parosteal osteochondromatous proliferation, the

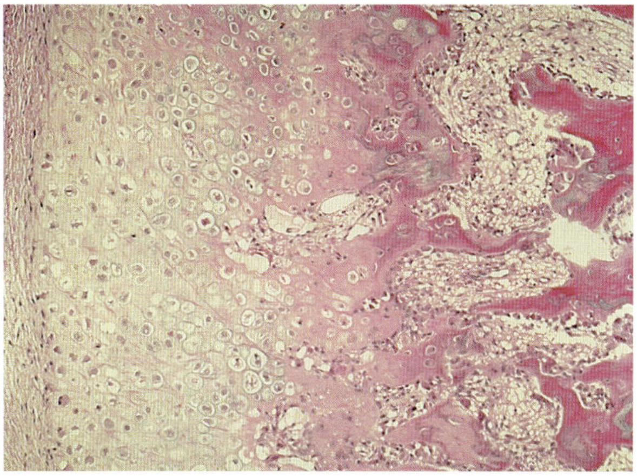

FIGURE 12.17 Dupuytren's subungual exostosis often closely resembles bizarre parosteal osteochondromatous proliferation with an overlying, hypercellular cartilaginous cap and underlying enchondral ossification. The latter is admixed with bland-appearing fibrous tissue. (H&E.)

cartilage cap may be alarmingly cellular, being composed of atypical and multinucleated chondrocytes. This appearance may cause diagnostic confusion with chondrosarcoma. Nevertheless the heterogeneity of the tumefaction, the overall exostotic features, and the benign-appearing radiographs militate against the latter diagnosis. Surgical excision is generally curative for Dupuytren's subungual exostosis.

Osteoma Cutis

Osteoma cutis is seen most often in young adults 30 to 40 years old. Trauma or scars or both are common antecedent events; however, similar-appearing cutaneous ossification also has been documented in association with melanocytic nevi, chondroid syringoma, hemangioma, basal cell carcinoma, and pilomatricoma and in the lower extremities of patients with venous stasis.[20,21] Most examples of osteoma cutis resemble mature or older cases of myositis ossificans, being composed of spicules or sheets of mature lamellar bone enclosing mature adipose tissue and, less commonly, bone marrow elements. Rarely, cartilage and enchondral ossification are evident.[20]

Bone Island (Enostosis)

Bone islands are ovoid-to-round intramedullary nodules of lamellar cortical bone, generally found incidentally in adults. Consequently, they are asymptomatic. It is possible that bone islands represent a developmental abnormality during skeletal growth. They may involve virtually any bone and, rarely, as in the hereditary syndrome, osteopoikilosis, involve virtually the entire skeleton. Conventional radiographs reveal well-circumscribed, sclerotic lesions without bone destruction or periosteal reaction (Fig. 12.18). Because these lesions are nonactive, bone islands are detected less commonly by bone scan.[22] Occasional bone islands may be large, exceeding 3 cm in greatest dimension.[23] Pathologically, bone islands are composed entirely of lamellar bone with a well-developed haversian system and a few vascular channels. Osteoblastic activity and fibroblastic stroma are distinctly absent. Recognition by an experienced radiologist is important to prevent surgical intervention. Nevertheless, larger lesions probably should be followed with serial radiographs and subsequently a biopsy if significant enlargement occurs (e.g., 25% in <6 months or 50% in <1 year).[24]

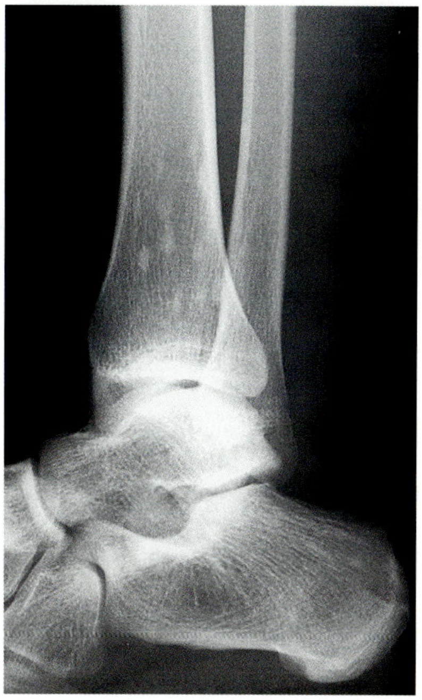

FIGURE 12.18 Bone islands in osteopoikilosis. A lateral radiograph of the ankle reveals many small, ovoid deposits of cortical bone density within the distal tibia and calcaneus. Each represents an individual bone island.

Osteoma

Clinical Features

Osteoma presents as an exophytic mass usually arising from the bones of the skull and paranasal sinuses. Although any age may be affected, most osteomas occur in adults between the ages of 30 and 50 years. Similar to bone islands, osteomas are often incidental, asymptomatic findings; however, some present with long-standing (often years) symptoms of sinus obstruction.[25] Rarely, extracranial extension or nerve compression or both may occur. Multiple osteomas, especially involving the long bones, suggest Gardner's syndrome and should prompt a thorough clinical history and physical examination for additional stigmata (e.g., colonic polyposis, pelvic fibromatosis, and epidermal inclusion cysts in the skin). The most common anatomic site is the frontal sinus, followed by the ethmoids and sphenoid sinuses.

Radiologically, osteomas generally appear as sharply demarcated ossified masses protruding from a bony surface (Fig. 12.19). Bony destruction and periosteal reaction are absent. Examples arising from the surface of the long bones of the extremities (parosteal osteomas) may mimic parosteal osteosarcoma.[26]

Pathologic Findings

Morphologically, osteomas usually consist of compact, lamellar cortical bone but may contain mixtures of medullary bone (Fig. 12.20). Small amounts of fibrofatty stroma or hematopoietic elements or both also may be present. The fibroblastic stroma typical of parosteal osteosarcoma is never observed, however.

Prognosis and Therapy

Simple excision is the treatment of choice for symptomatic lesions. Malignant transformation does not occur.

Osteoid Osteoma

Clinical Features

Osteoid osteoma is a benign osteoblastic lesion of bone, usually arising in children and adolescents, with a predilection for the second decade of life. Males are affected more commonly than females. Characteristically, patients complain of localized pain, generally worse at night and often relieved by salicylates.[27] This classic presentation is not always present, however, and night pain may be observed

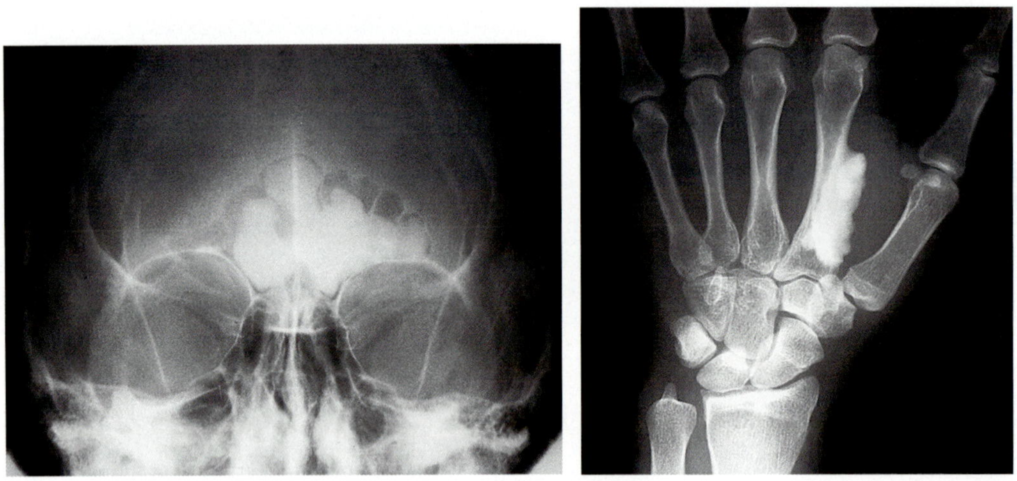

A B

FIGURE 12.19 Osteoma. A frontal view of the face shows a well-demarcated, homogeneously dense mass filling the frontal sinuses **(A)**. A posterior view of the hand in another patient shows a homogeneously dense, exophytic mass arising from the radial surface of the second metacarpal **(B)**.

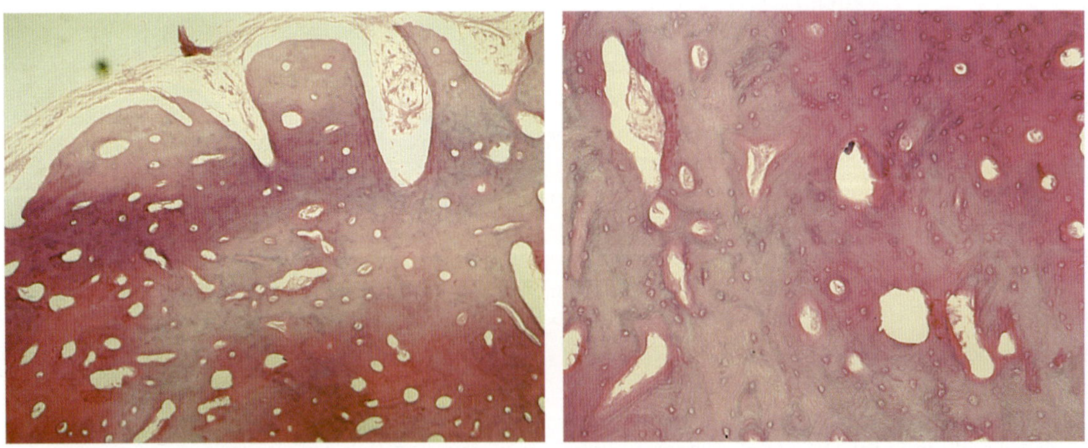

A B

FIGURE 12.20 Osteoma characterized by exophytic proliferation of dense and mature cortical bone (**A** and **B**).

with other bone tumors. More importantly, virtually all patients have progressive pain. Rare reports of nonpainful lesions have been documented.[28] Although virtually any bone may be affected, the intracortical, metaphyseal, and diaphyseal regions of the long bones, especially the lower extremities, are the most common anatomic sites. More specifically, in decreasing order of frequency, osteoid osteoma arises in the femur (especially proximal), tibia, spine, and humerus. When osteoid osteoma occurs in the spine, the dorsal elements (vertebral arches) are typically involved. These patients may present with neurologic impairment or scoliosis or both.

Radiologically, osteoid osteoma generally appears as a sharply demarcated, less than 1 cm, intracortical radiolucency (nidus) surrounded by markedly sclerotic and reactive bone (Figs. 12.21 and 12.22). With maturation, the nidus becomes progressively more radiodense and ultimately may disappear. Because ossification (maturation) of the nidus starts centrally, a ring of lucency immediately surrounding the nidus may develop, the so-called ring sequestrum. Occasionally, radiographs fail to show the nidus, necessitating the use of more sensitive techniques, including computed tomographic scans and magnetic resonance imaging.[29]

Pathologic Findings

Morphologically the well-circumscribed nidus comprises woven bone trabeculae and osteoid, lined by a prominent single layer of osteoblasts, and an intervening hypocellular but highly vascular stroma. The trabeculae are haphazardly arranged and thin. Hyaline cartilage is not present. Osteoclasts may be distributed randomly throughout the lesion (Fig. 12.23). Significant mitotic activity is usually absent and, when present, limited to the stromal cells. Mature osteoid osteomas may be composed virtually entirely of compact woven bone (Fig. 12.24). In all cases, the nidus is sharply demarcated from the surrounding, generally sclerotic, bone.

O'Connell and colleagues[30] showed the presence of "phosphorylated neurofilament-, neurofilament-, and/or S-100-positive nerve fibers in the reactive zone around the nidus and/or in the nidus." None of the control "bone tumors" (e.g., osteoblastomas, osteosarcomas, giant cell tumors) had detectable nerve fibers either within their substance or within the surrounding bone.[30]

Prognosis and Therapy

After radiographic and surgical localization, the nidus should be removed in its entirety. Complete surgical resection may necessitate bone grafting, depending on the size of the defect. Local recurrence is rare but may occur years after the initial surgery.[31] Some investigators have reported successful treatment of osteoid osteomas using computed tomography–guided excision or radiofrequency ablation.[32] Although not confirmed pathologically, spontaneous resolution has been reported.[33]

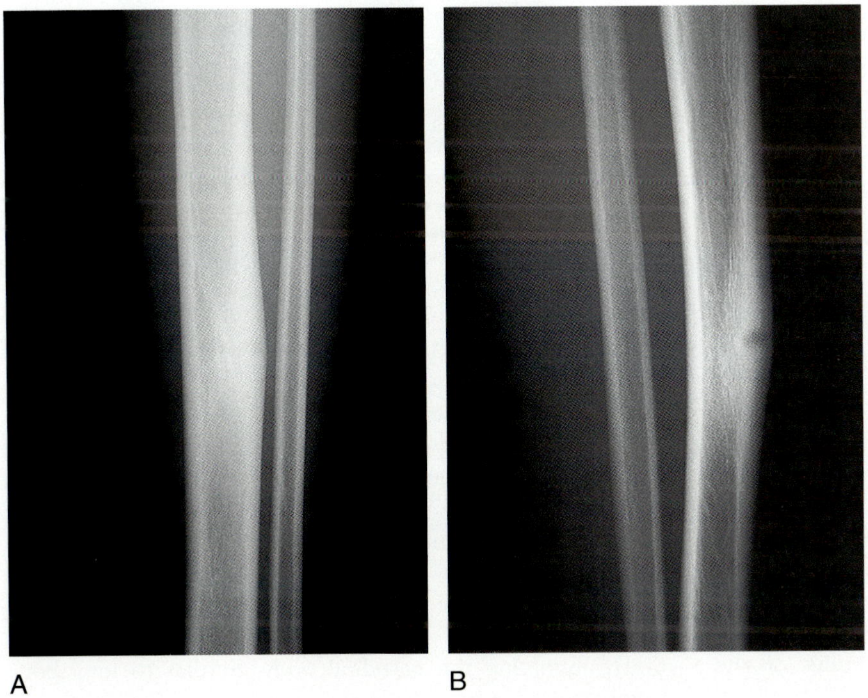

FIGURE 12.21 Osteoid osteoma. Anteroposterior **(A)** and lateral **(B)** radiographs of the tibia show a well-defined, lytic nidus within the cortex and associated with smooth thickening of the adjacent cortex and surrounding sclerosis.

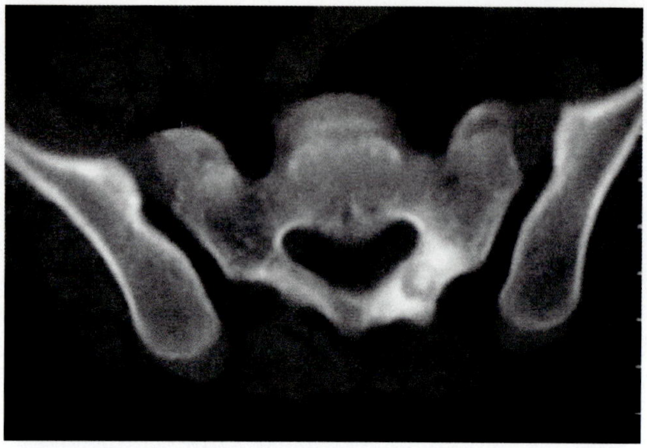

FIGURE 12.22 Osteoid osteoma. An axial computed tomographic scan of the sacrum shows a well-defined, lytic nidus in the posterior left sacrum. The nidus contains central calcification and is surrounded by dense medullary sclerosis and cortical thickening.

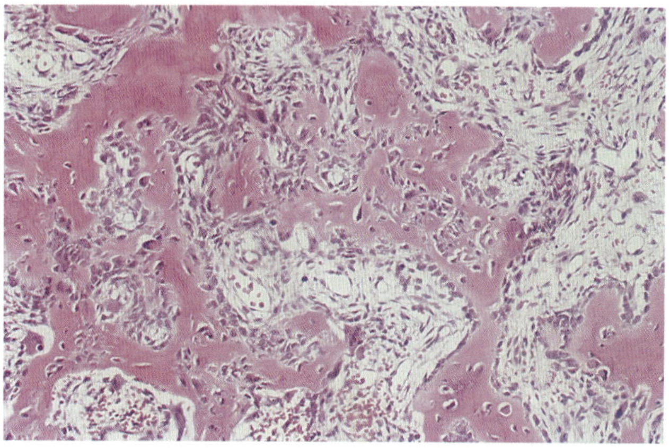

FIGURE 12.23 Osteoid osteoma characterized by anastomosing woven bone trabeculae, rimmed by a single layer of prominent osteoblasts. The intertrabecular spaces appear hypervascular and hypocellular. (H&E.)

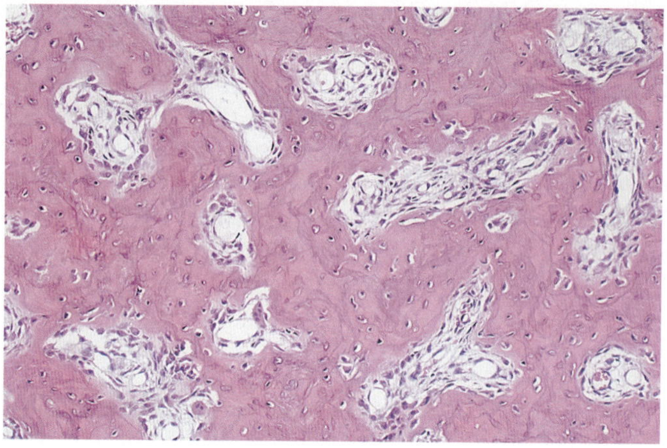

FIGURE 12.24 Occasional examples of osteoid osteoma may become progressively sclerotic, significantly diminishing the intertrabecular spaces. (H&E.)

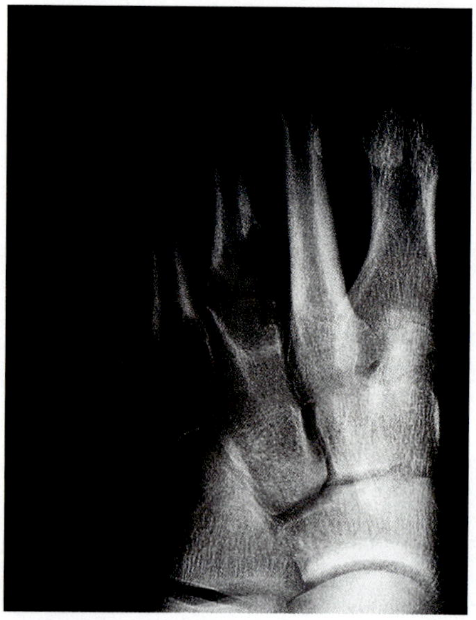

FIGURE 12.25 Osteoblastoma. An oblique radiograph of the foot reveals a lytic lesion involving the proximal end of the third metacarpal. The lesion is associated with periosteal new bone production distally but does not contain internal calcification.

Osteoblastoma

Clinical Features

Similar to osteoid osteoma, osteoblastoma is a benign osteoblastic lesion of bone, usually arising in children and adolescents, with a predilection for the second decade of life. Compared with osteoid osteoma, osteoblastoma has a wider age distribution and more commonly arises in young adults. Males are affected more commonly than females.[34] Most patients complain of localized pain, generally not responsive to salicylates. Although virtually any bone may be affected, the vertebral spine, especially the dorsal elements, is most commonly involved, followed by the long bones of the extremities and the craniofacial bones.

Radiologically, osteoblastomas usually form expansile, predominantly radiolucent but variably ossified and well-circumscribed lesions, ranging from 2 to greater than 10 cm in greatest dimension (Fig. 12.25).[34,35] Within the appendicular skeleton, most lesions involve the metaphyseal and diaphyseal regions, and localization within the cortex is more common than intramedullary areas. Cortical destruction and soft tissue extension may be present in one fourth of cases; other aggressive features, such as Codman's angle and pathologic fracture, also may suggest a malignant process.[34] Osteoblastomas arising in the vertebral column virtually always involve the dorsal elements, sometimes concomitantly involving the vertebral body. Similar to long bone involvement, most appear well marginated, but poor margination and more aggressive features, such as cortical destruction and pathologic fracture, may be present.

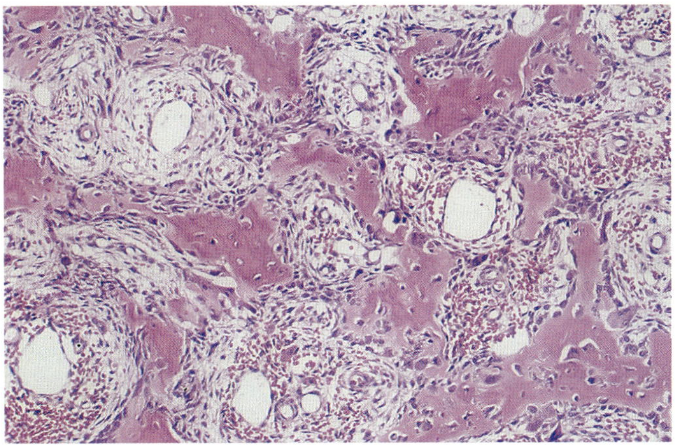

FIGURE 12.26 Osteoblastoma is histologically similar to osteoid osteoma, consisting of anastomosing woven bone trabeculae, lined by a single but prominent layer of osteoblasts, and intervening hypervascular, hypocellular intertrabecular spaces. (H&E.)

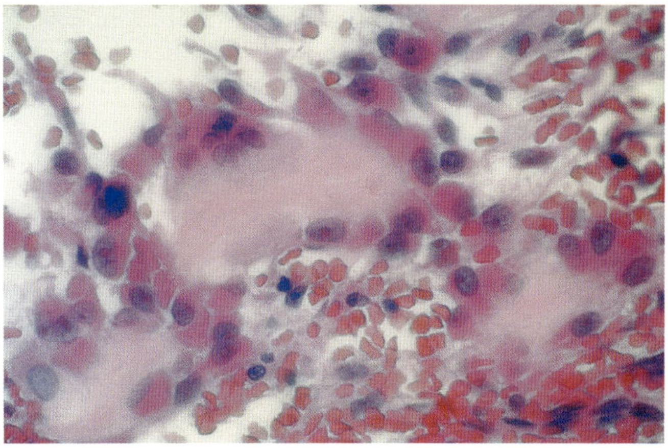

FIGURE 12.27 Some examples of osteoblastoma reveal enlarged, hypereosinophilic osteoblasts. (H&E.)

Pathologic Findings

Morphologically, osteoblastoma closely resembles osteoid osteoma, comprising woven bone trabeculae and osteoid, lined by a prominent, single layer of osteoblasts, and an intervening hypocellular but highly vascular stroma (Fig. 12.26). The clinicoradiologic and pathologic characteristics for osteoid osteoma and osteoblastoma are summarized in Table 12.4. The trabeculae are haphazardly arranged and irregular but generally sharply demarcated from the surrounding bone peripherally. Hyaline cartilage and a lace-like pattern of calcification/ossification may be present, mimicking osteosarcoma.[36] The osteoblasts are usually uniform and cytologically bland; however, about 10% of cases may be composed predominantly of "epithelioid" osteoblasts often proliferating in a multifocal pattern (e.g., forming more than one nidus within an area of tumefaction) (Fig. 12.27).[34] Less commonly, bizarre, degenerative-appearing cells with enlarged but dark, "smudgy" chromatin are observed, probably analogous to the so-called ancient change seen in schwannomas (Fig. 12.28). Osteoclasts often are distributed randomly throughout the lesion. Mitotic activity, usually within the stromal cells, is variably present, but atypical mitotic figures are never observed.

Prognosis and Therapy

When possible, en bloc resection is the therapy of choice, and bone grafting may be necessary, depending on location. Local recurrence is more likely to follow intralesional

TABLE 12.4 Clinicoradiologic and Pathologic Characteristics of Osteoid Osteoma and Osteoblastoma

	Osteoid Osteoma	Osteoblastoma
Peak Age	10-20 yr	10-20 yr
Gender	Males > females	Males > females
Symptoms	Localized pain, often worse at night, relieved by salicylates	Localized pain, usually no pattern
Involved Bones (Decreasing Order of Frequency)	Femur, tibia, spine	Spine, femur, jawbones
Lesion Size	<1 cm	>2 cm
Radiographic Features	Intracortical lucency (nidus) surrounded by sclerotic bone	Well-circumscribed, expansile lesion, variable ossification, may have aggressive features
Pathologic Features		
Woven Bone/Osteoid	Yes	Yes
Prominent Osteoblasts	Yes	Yes
Circumscription	Yes	Yes
Hyaline Cartilage	No	Sometimes

excisions and curettage and may occur in 10% to 20% of patients. Histologic features, including the presence of epithelioid osteoblasts or cartilage, do not predict prognosis.[34,35] Although considered a benign neoplasm, death rarely may result from "direct impingement of tumors on the central neuraxis."[34] Additionally, malignant transformation of a previously, histologically documented osteoblastoma occurs in less than 1% of cases.[34,37]

Fibrous Dysplasia

Clinical Features

The clinical, radiologic, and pathologic features of fibrous dysplasia are summarized in Table 12.5. Fibrous dysplasia is a benign proliferation of fibro-osseous tissue that may be detected at any age, but most manifest in the teens and 20s.

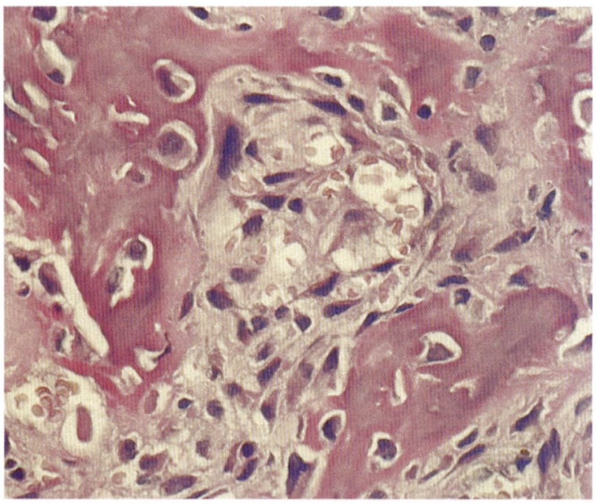

FIGURE 12.28 Rarely, scattered atypical and enlarged cells with dark, smudgy chromatin may be seen in osteoblastoma but are of no prognostic significance. (H&E.)

Males and females are affected equally. Whether fibrous dysplasia is a true neoplasm, a hamartoma, or a localized failure of bone maturation is unclear. Most cases are solitary (monostotic), but a few patients have multiple bone involvement (polyostotic). Although symptoms vary depending on anatomic site, most patients are asymptomatic, and, consequently, fibrous dysplasia is typically an incidental finding. Patients with polyostotic disease are more often symptomatic in childhood primarily owing to developmental malformations leading to complaints of pain or gait disturbances or both. In the more common monostotic form, fibrous dysplasia arises most commonly from the bones in the craniofacial region followed by the long bones of the lower extremities and ribs. Polyostotic fibrous dysplasia has a predilection for the pelvis and long bones of the lower extremities. Albright syndrome is polyostotic fibrous dysplasia in association with various stigmata, including pigmented skin lesions and precocious puberty. Mazabraud's syndrome presents as polyostotic fibrous dysplasia and intramuscular soft tissue myxomas.

The radiologic appearance of fibrous dysplasia is variable, but most examples show an expansile, sharply marginated, variably ossified lesion (Fig. 12.29). Fibrous dysplasia may be virtually completely lytic or significantly more dense than the surrounding bone. A sclerotic rim often is observed. With rib involvement, marked expansion of the affected bone typically is seen (Fig. 12.30). Intralesional densifications may impart a ground-glass appearance. Rarely, fibrous dysplasia may erode the overlying cortex.

Pathologic Findings

Morphologically, fibrous dysplasia is a fibro-osseous lesion, consisting of a variable mixture of haphazardly arranged bony trabeculae often in alphabet-like shapes embedded within a slightly to moderately cellular fibrous stroma (Fig. 12.31). In most cases, the bony trabeculae represent woven bone, but

TABLE 12.5 Clinicoradiologic and Pathologic Characteristics of Fibrous Dysplasia and Osteofibrous Dysplasia

	Fibrous Dysplasia	Osteofibrous Dysplasia
Peak Age	10-30 yr	1-10 yr
Gender	Males = females	Males = females
Symptoms	Painless soft tissue swelling, abnormal bone growth, Albright's syndrome (polyostotic lesions, pigmentation, precocious puberty), Mazabraud's syndrome (polyostotic lesions, myxomas)	Painless soft tissue swelling, bowing of the tibia/fibula
Involved Bones (Decreasing Order of Frequency)	Skull and craniofacial regions, femur, tibia, and ribs	Tibia (almost exclusively), fibula (rarely)
Radiographs	Metaphyseal/diaphyseal, lytic, expansile, sharply marginated; ground-glass appearance; may affect multiple bones (polyostotic)	Cortical diaphysis, lytic, expansile, multiloculated; no periosteal reaction
Osteoblastic Rimming	Usually absent; when present, typically minimal and focal	Present, prominent and diffuse
Hyaline Cartilage	May be present; rarely can predominate	Absent

more mature lamellar bone is usually at least focally present and may predominate, especially in the craniofacial region (Fig. 12.32). The presence of reversal lines mimicking Paget's disease is observed frequently. Calcified spherules (cementicles) are observed sometimes, especially in the craniofacial region, but also in the extremities (Fig. 12.33). Their presence in various anatomic sites has led some to postulate that cemento-ossifying fibroma and fibrous dysplasia represent a spectrum of similar disease and not specific clinicopathologic entities.[38] Although almost never conspicuous, osteoblastic rimming often is seen focally and does not preclude the diagnosis of fibrous dysplasia in the appropriate clinicoradiologic setting. Occasional examples of fibrous dysplasia contain aggregates of hyaline cartilage that may rarely be prominent, raising the differential diagnosis of enchondroma (Fig. 12.34).[39] Between the bony trabeculae, the fibrous stroma ranges from slightly cellular with abundant collagenization to highly cellular and minimal collagen deposition. Marked stromal myxoid or cystic changes potentially may confound the diagnosis (Fig. 12.35). Cytologically the individual fibroblasts are small and uniformly round to ovoid with plump-to-spindled, hyperchromatic nuclei. As with virtually all bone tumors, randomly distributed osteoclast-type giant cells are common. Mitotic activity is scant and never atypical. Xanthomatous changes frequently are present and, similar to hyaline cartilage, may obscure the more characteristic diagnostic features (Fig. 12.36). Meticulous sampling and attentively seeking more typical areas representative of fibrous dysplasia lead to the correct diagnosis. It is likely that many examples of the so-called xanthoma of bone represent forms of fibrous dysplasia.[40]

Prognosis and Therapy

The therapy of fibrous dysplasia is complex and depends on the anatomic location, extent of involvement, and symptoms. In some cases, simple observation is adequate. For cases that are symptomatic or extensive or both, curettage and bone grafting is often sufficient. Local recurrence may occur, especially if the extent of the lesion is underestimated at surgical resection.

Sarcomatous transformation of fibrous dysplasia is a well-recognized phenomenon but occurs in less than 1% of cases (Fig. 12.37). It is more likely to occur in previously irradiated lesions and in patients with polyostotic disease. Most appear as osteosarcomas followed by fibrosarcoma and chondrosarcoma, and the prognosis is poor.[41]

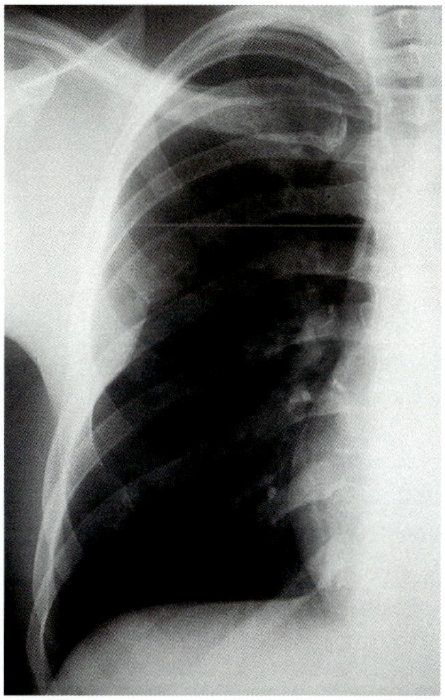

FIGURE 12.30 Fibrous dysplasia. An anteroposterior radiograph of the right ribs reveals an expansile lesion extending along the length of the sixth rib. The margins are sharply defined, but internal matrix calcification is not apparent.

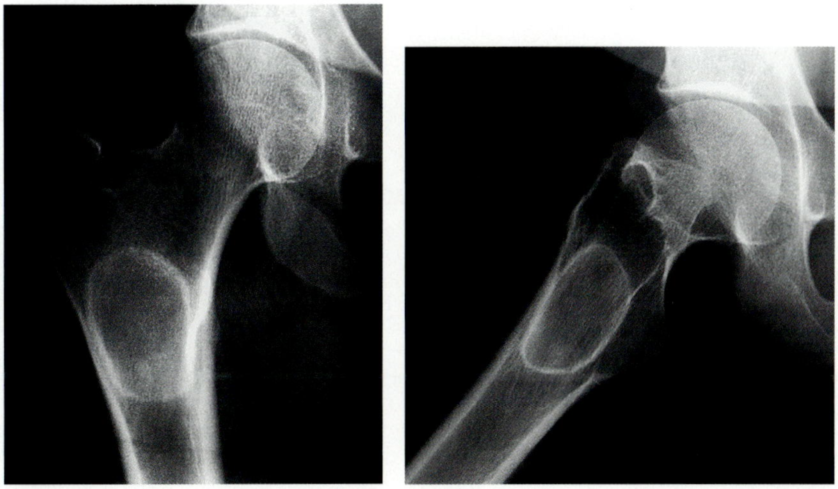

A B

FIGURE 12.29 Fibrous dysplasia. Anteroposterior **(A)** and abducted lateral **(B)** radiographs of the proximal femur show a well-demarcated lesion in the proximal femur. The margin of the lesion is thick and sclerotic, and the lesion contains smudgy, ground-glass calcification.

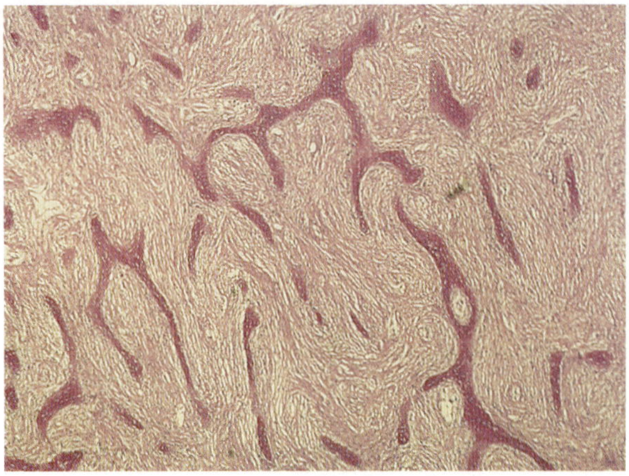

A

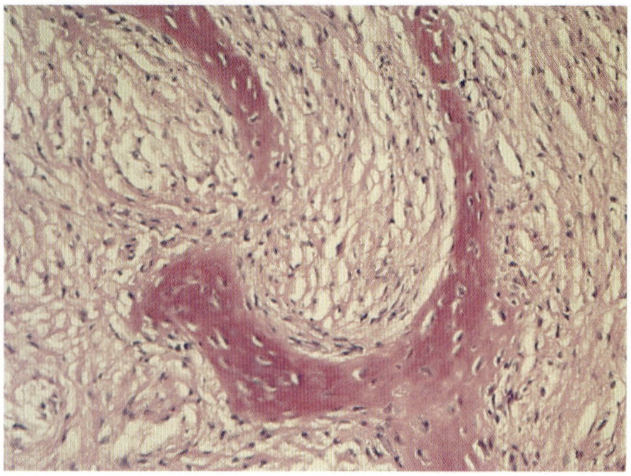

B

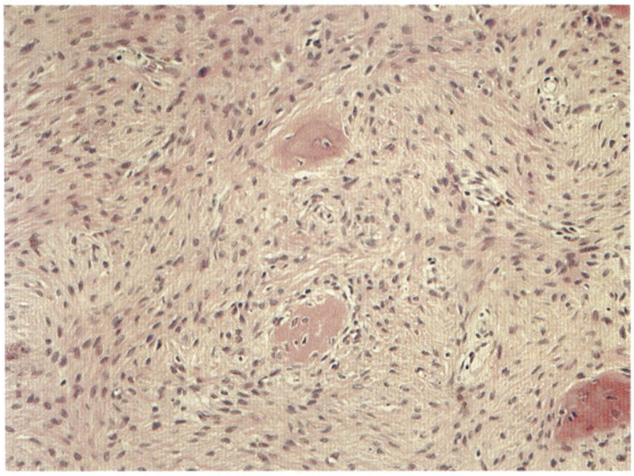

C

FIGURE 12.31 Classic fibrous dysplasia composed of spicules of woven bone, arranged in an alphabet-like pattern and emanating from a bland-appearing fibrous stroma **(A-C). (A**, Low power; **B** and **C**, high power, H&E.)

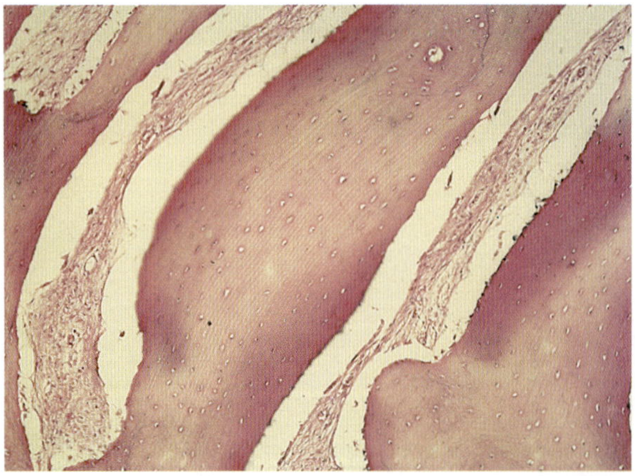

FIGURE 12.32 Fibrous dysplasia with thickened, mature lamellar bone trabeculae. (H&E.)

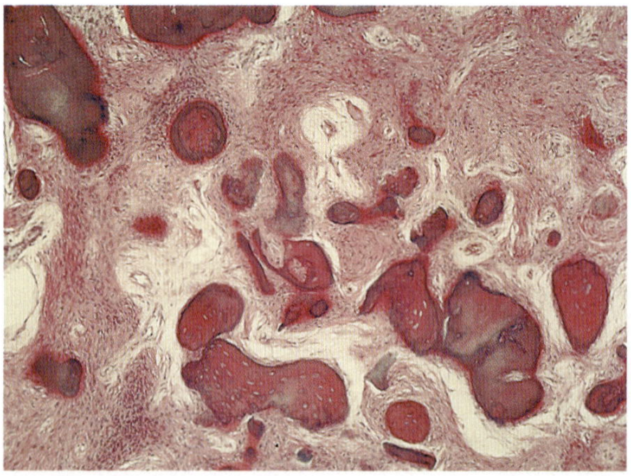

FIGURE 12.33 Calcified sphericles (cementicles) are a common finding in fibrous dysplasia, especially within the craniofacial regions. (H&E.)

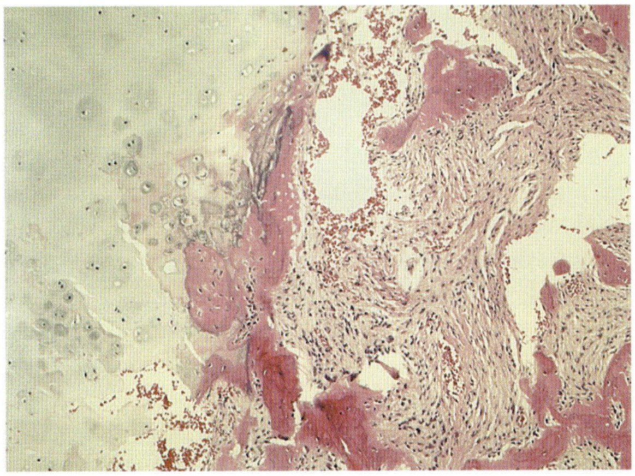

FIGURE 12.34 Fibrous dysplasia is rarely associated with abundant hyaline cartilage production, fibrocartilaginous dysplasia. (H&E.)

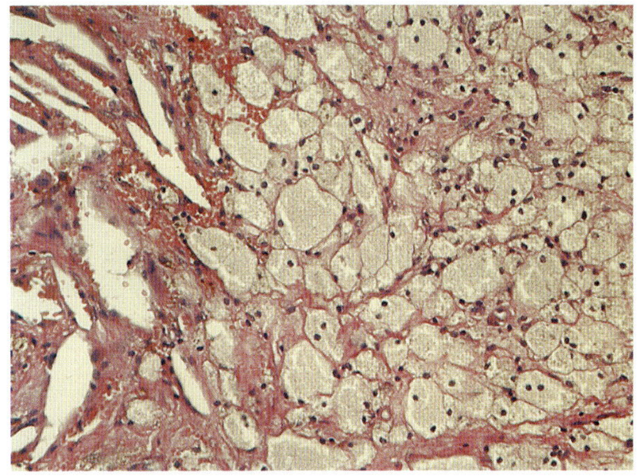

FIGURE 12.36 Fibrous dysplasia with xanthomatous changes, including abundant foamy histiocytes and cholesterol clefts. (H&E.)

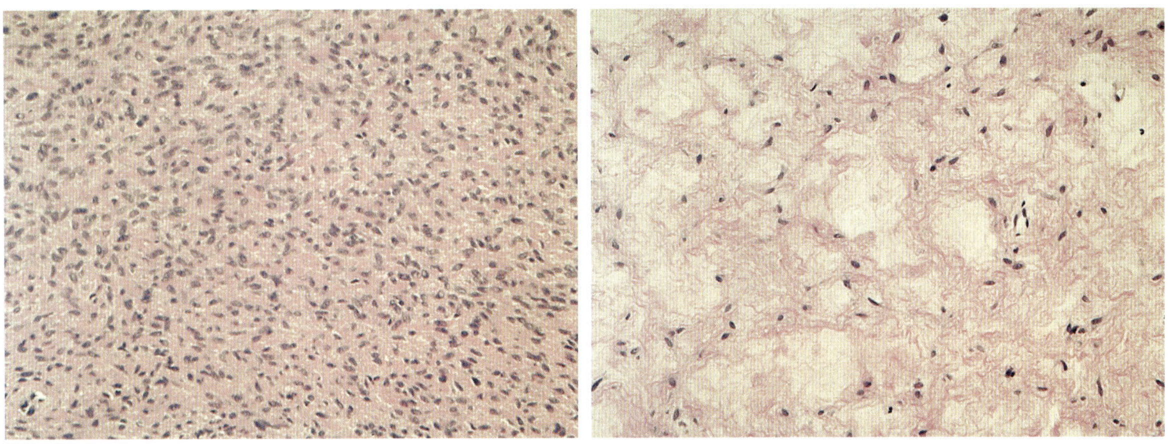

A B

FIGURE 12.35 The stroma of fibrous dysplasia ranges from a hypercellular, less collagenous background **(A)** to a hypocellular, "bubbly" myxoid stroma **(B).** Significant nuclear atypia is not observed, however. (H&E.)

Osteofibrous Dysplasia (Ossifying Fibroma)

Osteofibrous dysplasia is a rare but poorly understood lesion that has been referred to by a variety of confusing synonyms, including intracortical fibrous dysplasia and ossifying fibroma. Although malignant transformation has never been documented, it shares some clinicopathologic features with adamantinoma, but the nature of this relationship is unclear and controversial.

Clinical Features

The clinical and pathologic features of osteofibrous dysplasia compared with usual fibrous dysplasia are summarized in Table 12.5. Osteofibrous dysplasia generally presents in the first decade of life, and boys and girls are affected equally.[42] In most cases, osteofibrous dysplasia presents as a painless swelling of the anterior lower extremity and may be associated with bowing or pathologic fracture or both.

The radiographic appearance of osteofibrous dysplasia is highly characteristic and often diagnostic when observed by an experienced radiologist. The lesions almost always involve the tibial diaphysis (less often fibula) and are within an expanded cortex. Multiple areas of lucency with intervening bony sclerosis frequently are associated with a thinned-to-absent overlying cortical rim (Fig. 12.38). Periosteal reaction is not present, but severe bowing of the affected bone typically is observed. Osteofibrous dysplasia usually is confined to one tibia, but ipsilateral fibular or contralateral tibial and fibular involvement has been reported.[42]

Pathologic Findings

Similar to fibrous dysplasia, osteofibrous dysplasia is a fibro-osseous lesion but differs from fibrous dysplasia in the following aspects. First, the thin, woven bone trabeculae are arranged haphazardly within the center of the lesion but, as one moves toward the periphery, become progressively wider and mature, developing into lamellar bone and ultimately merging imperceptibly with the surrounding sclerotic and reactive bone. These features likely would be obvious only within intact lesional resection specimens. Second, the bony trabeculae are rimmed by plump and conspicuous osteoblasts, occasionally accompanied by osteoclasts, present throughout the entirety of the lesion (Fig. 12.39). The intervening fibrous stroma ranges from cellular to compact and collagenized, composed of a slightly to moderately cellular population of plump but uniform and benign-appearing fibroblasts, arranged in short fascicles and storiform patterns (Fig. 12.40).

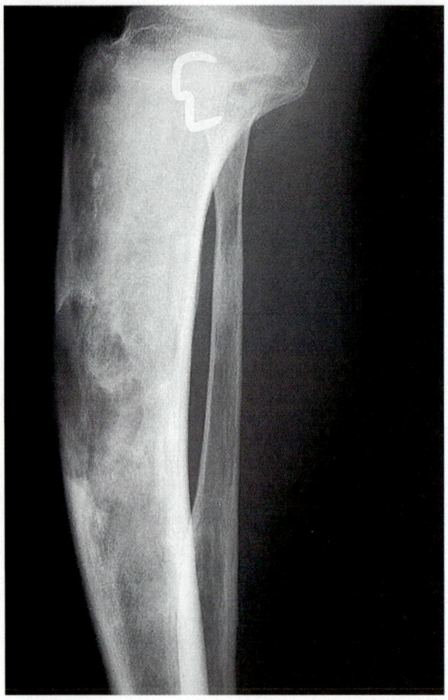

FIGURE 12.37 Secondary osteosarcoma arising in fibrous dysplasia. A lateral radiograph of the tibia shows fibrous dysplasia in the proximal tibia. A focal lytic lesion in the tibial shaft has resulted in destruction of the anterior tibial cortex and is associated with faint, immature, periosteal new bone production anteriorly.

Immunohistochemical studies have documented the presence of cytokeratin-positive cells in some cases, leading some to propose a causal relationship between osteofibrous dysplasia and adamantinoma.[42,43] In a review of more than 80 patients with osteofibrous dysplasia at the Mayo Clinic, Park and colleagues[42] documented no cases of osteofibrous dysplasia progression to adamantinoma.

Prognosis and Therapy

Asymptomatic lesions may be observed, and many show spontaneous regression. Because of the high incidence of recurrence and frequent disease progression, surgical excision and bone grafting probably should be avoided until after the age of 10 years and only if necessary.[44] Severe bowing deformities may require osteotomy and internal fixation.

Osteosarcoma (General Concepts)

The diagnosis of osteosarcoma encompasses a group of heterogeneous malignant neoplasms, all of which are linked by the production of osteoid/bone by the malignant cells.

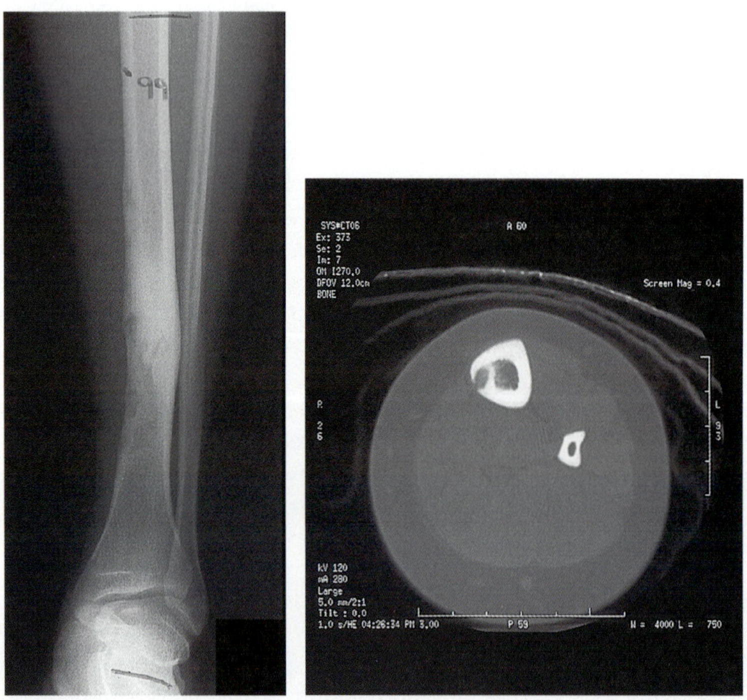

FIGURE 12.38 Osteofibrous dysplasia. An anteroposterior radiograph of the tibia shows a lytic lesion in the tibial cortex with surrounding sclerosis. There is moderate bowing of the tibia centered at the area of bone lysis **(A).** An axial computed tomographic scan shows a lytic lesion at the tibial cortex. The overlying cortical rim is absent **(B).**

Consequently the clinical and histologic spectrum of osteosarcoma is large and arguably exceeds that of any other primary bone tumor. The clinical and pathologic subtypes of osteosarcoma are summarized in Table 12.6. Although there is considerable clinicopathologic overlap among the various osteosarcoma subtypes, differences exist, and the variants are best discussed individually. The specific aspects of therapy, especially pathologic evaluation of postchemotherapy specimens, are discussed later in this chapter.

Histologic Grading in Osteosarcoma

The pretherapy grading of osteosarcoma is controversial. Consequently, no universally accepted criteria, applicable to the entire spectrum of osteosarcoma, exist for this determination. Taylor and coworkers[45] reported a multi-institutional study of 543 patients with osteosarcoma and found that the presence of high grade was only of borderline significance (P=.06) for death during the first 3 years after initial diagnosis but was highly significant (P=.0002) for disease progression within the same interval. The grading system used by the authors was the widely used Broders' system. This grading scheme is based primarily on a subjective assessment of the degree of cytologic atypia and anaplasia of the tumor cells.[46] It is summarized for various histologic subtypes in Table 12.7. Inwards and Unni[47] admitted that "'cytologic atypia' may be more subject to interobserver variation than any other feature." Additionally, the Broders system does not account for the degree of mitotic activity or the presence or absence of tumor necrosis; this may be shortsighted because the presence of spontaneous tumor necrosis has been shown by some authors to be prognostically significant.[48]

Patients with high-grade osteosarcoma (e.g., conventional, telangiectatic) usually receive preoperative chemotherapy, whereas patients with low-grade (e.g.,

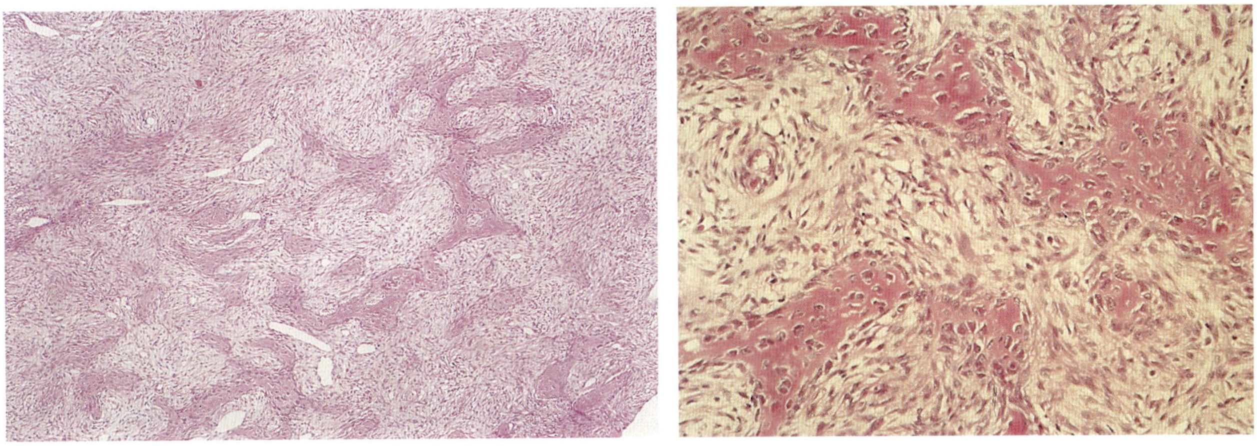

A B

FIGURE 12.39 Osteofibrous dysplasia may closely mimic fibrous dysplasia at low power **(A)**. A high-power view reveals that all of the woven bone trabeculae are rimmed by a single layer of osteoblasts. Additionally, the fibroblastic stroma tends to be more cellular **(B)**. **(A,** Low power; **B,** high power, H&E.)

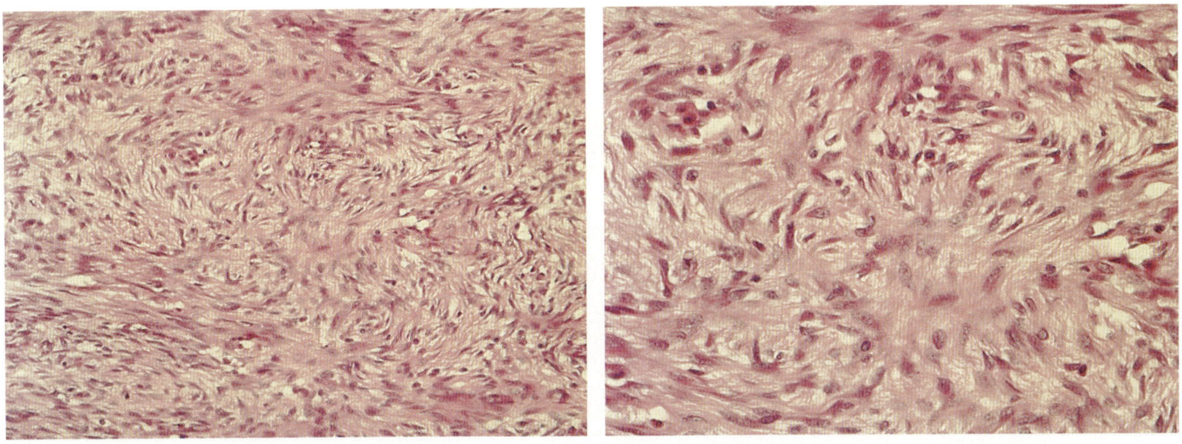

A B

FIGURE 12.40 The fibrous stroma within osteofibrous dysplasia may be quite cellular, composed of fascicles of bland-appearing, spindle-shaped cells occasionally exhibiting prominent storiform patterns **(A** and **B)**. **(A,** low power; **B,** high power, H&E.)

TABLE 12.6 Clinical and Pathologic Subtypes of Osteosarcoma

Pathologic Subtypes
Intramedullary osteosarcoma
  Conventional high-grade osteosarcoma (osteoblastic, fibroblastic, chondroblastic)
  Telangiectatic osteosarcoma
  Small cell osteosarcoma
  Low-grade intraosseous osteosarcoma (well differentiated)
Surface (juxtacortical) osteosarcoma
  Parosteal osteosarcoma
  Periosteal osteosarcoma
  High-grade surface osteosarcoma

Clinical Subtypes
Extraskeletal osteosarcoma
Osteosarcoma of the jawbones
Secondary osteosarcoma
  Postradiation
  Paget's disease
  Fibrous dysplasia

TABLE 12.7 Relationship of Established Histologic Osteosarcoma Subtypes to Broders' Grading System

Grade 1-2	Low-grade intraosseous osteosarcoma
	Parosteal osteosarcoma
Grade 2-3	Periosteal osteosarcoma
Grade 3-4	Conventional osteosarcoma
	High-grade surface osteosarcoma
	Extraskeletal osteosarcoma*
	"Secondary" osteosarcoma*
Grade 4	Telangiectatic osteosarcoma
	Small cell osteosarcoma

*Although rare examples of extraskeletal and secondary osteosarcomas represent low-grade varieties, most are high grade, resembling the conventional osseous form.

parosteal, low-grade intraosseous) histology do not. No universally accepted and well-established criteria exist, however, for determining which osteosarcoma patients should receive neoadjuvant chemotherapy. Although pathologists and clinicians seem to rely mainly on subtype or histologic grade or both to help make this decision, these subtyping and grading criteria are subjective and may vary widely from institution to institution. In most cases, the histologic grade of the tumor is reflected in part by the known biologic behavior, as illustrated in Table 12.7. Consequently, some advocate that the histologic grading of osteosarcoma is neither necessary nor reproducible and does not add significantly to treatment as long as the subtype is recognized.[49] What happens if the tumor appears to represent an osteosarcoma but does not "fit" into a recognizable subtype? Do any universally accepted, objective guidelines exist regarding applying a histologic grade to such a tumor? Over the course of 5 years, we encountered, among 50 consecutive osteosarcoma cases, 4 (10%) examples in which there was a significant, therapeutically altering discrepancy among expert orthopedic pathologists regarding the histologic grade of the tumor. For this reason, Kilpatrick and associates[50] undertook a study to investigate interobserver variability for histologic grading and the determination of chemotherapy. Eight expert orthopedic pathologists voluntarily reviewed the clinicoradiologic and histologic data from 12 selected cases coded as osteosarcoma over the past 7 years (procured from a total of 40 cases) from the files of the University of North Carolina and Wake Forest University. Uniform agreement regarding overall histologic grade and the necessity of chemotherapy was observed in only five cases (42%). In seven cases (58%), there was disagreement from at least one consultant regarding the necessity of chemotherapy. For the well-established and common osteosarcoma subtypes, a uniform consensus was usually observed.[50] An attempt should be made to provide reproducible and practical clinical and pathologic criteria, applicable to the entire spectrum of osteosarcoma, for the identification of patients who might benefit from adjuvant therapy. In the meantime, it is recommended that pathologists make a diligent effort to subtype osteosarcomas accurately, when possible, and at least attempt to categorize the tumor as either high or low grade. The latter usually is reflected by the histologic subtype.

Conventional Osteosarcoma

When most people think of osteosarcoma, the classic conventional intramedullary form usually comes to mind. Conventional osteosarcoma represents 80% to 90% of all osteosarcomas and is the most common primary bone sarcoma.

Clinical Features

Although conventional osteosarcoma may arise at any age, most present de novo before age 30. The peak incidence is the second decade of life, and males are affected more often than females. Pain of short duration, often accompanied by soft tissue swelling, is universally present, but fracture tends to be uncommon at initial presentation. Serum alkaline phosphatase frequently is elevated but is relatively nonspecific, occurring in other neoplastic and inflammatory processes. Virtually all sites of involvement have been reported; however, the metaphyseal regions of the long bones are affected most commonly. More specifically, conventional osteosarcoma involves, in decreasing order of frequency, the metaphyseal regions of the distal femur, proximal tibia, and proximal humerus. Involvement of the flat bones is observed more commonly in patients older than age 30 in whom osteosarcoma often arises in a pre-existing bone lesion or irradiated bone.

Radiologically, conventional osteosarcoma is a permeative lesion, usually metaphyseal-centered and associated with a periosteal reaction and soft tissue extension. Depending on the degree of mineralization, the lesion ranges from purely lytic to densely sclerotic or a combination of sclerotic/lytic areas (Fig. 12.41). Whether mineralization is present or not, the radiographic appearance of conventional osteosarcoma is that of an aggressive lesion. Magnetic resonance imaging is helpful in defining the full extent of the lesion, which often is underestimated by conventional radiographs (Fig. 12.42).

Pathologic Findings

Histology

Despite the varied appearance, all show frankly high-grade, sarcomatous features and the production of malignant osteoid/bone. The stroma may range from osteoblastic (or

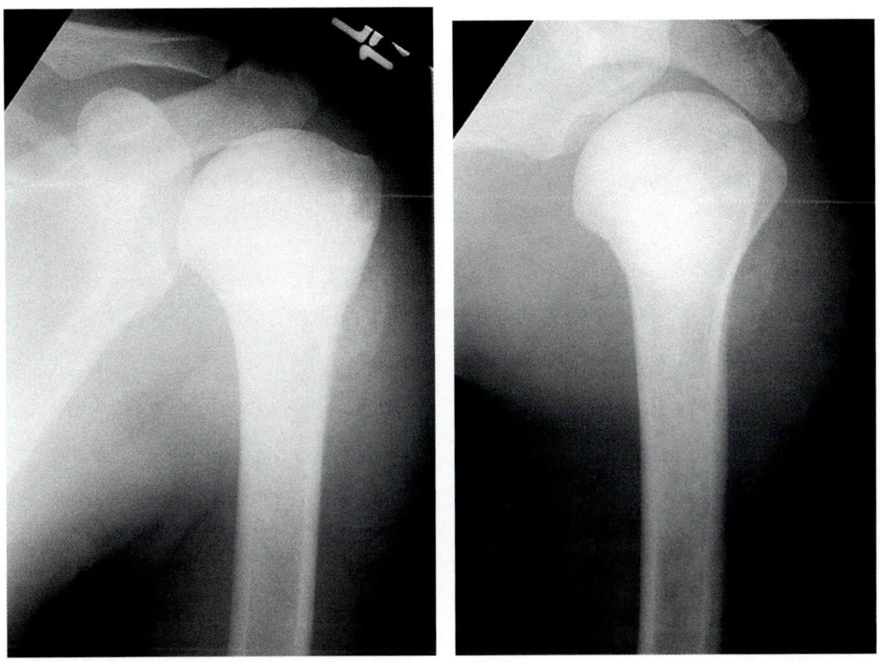

A B

FIGURE 12.41 Conventional osteosarcoma. Anteroposterior **(A)** and lateral **(B)** radiographs of the proximal humerus show a poorly marginated, dense lesion in the proximal humerus. Soft tissue extension is evident by the ill-defined, immature periosteal new bone production adjacent to the lateral aspect of the humerus just distal to the greater tuberosity.

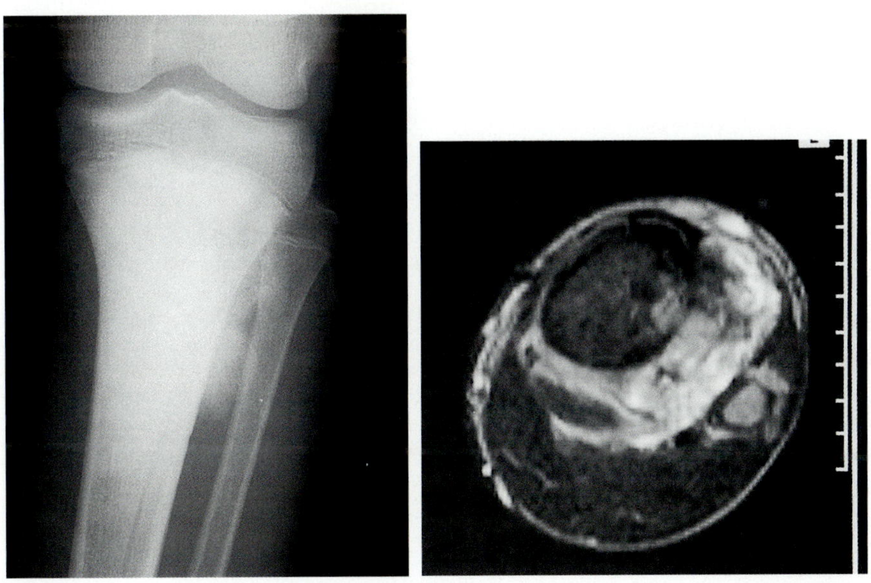

A B

FIGURE 12.42 Conventional osteosarcoma. An anteroposterior radiograph of the proximal tibia shows a poorly marginated, sclerotic lesion in the metaphysis. Soft tissue calcification extending laterally indicates cortical penetration and soft tissue extension of the tumor **(A)**. An axial magnetic resonance image shows the osteosclerotic intramedullary tumor (dark on this scan) with extensive soft tissue involvement (heterogeneously bright on this scan) extending anteriorly and posteriorly and abutting the proximal fibula laterally **(B)**.

sclerotic), fibroblastic, or chondroblastic; varying proportions of all of these stromal components may be seen but do not appear to be of any prognostic significance (Fig. 12.43). Rarely, malignant osteoid may be difficult to find, raising the differential diagnosis of fibrosarcoma or malignant fibrous histiocytoma. Such a distinction is of more academic importance than therapeutic significance because most clinicians advocate similar therapy for all of these tumors.[51-53] The malignant osteoid is often laid down in a lace-like pattern, with or without mineralization (calcification). Some conventional high-grade osteosarcomas, so-called sclerosing osteoblastic variant, consist of anastomosing trabeculae of woven bone within which are malignant osteoblasts showing minimal nuclear pleomorphism. Permeation and entrapment of lamellar bone by the neoplastic bone is a helpful feature in establishing the diagnosis (Fig. 12.44). Cytologically, the neoplastic cells range from spindled to epithelioid with round-to-ovoid, sometimes anaplastic nuclei and small-to-prominent nucleoli (Fig. 12.45). In rare cases, the epithelioid cells may appear remarkably uniform, mimicking a carcinoma (Fig. 12.46).[54] The cytoplasm varies from clear to basophilic and abundant. Mitotic figures are often numerous and frequently atypical. As with most primary bone tumors, randomly distributed osteoclast-type giant cells are often present and should not be confused with tumor giant cells, also typically seen in conventional osteosarcoma.

Fine Needle Aspiration Biopsy

Despite the presence of mineralization, most osteosarcomas, especially the conventional variant, are amenable to FNAB. The accuracy rates for establishing the diagnosis of conventional osteosarcoma exceed 90%.[55,56] Cytologic smears are generally moderately to markedly cellular comprising small aggregates and solitary, polygonal-shaped tumor cells, usually exhibiting plasmacytoid features with eccentric, round-to-ovoid nuclei; one or more nucleoli; and abundant cytoplasm (Fig. 12.47). The cytoplasm may contain minute vacuoles. By Diff-Quik stain, at least focal aggregates of metachromatic matrix material typically are observed (Fig. 12.48). Osteoid/bone, chondroid, and hyaline cartilage appear tinctorially similar, and absolute distinction is not always possible. This situation is rarely problematic because correlation with the clinical and radiologic findings almost always yields the correct diagnosis.[55]

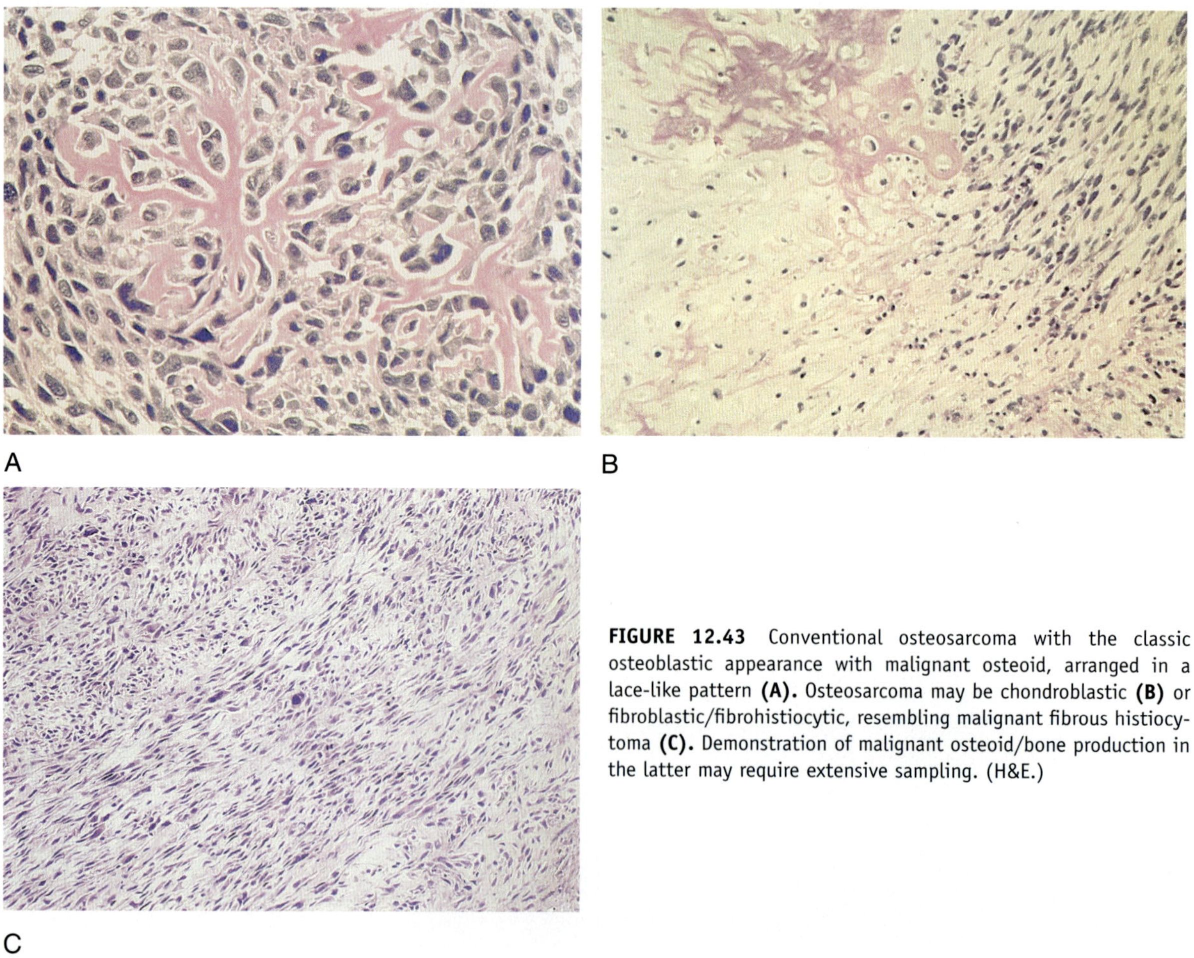

FIGURE 12.43 Conventional osteosarcoma with the classic osteoblastic appearance with malignant osteoid, arranged in a lace-like pattern **(A).** Osteosarcoma may be chondroblastic **(B)** or fibroblastic/fibrohistiocytic, resembling malignant fibrous histiocytoma **(C).** Demonstration of malignant osteoid/bone production in the latter may require extensive sampling. (H&E.)

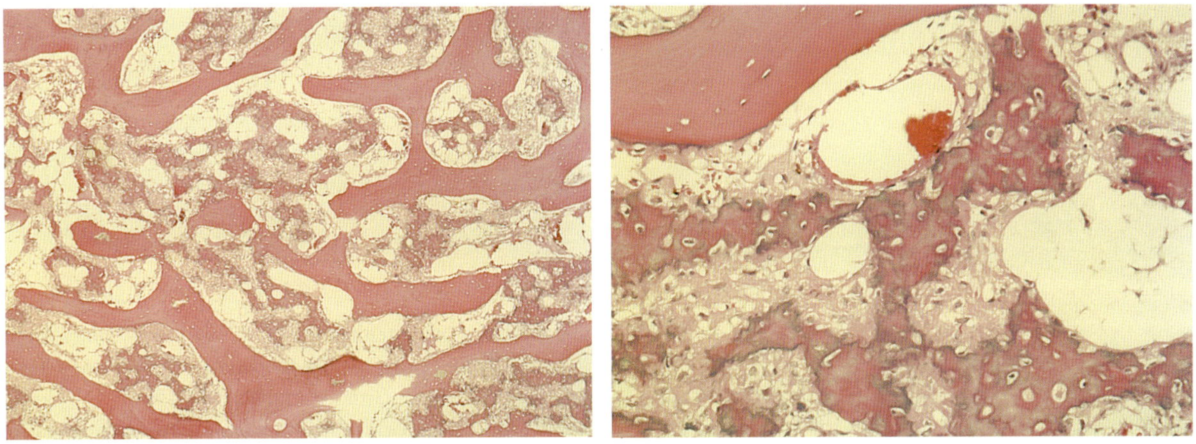

A B

FIGURE 12.44 Osteoblastic "sclerosing" osteosarcoma with extensive permeation of intramedullary bone **(A).** Note the absence of significant atypia at high power **(B).** Despite the absence of atypia, "sclerosing" osteosarcoma should be considered a form of high-grade conventional osteosarcoma and treated accordingly. (H&E.)

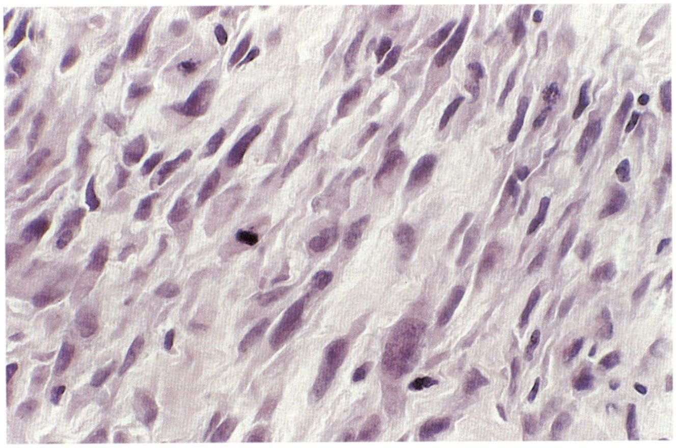

FIGURE 12.45 Spindled, sarcomatous appearance of osteosarcoma with marked anaplasia and mitotic activity. (H&E.)

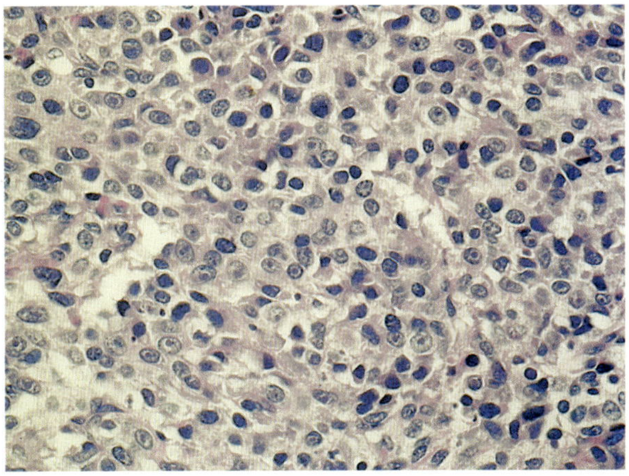

FIGURE 12.46 Osteosarcoma with epithelioid features. (H&E.)

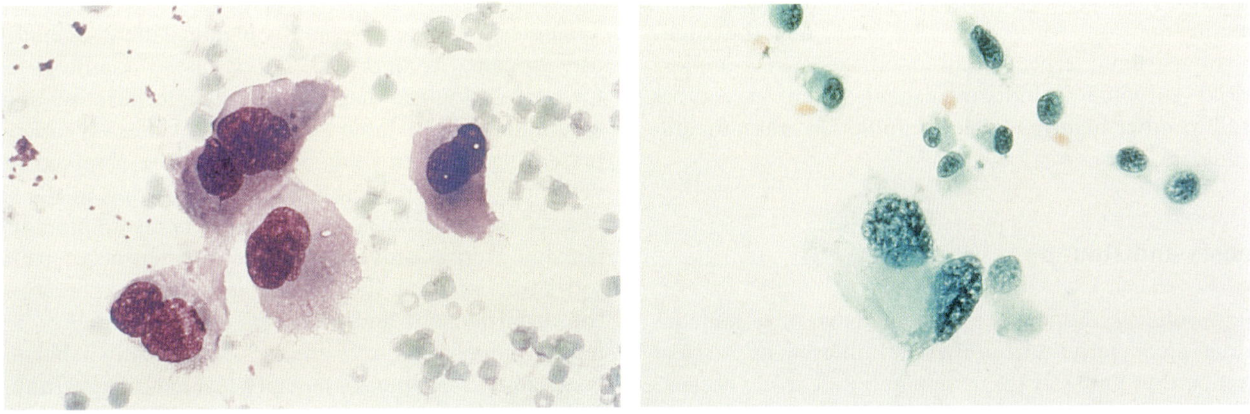

A B

FIGURE 12.47 Fine needle aspiration biopsy of conventional osteosarcoma is characterized by moderate to highly cellular smears with a population of mostly discohesive tumor cells with round-to-ovoid, eccentrically placed nuclei; one or more prominent nucleoli; and abundant cytoplasm. Note the occasional binucleated forms and significant nuclear pleomorphism **(A** and **B). (A,** Diff-Quik; **B,** Papanicolaou.)

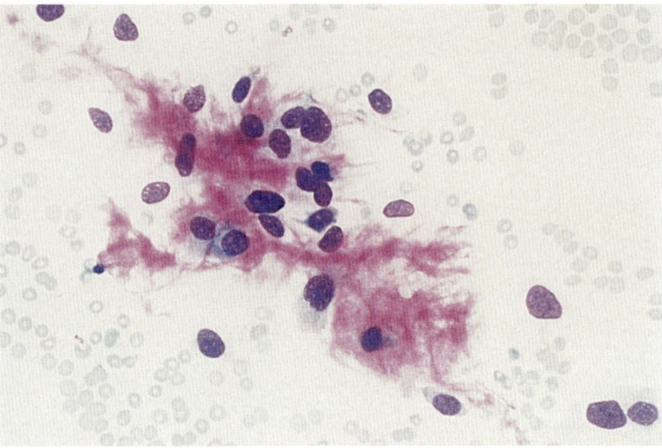

FIGURE 12.48 In most cases, a magenta-appearing matrix intimately associated with the tumor cells is identified, at least focally. Such matrix material is best observed in Romanowsky preparations. (Diff-Quik.)

Ancillary Studies

Ultrastructural examination shows features of atypical osteoblasts with abundant cytoplasm, desmosome-like cell junctions, dilated rough endoplasmic reticulum, calcific inclusions within mitochondria, and cytoplasmic processes. Multilobated nuclei are observed occasionally. Calcium deposits are noted between matrix collagen fibers.[57]

Because of the occasional difficulty of distinguishing osteoid from hyalinized, dense collagen, some investigators have explored the role of osteocalcin and osteonectin immunohistochemistry in helping to establish the diagnosis of osteosarcoma.[58] Although not entirely specific, osteocalcin seems to be the more useful marker, present in virtually all osteosarcomas. The low specificity of osteonectin likely renders it impractical for routine use. Nevertheless, most authors agree that most osteosarcomas are diagnosed easily by light microscopy alone.[55,58]

Cytogenetic analysis of osteosarcoma has yielded mostly nonspecific findings. Most examples, especially the high-grade conventional type, reveal nondiagnostic, complex, aneuploid karyotypes, indistinguishable from karyotypes observed in other high-grade pleomorphic sarcomas, including malignant fibrous histiocytoma.[59]

Prognosis and Therapy

Standard surgical therapy for osteosarcoma now includes multidrug preoperative chemotherapy followed by surgical resection, either limb salvage or amputation. Largely because of multidrug chemotherapy, survival for high-grade conventional osteosarcoma approaches "77% and 73% at 5 and 10 years, respectively, with continuously disease-free survival being 70% and 69%."[60] Adverse prognostic variables in conventional osteosarcoma include advanced stage and proximal anatomic location. Conventional-appearing osteosarcomas that arise as secondary tumors tend to fare worse than tumors that arise de novo.[61] As discussed later in this chapter, response to chemotherapy as measured by pathologic evaluation of preoperative chemotherapy effect may be the most important prognostic variable.[51,60] There is good evidence that resection of pulmonary metastases is associated with improved survival.[62,63] A strong correlation is apparent between the observed degree of necrosis in the primary tumor and that seen in the metastatic foci.[63]

In the 1990s, a variety of molecular markers were investigated in osteosarcoma. Alterations of p53 in osteosarcoma are relatively common but, at present, do not seem to correlate with survival.[64] Kloen and associates[65] examined transforming growth factor-β and found a strong correlation between immunoexpression of transforming growth factor-β and disease progression. Earlier studies suggested that expression of *c-erbB-2* (*HER-2/neu*) was associated with poor survival.[66,67] More recent studies have not observed this correlation, however.[68,69] Different antibodies and variable scoring systems (e.g., cytoplasmic versus membranous staining) may contribute to discrepant results among various studies. To date, no evidence of gene amplification or mutation of the *HER-2/neu* oncogene has been documented in osteosarcoma.[67,68]

TABLE 12.8 Clinical and Pathologic Diagnostic Criteria for Telangiectatic Osteosarcoma

Presence of a purely lytic lesion radiographically
Gross examination revealing a multicystic, blood-filled cavity
Histologic features of aneurysmal bone cyst

Telangiectatic Osteosarcoma

Telangiectatic osteosarcoma is a rare variant of high-grade osteosarcoma, comprising 10% of cases.[70] Cardinal features for establishing the diagnosis of telangiectatic osteosarcoma are summarized in Table 12.8.[71] Ages of affected patients and presenting symptoms are similar to those observed in conventional osteosarcoma, with most occurring in the second decade of life. Males are affected more commonly than females. Pain is universally present, often accompanied by soft tissue swelling. The bones around the knee, especially the distal femoral and proximal tibial metaphyses, are the most common anatomic areas. Radiologically, telangiectatic osteosarcoma is typically metaphyseal-centered within a long bone, purely lytic, and large and poorly marginated with extensive permeation (Fig. 12.49). Periosteal new bone formation is common, and soft tissue extension usually is observed. Occasionally, telangiectatic osteosarcoma may mimic closely an aneursymal bone cyst.

Morphologically the low-power appearance ranges from a multicystic, aneurysmal bone cyst–like tumor to a hemorrhagic, largely necrotic neoplasm. In all cases, markedly anaplastic, spindled-to-polygonal tumor cells are found within the cyst walls or randomly distributed within the hemorrhagic and necrotic areas (Fig. 12.50). Mitotic activity is prominent, and atypical mitotic figures are present (Fig. 12.51). Accompanying the frankly malignant cells are variable numbers of osteoclast-type giant cells. Osteoid, usually arranged in a lace-like appearance, is focally present but may require extensive sampling to demonstrate (Fig. 12.52). FNAB reveals obviously malignant cells without associated matrix material (Fig. 12.53).

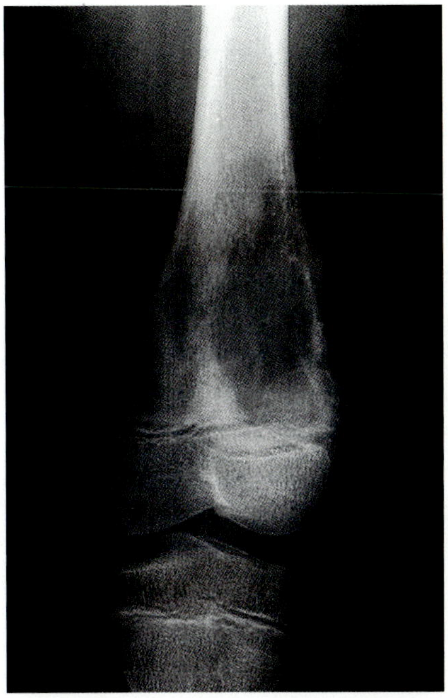

FIGURE 12.49 Telangiectatic osteosarcoma. An oblique radiograph of the distal femur shows a poorly demarcated, permeative, purely lytic lesion in the distal femoral metaphysis. No sclerotic density is apparent within the lesion.

Before the modern age of chemotherapy, the prognosis of telangiectatic osteosarcoma was considered poor. More recent evidence suggests, however, that neoadjuvant chemotherapy as applied to conventional osteosarcoma results in similar survival rates.[70,71] In most cases, the postchemotherapy resection specimen is virtually entirely necrotic with few if any anaplastic cells remaining.

Small Cell Osteosarcoma

By definition, small cell osteosarcoma is a tumor composed of cells closely resembling Ewing's sarcoma but clearly associated with osteoid/bone production. Small cell osteosarcoma is a rare variant of osteosarcoma, accounting for 1% to 2% of all osteosarcomas. Similar to conventional osteosarcoma, most patients present with pain and soft tissue swelling, usually manifesting within the first and second decades of life.

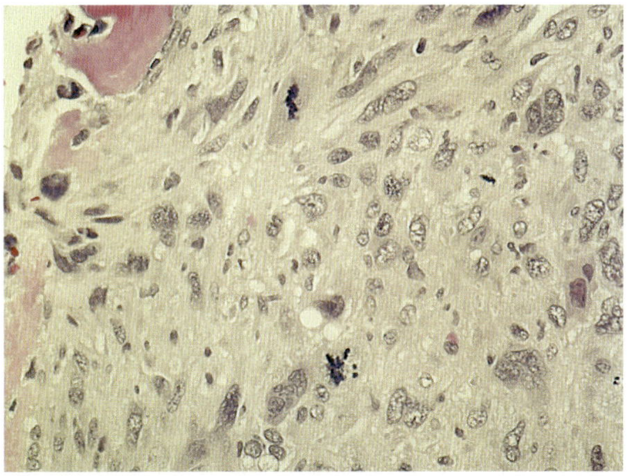

FIGURE 12.51 Telangiectatic osteosarcoma with markedly atypical and multinucleated tumor giant cells and scattered mitotic figures. (H&E.)

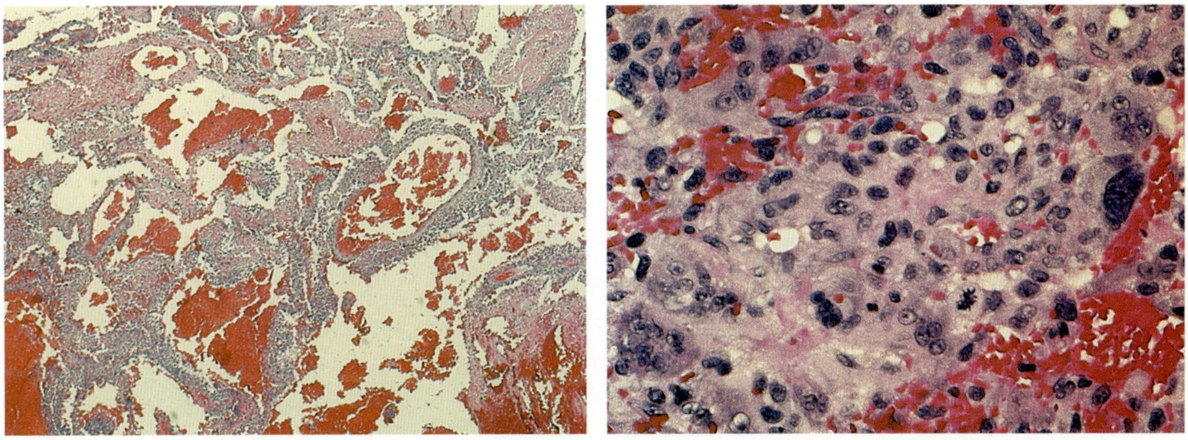

A B

FIGURE 12.50 Telangiectatic osteosarcoma is composed of variably sized cystic spaces, filled with blood and resembling an aneurysmal bone cyst **(A)**. Closer inspection of the fibrous cyst walls reveals scattered, markedly atypical and hyperchromatic tumor cells **(B)**. (H&E.)

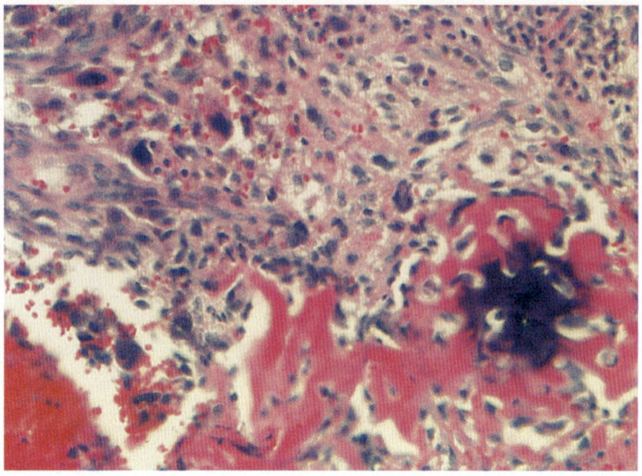

FIGURE 12.52 Telangiectatic osteosarcoma with osteoid/bone production by the malignant tumor cells. (H&E.)

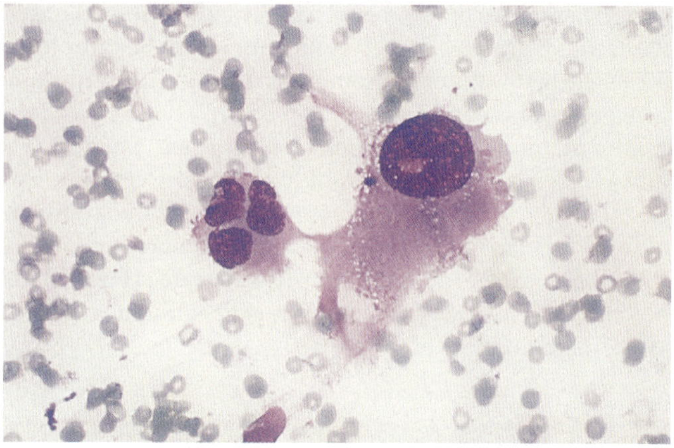

FIGURE 12.53 Fine needle aspiration biopsy of telangiectatic osteosarcoma generally yields markedly atypical tumor cells, some of which appear multinucleated. Metachromatic matrix is generally not observed. (Diff-Quik.)

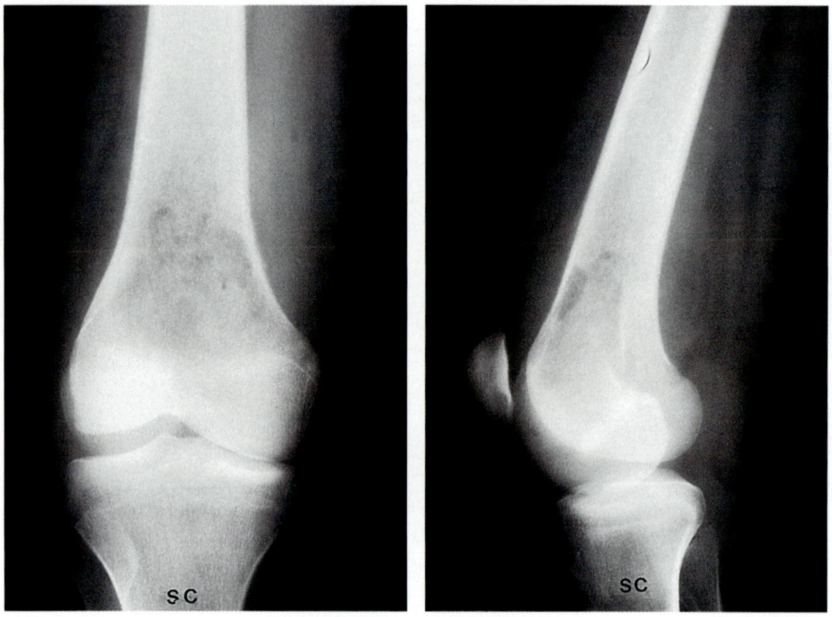

A B

FIGURE 12.54 Small cell osteosarcoma. Anteroposterior **(A)** and lateral **(B)** radiographs of the distal femur show a lytic lesion in the metaphyseal portion of the distal femur. The proximal margins are poorly defined.

There seems to be a slight male predominance. Favored anatomic sites include the distal and proximal femur, pelvis, and proximal humerus.[72] Radiologically, small cell osteosarcoma generally has an aggressive, at least focally, lytic appearance with variable amounts of mineralization and sclerosis (Fig. 12.54). Rarely the entire lesion may be osteoblastic. Soft tissue extension is observed frequently. Within the long bones, most are metaphyseal but occasionally may present solely diaphyseal.

Histologically, small cell osteosarcoma consists of sheets, nests, or cords of mostly uniform, round to slightly spindled tumor cells with oval-to-round, hyperchromatic nuclei, high nuclear-to-cytoplasmic ratios, and variable but generally scant cytoplasm (Fig. 12.55). Nucleoli range from inconspicuous to prominent. Reports of glandular structures and rosettes have been described. Although closely resembling Ewing's sarcoma, most cases of small cell osteosarcoma show more morphologic variation than typically is observed in Ewing's sarcoma. The amount of osteoid varies from case to case but is rarely prominent, requiring meticulous sampling and correlation with clinicoradiologic features to establish the diagnosis. FNAB findings are similar with moderately to highly cellular smears composed of mostly discohesive, uniform-appearing tumor cells with high nuclear-to-cytoplasmic ratios, round-to-ovoid nuclei, inconspicuous-to-small nucleoli, and scant cytoplasm (Fig. 12.56).[56] There are no reliable immunohistochemical markers for small cell osteosarcoma. Further confusing the matter, occasional examples of small cell osteosarcoma express CD99.[73] The diagnosis of small cell osteosarcoma should rest on the light

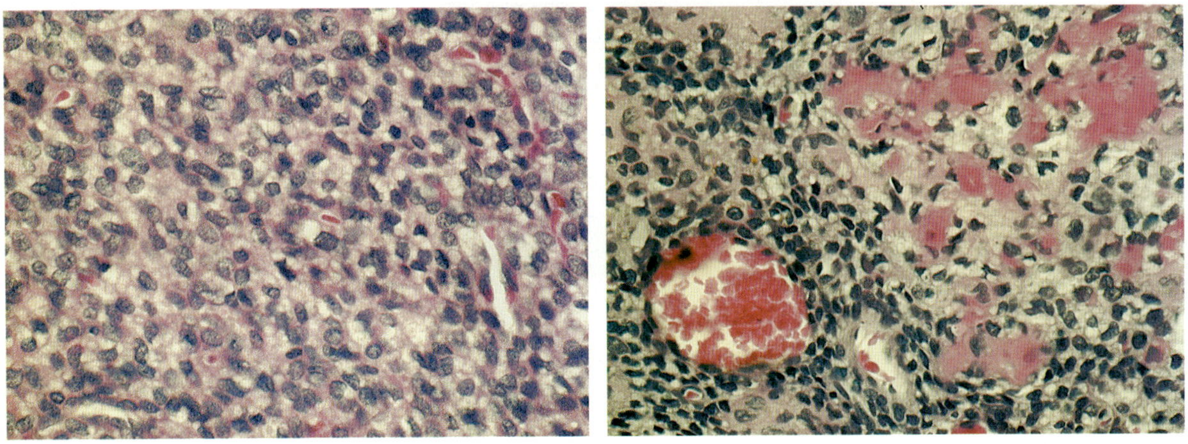

A B

FIGURE 12.55 Small cell osteosarcoma is composed of cells that morphologically appear similar to Ewing's sarcoma **(A).** The presence of osteoid production by the malignant tumor cells confirms the diagnosis of osteosarcoma **(B).** (H&E.)

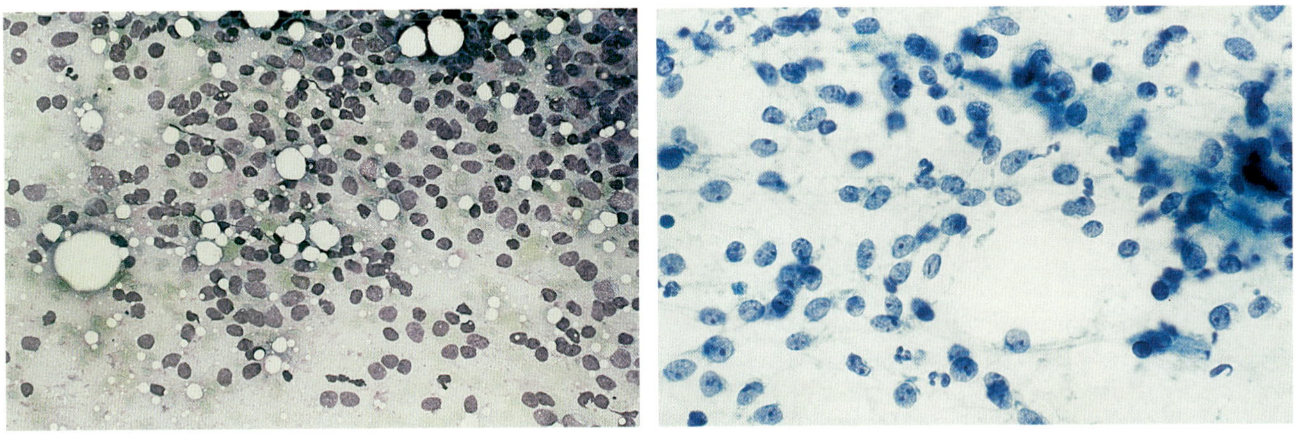

A B

FIGURE 12.56 Fine needle aspiration biopsy of small cell osteosarcoma yields highly cellular smears, composed of Ewing's sarcoma–like tumor cells with round-to-ovoid nuclei, high nuclear-to-cytoplasmic ratios, and inconspicuous-to-small nucleoli **(A** and **B). (A,** Diff-Quik; **B,** Papanicolaou.)

microscopic finding of at least focal osteoid/bone production by the malignant tumor cells. The overall prognosis of small cell osteosarcoma seems to be slightly worse than that observed with conventional osteosarcoma but has improved dramatically with the use of preoperative chemotherapy.[72]

Low-Grade Intraosseous (Well-Differentiated) Osteosarcoma

Low-grade intraosseous osteosarcoma, also known as well-differentiated intramedullary osteosarcoma, accounts for 1% to 2% of all osteosarcomas. Compared with conventional osteosarcoma, patients tend to be older, with most presenting between 20 and 40 years of age. There is no gender predilection. The metaphyseal region of the long bones, especially the distal femur, proximal tibia, and distal tibia, are most commonly involved.[74] Radiologically, low-grade intraosseous osteosarcoma is generally a metaphyseal, centrally located but poorly marginated lesion with variable amounts of ossification and cortical destruction (Fig. 12.57). Although most appear aggressive radiologically, 20% of cases may have deceptively circumscribed margins. Soft tissue extension is frequently present but is observed less commonly than in high-grade osteosarcomas.

Histologically, low-grade intraosseous osteosarcoma is a fibro-osseous lesion, bearing close resemblance to fibrous dysplasia or parosteal osteosarcoma. Variably thickened and randomly distributed, woven-to-lamellar bone trabeculae are embedded in a fibroblastic stroma, often resembling desmoid tumor. The bone trabeculae may resemble Paget's disease with irregular cement lines. Cytologically the individual cells within the fibroblastic stroma show minimal nuclear pleomor-

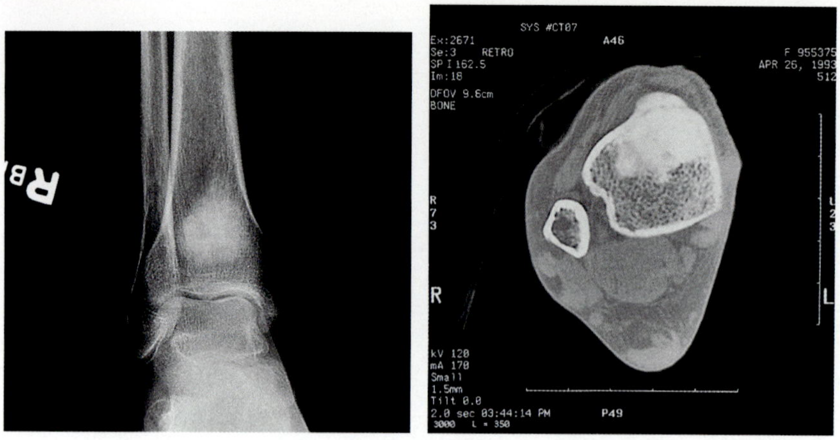

A B

FIGURE 12.57 Low-grade intraosseous osteosarcoma. An anteroposterior radiograph of the distal tibia shows a sclerotic lesion in the medullary canal of the distal tibia. No cortical penetration or soft tissue extension is evident **(A).** An axial computed tomographic scan shows a sclerotic medullary lesion with cortical penetration and periosteal new bone production anteriorly **(B).**

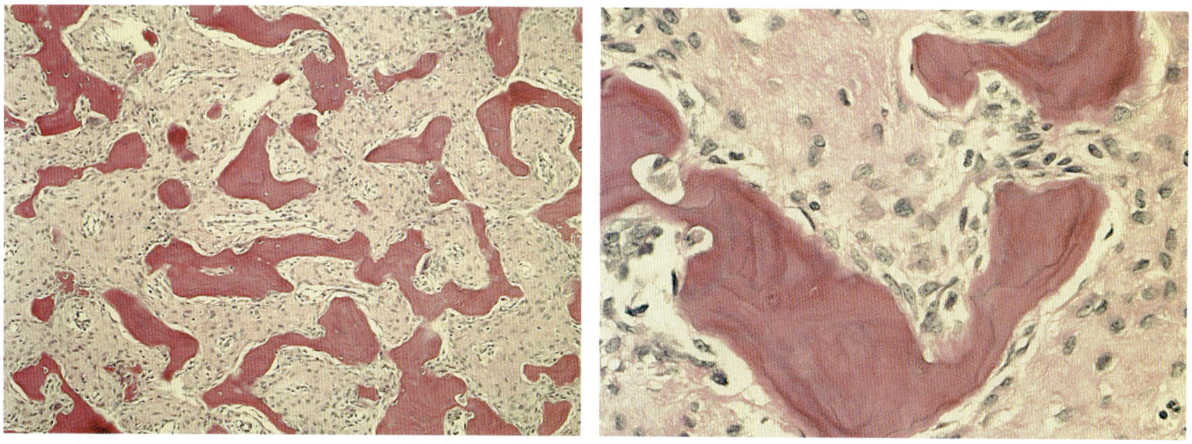

A B

FIGURE 12.58 Low-grade intraosseous osteosarcoma with haphazardly arranged, variably sized woven bone trabecula admixed with a dense, mildly to moderately cellular fibrous stroma. Irregular cement lines within the woven bone trabeculae may impart a pagetoid appearance. Clinical and radiologic correlation is essential for distinguishing low-grade interosseous osteosarcoma from fibrous dysplasia **(A** and **B). (A,** low power; **B,** high power, H&E.)

phism, and mitotic activity rarely exceeds 2 mitotic figures per 10 high-power fields (Fig. 12.58). Perhaps the most reliable feature separating low-grade intraosseous osteosarcoma from fibrous dysplasia is the presence of permeation of surrounding bone and, when present, invasion of periosteum and adjacent soft tissues. Most cases of low-grade intraosseous osteosarcoma are not amenable to FNAB analysis.

Wide surgical resection is the therapy of choice and usually results in a cure; curettage and marginal resection virtually always are followed by local recurrence. Chemotherapy and radiation therapy are generally not necessary. With each local recurrence, 15% of cases become progressively higher grade (dedifferentiation).[74] The latter finding requires adjuvant therapy and often results in death.

Surface Osteosarcoma

Most osteosarcomas arise from the intramedullary compartment of bone; however, occasional examples may originate from the adjacent periosteum or cortical bone surface or both, so-called surface osteosarcomas. The distinction between intramedullary and surface osteosarcomas is confounded by the fact that the former may have a significant extraosseous soft tissue component. By definition, surface osteosarcomas have little to no intramedullary extension. Substantial intramedullary extension (>10% of volume) excludes the diagnosis. The surface osteosarcoma subtypes, in decreasing order of frequency, include parosteal, periosteal, and high-grade surface osteosarcomas. The clinicoradiologic and pathologic features of these osteosarcoma subtypes are summarized in Table 12.9. Except in reference to osteosarcoma, the designations *parosteal* and *periosteal* are relatively nonspecific terms and refer to lesions arising adjacent to (e.g., juxtacortical) or from periosteum. Because the origin of juxtacortical lesions is largely unknown, the terms may be used interchangeably. In osteosarcoma, the terms *parosteal* and *periosteal* refer to biologically and pathologically distinct entities. The lower grade surface osteosarcoma subtypes, parosteal and periosteal forms, are generally not amenable to FNAB analysis because of extensive mineralization. The cytologic

TABLE 12.9 Clinicoradiologic and Pathologic Distinguishing Features of Various Surface Osteosarcoma Subtypes

	Parosteal Osteosarcoma	Periosteal Osteosarcoma	High-Grade Surface Osteosarcoma
Peak Age	20-30 yr	15-25 yr	10-20 yr
Location	Posterior distal femur (60%-75%), proximal tibia, proximal humerus	Tibial shaft, femur, and humerus	Midshaft and distal femur, midshaft of tibia
Symptoms	Painless swelling	Painful swelling	Painful swelling
Radiographs	Densely mineralized; broad attachment but lucent zone between tumor and bone; metaphyseal	Spiculated matrix pattern; more dense at the base; no intramedullary extension; diaphyseal or metadiaphyseal	Densely mineralized, base greater than periphery, with a "fluffy" immature appearance; diaphyseal, metaphyseal, or metadiaphyseal
Histology	Low-grade fibro-osseous lesion; may have cartilage cap	Intermediate-grade chondroblastic lesion with osteoid often most obvious at the base	Conventional osteosarcoma
Therapy	Surgical resection; chemotherapy for dedifferentiation	Surgical resection; chemotherapy for metastatic lesions	Preoperative chemotherapy followed by surgical resection

features of the high-grade form are essentially indistinguishable from conventional osteosarcoma.

Parosteal Osteosarcoma

Parosteal osteosarcoma is the most common form of surface osteosarcoma, accounting for 1% to 2% of all osteosarcomas. As with low-grade intraosseous osteosarcoma, patients tend to be a decade older than patients with conventional osteosarcoma. Clinically, most patients present with painless soft tissue swelling or mass.[75] Of cases, 75% involve the distal femoral metaphysis, especially the posterior aspect. Second in frequency is the proximal tibial metaphysis followed by the proximal humeral metaphysis. Involvement of the small tubular bones of the digits is extraordinarily rare; most cases likely represent one of the various forms of myositis ossificans (e.g., florid reactive periostitis). Radiologically, parosteal osteosarcomas form densely mineralized lesions with broad attachment to the underlying bony cortex (Fig. 12.59). Characteristically a thin lucent zone separates the tumor from the cortical bone, best visualized on CT scan. Intramedullary involvement may be observed in 20% of patients but is not prognostically significant.[75]

Parosteal osteosarcoma is a low-grade fibro-osseous lesion composed of a cytologically bland, spindle cell fibroblastic stroma and randomly distributed woven to lamellar bony trabeculae (Fig. 12.60). More ossified examples may mimic parosteal osteoma (Fig. 12.61). Osteoblastic rimming is generally not a prominent feature. Mitotic activity is minimal. One third of cases have cartilaginous differentiation, usually at the periphery (cartilage cap), that initially may cause confusion with a primary cartilaginous lesion or periosteal osteosarcoma, especially in needle or superficial incisional biopsy specimens (Fig. 12.62). Dedifferentiation to a high-grade osteosarcoma, an ominous prognostic feature, occurs in 16% of parosteal osteosarcomas and is especially likely to occur in locally recurrent lesions (Fig. 12.63).[75] Therapy involves complete resection and, depending on the size of the tumor, includes en bloc resection or amputation. Less than complete resection invariably results in local recurrence. Because the lesion is "biologically" and pathologically low grade, chemotherapy is generally not indicated, and metastases, with the exception of dedifferentiated tumors, are rare. Dedifferentiation requires chemotherapy, and response rates seem similar to that observed in conventional osteosarcoma.[76]

Periosteal Osteosarcoma

Periosteal osteosarcoma is the second most common form of surface osteosarcoma but is exceedingly rare (<1% of all osteosarcomas).[77] Most patients are between 10 and 25 years old, slightly younger than patients with parosteal osteosarcoma. Clinically, most patients present with symptoms of pain and soft tissue swelling. The shaft and proximal metaphyseal regions of the tibia are the most common anatomic locations, followed by the femur. For unknown reasons, periosteal osteosarcoma has a predilection for the shaft (diaphyseal region) of the long bones. Radiologically, periosteal osteosarcoma differs from parosteal osteosarcoma and tends to be smaller and significantly radiolucent with mineralization more obvious near the base of the tumor, adjacent to the cortex (Fig. 12.64). Additionally, the mineralization may exhibit a spiculated appearance. Although the underlying cortex may be variably thickened, intramedullary involvement is not observed, and, in our opinion, its presence excludes the diagnosis of periosteal osteosarcoma.

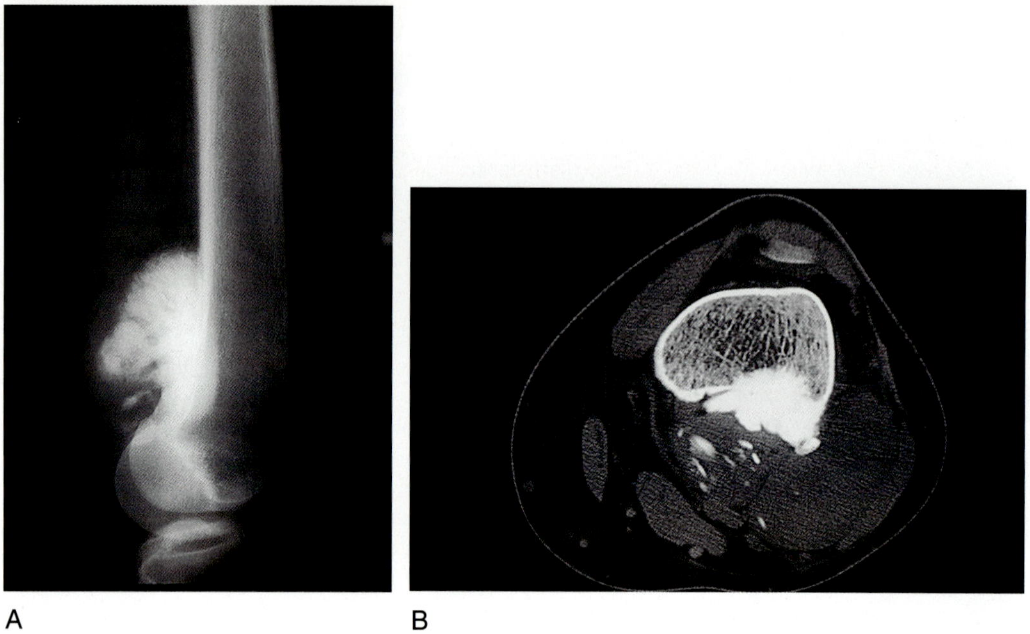

FIGURE 12.59 Parosteal osteosarcoma. A lateral radiograph of the distal femur shows a densely calcified, exophytic mass abutting the posterior surface of the distal femur. Medullary invasion is apparent just proximal to the femoral condyle **(A).** An axial computed tomographic scan shows the exophytic, solidly calcified mass and confirms medullary invasion **(B).**

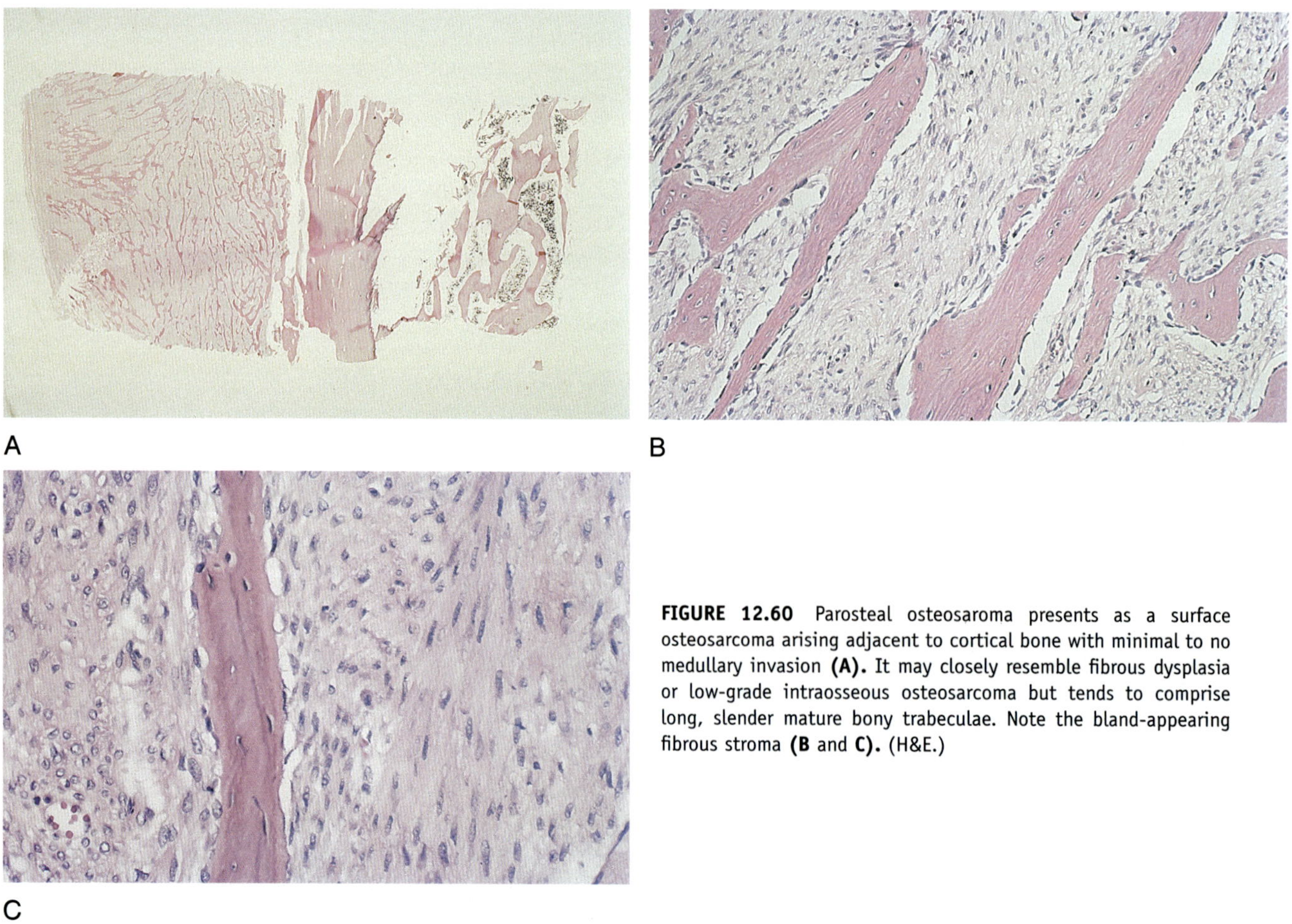

FIGURE 12.60 Parosteal osteosaroma presents as a surface osteosarcoma arising adjacent to cortical bone with minimal to no medullary invasion **(A).** It may closely resemble fibrous dysplasia or low-grade intraosseous osteosarcoma but tends to comprise long, slender mature bony trabeculae. Note the bland-appearing fibrous stroma **(B** and **C).** (H&E.)

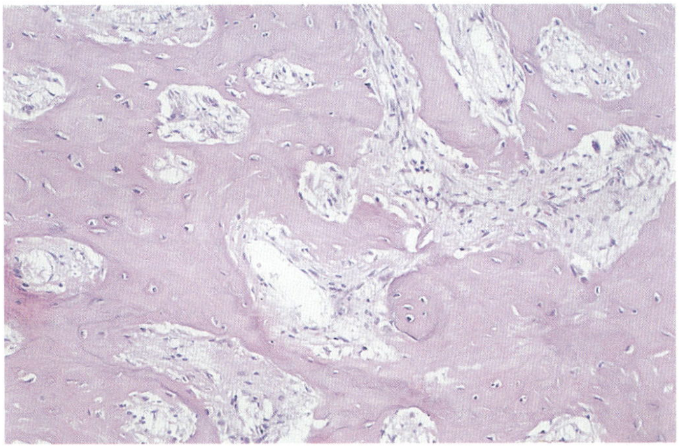

FIGURE 12.61 Parosteal osteosarcoma may become progressively more ossified and the fibrous stroma less apparent. (H&E.)

Histologically, periosteal osteosarcoma is a chondroblastic osteosarcoma, predominantly composed of lobules of low-grade to intermediate-grade hyaline cartilage; the peripheral portions of the cartilaginous lobules often appear cellular and spindled with moderate nuclear pleomorphism (Fig. 12.65). The border between the tumor and adjacent soft tissues is typically pushing and well defined. Malignant bone or lace-like osteoid or both is always present, however, typically more central in location, imparting a "feathery" appearance. Because periosteal osteosarcoma is considered a "biologically" higher grade lesion than parosteal osteosarcoma, metastases are more likely to occur (approximately 15% of cases) but are far less frequent than in conventional osteosarcoma.[77] Complete surgical resection with resulting negative margins is the therapy of choice. Chemotherapy is indicated for metastatic lesions, but at present, its effectiveness is unclear.

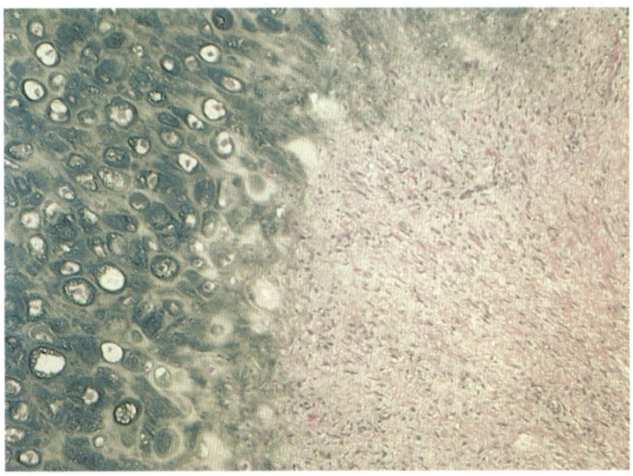

FIGURE 12.62 Parosteal osteosarcoma frequently has an overlying, mildly to moderately cellular cartilaginous cap. (H&E.)

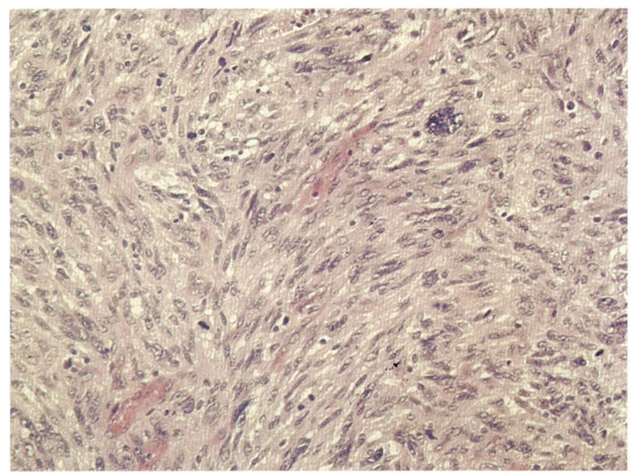

FIGURE 12.63 Dedifferentiated parosteal osteosarcoma with a high-grade, malignant fibrous histiocytoma–like component. (H&E.)

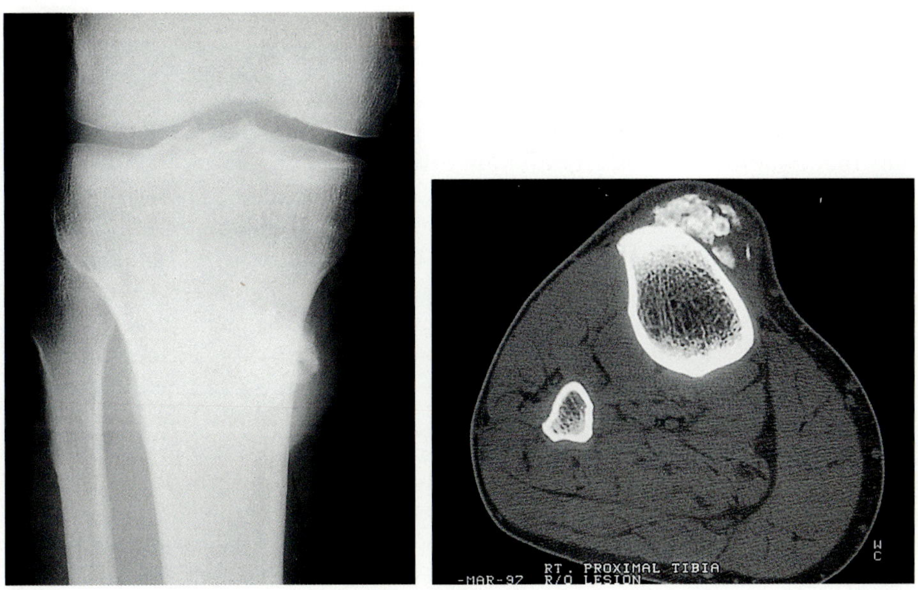

A B

FIGURE 12.64 Periosteal osteosarcoma. An anteroposterior radiograph of the proximal tibia reveals an irregularly calcified mass abutting the tibia **(A).** An axial computed tomographic scan shows irregular calcification abutting the proximal tibia. Although most of the calcification is amorphous, suggesting osteoid matrix calcification, other, more circular calcifications are typical of chondroid matrix calcification **(B).**

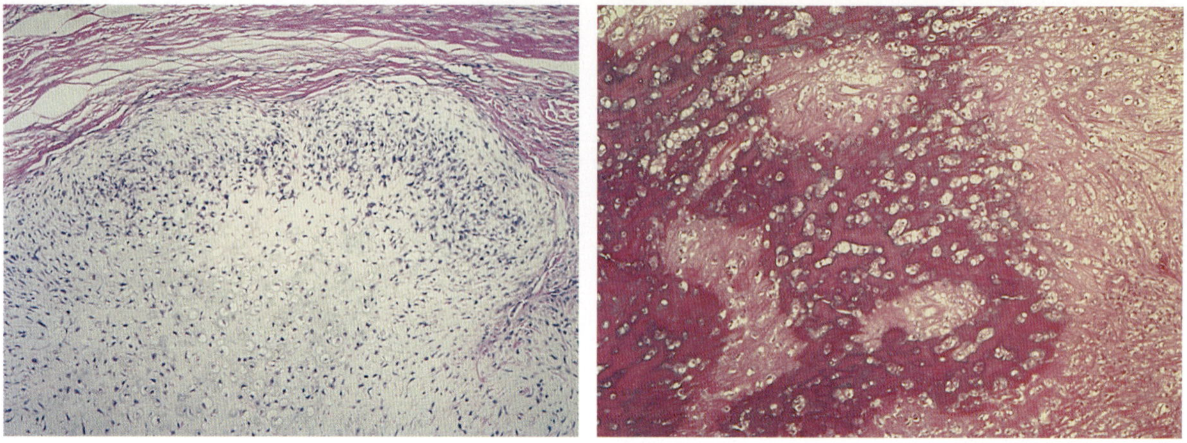

A B

FIGURE 12.65 Periosteal osteosarcoma is a surface chondroblastic osteosarcoma that usually appears sharply circumscribed from the adjacent soft tissues. Note the increased cellularity at the periphery of the cartilaginous lobule **(A).** Elsewhere, more centrally within the lesion, ossification is readily apparent **(B).** (H&E.)

High-Grade Surface Osteosarcoma

High-grade surface osteosarcoma is the rarest form of surface osteosarcoma. Similar to conventional osteosarcoma, most patients initially are diagnosed between ages 10 and 20; the most frequent anatomic sites are the midshaft and distal femoral metaphysis, followed by the tibial diaphysis.[78] Soft tissue swelling is the most common presenting complaint. Radiologically, most cases show extensive mineralization with a "fluffy, immature appearance."[78] The morphologic features of high-grade surface osteosarcoma are identical to features observed in conventional osteosarcoma. To establish the diagnosis of high-grade surface osteosarcoma, the tumor should meet the following criteria: (1) clinically present as a surface bone lesion and (2) absent-to-minimal (<10%) medullary involvement, clinically and pathologically.

The degree of medullary involvement permissible to establish a diagnosis of high-grade surface osteosarcoma is controversial, but all agree that it should be minimal. Dedifferentiated parosteal osteosarcoma may closely mimic high-grade surface osteosarcoma; meticulous sampling of the resection specimen is required to exclude fully the low-grade parosteal osteosarcoma component. Proper therapy for high-grade surface osteosarcoma includes complete excision and systemic chemotherapy; postchemotherapy response rates appear similar to that observed with conventional osteosarcoma.[78]

Osteosarcoma of the Jaw

Because of its unusual histologic features and tendency toward favorable biologic behavior, osteosarcoma of the jaw is considered as a diagnostically distinct entity. Compared with conventional osteosarcoma, patients are typically older, generally between ages 20 and 50 (average age 34 years) at initial presentation.[79] Soft tissue swelling and localized pain are the most common initial complaints. The maxilla and mandible are involved roughly equally. Radiologically, most tumors appear aggressive and permeative but may range from purely lytic lesions to virtually sclerotic forms (Fig. 12.66). Overall the morphologic features of osteosarcoma of the jaw are essentially identical to features observed in the long bone. The chondroblastic subtype tends to predominate, however, and a higher percentage of tumors present with a lower histologic grade (Fig. 12.67). Improved survival has been reported with the lower grade chondroblastic subtype. Radical surgery offers the best chance for long-term survival. The local recurrence rate for most treatment modalities ranges up to 70%.[79] Death is usually secondary to uncontrolled local disease and not metastatic spread. The role of chemotherapy for osteosarcoma of the jaw is unclear.

Secondary Osteosarcoma

The term *secondary osteosarcoma* refers to osteosarcomas arising from a pre-existing bone condition or after therapy, usually radiation, for a prior malignancy. Pre-existing bone lesions that rarely may undergo malignant transformation to osteosarcoma include Paget's disease (Fig. 12.68), fibrous dysplasia (see Fig. 12.37), and bone infarcts.[80-83] Osteosarcoma arising in association with orthopedic implants also has been documented.[84] Compared with primary osteosarcoma, secondary osteosarcomas are more likely to involve the axial skeleton and flat bones. Patients who have received ionizing radiation rarely develop osteosarcoma within the radiation field. To establish such a diagnosis, there should be no initial evidence of an unrelated neoplasm within the radiated field, and a latency period of at least 2 years (between the radiation exposure and development of the sarcoma) must be present. Histologically, osteosarcomas arising from any pre-existing bone lesion or previously irradiated bone tend to be high-

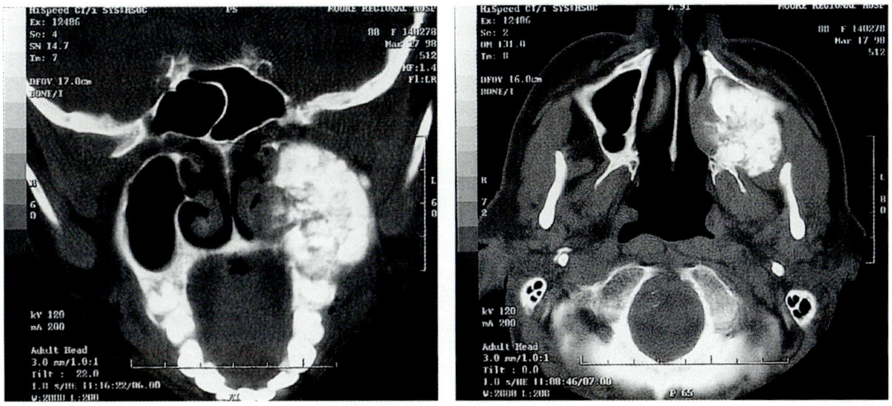

A B

FIGURE 12.66 Osteosarcoma of the jaw. Coronal **(A)** and axial **(B)** computed tomographic scans show a lobulated, dense tumor arising from the maxilla and extending into the left maxillary sinus. The sarcoma has eroded the maxillary sinus walls medially and laterally and abuts the turbinates.

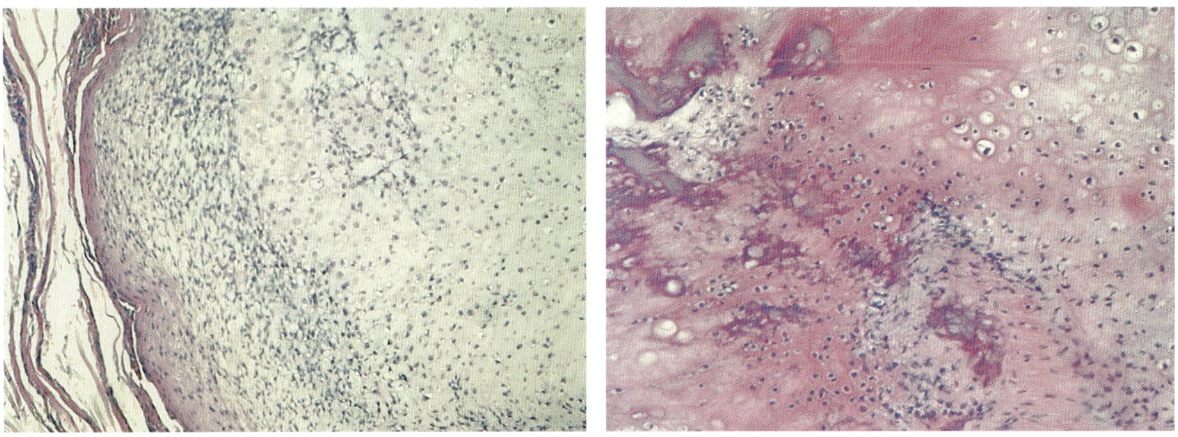

A B

FIGURE 12.67 Osteosarcoma of the jaw most frequently manifests as a chondroblastic osteosarcoma. Note the sharply circumscribed borders and the increased cellularity at the periphery of the cartilaginous lobule **(A).** Although predominantly composed of cartilage, such tumors always show at least focal malignant bone production **(B).** (H&E.)

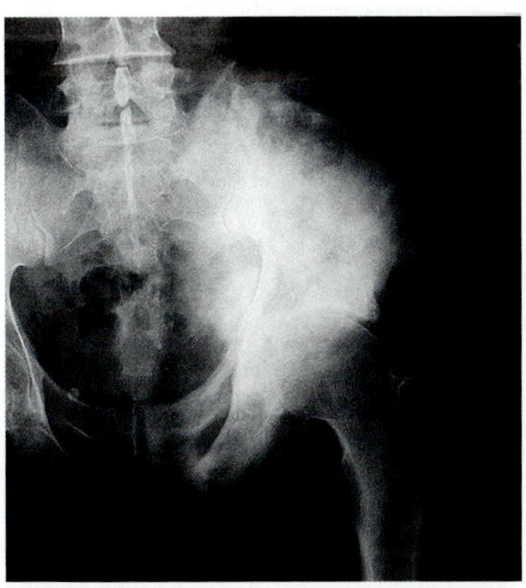

FIGURE 12.68 Secondary osteosarcoma. An anteroposterior radiograph of the left hemipelvis shows typical radiographic manifestations of long-standing Paget's disease; the ilium, ischium, and pubis are enlarged with thickened cortex and coarsened trabeculae. There is a large calcified soft tissue mass overlying the supra-acetabular ilium, extending toward the sciatic notch and containing dense osteoid matrix calcification, representing a secondary osteosarcoma.

grade, aggressive neoplasms. As expected, most patients are older (>40 years old) than the typical osteosarcoma patient, and despite modern chemotherapy, overall prognosis is poor.[80,83,84]

Certain malignancies, such as retinoblastoma, predispose patients to other malignancies, including osteosarcoma. Some patients with retinoblastoma contain a 13q deletion of the tumor-suppressor gene *RB* and are at increased risk for the development of osteosarcoma. This risk seems to increase with the use of radiation or chemotherapy.[81]

Extraskeletal Osteosarcoma

Extraskeletal osteosarcomas are extraordinarily rare lesions, generally accounting for only 1% of all soft tissue sarcomas. Most patients are older than 40 years of age at diagnosis, and the lower limbs, especially the thigh, are most commonly affected. Patients generally present with an enlarging soft tissue mass. To establish a diagnosis of extraskeletal osteosarcoma,

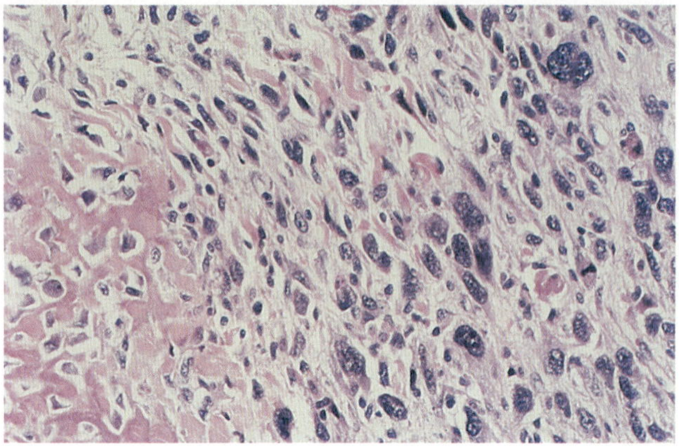

FIGURE 12.69 Extraskeletal osteosarcoma with a malignant fibrous histiocytoma–like stroma and obvious lace-like osteoid production by the tumor cells. (H&E.)

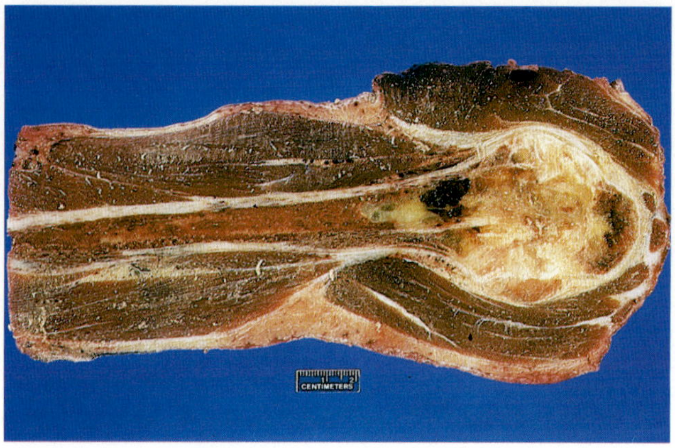

FIGURE 12.70 Postchemotherapy resection specimen for evaluation of extent of necrosis should include sampling of a complete cross section of tumor.

there should be no involvement of the underlying bone or periosteum. Histologically, malignant osteoid must be produced by the sarcomatous tumor cells. Similar to secondary osteosarcomas, extraskeletal osteosarcomas are virtually always high grade, closely resembling conventional "bone" osteosarcoma. Although the distinction between extraskeletal osteosarcoma and malignant fibrous histiocytoma may be difficult, we consider the presence of even minimal (<1%) osteoid production by the sarcomatous tumor cells as sufficient to render the diagnosis of extraskeletal osteosarcoma (Fig. 12.69). Establishing the diagnosis, especially in small biopsy specimens, often is difficult. In one study of 25 cases of extraskeletal osteosarcoma, the correct initial diagnosis was rendered in only 8 cases.[85] Although FNAB appears accurate for establishing the diagnosis of skeletal osteosarcoma, it has not performed as well for the extraskeletal form.[56] In most cases, the diagnosis of "pleomorphic sarcoma, not otherwise specified" is rendered. At present, immunohistochemistry does not seem helpful. Occasional examples of extraskeletal osteosarcoma may express cytokeratin and epithelial membrane antigen, confounding the diagnosis.[85] Although the prognosis of primary skeletal osteosarcoma is related to histologic grade and response to adjuvant therapy, histologic grade does not correlate significantly with survival in patients with extraskeletal osteosarcoma. This situation results partly from the fact that extraskeletal osteosarcomas are almost invariably high-grade lesions.[86,87] Chung and Enzinger[86] reported that no distinct histologic parameters seemed to correlate significantly with clinical behavior; however, extraskeletal osteosarcomas that were predominantly fibroblastic seemed to have a slightly better prognosis than osteoblastic, chondroblastic, or telangiectatic subtypes. Lee and colleagues[87] found that patients with extraskeletal chrondroblastic osteosarcomas survived longer than patients with the osteoblastic subtype. The therapy of choice seems to be radical resection followed by chemotherapy.

Pathologic Evaluation of Osteosarcoma after Chemotherapy

The therapy of high-grade intramedullary osteosarcomas has improved dramatically through the use of chemotherapeutic regimens. Consequently the role of the pathologist has evolved. Traditional prognostic factors for osteosarcoma include age at presentation, stage, anatomic localization (proximal versus distal), and histologic grade/subtype. The most important prognostic feature may be histologic response to preoperative chemotherapy, however. The extent of tumor necrosis in the postchemotherapy resection specimen correlates strongly with patient survival. Patients with 90% or more postchemotherapy tumor necrosis have a reported 91% survival rate compared with 14% in patients with less than 90% necrosis.[51] The best clinical outcome is observed in patients with greater than 95% necrosis. These observations have led to therapy intensification, however, for patients deemed "poor responders." Consequently, survival for patients with 80% to 89% necrosis is similar to that observed in patients with 90% to 95% necrosis.[88]

Evaluation of postchemotherapy tumor necrosis generally is carried out by a complete cross section of tumor obtained from a limb salvage procedure or amputation (Fig. 12.70). This representative section is sampled and "blocked in" completely using a grid pattern diagram or radiographs indicating the site of each numbered block. Blocks not only should be taken from the main tumor, but also should include areas "shielded" from chemotherapy effect, including adjacent soft tissue, tumor/normal tissue interface, cortical bone and subcortical marrow, periarticular regions, and areas surrounding ligaments.

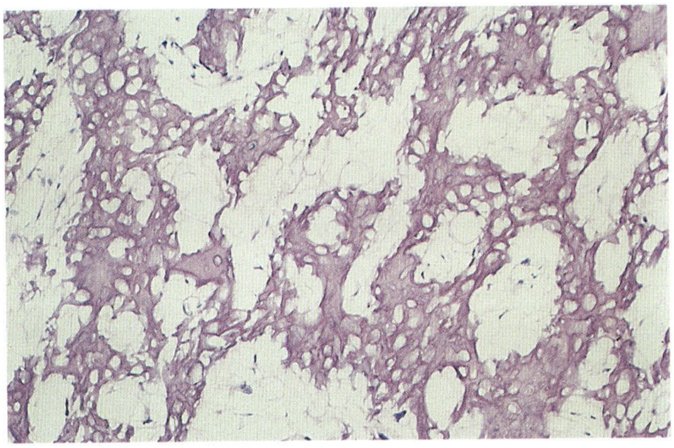

FIGURE 12.71 Postchemotherapy effect in osteoblastic and chondroblastic osteosarcomas is manifested by cellular dropout (empty lacunae). (H&E.)

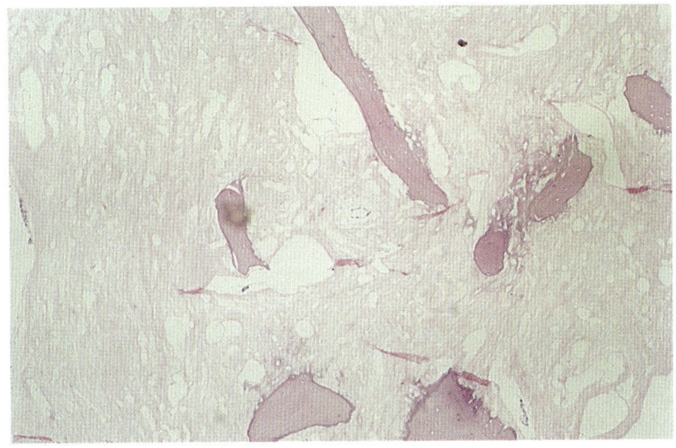

FIGURE 12.72 Postchemotherapy effect in fibroblastic osteosarcoma characterized by acellular fibrous tissue with entrapped mature, lamellar bony trabeculae. (H&E.)

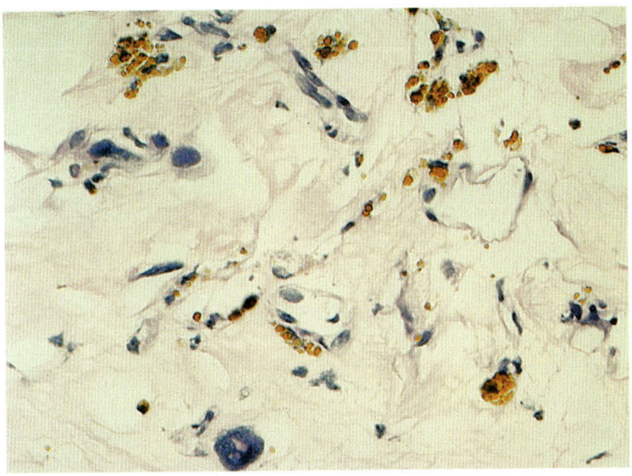

FIGURE 12.73 Postchemotherapy osteosarcoma characterized by scattered atypical cells with smudgy chromatin and rare multinucleation. Although such cells may not be "viable," they should not be considered as evidence of "necrosis." (H&E.)

TABLE 12.10 Grading System for Treated Osteosarcomas

Grade	Definition
1	No effect (necrosis)
2	Focal necrosis
A	>50% viable tumor remaining (<50% necrosis)
B	5-50% viable tumor remaining (50%-95% necrosis)
3	Rare foci of viable tumor, <5% (>95% necrosis)
4	No viable tumor identified (100% necrosis)

Defining tumor necrosis is difficult and subjective, but specific guidelines are applicable to certain osteosarcoma subtypes. For osteoblastic and chondroblastic osteosarcomas, tumor necrosis is best defined by "cell dropout" (empty lacunae) (Fig. 12.71). Remnants of neoplastic cells appearing as minute pyknotic structures of ill-defined basophilia, so-called ghost cells, also are observed sometimes within the lacunae of postchemotherapy chondroblastic osteosarcomas. In fibroblastic and small cell osteosarcomas, postchemotherapy tumor necrosis generally is manifested by replacement of the tumor with acellular fibrous tissue or granulation tissue with scattered chronic inflammatory cells (Fig. 12.72). Postchemotherapy specimens of telangiectatic osteosarcoma often reveal residual, blood-filled cystic spaces with randomly distributed hemosiderin deposition. Residual but rare atypical cells also may be evident. In all of these specimens, a population of cells may exist that probably represents postchemotherapy effect, but its significance is unclear. These cells often show marked nuclear atypia, a smudgy nuclear chromatin pattern, and cytoplasmic vacuolization (Fig. 12.73). To reduce the subjectivity of determining tumor necrosis, we recommend that such cytologic changes not be considered necrosis. Taking into account all subtypes of osteosarcoma, postchemotherapy tumor necrosis is assessed most accurately and reproducibly by the presence or absence of neoplastic cells. A variety of grading systems for the postchemotherapy evaluation of osteosarcomas exist. We endorse the system used by the Children's Cancer Group and Pediatric Oncology Group (Table 12.10).[89]

Differentiating spontaneous tumor necrosis from postchemotherapy tumor necrosis is not always possible, but features such as the absence of tumor cells, fibroblastic ingrowth, and hemosiderin deposition are more likely to be the result of chemotherapy and not spontaneously induced.

Hamartoma (Mesenchymoma) of the Chest Wall

Chest wall hamartoma of infancy is a rare lesion usually observed at birth or shortly thereafter. It may be asymptomatic, cause respiratory difficulties, or cause swelling of the chest wall. Radiologically a large, well-circumscribed but focally mineralized mass involves one or more ribs; varying degrees of erosion and destruction may be present (Fig. 12.74).[90] Morphologically the lesion appears well circumscribed and consists of islands of mature hyaline cartilage, resembling epiphyseal growth plate, admixed with bland-appearing fibroblasts and bony trabeculae (Fig. 12.75). Mitotic figures may be observed but are never atypical. Adequate therapy includes complete surgical excision; some lesions may regress spontaneously.

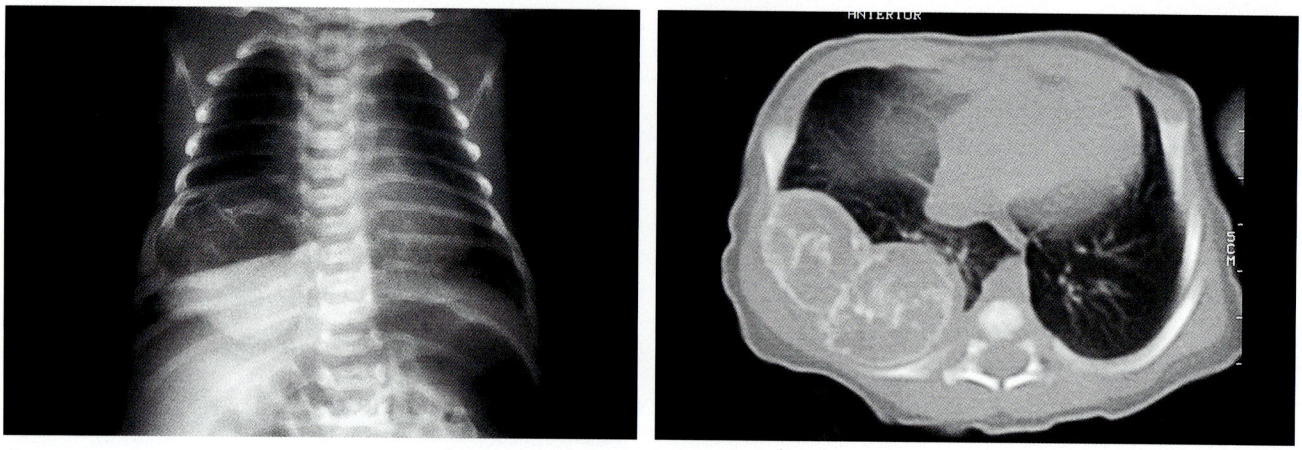

A B

FIGURE 12.74 Hamartoma of the chest wall. A frontal radiograph of the chest in a neonate shows a lobulated, soft tissue mass in the right hemithorax. The right seventh and eighth posterior ribs are largely eroded **(A).** A computed tomographic scan reveals the large intrathoracic mass containing irregular calcifications **(B).**

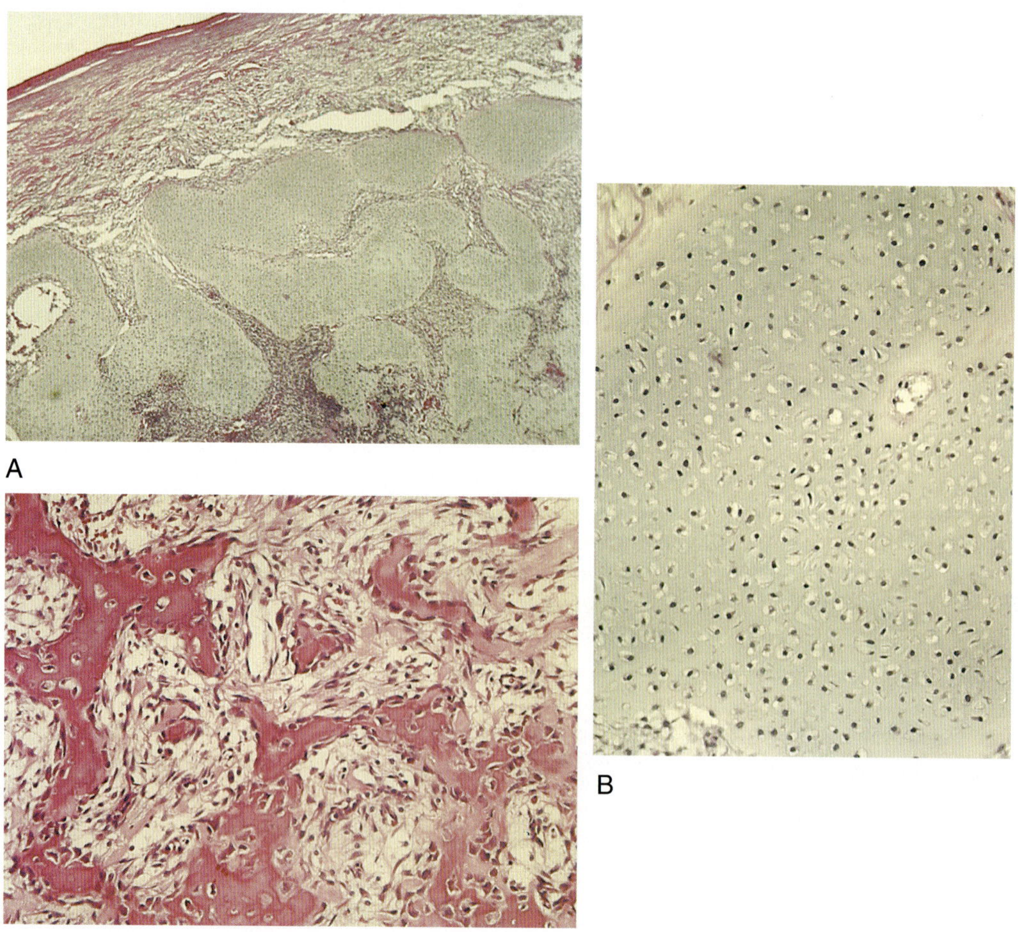

A B C

FIGURE 12.75 Hamartoma of the chest wall is usually well circumscribed and sharply demarcated from the surrounding soft tissues. It is composed of islands of moderately cellular cartilage admixed with bland-appearing fibrous stroma and mature bony trabeculae **(A-C). (A-C,** H&E.)

REFERENCES

Myositis Ossificans and Variants

1. Kilpatrick SE, Koplyay P, Pope TL Jr, et al: Clinical, radiologic, and pathologic spectrum of myositis ossificans and related lesions: A unifying concept. Adv Anat Pathol 1997;4:277.
2. Ackerman LV: Extra-osseous localized non-neoplastic bone and cartilage formation (so-called myositis ossificans): Clinical and pathological confusion with malignant neoplasms. J Bone Joint Surg Am 1958;40:279.
3. Monu JUV, Pope TL, Ward WG, et al: Magnetic resonance imaging of myositis ossificans. J South Orthop Assoc 1993;2:67.
4. Norman A, Dorfman HD: Juxtacortical circumscribed myositis ossificans: Evolution and radiographic features. Radiology 1970;96:301.
5. Nuovo MA, Norman A, Chumas J, et al: Myositis ossificans with atypical clinical, radiologic or pathologic findings: A review of 23 cases. Skeletal Radiol 1992;21:87.
6. Mirra JM, Picci P, Gold RH: Parosteal tumors. In: Bone Tumors: Clinical, Radiologic, and Pathologic Correlations. Philadelphia: Lea & Febiger, 1989, pp 1599-1612.
7. Reiman HM, Dahlin DC: Cartilage- and bone-forming tumors of soft tissues. Semin Diagn Pathol 1988;3:288.
8. Rodriquez-Peralto JL, Lopez-Barea F, Sanchez-Herrera S, et al: Primary aneurysmal bone cyst of soft tissues (extraosseous aneurysmal cyst). Am J Surg Pathol 1994;18:632.
9. Amir G, Mogle P, Sucher E: Case report 729: Myositis ossificans and aneurysmal bone cyst. Skeletal Radiol 1992;21:257.
10. Daroca PJ, Pulitzer DR, LeCicero J: Ossifying fasciitis. Arch Pathol Lab Med 1982;106:682.
11. Chung EB, Enzinger FM: Proliferative fasciitis. Cancer 1975;36:1450.
12. Dupree WB, Enzinger FM: Fibro-osseous pseudotumor of the digits. Cancer 1986;58:2103.
13. Spjut HJ, Dorfman HD: Florid reactive periostitis of the tubular bones of the hands and feet: A benign lesion which may simulate osteosarcoma. Am J Surg Pathol 1981;5:423.
14. Holmes WS, Pope TL Jr, deLange EE, et al: Case report 413: Florid reactive periostitis of the proximal phalanx of the fourth finger (parosteal fasciitis, pseudosarcomatous fibormatosis, fasciitis ossificans). Skeletal Radiol 1987;16:163.
15. Nora FE, Dahlin DC, Beabout JW: Bizarre parosteal osteochondromatous proliferations of the hands and feet. Am J Surg Pathol 1983;7:245.
16. deLange EE, Pope TL Jr, Fechner RE, et al: Case report 428: Bizarre parosteal osteochondromatous proliferation (BPOP). Skeletal Radiol 1987;16:481.
17. Meneses MF, Unni KK, Swee RG: Bizarre parosteal osteochondromatous proliferation of bone (Nora's lesions). Am J Surg Pathol 1993;17:691.
18. Landon GC, Johnson KA, Dahlin DC: Subungual exostosis. J Bone Joint Surg Am 1979;61:256.
19. Miller-Breslow A, Dorfman HD: Dupuytren's (subungual) exostosis. Am J Surg Pathol 1988;12:368.
20. Roth SI, Stowell RE, Helwig EB: Cutaneous ossification: Report of 120 cases and review of the literature. Arch Pathol 1963;76:44.
21. Becker SW: Osteosis cutis: Case report. Arch Dermatol Syph 1924;10:163.

Bone Island (Enostosis)

22. Greenspan A, Steiner G, Knutzon R: Bone island (enostosis): Clinical significance and radiologic and pathologic correlations. Skeletal Radiol 1991;20:85.
23. Greenspan A, Klein MJ: Giant bone island. Skeletal Radiol 1996;25:67.
24. Mirra JM, Picci P, Gold RH: Osseous tumors of intramedullary origin. In: Bone Tumors: Clinical, Radiologic, and Pathologic Correlations. Philadelphia: Lea & Febiger, 1989, pp 182–190.

Osteoma

25. Hallberg OE, Begley JW Jr: Origin and treatment of osteomas of the paranasal sinuses. Arch Otolaryngol 1950;51:750.
26. Peyser AB, Makley JT, Callewart CC, et al: Osteoma of the long bones and the spine: A study of eleven patients and a review of the literature. J Bone Joint Surg Am 1996;78:1172.

Osteoid Osteoma

27. Klein MH, Shankman S: Osteoid osteoma: Radiologic and pathologic correlation. Skeletal Radiol 1992;21:23.
28. McDermott MB, Kyriakos M, McEnery K: Painless osteoid osteoma of the rib in an adult: A case report and a review of the literature. Cancer 1996;77:1442.
29. Bell RS, O'Connor GD, Waddell JP: Importance of magnetic resonance imaging in osteoid osteoma: A case report. Can J Surg 1989;32:276.
30. O'Connell JX, Nanthakumar SS, Nielsen GP, et al: Osteoid osteoma: The uniquely innervated bone tumor. Mod Pathol 1998;11:175.
31. Regan MW, Galey JP, Oakeshott RD: Recurrent osteoid osteoma: Case report with a ten-year asymptomatic interval. Clin Orthop 1990;253:221.
32. Voto SJ, Cook AJ, Weiner DS, et al: Treatment of osteoid osteoma by computed tomography guided excision in the pediatric patient. J Pediatr Orthop 1990;10:510.
33. Vickers CW, Pugh DC, Ivins JC: Osteoid osteoma: A 15 year follow-up of an untreated patient. J Bone Joint Surg Am 1959;41:357.

Osteoblastoma

34. Lucas DR, Unni KK, McLeod RA, et al: Osteoblastoma: A clinicopathologic study of 306 cases. Hum Pathol 1994;25:117.
35. Rocca CD, Huvos AG: Osteoblastoma: Varied histological presentations with a benign clinical course: An analysis of 55 cases. Am J Surg Pathol 1996;20:841.
36. Bertoni F, Unni KK, Lucas DR, McLeod RA: Osteoblastoma with cartilaginous matrix: An unusual morphologic presentation in 18 cases. Am J Surg Pathol 1993;17:69.
37. Seki T, Fukuda H, Ishii Y, et al: Malignant transformation of benign osteoblastoma. J Bone Joint Surg Am 1975;57:424.

Fibrous Dysplasia

38. Voytek TM, Ro JY, Edeiken J, et al: Fibrous dysplasia and cemento-ossifying fibroma: A histologic spectrum. Am J Surg Pathol 1996;19:775.
39. Ishida T, Dorfman HD: Massive chondroid differentiation in fibrous dysplasia of bone (fibrocartilaginous dysplasia). Am J Surg Pathol 1993;17:924.
40. Bertoni F, Unni KK, McLeod RA, et al: Xanthoma of bone. Am J Clin Pathol 1988;90:377.
41. Yabut SM Jr, Kenan S, Sissons HA, et al: Malignant transformation of fibrous dysplasia: A case report and review of the literature. Clin Orthop 1988;228:281.

Osteofibrous Dysplasia

42. Park Y-K, Unni KK, McLeod RA, et al: Osteofibrous dysplasia: Clinicopathologic study of 80 cases. Hum Pathol 1993;24:1339.
43. Sweet DR, Vinh TN, Devaney K: Cortical osteofibrous dysplasia of long bone and its relationship to adamantinoma: A clinicopathologic study of 30 cases. Am J Surg Pathol 1992;16:282.
44. Campanacci M, Laus M: Osteofibrous dysplasia of the tibia and fibula. J Bone Joint Surg Am 1981;63:367.

Osteosarcoma

45. Taylor WF, Ivins JC, Unni KK, et al: Prognostic variables in osteosarcoma: A multi-institutional study. J Natl Cancer Inst 1989;81:21.
46. Unni KK, Dahlin DC: Grading of bone tumors. Semin Diagn Pathol 1984;1:165.

47. Inwards CY, Unni KK: Classification and grading of bone sarcomas. Hematol Oncol Clin N Am 1995;9:541.
48. Bjornsson J, Inwards CY, Wold LE, et al: Prognostic significance of spontaneous tumor necrosis in osteosarcoma. Virchow Arch A Pathol Anat 1993;423:195.
49. Huvos AG: Bone Tumors: Diagnosis, Treatment and Prognosis, 2nd ed. Philadelphia: WB Saunders, 1991, pp 85-155.
50. Kilpatrick SE, Abdul-Karim FW, Renner JB, et al: Interobserver variability among expert orthopedic pathologists for diagnosis, histologic grade, and determination of necessity for chemotherapy in osteosarcoma. Pediatr Pathol Mol Med 2000;19:337.
51. Raymond AK, Sant CP, Carrasco CH, et al: Osteosarcoma chemotherapy effect: A prognostic factor. Semin Diagn Pathol 1987;4:212.
52. Nishida J, Sim FH, Wenger DE, Unni KK: Malignant fibrous histiocytoma of bone: A clinicopathologic study of 81 patients. Cancer 1997;79:482.
53. Urban C, Rosen G, Huvos AG, et al: Chemotherapy of malignant fibrous histiocytoma of bone: A report of five cases. Cancer 1983;51:795.
54. Inwards C, Bertoni F, Unni KK, et al: Epithelioid osteosarcoma: A clinicopathologic and immunohistochemical study (abstract). Mod Pathol 1997;10:11A.
55. Kilpatrick SE, Ward WG, Bos GD, et al: The role of fine needle aspiration biopsy in the diagnosis and management of osteosarcoma. Pediatr Pathol Mol Med 2001;20:175.
56. Nicol KK, Ward WG, Savage PD, et al: Fine needle aspiration biopsy of skeletal versus extraskeletal osteosarcoma. Cancer 1998;84:176.
57. Garbe LR, Monges GM, Pellegrin EM, et al: Ultrastructural study of osteosarcomas. Hum Pathol 1981;12:891.
58. Fanburg JC, Rosenberg AE, Weaver DL, et al: Osteocalcin and osteonectin immunoreactivity in osteosarcoma. Am J Clin Pathol 1997;108:464.
59. Bridge JA, Nelson M, McComb E, et al: Cytogenetic findings in 73 osteosarcoma specimens and a review of the literature. Cancer Genet Cytogenet 1997;95:74.
60. Glasser DB, Lane JM, Huvos AG, et al: Survival, prognosis, and therapeutic response in osteogenic sarcoma: The Memorial Hospital experience. Cancer 1992;69:698.
61. Pratt CB, Meyer WH, Rao BN, et al: Comparison of primary osteosarcoma of flat bones with secondary osteosarcoma of any site. Cancer 1997;80:1171.
62. Ward WG, Mikaelian K, Dorey F, et al: Pulmonary metastases of stage IIB extremity osteosarcoma and subsequent pulmonary metastases. J Clin Oncol 1994;12:1849.
63. Bacci G, Mercuri M, Briccoli A, et al: Osteogenic sarcoma of the extremity with detectable lung metastases at presentation: Results of treatment of 23 patients with chemotherapy followed by simultaneous resection of primary and metastatic lesions. Cancer 1997;79:245.
64. Lonardo F, Ueda T, Huvos AG, et al: p53 and MDM2 alterations in osteosarcomas: Correlation with clinicopathologic features and proliferative rate. Cancer 1997;79:1541.
65. Kloen P, Gebhart M, Perez-Atayde A, et al: Expression of transforming growth factor-β (TGF-β) isoforms in osteosarcoma. Cancer 1997;80:2230.
66. Gorlick R, Huvos AG, Aledo A, et al: Expression of HER2/erbB-2 correlates with survival in osteosarcoma. J Clin Oncol 1999;17:2781.
67. Onda M, Matsuda S, Higaki S, et al: ErbB-2 expression is correlated with poor prognosis for patients with osteosarcoma. Cancer 1996;77:71.
68. Maitra A, Wanzer DM, Weinberg AG, et al: Amplification of the HER-2/neu ocogene is uncommon in pediatric osteosarcomas. Cancer 2001;92:677.
69. Kilpatrick SE, Geisinger KR, King TS, et al: Clinicopathologic analysis of HER-2/neu immunoexpression among various histologic subtypes and grades of osteosarcoma. Mod Pathol 2001;14:1277.
70. Huvos AG, Rosen G, Bretsky SS, et al: Telangiectatic osteogenic sarcoma: A clinicopathologic study of 124 patients. Cancer 1982;49:1679.
71. Mervak TR, Unni KK, Pritchard DJ, et al: Telangiectatic osteosarcoma. Clin Orthop 1991;270:135.
72. Nakajima H, Sim FH, Bond JR, et al: Small cell osteosarcoma of bone: Review of 72 cases. Cancer 1997;79:2095.
73. Stevenson AJ, Chatten J, Bertoni F, et al: CD99(p30/32 MIC2) neuroectodermal/Ewing's sarcoma antigen as an immunohistochemical marker: Review of more than 600 tumors and the literature experience. Appl Immunohistochem 1994;2:231.
74. Kurt A-M, Unni KK, McLeod RA, et al: Low-grade intraosseous osteosarcoma. Cancer 1990;65:1418.
75. Okada K, Frassica FJ, Sim FH, et al: Parosteal osteosarcoma: A clinicopathologic study. J Bone Joint Surg Am 1994;76:366.
76. Sheth DS, Yasko AW, Raymond AK, et al: Conventional and dedifferentiated parosteal osteosarcoma: Diagnosis, treatment, and outcome. Cancer 1996;78:2136.
77. Unni KK, Dahlin DC, Beabout JW: Periosteal osteosarcoma. Cancer 1976;37:2476.
78. Okada K, Unni KK, Swee RG, et al: High grade surface osteosarcoma: A clinicopathologic study of 46 cases. Cancer 1999;85:1044.
79. Clark JL, Unni KK, Dahlin DC, et al: Osteosarcoma of the jaw. Cancer 1983;51:2311.
80. Huvos AG, Butler A, Bretsky SS: Osteogenic sarcoma associated with Paget's disease of bone: A clinicopathologic study of 65 patients. Cancer 1983;52:1489.
81. Mark RJ, Poen J, Tran LM, et al: Postirradiation sarcomas: A single-institution study and review of the literature. Cancer 1994;73:2653.
82. Jacobs B, Huvos AG: Malignant fibrous histiocytoma and osteosarcoma in association with bone infarcts: Report of four cases, two in caisson workers. J Bone Joint Surg Am 1974;56:932.
83. Taconis WK: Osteosarcoma in fibrous dysplasia. Skeletal Radiol 1988;17:163.
84. Keel SB, Jaffe KA, Nielsen GP, et al: Orthopaedic implant-related sarcoma: A study of twelve cases. Mod Pathol 2001;14:969.
85. Jensen ML, Schumacher B, Jensen OM, et al: Extraskeletal osteosarcomas: A clinicopathologic study of 25 cases. Am J Surg Pathol 1998;22:588.
86. Chung EB, Enzinger FM: Extraskeletal osteosarcoma. Cancer 1987;60:1132.
87. Lee JSY, Fetsch JF, Wasdahl DA, et al: A review of 40 patients with extraskeletal osteosarcoma. Cancer 1995;76:2253.
88. Raymond AK, Ayala AG, Patel S, et al: Osteosarcoma (OS): Chemotherapy-induced tumor necrosis: Threshold tumor necrosis...prognostic factor in dynamic evolution (abstract). Mod Pathol 1997;10:13A.
89. Wold LE: Practical approach to processing osteosarcomas in the surgical pathology laboratory. Pediatr Dev Pathol 1998;1:449.

Hamartoma of the Chest Wall

90. McLeod RA, Dahlin DC: Hamartoma (mesenchymoma) of the chest wall in infancy. Radiology 1979;131:657.

CHAPTER 13

Chondroid Tumors of Bone and Soft Tissue

Chondroid tumors of bone and soft tissue include lesions that definitionally produce, at least focally, chondroid and/or hyaline cartilage. Table 13.1 summarizes the lesions included in this categorization. Mesenchymal chondrosarcoma is discussed with other small round cell tumors (see Chapter 3), and dedifferentiated chondrosarcoma is discussed with pleomorphic sarcomas (see Chapter 11). Because extraskeletal myxoid chondrosarcoma only rarely has definite hyaline cartilage differentiation, it is not included with these tumors. Table 13.2 lists the tumors that occasionally exhibit chondroid metaplasia but are not considered true cartilaginous neoplasms.

Nowhere is the correlation of pathologic with clinical and radiographic findings more necessary than in the differentiation of enchondroma from chondrosarcoma; this is not to say that specific morphologic findings do not exist for these entities. Histologic features supporting a diagnosis of chondrosarcoma include enlarged chondrocytes with atypical nuclei, hypercellularity, myxoid changes, and permeation (and entrapment) of medullary bone. In most cases of chondrosarcoma, the degree of cellularity is not appreciably different, however, from that observed with enchondroma. The presence of permeation and bone entrapment often is not obvious in small biopsy or curettage specimens. Binucleated chondrocytes may be observed in enchondroma and chondrosarcoma. Complicating matters further, the degree of acceptable cellularity in enchondroma depends, at least in part, on anatomic site (origin). Enchondromas of the phalanges and soft tissue chondromas of the distal extremities are often significantly hypercellular, with the latter frequently displaying bizarre and atypical chondrocytes. Similar findings within the femoral medullary canal would constitute a diagnosis of chondrosarcoma. Likewise, periosteal chondromas tend to be more cellular than their classic intramedullary counterparts. All of these entities are discussed separately in greater detail.

TABLE 13.1 Chondroid/Cartilage Lesions of Bone and Soft Tissue

Bone Origin	Soft Tissue Origin
Enchondroma	Chondroma
Conventional chondrosarcoma	Synovial chondromatosis
Osteochondroma	
Chondrosarcoma	
Chondromyxoid fibroma	
Clear cell chondrosarcoma	
Mesenchymal chondrosarcoma	
Dedifferentiated chondrosarcoma	

Osteochondroma

Osteochondroma is a benign bony projection arising from the surface of the bone and remaining in continuity with the bone of origin. It may occur as a solitary process, or it may be familial and associated with multiple osteochondromas (osteochondromatosis or hereditary multiple exostoses).

TABLE 13.2 Bone and Soft Tissue Tumors Frequently Containing Chondroid Metaplasia

Myositis ossificans
Mixed tumor/myoepithelioma
Calcifying aponeurotic fibroma
Osteosarcoma

Clinical Features

Most cases of osteochondroma present within the first 2 decades of life. Mayo Clinic data indicate that males are affected more often than females.[1] In decreasing order of frequency, the common anatomic locations include the metaphyseal regions of the distal femur, proximal humerus, and proximal tibia.[1] Involvement of the digits is extraordinarily rare. Many lesions are probably asymptomatic. Patients seeking medical attention usually report symptoms related to the size and anatomic location of the osteochondroma. Consequently, clinical symptoms may include the presence of a mass, localized pain resulting from nerve impingement, or limitation of movement.

Although sometimes present at birth, patients with osteochondromatosis usually come to clinical attention early in the first decade of life. Because of the multiple osteochondromas, affected individuals may develop growth retardation, joint deformities, or premature osteoarthrosis.[2] Hereditary osteochondromatosis is transmitted among family members as an autosomal dominant trait.

The risk of malignant transformation is reportedly 1% to 2% for patients with a solitary osteochondroma and 5% to 25% for patients with osteochondromatosis.[3] These estimates may be artificially high, however, because most of the reports are from tertiary care centers and reflect a higher proportion of referral patients. Not all osteochondromas require surgical intervention, and some likely remain undiscovered. Patients with secondary chondrosarcoma are usually between 20 and 40 years old, significantly younger than patients with de novo forms.

Radiographically, osteochondromas present as pedunculated or sessile bony projections in continuity with the underlying bone of origin (Fig. 13.1). The cartilage cap often appears lobulated and variably calcified. The presence of a thickened cartilage cap with extensive calcifications alternating with radiolucent areas should raise the possibility of chondrosarcomatous change (Fig. 13.2). Destruction of the underlying bone indicates a high-grade malignancy. Computed tomography and magnetic resonance imaging may be useful for estimating the cartilage cap thickness but are generally not precise for cartilage caps less than 2.5 cm in thickness.[4] The radiographic features of osteochondromatosis are similar, but additional remodeling defects of bone also may be seen (Fig. 13.3).

Pathologic Findings

Histology

In most cases, osteochondromas exhibit normal-appearing medullary bone and marrow fat/elements surrounded, peripherally, by a variably thickened cartilaginous cap (usually <1 cm in thickness). Within the cartilaginous cap, individual chondrocytes may be solitary or clustered; where adjacent to the medullary bone, chondrocytes often are arranged in rows, undergoing enchondral ossification, resembling the epiphyseal growth plate (Fig. 13.4).

Malignant transformation generally takes the form of a low-grade chondrosarcoma. Rare examples of dedifferentiated chondrosarcoma have been described.[5] A cartilage cap exceeding 2 cm in thickness almost always indicates chondrosarcomatous transformation (Fig. 13.5). Additional worrisome features include nodules of invasive cartilage within adjacent soft tissues separate from the main tumor, myxoid stromal changes, hypercellularity, mitotic activity, and chondrocyte atypia (Fig. 13.6). Table 13.3 summarizes the clinical, radiographic, and pathologic features that suggest

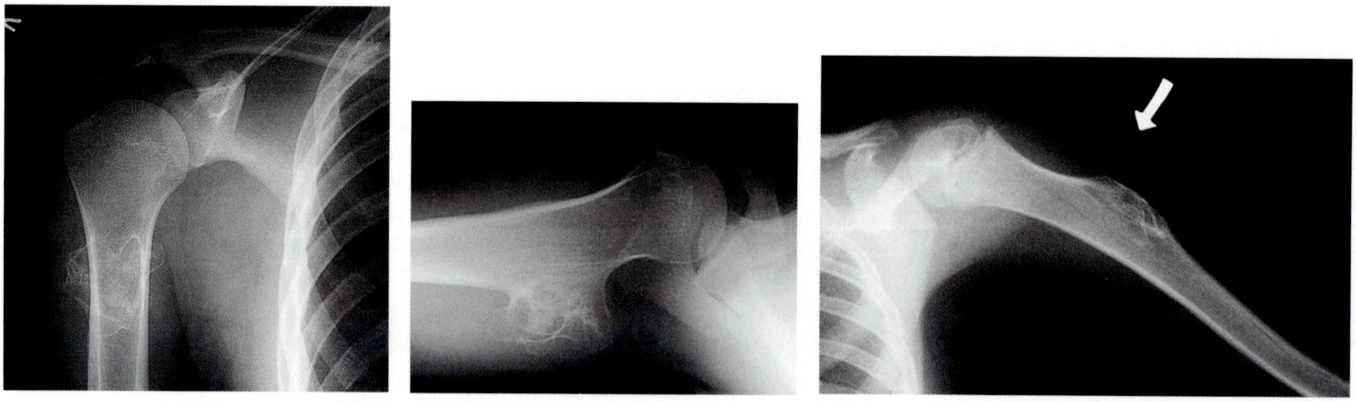

A B C

FIGURE 13.1 Osteochondroma. Anteroposterior **(A)** and axillary **(B)** views of the proximal humerus show a pedunculated osseous excrescence arising from the humerus and projecting posteriorly. The cortex of the humerus extends smoothly onto the surface of the excrescence, and the trabeculae of the humerus extend out into the lesion. In another patient, a sessile osteochondroma projects from the lateral surface of the humerus at the attachment of the deltoid muscle (**C**, *arrow*).

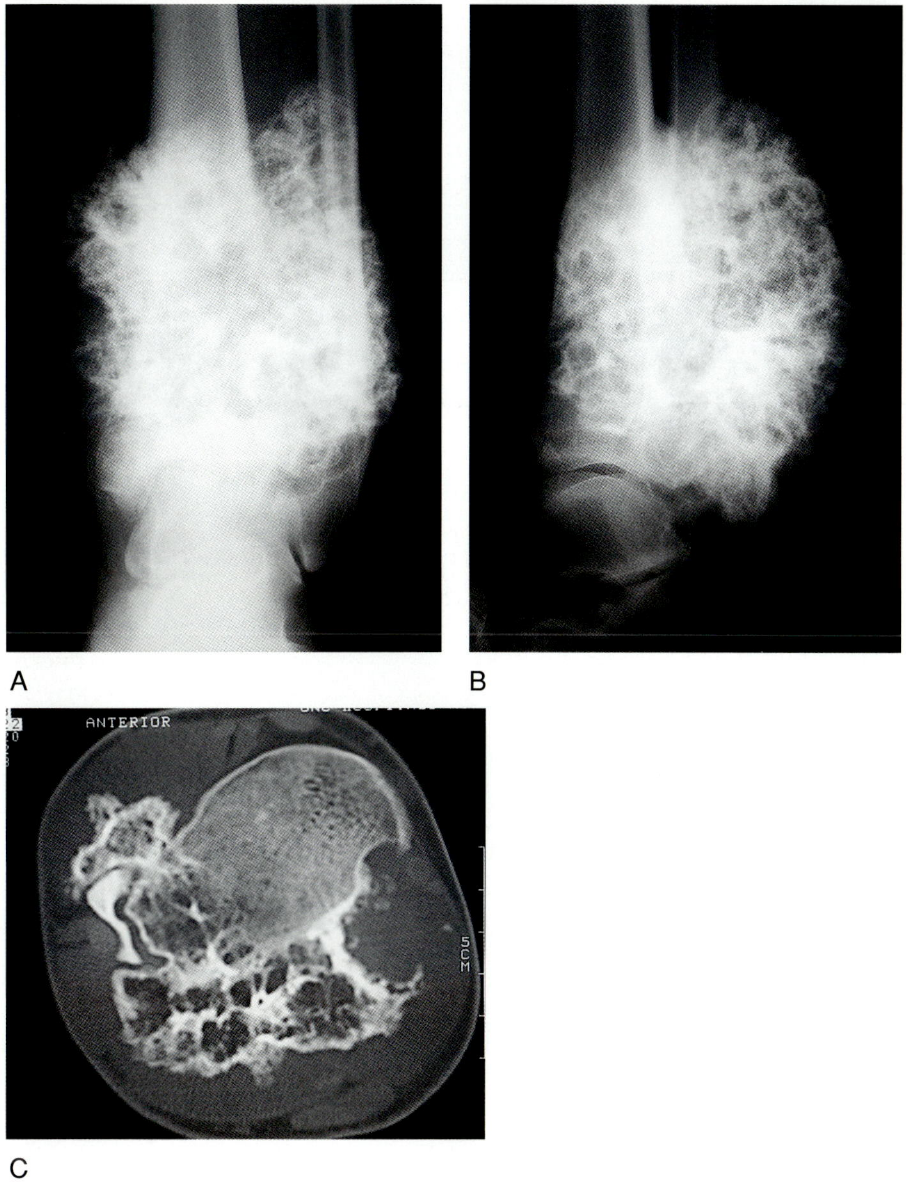

FIGURE 13.2 Malignant degeneration of osteochondroma. Anteroposterior **(A)** and lateral **(B)** projections of the distal tibia show a large, verrucous, densely calcified lesion overlying the distal tibia and fibula. An axial computed tomographic scan of the distal tibia **(C)** shows the large, exophytic lesion arising from the distal tibia, extending laterally and enveloping the distal fibula. Cortical and medullary bone destruction along the posteromedial surface of the tibia indicates chondrosarcomatous degeneration of the osteochondroma.

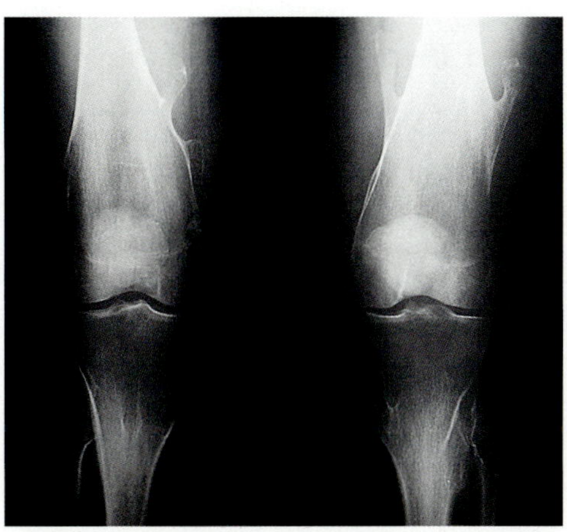

FIGURE 13.3 Osteochondromatosis. An anteroposterior radiograph of the knees reveals bilateral exostoses arising from the distal femora and tibiae.

chondrosarcomatous transformation. It is inevitable that some osteochondromas may show borderline features with cartilaginous caps measuring between 1 and 2 cm in thickness. In these cases, it is appropriate to render the diagnosis of osteochondroma with "atypical" or "borderline" features and to recommend complete excision and close clinical follow-up.

Ancillary Studies

Cytogenetic analysis has revealed structural aberrations involving 8q22-24 (*EXT1* gene) in 10 (of 30) sporadic osteochondromas and 1 (of 13) hereditary osteochondromatosis case.[6,7]

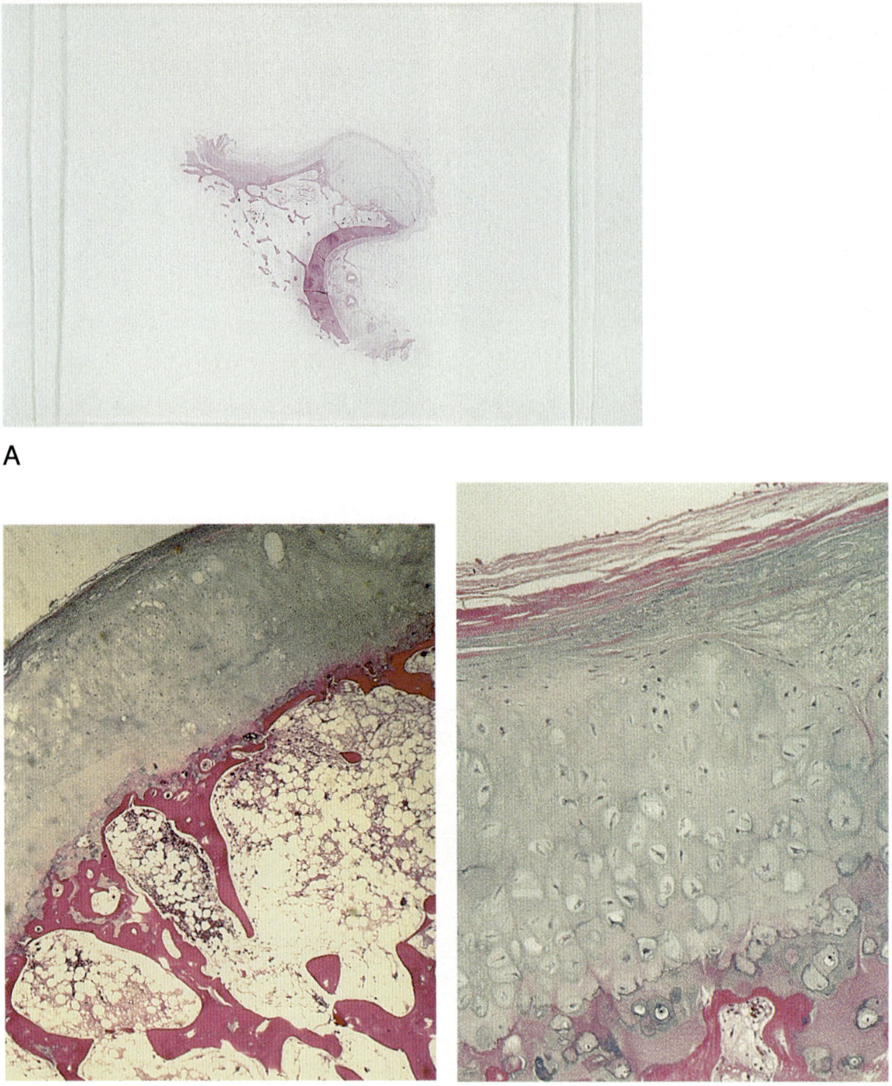

A

B

C

FIGURE 13.4 Osteochondroma with a typical pedunculated appearance, capped by a layer of hyaline cartilage and surrounding bone, fat, and marrow elements contiguous with the bone of origin **(A)**. The hyaline cartilage cap usually appears bland and hypocellular. Individual chondrocytes lack significant nuclear atypia and may show a vague single-file arrangement before enchondral ossification **(B** and **C)**. **(A,** H&E; **B,** low power, H&E; **C,** high power, H&E.)

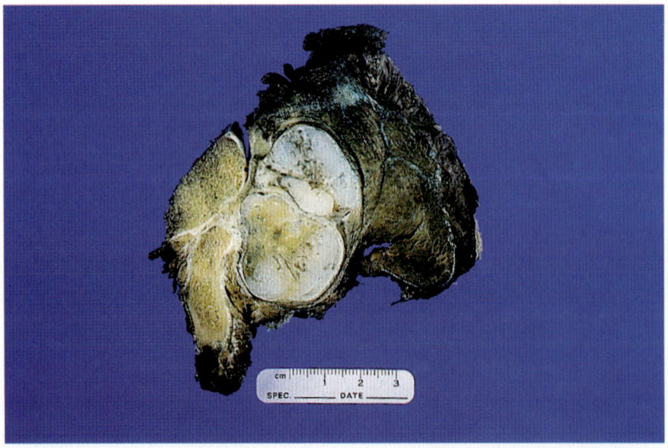

FIGURE 13.5 Chondrosarcoma arising in osteochondroma. Note the irregular and lobulated cartilage cap, which exceeds 2 cm in thickness.

Prognosis and Therapy

Surgical resection of osteochondromas is recommended for symptomatic cases. Local recurrence may occur with less than complete excision but tends to be rare. For chondrosarcomas arising in osteochondromas, complete resection is usually curative. Distant metastasis is rare; most patients die as a result of complications of local recurrence.[3]

Enchondroma

Enchondroma is a benign hyaline cartilage neoplasm arising within the medullary canal of a bone. Most are solitary, but

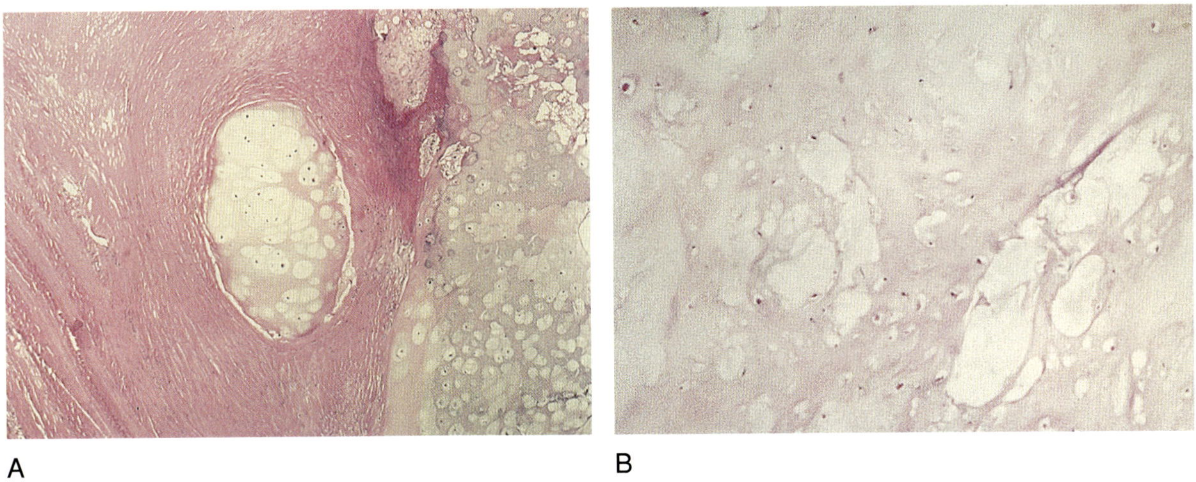

FIGURE 13.6 Chondrosarcoma arising in osteochondroma is usually low grade. Helpful diagnostic features include a cartilage cap greater than 2 cm in thickness, nodules of cartilage within soft tissues clearly separate from the main tumor mass **(A)**, and myxoid changes **(B)**. (**A** and **B**, H&E.)

multiple bone involvement (enchondromatosis) occurs rarely.

Clinical Features

Enchondromas may arise at any age; however, most arise in individuals between the second and fourth decades of life. Males and females are affected roughly equally. The small tubular bones of the hands and feet are the most common anatomic location followed by the proximal humerus and distal femur. Enchondroma is the most common bone tumor of the hand.[8] Involvement of the pelvis, scapula, and vertebral spine are extraordinarily rare. For practical purposes, cartilaginous tumors of the sternum represent chondrosarcomas. When enchondroma arises within the small tubular bones of the hands and feet, most patients complain of soft tissue swelling, sometimes associated with pain and pathologic fracture. Enchondromas within the long bones are usually asymptomatic, incidental findings.[9]

TABLE 13.3 Clinical, Radiographic, and Pathologic Features Suggestive of Chondrosarcomatous Change in Osteochondroma

Clinical and Radiographic Features
Presence of localized pain
Recent growth in an adult patient
Irregularly thickened cartilage cap with areas of lucency
Pathologic Features
Cartilage cap >2 cm
Nodules of invasive cartilage within adjacent soft tissues separate from the main tumor
Myxoid stromal changes
Necrosis
Loss of single file arrangement at zone of enchondral ossification
Hypercellularity and atypia*

* Least sensitive; most chondrosarcomas with hypercellularity and atypia are high grade and less frequently seen in osteochondromas.

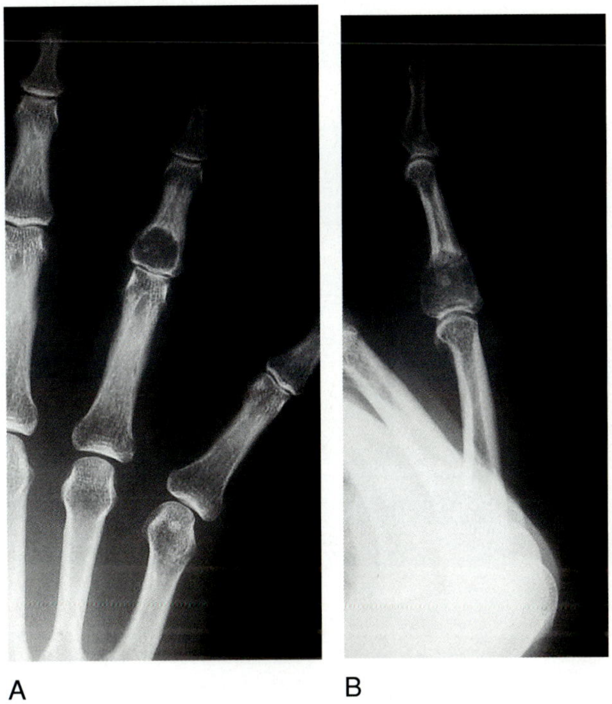

FIGURE 13.7 Enchondroma. Posteroanterior **(A)** and lateral **(B)** projections of the ring finger show a lytic lesion in the middle phalanx. A single rounded calcification within the lesion indicates chondroid calcification. A pathologic fracture has developed through the distal end of the lesion.

Radiographically, enchondromas are generally well-marginated, metaphyseal/diaphyseal lesions with varying amounts of mineralization, arranged in punctate or ring and arc-type patterns. Within the small tubular bones, enchondromas are often expansile and may show cortical erosion and thinning (Fig. 13.7). Conversely, within the

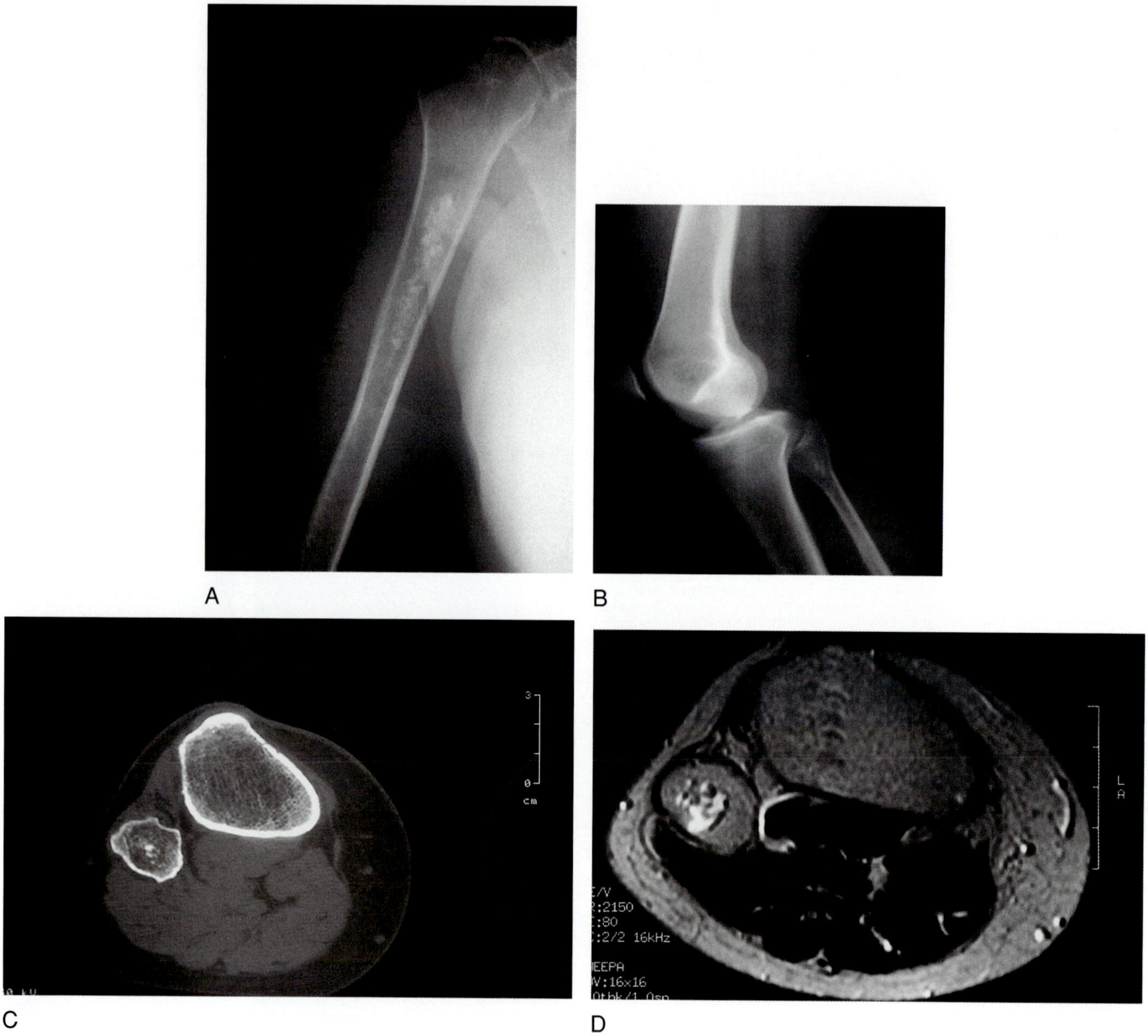

FIGURE 13.8 Enchondroma. An anteroposterior radiograph **(A)** of the proximal humerus reveals a calcified lesion in the proximal humerus. The flocculent, lobulated calcifications are typical of those associated with a chondroid lesion. The lack of bone destruction and periosteal new bone formation indicates a nonaggressive lesion. In another patient, a lateral radiograph of the knee **(B)** shows a faintly calcified lesion in the proximal fibula. An axial computed tomographic scan **(C)** and magnetic resonance image **(D)** of the fibula show the lesion in the proximal fibula without bone destruction or soft tissue extension.

long bones, enchondromas show only minimal bone expansion and virtually no endosteal erosion (Fig. 13.8). Soft tissue extension indicates chondrosarcoma, regardless of origin.

Pathologic Findings

Histology

Morphologically, enchondroma consists of sharply marginated lobules of mature, hypocellular hyaline cartilage that appear at least partially surrounded by shells of lamellar bone.[10] Individual chondrocytes are usually solitary, uniformly distributed or arranged in small clusters, and show minimal variation in size and shape from one cell to the next. The cells have small, round-to-ovoid nuclei and granular, often vacuolated cytoplasm (Fig. 13.9). Occasional binucleated cells may be observed. Mitotic figures are virtually never seen. Myxoid change within the hyaline cartilage matrix may be focally present but should never be a prominent feature of enchondroma.[9] The clinical, radiographic, and histologic features of enchondroma versus chondrosarcoma are compared in Table 13.4.

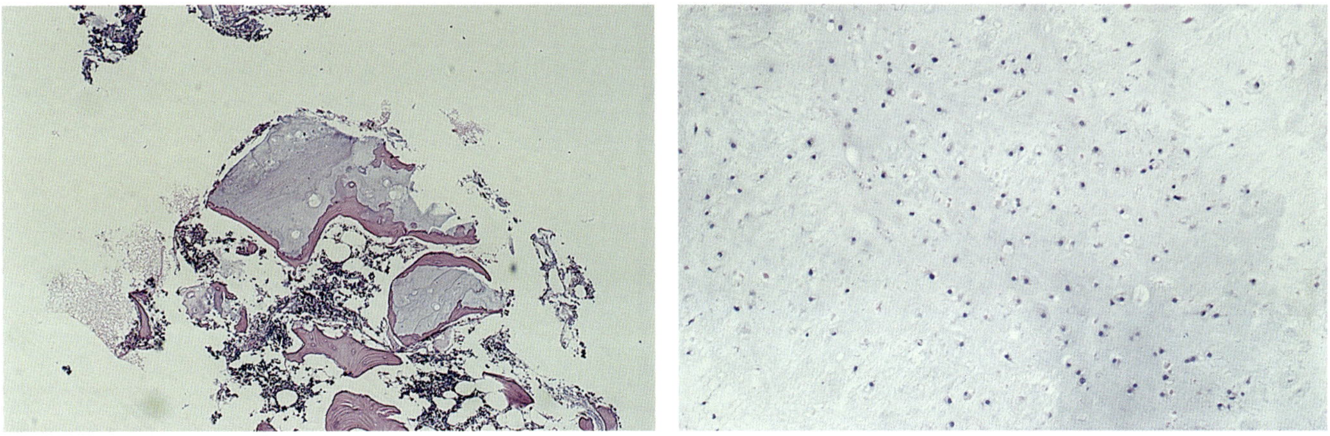

A B

FIGURE 13.9 Enchondroma in a curettage specimen. Lobules of bland-appearing hyaline cartilage are surrounded at least partially by lamellar bone shells **(A)**. At high power, individual chondrocytes are bland and mostly uniform with small nuclei **(B)**. (**A** and **B**, H&E.)

The degree of acceptable cellularity and chondrocyte atypia within enchondromas arising from the small tubular bones of the hands and feet is significantly higher than that observed in the extremity long bones (Fig. 13.10). Consequently, hypercellularity is not a reliable feature for distinguishing digital enchondroma from digital chondrosarcoma. Features favoring a diagnosis of chondrosarcoma of the digits are summarized in Table 13.5. Extension into soft tissues or permeation of medullary bone is diagnostic of chondrosarcoma (Fig. 13.11).[11]

Fine Needle Aspiration Biopsy

Because the cortex surrounding enchondromas is generally intact, sampling by conventional fine needle aspiration biopsy (FNAB) is usually not possible. On Diff-Quik staining, reported acceptable examples (usually involving intermediate-bore cutting needles with fluoroscopic guidance) of enchondroma show lobules of matrix and scattered small and uniform-appearing chondrocytes within distinct lacunae. Binucleated cells and mitotic figures are generally absent.[12] Correlation with radiographic findings is essential to exclude low-grade chondrosarcoma. We do not analyze suspected cases of enchondroma by FNAB.

Ancillary Studies

Immunohistochemistry is not helpful in the differential diagnosis of enchondroma. Cytogenetic analysis has revealed mostly diploid tumors with occasional structural anomalies, most commonly involving chromosome 6 and 12.[13,14]

TABLE 13.4 Clinical, Radiographic, and Pathologic Characteristics of Enchondroma versus Chondrosarcoma

	Enchondroma	Chondrosarcoma
Peak Age (yr)	10-30	40-60
Gender	Males = females	Males > females
Symptoms	Usually incidental finding; localized pain rare	Localized pain universally present; rarely soft tissue swelling
Involved Bones (Decreasing Order of Frequency)	Tubular bones of the hands and feet, proximal humerus	Pelvis, extremity long bones, especially proximal femur
Radiographic Features	Metaphyseal in long bones, lytic, sharply marginated, punctate calcifications	Metaphyseal or diaphyseal, lytic, cortical (endosteal) erosion or thickening; variable calcifications; soft tissue extension
Pathologic Features	Mature, hypocellular, cartilage-forming multiple nodules separated by normal marrow; lamellar bony shells; minimal atypia*	Mature, variably cellular confluent sheets of hyaline cartilage; permeation of medullary bone; myxoid stromal changes; minimal-to-marked atypia (depending on histologic grade)

* Enchondromas of the digits may exhibit hypercellularity and significant atypia.

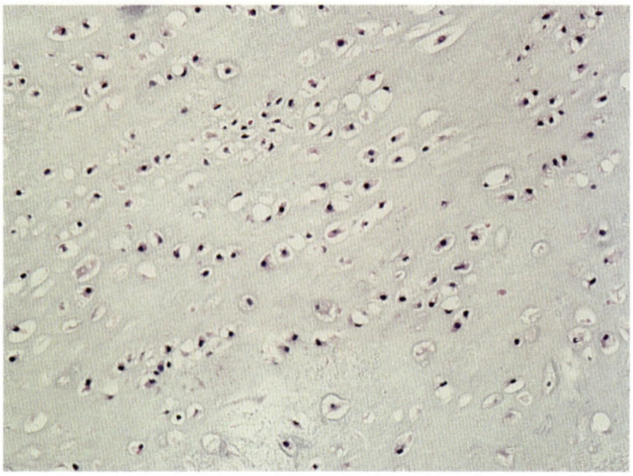

A

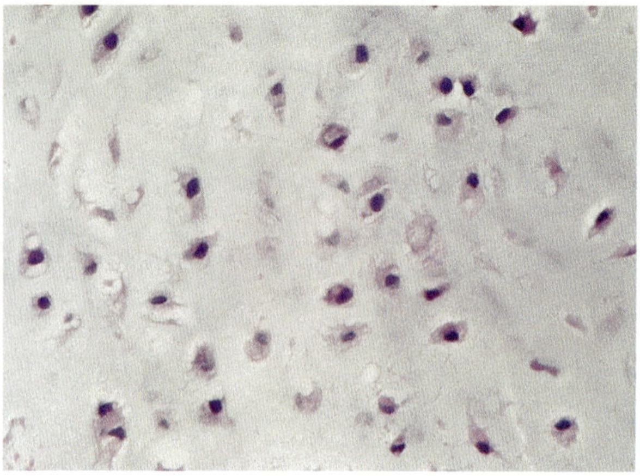

B

FIGURE 13.10 Enchondromas of the digits often show greater cellularity and atypia than their long bone counterparts **(A** and **B)**. (**A,** low power, H&E; **B,** high power, H&E.)

Prognosis and Therapy

Most enchondromas are cured by simple curettage. Local recurrences are rare.

Enchondromatosis

Enchondromatosis (Ollier's disease) is a developmental disorder, possibly a failure of normal enchondral ossification, characterized by the presence of multiple cartilaginous lesions (enchondromas), preferentially affecting the small tubular bones of the hands and feet. Rarely, it may be associated with soft tissue and visceral hemangiomas (Maffucci's syndrome). Most patients develop clinical manifestations at a younger age than those seen with the solitary form of the disease. Most patients present before age 20. Males and females are affected equally. The severity of the disease varies among individual patients, ranging from involvement of a single extremity to multifocal, widespread disease with severe osseous deformities. Regardless of the extent of disease, the small tubular bones of the hand most commonly are affected, followed by the feet and extremity long bones. In Maffucci's syndrome, the hemangiomas are multiple and typically located in the soft tissues of the distal extremities. In 30% of patients, the enchondromas and hemangiomas localize exclusively to the same extremity.[15] Most examples of enchondromatosis are sporadic (nonhereditary), but rare examples appear familial with an autosomal dominant inheritance pattern.[16] The clinical features of enchondromatosis vary depending on the extent of the disease. Severe cases are associated with significant skeletal abnormalities, secondary to pathologic fractures and bowing deformities. Radiographically, lesions of enchondromatosis resemble lesions observed with solitary enchondroma; however, the tumors may be intramedullary, subperiosteal, or intracortical (Fig. 13.12). Hemangiomas frequently contain radiographically visible, calcified phleboliths (Fig. 13.13).

Compared with solitary enchondroma, enchondromatosis shows significantly greater cellularity and cytologic atypia (Fig. 13.14). The hemangiomas of Maffucci's syndrome may represent capillary, cavernous, or spindle cell subtypes.[15] The diagnosis of chondrosarcomatous transformation is heralded by the presence of significant myxoid changes, permeation of medullary bone, and/or cortical destruction with soft tissue extension (Fig. 13.15).

TABLE 13.5 Clinical, Radiographic, and Pathologic Features Characteristic of Chondrosarcoma of the Digits

Clinical and Radiographic Features
Cortical destruction with soft tissue extension
Pathologic Features
Permeation of pre-existing bone
Soft tissue extension
Extensive myxoid stromal changes

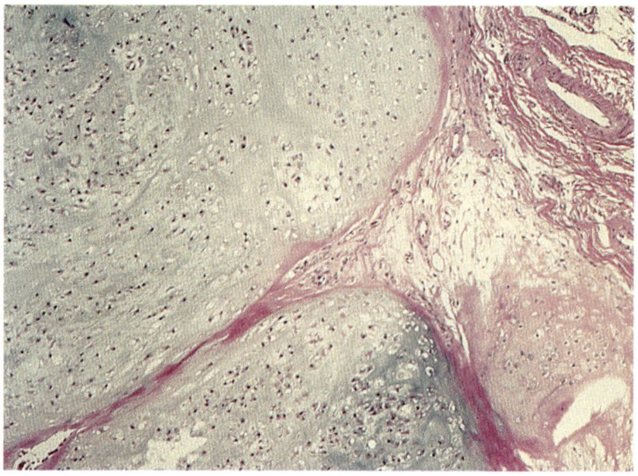

FIGURE 13.11 Chondrosarcoma of the digits with nodules of cartilage extending through the bone and into adjacent soft tissues. (H&E.)

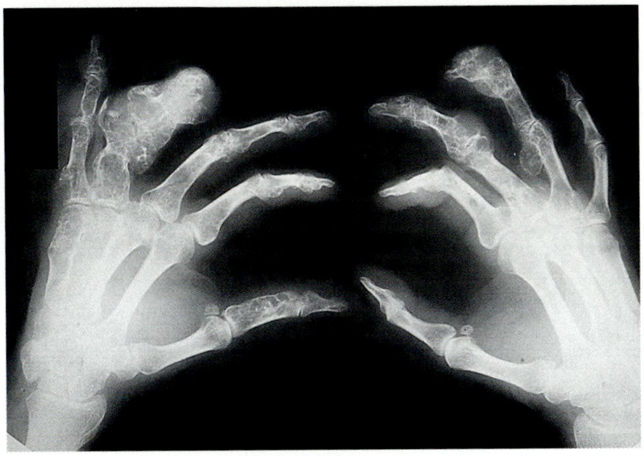

FIGURE 13.12 Enchondromatosis (Ollier's disease). An oblique view of the hands shows multiple, intraosseous expansile lesions. There is marked deformity of multiple phalanges.

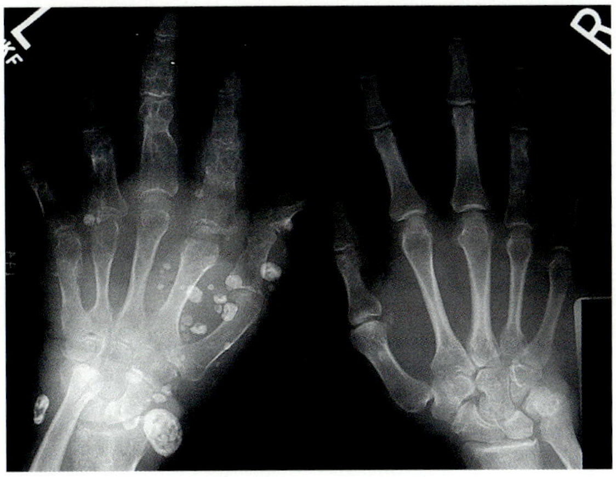

FIGURE 13.13 Maffucci's syndrome. A posteroanterior radiograph of the hands shows multiple phalangeal deformities typical for enchondromas. There are rounded soft tissue calcifications bilaterally, however, that are typical for phleboliths (indicate soft tissue hemangiomas).

As expected, the prognosis of enchondromatosis depends on the extent and severity of the underlying disease. It is estimated that malignant transformation may occur in 15% to 30% of cases, usually in the form of a low-grade chondrosarcoma.[17,18] The prognosis of most patients with Ollier's disease with chondrosarcomatous transformation is good.[17] Conversely, when chondrosarcoma develops in patients with Maffucci's syndrome, the prognosis generally is considered poor.[18] Dedifferentiated chondrosarcoma is a rare complication and almost always fatal.

Chondrosarcoma

Chondrosarcoma is a malignant neoplasm of hyaline cartilage. It may arise as a primary condition (conventional or classic chondrosarcoma) or be secondary to a precursor lesion (e.g., enchondroma or osteochondroma).

Clinical Features

Chondrosarcoma is the third most common primary malignancy of bone. Most patients are between 40 and 60 years old at clinical presentation. There appears to be slight male predominance. The pelvis is the most common anatomic site, followed by the proximal long bones of the extremities, especially the femur and humerus. In contrast to enchondroma, the small tubular bones of the hands and feet rarely are involved.[11,19] Patients with chondrosarcoma usually complain of localized pain in the affected region. Some patients report soft tissue swelling. Clinical symptoms are usually of long duration. Skeletal chondrosarcomas rarely are observed in children (usually 10 to 16 years old). The most common anatomic sites are the humerus and femur. Most are low-grade lesions.[20]

Radiographically, most chondrosarcomas appear variably calcified with poor margination, although purely lytic

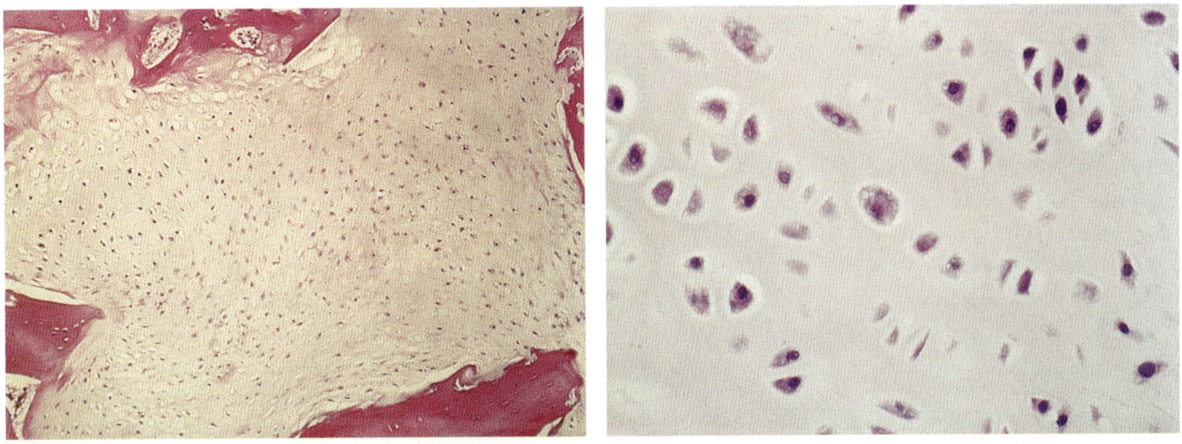

A B

FIGURE 13.14 Enchondromatosis is characterized by cellular hyaline cartilage nodules that may be intramedullary, intracortical, or subperiosteal **(A)**. Closer inspection often reveals significant chondrocyte atypia that, outside of the clinical context, could result in a misdiagnosis of chondrosarcoma **(B)**. **(A,** low power, H&E; and **B,** high power, H&E.)

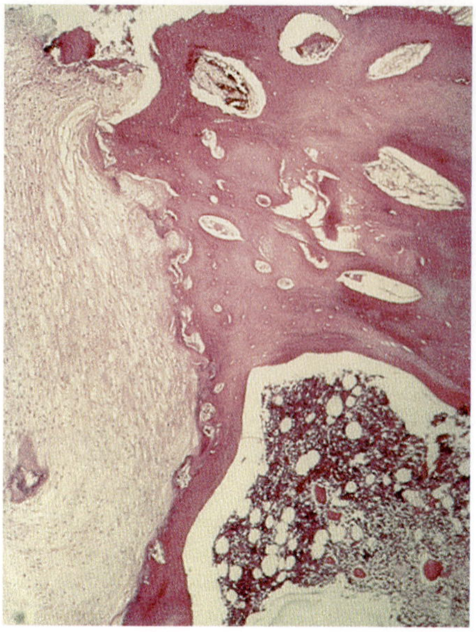

FIGURE 13.15 Chondrosarcoma arising in a patient with enchondromatosis. The cartilage extends through the cortex and into adjacent soft tissues. Correlation with clinical and radiographic features is essential to establish this diagnosis. (H&E.)

examples occasionally occur. Within the long bones, chondrosarcomas arise within the metaphysis or diaphysis, frequently showing areas of bone expansion, cortical thickening, or cortical endosteal erosion (Figs. 13.16 and 13.17). The most reliable radiographic features of malignancy are cortical erosion and poor margination.[19] Varying amounts of punctate and ring-like calcified densities are present in most tumors. Periosteal reaction is observed in only about 20% of patients; however, soft tissue extension is present in 50% of cases.[19]

Pathologic Findings

Histology

Conventional chondrosarcoma is a pure hyaline cartilage tumor. The morphologic features depend in part on the histologic grade of the tumor. Chondrosarcomas are graded according to a three-tiered system, based predominantly on cellularity (which is inversely related to quantity of matrix) and to a lesser extent on nuclear features.[21] In an evaluation of 338 patients with chondrosarcoma of the pelvic girdles and long bones of the extremities, Bjornsson and colleagues[19] reported that most cases (61%) were grade 1 lesions; approximately 36% of the tumors were grade 2, and only 3% were grade 3 chondrosarcomas.

Grade 1 chondrosarcomas are one of the most challenging diagnoses in bone pathology. The tumors generally are composed of confluent sheets of well-developed hyaline cartilage with mild-to-moderate cellularity; overlapping degrees of cellularity are observed in enchondroma.[10] Individual chondrocytes may be seen solitarily and in small clusters but generally show only minimal atypia with slightly enlarged, hyperchromatic nuclei. Binucleated chondrocytes may be observed, but these cells also may be seen in enchondroma. The clinical, radiographic, and pathologic features of enchondroma versus chondrosarcoma are compared in Table 13.4. Perhaps the most helpful diagnostic feature for chondrosarcoma is the presence of permeation of cortical or medullary bone (Fig. 13.18).[10,11] This permeation may be difficult to establish in curettage specimens but is found easily in resections. Permeation is defined as the presence of lobules of hyaline cartilage that infiltrate and replace portions of medullary or cortical bone, entrapping residual lamellar bone within the cartilaginous matrix. Frequently, enchondromas may exhibit nodules of hyaline cartilage clearly separated from the main tumor mass; however, these nodules are virtually always at least partially encircled by a shell of lamellar bone, without such bone entrapped in its matrix.[10] The presence of myxoid change tends to be more prominent in chondrosarcoma than in enchondroma (Fig. 13.19). Tumor necrosis, high cellularity, and mitotic activity are features usually seen in higher grade lesions and are generally not helpful in the differential diagnosis of grade 1 chondrosarcoma and enchondroma. Permeation of tumor into adjacent soft tissues generally is required to establish a diagnosis of grade 1 chondrosarcoma of the digits. It is essential that clinical and radiographic correlation be done. Table 13.5 summarizes the clinical and pathologic features of chondrosarcoma of the digits.

Within the long bones and limb girdles, grade 2 chondrosarcomas are recognized easily as malignant. The tumors are moderately cellular and tend to show greater nuclear atypia and pleomorphism. Nevertheless, the hyaline cartilage matrix remains well differentiated and easily recognizable (Fig. 13.20). Rarest of all are grade 3 chondrosarcomas. These tumors are highly cellular with a tendency toward spindling of the tumor cells. The hyaline cartilage differentiation tends to be less well developed than seen in the lower grade forms (Fig. 13.21). Mitotic figures are detected easily.[19]

Fine Needle Aspiration Biopsy

Sampling by FNAB is possible only when sufficient cortical thinning is present. Cytologic smears of low-grade chondrosarcomas typically show abundant amounts of mostly hypocellular matrix material, accompanied by scattered, mostly uniform chondrocytes, often showing little or no nuclear atypia. Most tumor cells appear uninucleated and larger than cells seen in enchondroma and contain an oval-to-round, slightly hyperchromatic nucleus (Fig. 13.22).[12] Binucleated forms rarely are observed. Nucleoli range from small to inconspicuous. Myxoid change or degeneration is a helpful diagnostic feature in the cytologic smears of

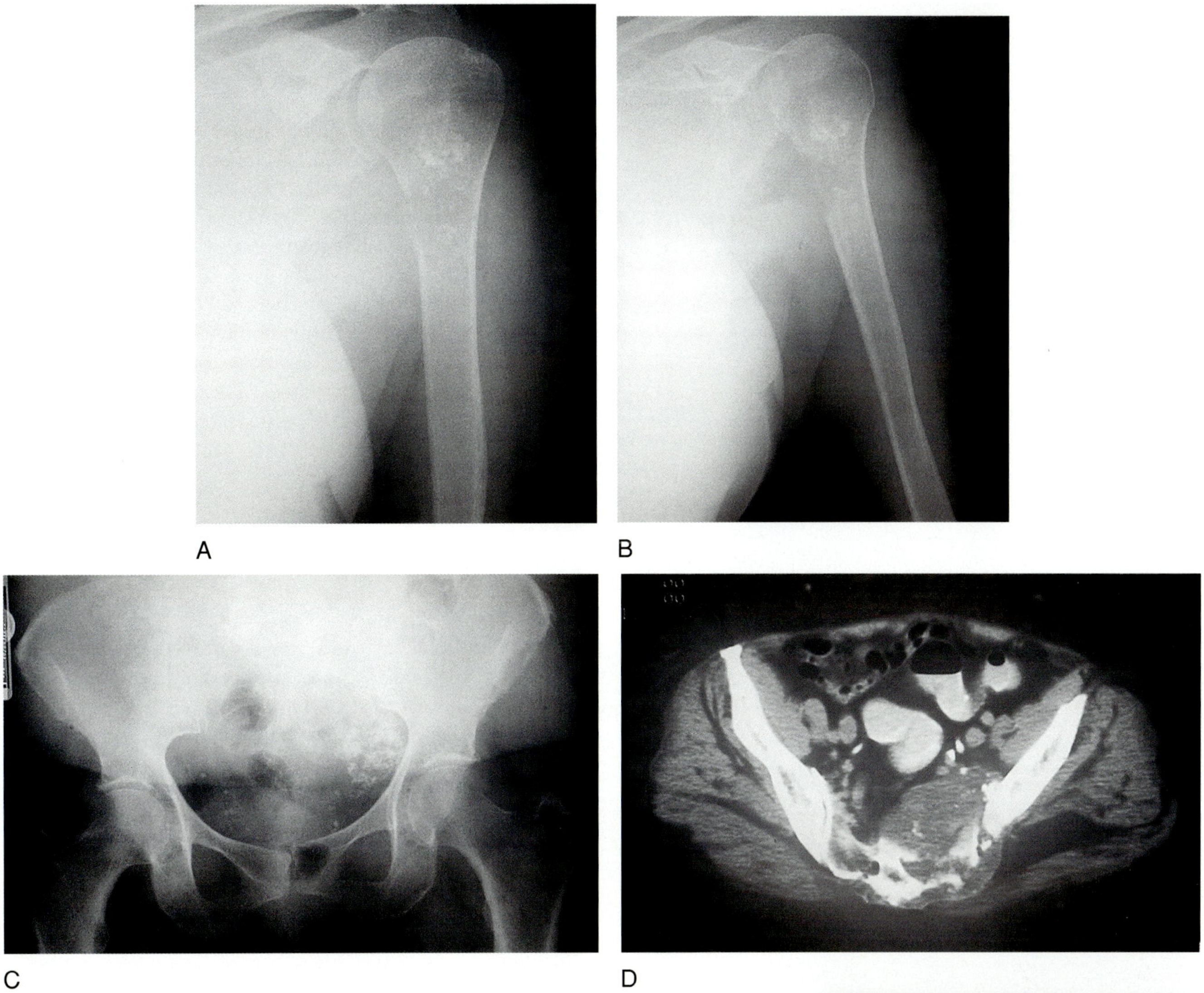

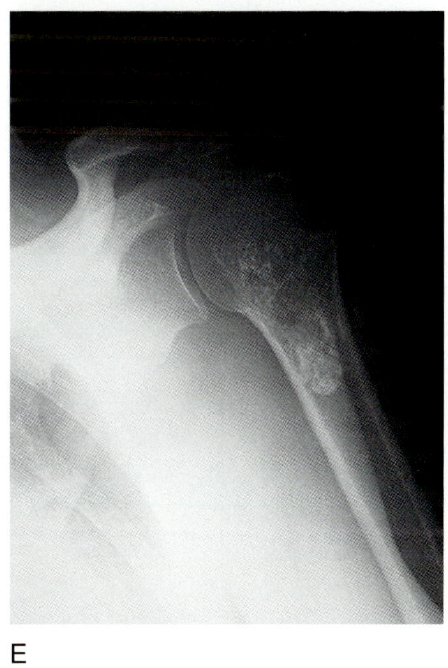

FIGURE 13.16 Chondrosarcoma. Anteroposterior **(A)** and oblique **(B)** views of the proximal humerus reveal a destructive lesion in the proximal humerus. Intraosseous chondroid calcifications are associated with periosteal new bone production and cortical bone destruction medially, indicating an aggressive lesion. In another patient, an anteroposterior view of the pelvis **(C)** shows an irregular, calcified lesion in the left hemipelvis. Although reminiscent of the calcification associated with a degenerating uterine leiomyoma, the eccentric position of the lesion should suggest another diagnosis. An axial computed tomographic scan of the pelvis **(D)** shows the destructive lesion centered at the sacrum and extending anteriorly and posteriorly and containing soft tissue calcifications. An oblique radiograph of the shoulder in another patient **(E)** reveals chondroid calcifications in the proximal humerus. There is no obvious bone destruction or periosteal new bone production associated with this lesion, a low-grade chondrosarcoma. The appearances of this lesion are indistinguishable from those of an enchondroma.

chondrosarcoma. It appears as a metachromatic granular background film or precipitant (Fig. 13.23). Nevertheless, clinical and radiographic correlation is important in establishing a diagnosis. Higher grade (grade 2 or 3) examples of chondrosarcoma are generally more cellular, exhibit more nuclear pleomorphism and atypia, and are recognized much more easily as malignant (Fig. 13.24). The main differential diagnosis in the latter includes chondroblastic osteosarcoma. Layfield and coworkers[22] documented one example of chondroblastic osteosarcoma initially misdiagnosed as chondrosarcoma. Nevertheless, we believe this diagnostic pitfall generally can be avoided if one pays attention to the older age of most patients with chondrosarcoma and the distinctive radiographic features. In limited histologic specimens (e.g., cell block), chondroblastic osteosarcomas show increased cellularity at the periphery of the cartilaginous lobules and greater nuclear atypia compared with most chondrosarcomas (Fig. 13.25).

Ancillary Studies

Electron microscopy and immunohistochemistry are not needed to establish a diagnosis of chondrosarcoma in most cases. Immunohistochemistry may be useful, however, for differentiating skull-based chondrosarcoma from chordoma. Typically, chondrosarcomas appear positive for S-100 protein but negative for cytokeratin. Chordomas coexpress S-100 protein and cytokeratin.[23]

Prognosis and Therapy

The most important predictor of local recurrence and distant metastases is histologic grade. In the study by Bjornsson and colleagues,[19] patients with grade 1 chondrosarcoma had a 5-year survival rate of approximately

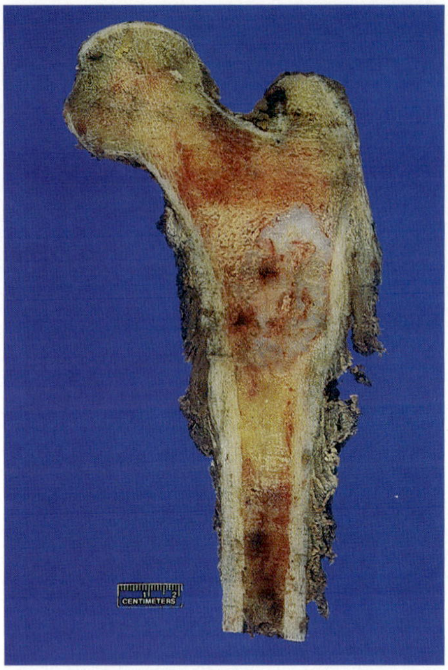

FIGURE 13.17 Chondrosarcoma arising in the femoral metaphysis producing a confluent mass of glistening cartilage with destruction of the overlying cortex.

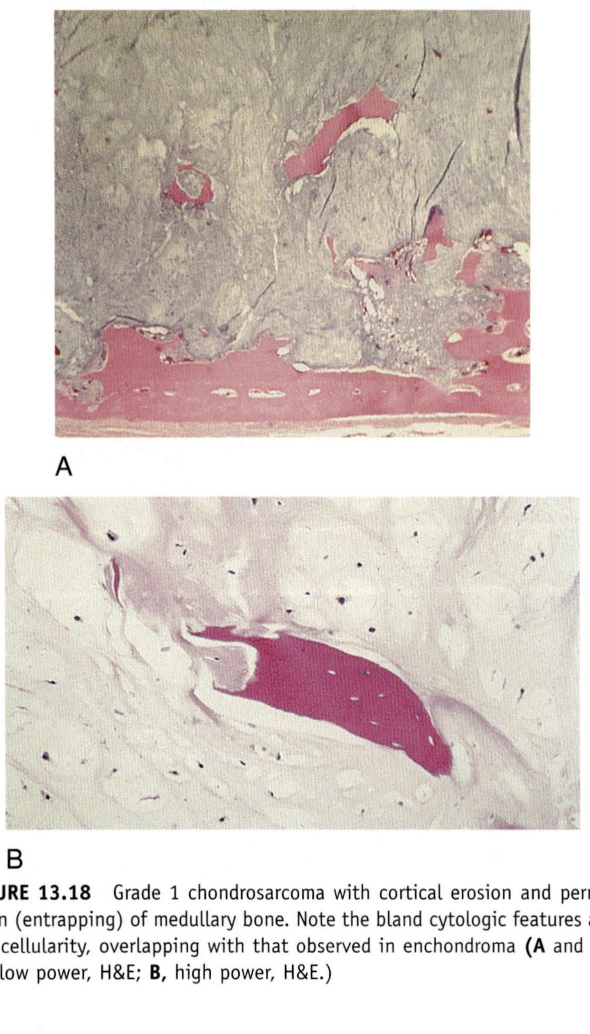

FIGURE 13.18 Grade 1 chondrosarcoma with cortical erosion and permeation (entrapping) of medullary bone. Note the bland cytologic features and low cellularity, overlapping with that observed in enchondroma **(A** and **B)**. **(A,** low power, H&E; **B,** high power, H&E.)

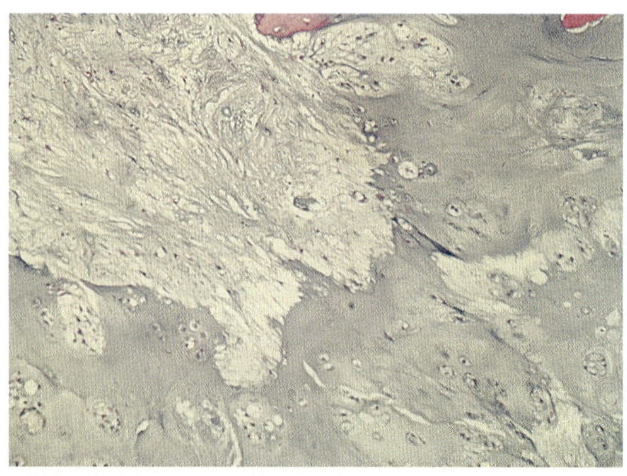

FIGURE 13.19 Grade 1 chondrosarcoma with paler staining areas of myxoid degeneration of the hyaline cartilage matrix, a feature that should never be prominent in enchondroma. (H&E.)

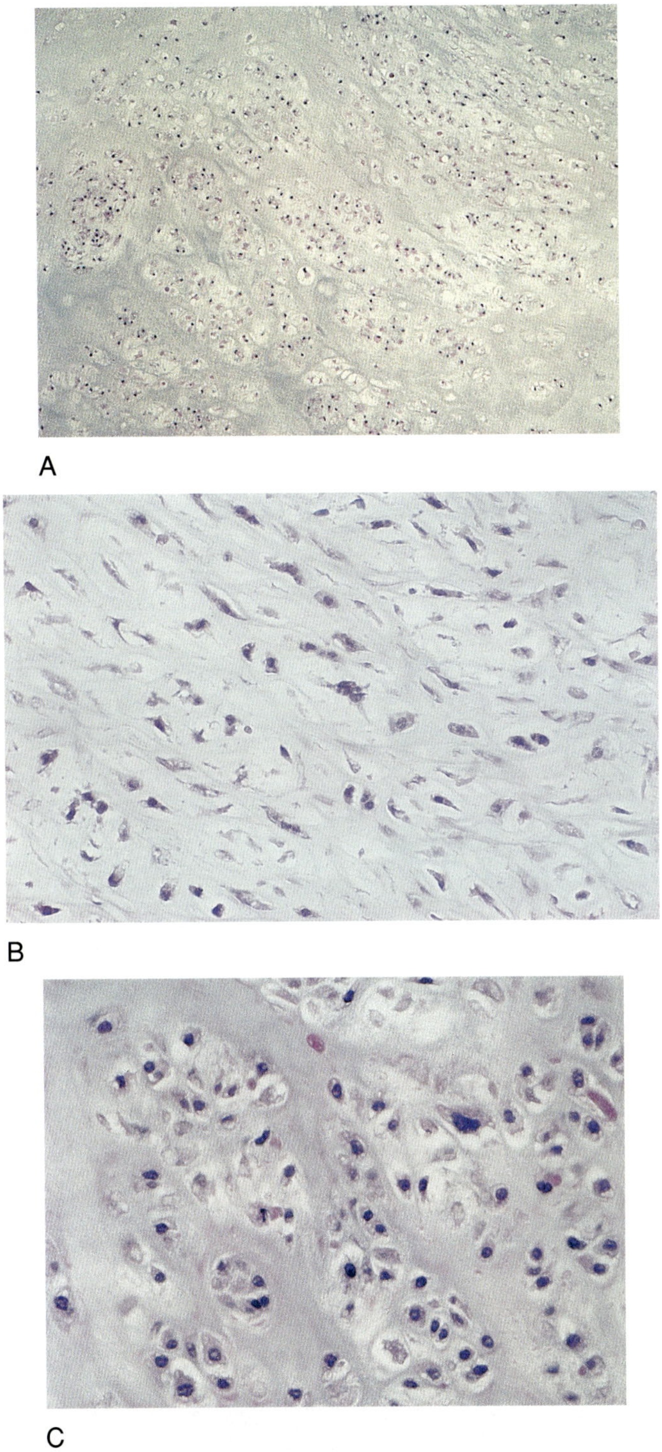

FIGURE 13.20 Grade 2 chondrosarcomas show significantly greater cellularity and atypia compared with grade 1 types and are recognized easily as malignant. Hyaline cartilage differentiation is still evident **(A-C)**. (**A,** low power, H&E; **B** and **C,** high power, H&E.)

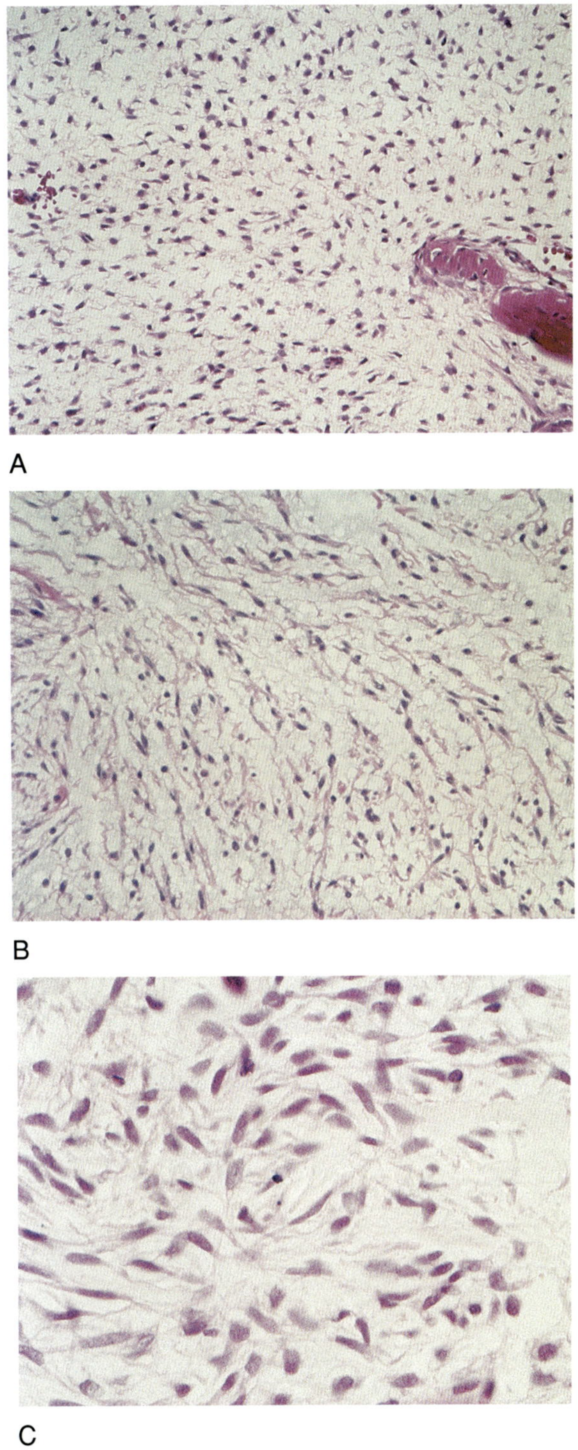

FIGURE 13.21 Grade 3 chondrosarcomas are rare. The tumors are highly cellular, and individual chondrocytes show a tendency toward spindling. The matrix also tends to be more myxoid, and well-developed hyaline cartilage differentiation is less obvious **(A-C)**. (**A,** low power, H&E; **B,** low power, H&E; **C,** high power, H&E.)

89%, whereas patients with grade 2 and 3 tumors had a reported 5-year survival rate of 53%. Histologic grade seems to be the most important predictor of distant metastasis and survival.[19,24] Chondrosarcomas arising in the digits are less likely to metastasize than tumors occurring more proximally.[25] Surgical resection is the treatment of choice. A higher risk of local recurrence is associated significantly with inadequate surgical margins. Approximately 10% of patients develop dedifferentiated chondrosarcoma, a lethal complication.

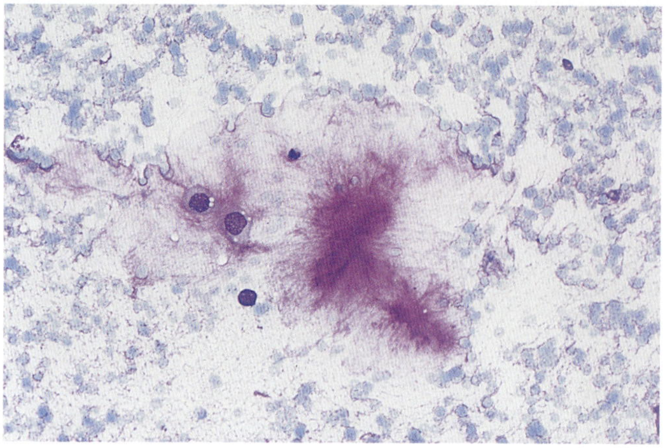

A

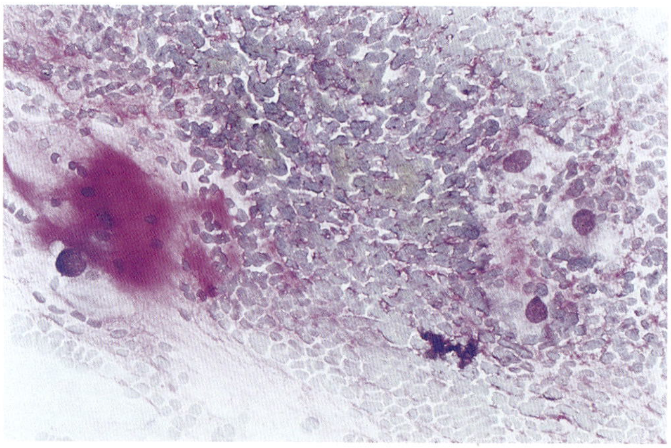

B

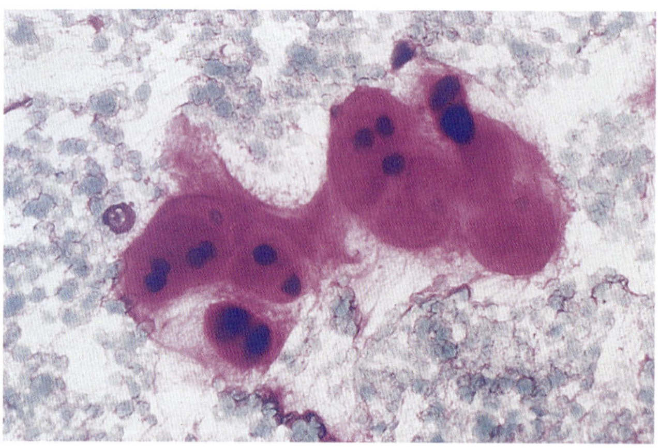

C

FIGURE 13.22 Fine needle aspiration biopsy of low-grade chondrosarcoma generally yields hypocellular smears with scattered metachromatic stromal fibrillary fragments. Individual cells appear mostly uniform and round to polygonal, with enlarged, ovoid-to-round nuclei **(A** and **B)**. Well-developed hyaline cartilage containing individual cells in lacunae is observed less commonly **(C)**. **(A,** intermediate power, Diff-Quik; **B,** high power, Diff-Quik; **C,** Diff-Quik.)

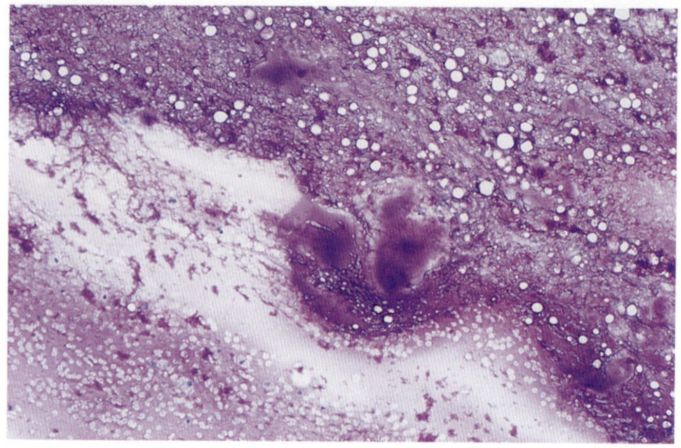

FIGURE 13.23 A helpful feature in fine needle aspiration biopsy specimens of low-grade chondrosarcoma is the presence of a myxoid granular metachromatic film, a feature not observed in enchondroma. (Diff-Quik.)

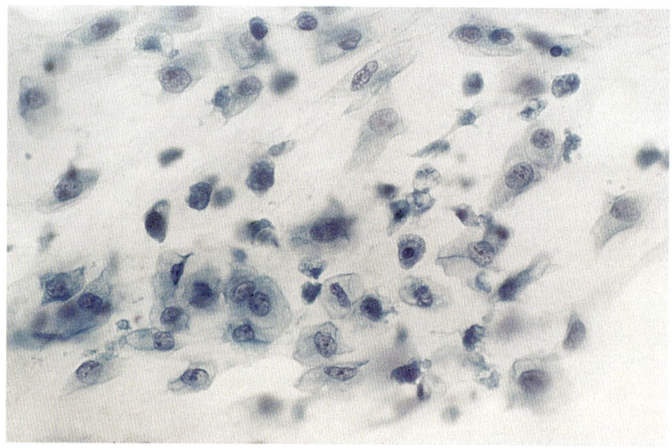

FIGURE 13.24 High-grade chondrosarcomas show greater cellularity and comparatively less background matrix material. (Papanicolaou.)

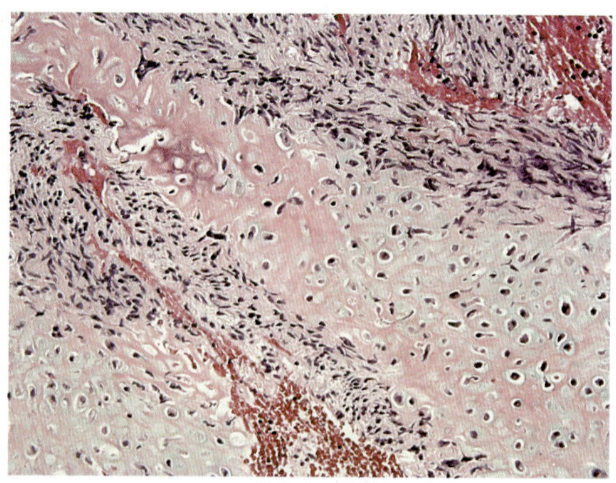

FIGURE 13.25 Cell block from a chondroblastic osteosarcoma. Note the hypercellularity and spindling of the tumor cells at the periphery of the cartilaginous lobule. (H&E.)

Periosteal Chondroma/ Chondrosarcoma

Clinical Features

Periosteal chondromas are rare lesions, most commonly occurring in patients between 10 and 30 years old. Males are affected more commonly than females.[26] The most common anatomic location is the long bones of the extremities, principally the proximal humerus, followed by the proximal and distal femur and the small tubular bones of the hands and feet. Pain and limitation of movement are common initial complaints.

Radiographically, periosteal chondromas are typically well-marginated, juxtacortical, metaphyseal or diaphyseal lesions with variable amounts of calcifications and associated underlying bone erosion (saucerization) of the cortex (Fig. 13.26). In response, the underlying cortex often is thickened with elevated edges and marginal buttressing. Magnetic resonance imaging frequently reveals intact periosteum overlying the lesion.

Periosteal chondrosarcoma is distinguished from periosteal chondroma by its large size (>5 cm), absence of a limiting periosteum and buttressing at the margins, and the presence of soft tissue invasion.[26,27] Medullary involvement tends to be rare. Table 13.6 compares the clinical and radiographic features of periosteal chondroma and periosteal chondrosarcoma.

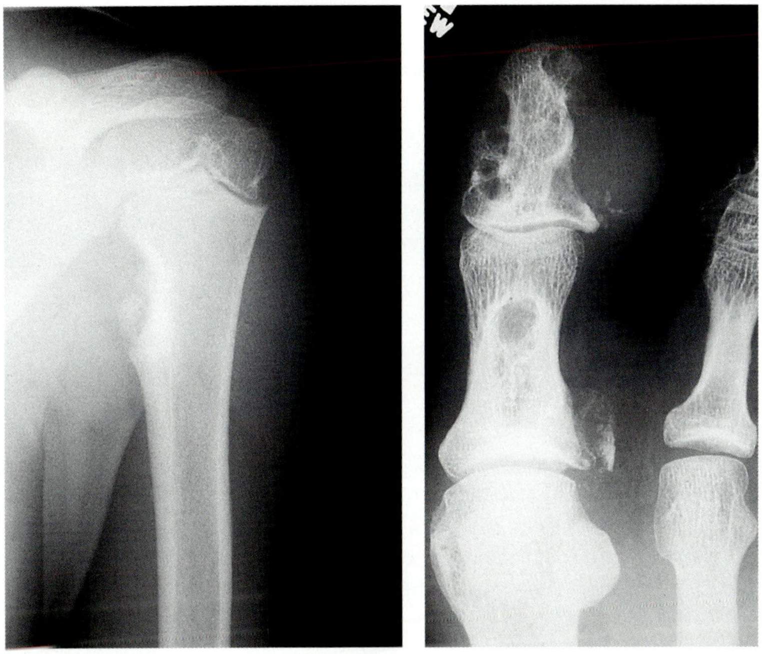

A B

FIGURE 13.26 Periosteal chondroma. An anteroposterior radiograph **(A)** of the proximal humerus reveals an erosive lesion arising along the medial, subperiosteal surface of the proximal humerus. Chondroid soft tissue calcifications are evident within the distal aspect of the tumor. The underlying cortex, although saucerized, is thickened. In another patient, an anteroposterior radiograph of the great toe **(B)** shows a soft tissue mass with subjacent bone erosion along the medial surface of the distal phalanx of the great toe. A lytic lesion in the proximal phalanx of the great toe represents an enchondroma.

TABLE 13.6 Clinical, Radiographic, and Pathologic Characteristics of Periosteal Chondroma versus Periosteal Chondrosarcoma

	Periosteal Chondroma	Periosteal Chondrosarcoma
Peak Age (yr)	5-30	20-50
Gender	Males > females	Males > females
Symptoms	Localized pain and/or soft tissue swelling	Localized pain and/or soft tissue swelling
Involved Bones (Decreasing Order of Frequency)	Femur, humerus	Femur, humerus
Lesion Size	<3 cm	>5 cm
Radiographic Features	Juxtacortical, metaphyseal, or diaphyseal; well-defined margination with buttresses at the tumor edge; cortical erosion	Juxtacortical, metaphyseal, or diaphyseal; poorly marginated; periosteal buttresses absent
Pathologic Features	Well demarcated from underlying cortex; no medullary invasion; hypercellularity and atypia	Well demarcated from underlying cortex; no medullary invasion; hypercellularity and atypia

Pathologic Findings

Histology

Periosteal chondromas show sharp margination from the underlying cortical bone without evidence of permeation. Although the hyaline cartilage matrix is well developed, periosteal chondromas often show greater cellularity than that observed with long bone enchondromas.[26] Additionally, nuclear atypia and binucleated chondrocytes frequently are observed (Fig. 13.27). Periosteal chondrosarcoma shows an even higher degree of cellularity and chondrocyte atypia than periosteal chondroma. Soft tissue invasion is observed frequently, but medullary involvement is seen only rarely.[26,27] The clinical and radiographic features are more reliable for establishing the diagnosis than the histologic findings.

Ancillary Studies

Immunohistochemistry is not helpful in the diagnosis of periosteal chondroma. Only one case of periosteal chondroma has been examined by cytogenetic analysis. Structural changes involving band q13 were observed involving the same band of both chromosomes 12.[28]

Prognosis and Therapy

Complete local excision of periosteal chondroma is almost always curative; local recurrence is seen rarely. Periosteal chondrosarcomas require wide resection. Among 14 patients with periosteal chondrosarcoma reported by Nojima and associates,[26] 2 patients had local recurrence and 2 developed distant metastasis. Dedifferentiated chondrosarcoma is a rare complication.[29]

Synovial Chondromatosis/ Chondrosarcoma

Synovial chondromatosis, also known as *synovial osteochondromatosis* or *primary synovial chondromatosis*, is a benign-appearing hyaline cartilage proliferation occurring within the synovium, bursa, or tendon sheaths surrounding joints. Chondrosarcoma of the synovium occurring either de novo or secondary to synovial chondromatosis is extraordinarily rare.[30,31]

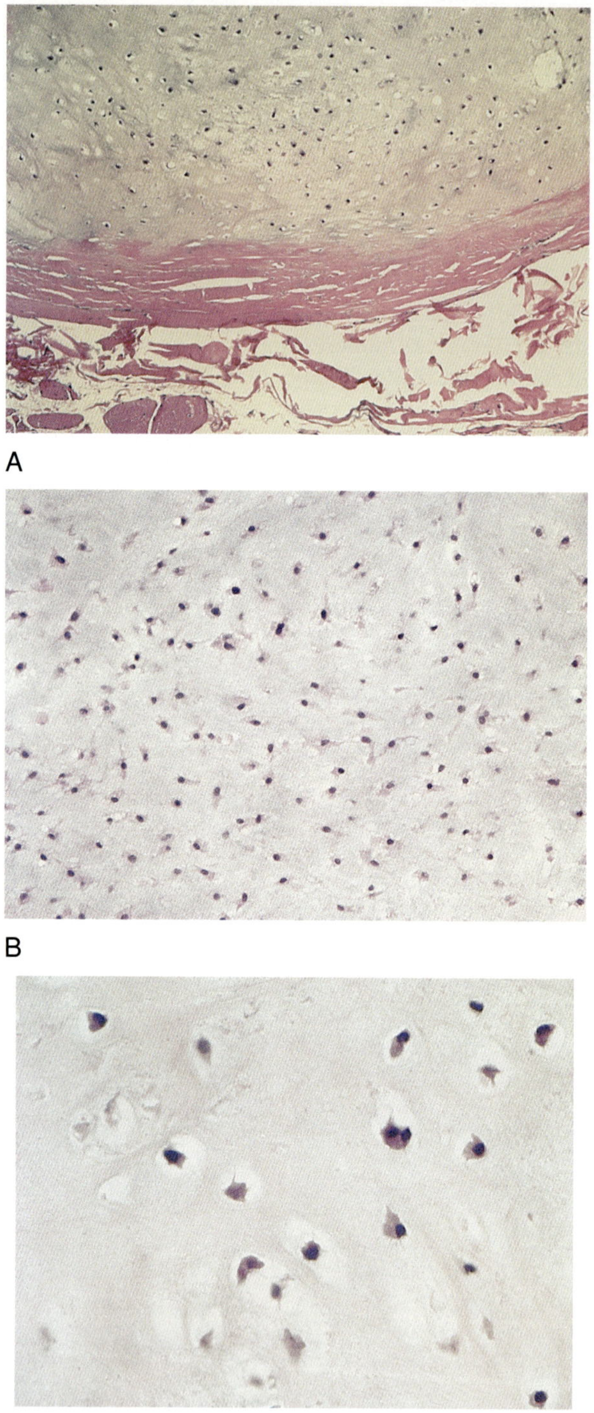
A
B
C

FIGURE 13.27 Periosteal chondromas often show significantly higher cellularity and nuclear atypia compared with enchondromas. Clinical and radiographic correlation is essential to establish the diagnosis and exclude periosteal chondrosarcoma **(A-C)**. **(A,** low power, H&E; **B,** intermediate power, H&E; **C,** high power, H&E.)

Clinical Features

Synovial chondromatosis may develop at any age but is seen most commonly between 30 and 50 years of age. Men are affected twice as often as women. The process typically involves only one joint, most commonly the knee, followed in frequency by the hip, elbow, and wrist. Clinical symptoms include localized pain, swelling, and limitation of joint movement. Often the symptoms have been present for several months to years before presentation.

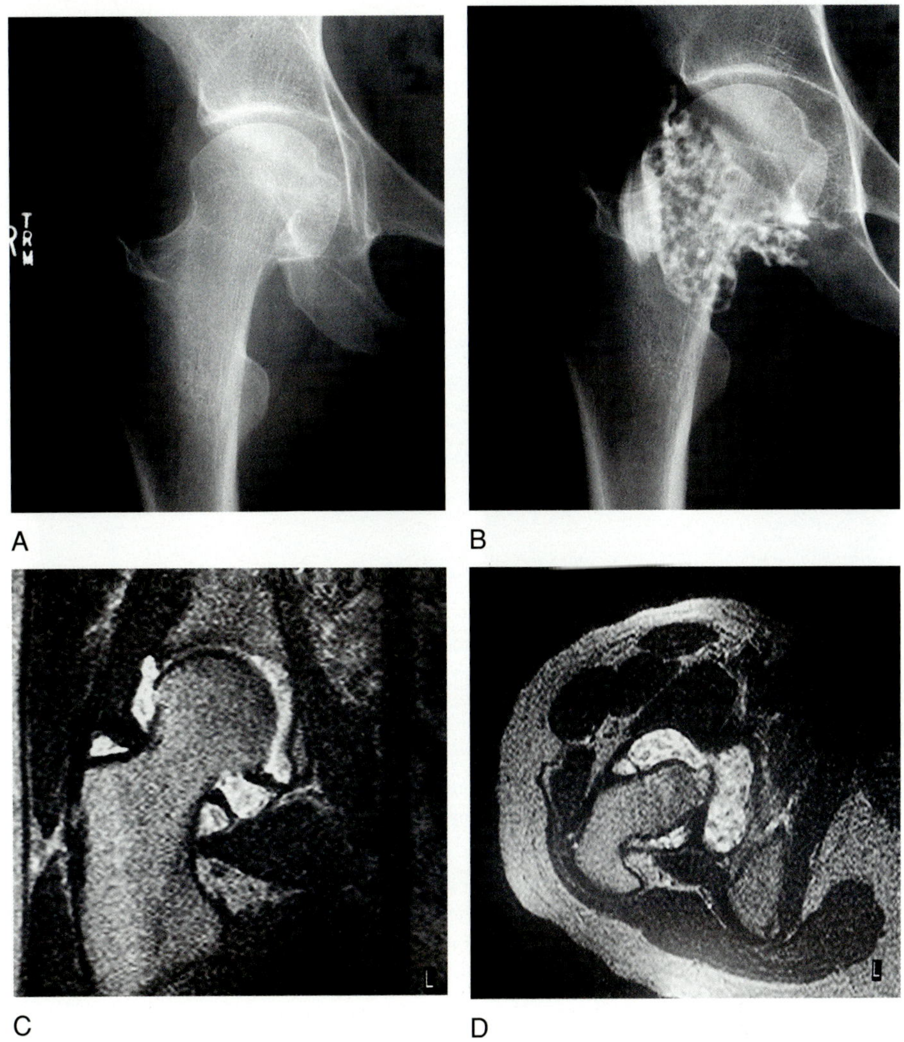

FIGURE 13.28 Synovial chondromatosis. An anteroposterior radiograph of the hip **(A)** shows a small lateral femoral osteophyte and the suggestion of diffuse soft tissue swelling about the knee. After intra-articular injection of iodinated contrast medium, a repeat radiograph of the hip **(B)** shows multiple filling defects in the hip joint. Coronal **(C)** and axial **(D)** T2-weighted magnetic resonance images of the hip reveal a large hip joint effusion and multiple filling defects within the distended hip joint.

Radiographically, synovial chondromatosis usually presents as multiple, articular and periarticular nodules with varying degrees of calcification (Fig. 13.28). Linear calcifications are evident in cases that have undergone enchondral ossification (Fig. 13.29). Less frequently, synovial chondromatosis may show involvement of multiple joints and/or tendons within the same anatomic region, suggesting more aggressive behavior. Erosion of adjacent bony cortex is observed sometimes.

Synovial chondrosarcoma may develop as a primary (de novo) process or may be secondary to pre-existing primary synovial chondromatosis. Most cases represent the latter. The most frequent anatomic location is the knee. A long-standing clinical history of localized pain of the affected joint may suggest the diagnosis of synovial chondrosarcoma, but similar findings may be observed in synovial chondromatosis. Likewise, the radiographic features are not entirely specific but include the presence of a "consolidated" calcified mass within the joint area, associated with erosion of adjacent bone.[31]

Pathologic Findings

Histology

The nodules of synovial chondromatosis are mildly to moderately cellular and often at least partially covered by a synovial lining. Individual chondrocytes are arranged in small clusters and show greater cytologic atypia than those observed in conventional enchondroma. Moderate nuclear pleomorphism and binucleated cells are usually present and do not indicate malignancy (Fig. 13.30). Mitotic figures are not found easily, however. Varying degrees of ossification may be superimposed on the cartilaginous lobules, most often at the periphery.

Primary synovial chondromatosis should be separated from secondary synovial chondromatosis, a process associated with severe degenerative joint disease. The cartilaginous nodules of secondary synovial chondromatosis often undergo enchondral ossification centrally and lack the clustering chondrocyte growth pattern observed in the primary form (Fig. 13.31).

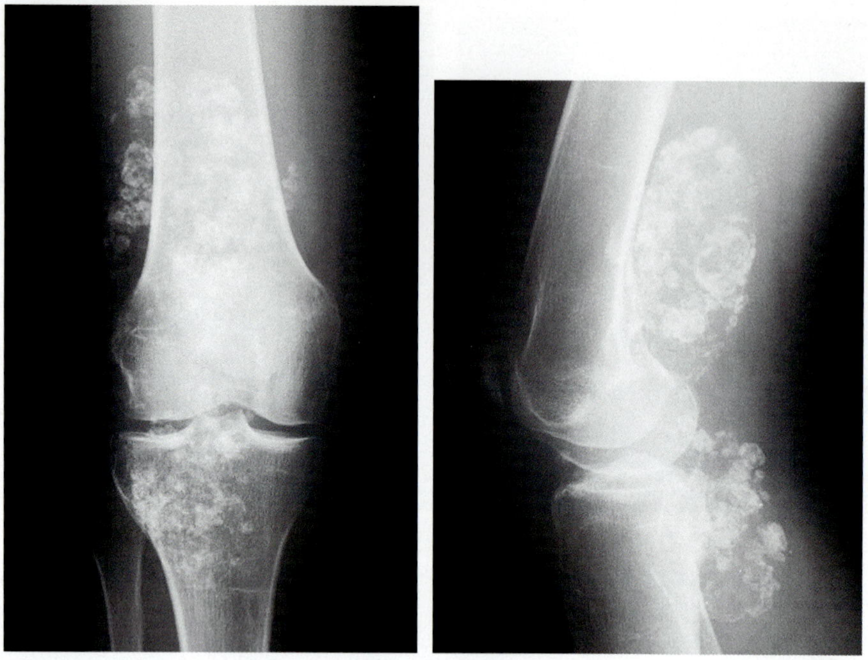

A B

FIGURE 13.29 Synovial chondromatosis. Anteroposterior **(A)** and lateral **(B)** radiographs of the knee reveal multiple, densely calcified fragments in the knee, positioned within a large popliteal cyst posteriorly.

The presence of prominent myxoid degeneration, loss of a clustered chondrocyte growth pattern, and spindling of the tumor cells at the periphery of the nodules are features of chondrosarcomatous transformation.[31] Permeation of bone may be evident (Fig. 13.32). Nevertheless, the diagnosis of synovial chondrosarcoma should be based on a combination of clinical, radiographic, and histologic findings. Table 13.7 summarizes the histologic features of synovial chondrosarcoma.

TABLE 13.7 Histologic Features of Synovial Chondrosarcoma

Loss of clustering growth pattern typical of synovial chondromatosis
Significant myxoid stromal changes
Hypercellularity and spindling of the tumor cells at the periphery of the nodules
Permeation of underlying bone

Ancillary Studies

Immunohistochemistry is not helpful in establishing a diagnosis of synovial chondromatosis. Reports of cytogenetic analysis of synovial chondromatosis have revealed clonal aberrations in six tumors, all associated with the knee. The most common structural aberration involves rearrangements of chromosome bands 1p13-p22.[32]

Prognosis and Therapy

With complete surgical excision, synovial chondromatosis usually pursues a self-limited course. Local recurrence may occur, however, especially after incomplete synovectomy or removal of the loose bodies in the early phase of the disease. Over time, most cases enter a quiescent stage. The presence of multiple local recurrences occurring within short intervals should raise the suspicion of synovial chondrosarcoma. When the diagnosis of synovial chondrosarcoma is established, aggressive therapy is required, sometimes including amputation. Pulmonary metastases develop in 50% of affected patients.[31]

Soft Tissue Chondroma

Soft tissue chondromas are benign, myxoid to hyaline cartilage–producing tumors arising in extra-articular locations. There is no malignant soft tissue counterpart.

Clinical Features

Although soft tissue chondroma may arise at any age, most patients are middle-aged at diagnosis. Men are affected slightly more commonly than women. Most cases involve the digits of the hands and feet, especially the fingers. Origin with the head and neck is extraordinarily rare. The most common presenting complaint is painless soft tissue swelling.[33,34] Radiographically, soft tissue chondromas appear well circumscribed and lobulated but variably calcified. There is no involvement of underlying bone.

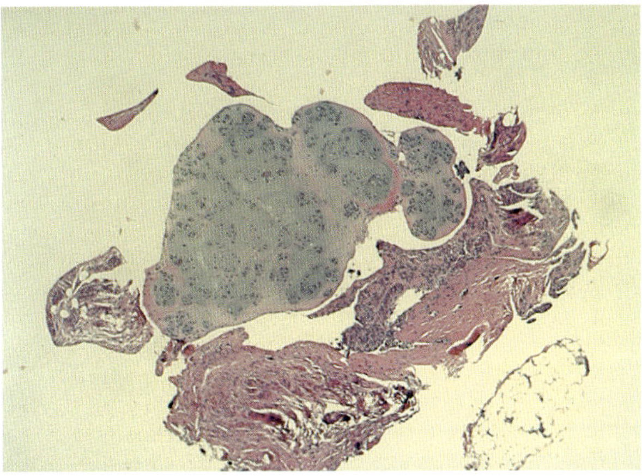
A

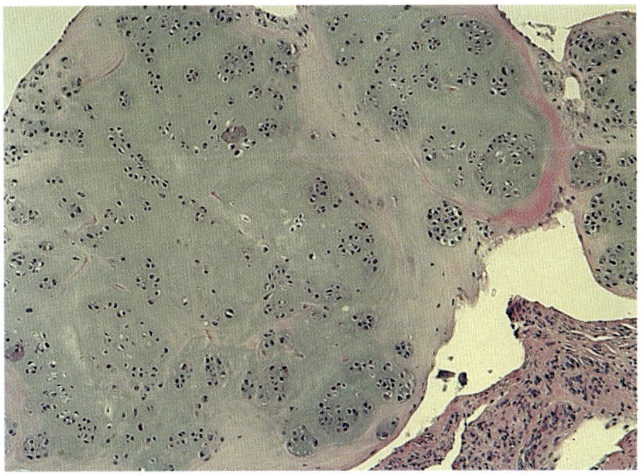
B

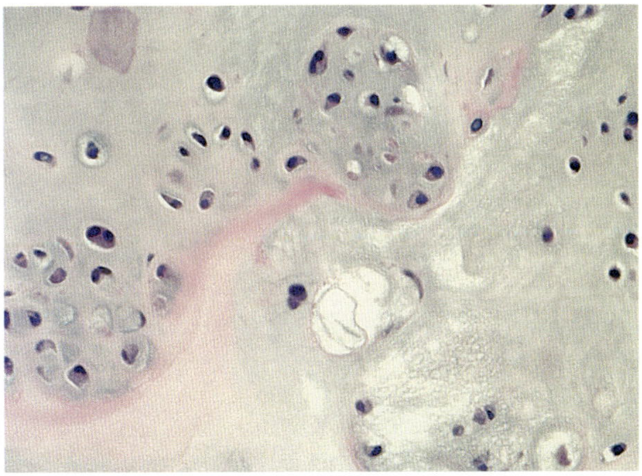
C

FIGURE 13.30 Primary synovial chondromatosis characterized by nodules of mature hyaline cartilage within the synovium. These nodules often appear quite cellular. Individual chondrocytes proliferate in clusters and may show nuclear atypia **(A-C)**. (**A,** low power, H&E; **B,** intermediate power, H&E; **C,** high power, H&E.)

Pathologic Findings

Histology

Soft tissue chondromas are well-circumscribed, lobulated lesions. The stroma within the lobules ranges from well-developed hyaline cartilage to entirely myxoid; foci of dystrophic calcifications or metaplastic bone are often present. Tumor cellularity may be high with individual chondrocytes displaying significant atypia, enlarged round-to-ovoid nuclei, and abundant eosinophilic cytoplasm (Fig. 13.33). In some cases, individual cells bear a striking resemblance to chondroblasts.[35] Binucleated forms are observed frequently. The finding of rare mitotic figures is considered normal; however, atypical forms are never observed. Necrosis is not a feature of soft tissue chondroma.[33] A significant histiocytic response, sometimes accompanied by osteoclast-type giant cells, should be expected at the periphery of the cartilaginous/myxoid lobules.

Fine Needle Aspiration Biopsy

FNAB of soft tissue chondromas yields moderately cellular smears with abundant myxoid granular film and stromal fragments. Individual cells are arranged solitarily and within the matrix clusters. The lesional cells often show significant nuclear pleomorphism and atypia (Fig. 13.34). Correlation with clinical and radiographic features prevents a misdiagnosis of malignancy.

Ancillary Studies

Immunohistochemistry is generally not helpful for the diagnosis of soft tissue chondroma. Individual tumor cells express vimentin and S-100 protein. Only four examples of soft tissue chondroma have been evaluated by cytogenetic analysis. Although clonal abnormalities were observed in all four cases, no reproducible or specific structural rearrangements have been identified.[36]

Prognosis and Therapy

Local excision usually is curative. Studies with prolonged follow-ups revealed local recurrence rates of 10% to 20%.[33,34,37] Distant metastasis has not been reported.

Chondroblastoma

Clinical Features

Most patients with chondroblastoma are between 10 and 25 years old at diagnosis, and there is a male predominance. Patients with skull and temporal bone involvement tend to present at 40 to 50 years of age.[38] More than 75% involve the extremity long bones; the most common anatomic sites are the epiphyseal and epimetaphyseal regions of the distal and proximal femur, proximal tibia, and proximal humerus.[38,39] Equivalent sites within flat bones, such as the acetabulum

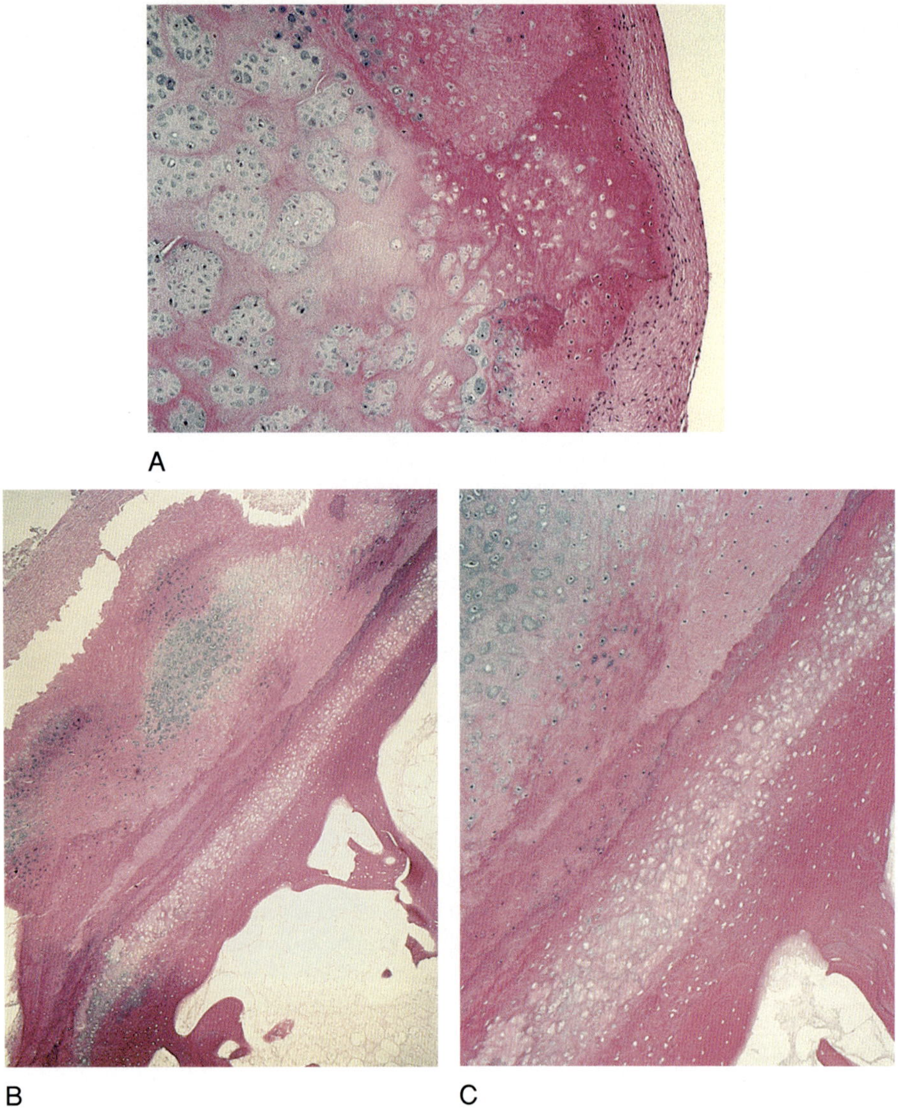

FIGURE 13.31 Primary synovial chondromatosis with the distinct clustering proliferation of chondrocytes and ossification at the periphery of the nodule, a common finding **(A)**. Secondary synovial chondromatosis lacks the clustering chondrocyte pattern and shows ossification more centrally, the result of enchondral ossification. Consequently the secondary form has a more layered appearance **(B** and **C)**. **(A,** H&E; **B,** low power, H&E; **C,** high power, H&E.)

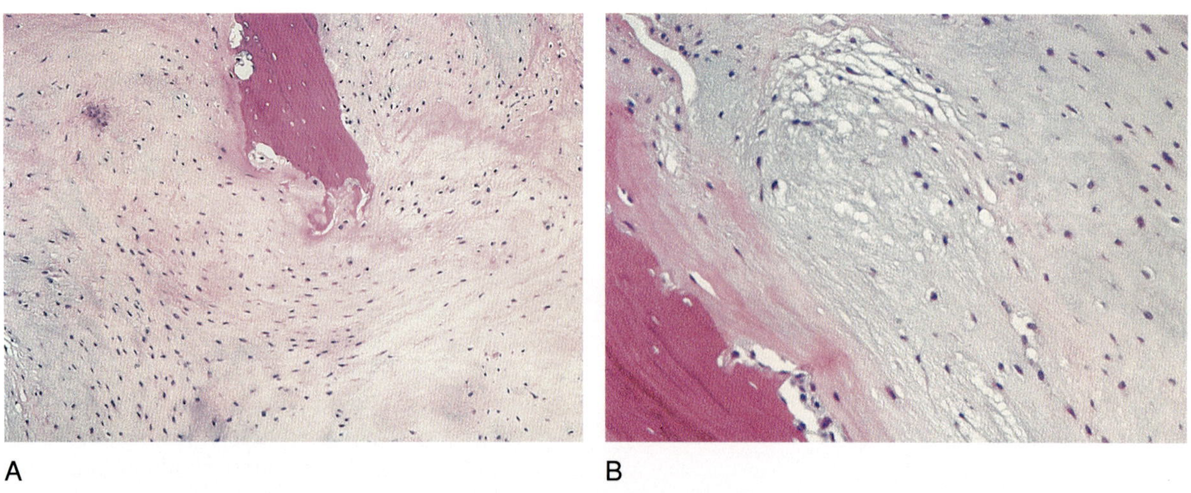

FIGURE 13.32 Synovial chondrosarcoma showing absence of clustering, permeation of underlying bone, and focal stromal myxoid changes **(A** and **B)**. **(A,** low power, H&E; **B,** high power, H&E.)

and ilium, are common. Additional unusual but classic sites of involvement include the talus, calcaneus, and patella. Within the craniofacial region, the temporal bone is affected most frequently. Chondroblastomas almost invariably involve a single bone, but multifocal lesions arising in two separate bones have been reported.[40] Most patients complain of localized pain, sometimes of many years' duration. Soft tissue swelling, joint stiffness and limitation of movement, and joint effusion are reported less commonly. Temporal bone involvement may be associated with hearing loss, tinnitus, or vertigo.[38,41]

Radiographically, chondroblastomas are generally lytic, centrally or eccentrically placed, relatively small lesions (3 to 6 cm), occupying less than 50% of the epiphysis (Fig. 13.35). They are sharply demarcated, with or without a sclerotic rim. There generally is no expansion of the bone. Larger lesions involving flat bones or small tubular bones may exhibit a periosteal reaction, however. Concomitant involvement of the metaphysis commonly is observed. Although often helpful, matrix calcifications are visible only in about one third of patients.[38]

Pathologic Findings

Histology

Histologically the characteristic chondroblast is a remarkably uniform, round-to-polygonal cell with well-defined cytoplasmic borders, clear to slightly basophilic cytoplasm, and a round-to-ovoid nucleus. The nucleus often displays clefts or longitudinal grooves and contains one or more small-to-inconspicuous nucleoli. Chondroblasts are packed in pseudolobulated sheets often showing a pavement-like pattern, accompanied by randomly distributed osteoclast-type giant cells (Fig. 13.36). Variably sized nodules of light-staining, amorphous, brownish-to-eosinophilic material (chondroid) accompany the chondroblasts (Fig. 13.37).[38] Mature,

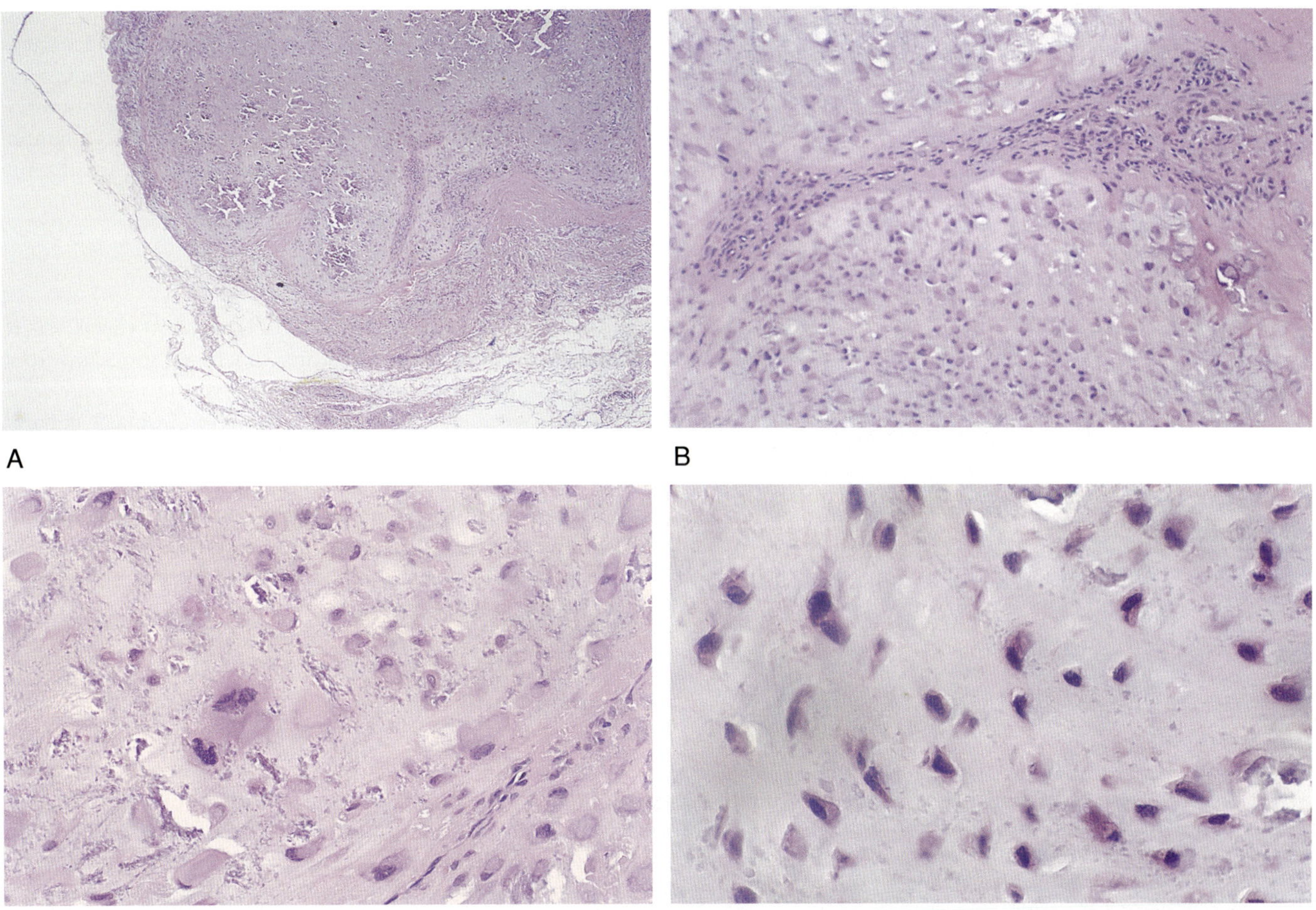

A B C D

FIGURE 13.33 Soft tissue chondroma is characteristically well circumscribed, lobulated, and myxoid. Calcifications may be evident. The stroma appears more cellular at the periphery of the lobules (**A** and **B**). Individual cells within the myxochondroid stroma show variation ranging from chondroblast-like cells with abundant cytoplasm to cells resembling chondrosarcoma. Significant nuclear atypia is often present but of no concern in the appropriate clinical context (**C** and **D**). (**A,** low power, H&E; **B,** intermediate power, H&E; **C** and **D,** high power, H&E.)

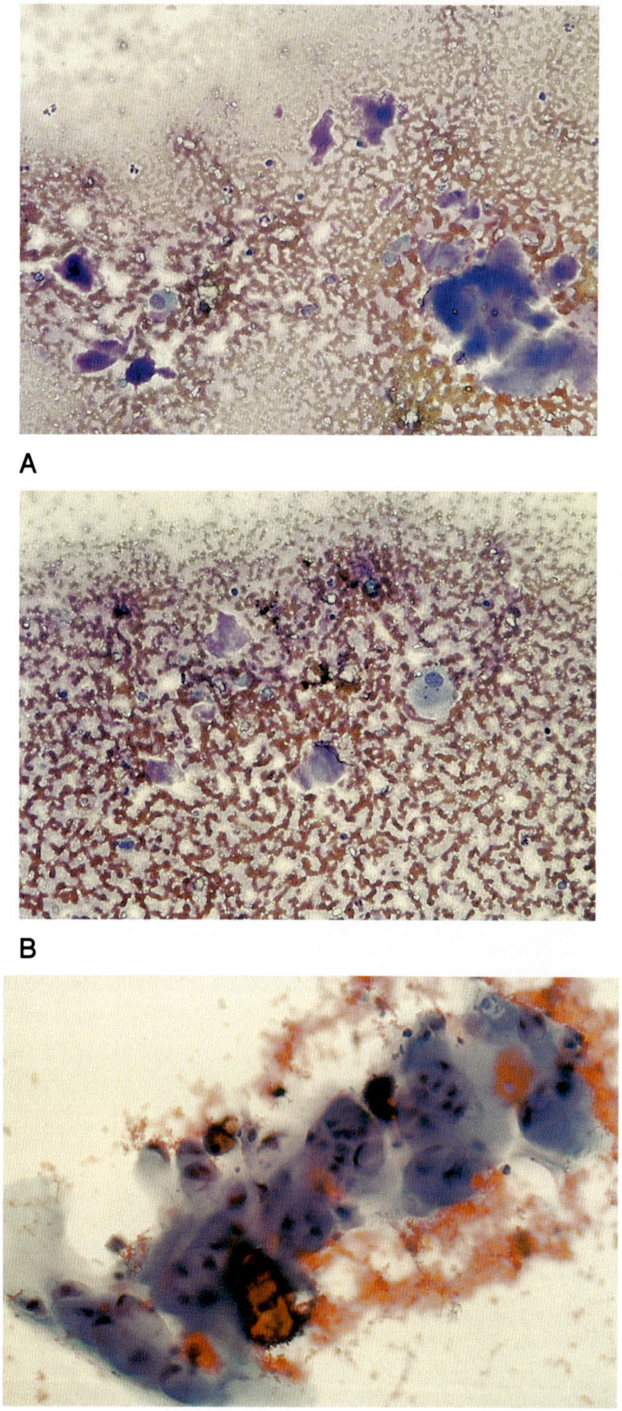

FIGURE 13.34 Fine needle aspiration biopsy of soft tissue chondroma yields moderately cellular smears dominated by clumps and a background film of metachromatic matrix material. Individual tumor cells are arranged singly and within the matrix material as clusters. The cells appear mostly polygonal with round-to-ovoid nuclei but may show significant nuclear atypia. The presence of a soft tissue mass involving the distal extremities without underlying bone abnormalities helps establish the diagnosis **(A-C)**. **(A** and **B,** Diff-Quik; **C,** Papanicolaou.)

basophilic, hyaline cartilage is relatively uncommon. A fine network of pericellular calcification defines the "chicken wire calcification," seen in most cases (Fig. 13.38). Individual chondroblasts may exhibit cytologic atypia most often represented by large, hyperchromatic nuclei; nevertheless, these features do not adversely affect prognosis. Mitoses are observed frequently, but atypical forms are never seen. Aneurysmal bone cysts may be found in one third of cases. In contrast to Langerhans' cell histiocytosis, inflammatory cells, such as lymphocytes or eosinophils, are conspicuously absent.

Fine Needle Aspiration Biopsy

FNAB of chondroblastoma yields hypercellular smears composed of uniform-appearing, round-to-polygonal chondroblasts with centrally to eccentrically located nuclei, often displaying prominent nuclear grooves and inconspicuous nucleoli. The matrix material (chondroid) appears tinctorially similar to osteoid but tends to be arranged in more well-defined nodules and plates reminiscent of mature hyaline cartilage.[42] In our experience, the matrix material is not a prominent feature in cytologic smears and is not necessary to establish the diagnosis (Fig. 13.39). Scattered osteoclast-type giant cells are usually present and may be numerous. Inflammatory cells (e.g., eosinophils, neutrophils, or lymphocytes), as seen in Langerhans' cell histiocytosis, are absent.

Ancillary Studies

Ultrastructural studies reveal deep indentations of the nuclear membrane and features, such as abundant rough endoplasmic reticulum and long cytoplasmic processes, typical of fetal chondroblasts.[43] The chondroblasts generally express S-100 protein and vimentin. More recently, the expression of other antigens has been reported, with cytokeratin being among the most commonly observed.[44,45] Immunohistochemical stains are rarely needed to establish the diagnosis, however, especially if meticulous attention is paid to clinical and radiographic features.

Prognosis and Therapy

Between 80% and 90% of chondroblastomas are treated successfully by simple curettage with bone grafting. Local recurrence rates range from 14% to 18%.[38,39] Probably because of anatomic localization and the difficulty of surgical extirpation, temporal bone lesions may recur in 50% of cases.[41] The rare development of pulmonary metastases in histologically benign chondroblastoma is well

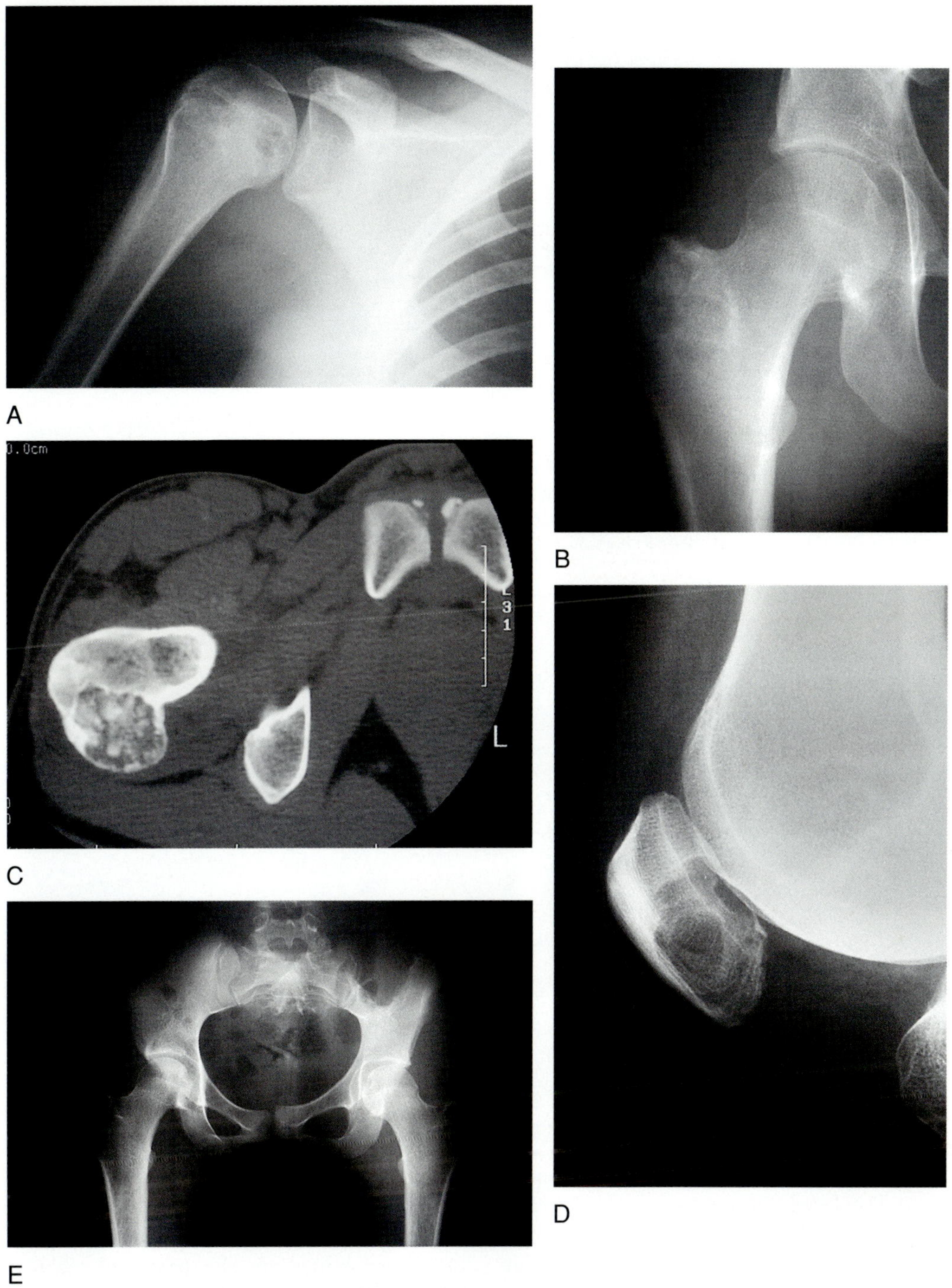

FIGURE 13.35 Chondroblastoma. An anteroposterior radiograph of the shoulder **(A)** shows a lytic lesion in the epiphyseal portion of the proximal humerus. The lesion is bounded by sclerosis, and there is periosteal new bone production along the surgical neck of the proximal humerus. In another patient, an anteroposterior radiograph of the proximal femur **(B)** shows a lytic lesion in the greater trochanter of the proximal femur. An axial computed tomographic scan **(C)** reveals that the greater trochanter lesion is associated with enlargement of the bone and intralesional chondroid soft tissue calcifications. In another patient, a lateral radiograph of the femur **(D)** shows a destructive lesion in the inferior pole of the patella. An anteroposterior radiograph of the pelvis **(E)** in another patient shows an extensive destructive lesion in the left iliac wing.

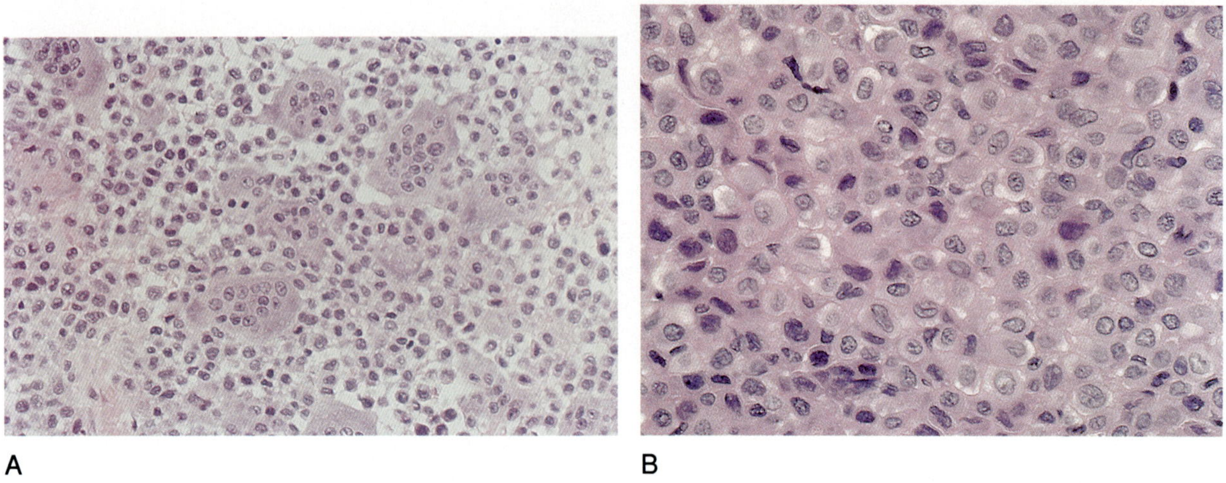

FIGURE 13.36 Chondroblastoma with sheets of mostly uniform-appearing chondroblasts and numerous randomly distributed osteoclast-type giant cells **(A)**; the individual chondroblasts are round to polygonal with sharply defined cytoplasmic borders, round-to-ovoid nuclei, and occasional small nucleoli. Nuclear grooves and indentations are seen frequently **(B)**. (**A**, low power, H&E; **B**, high power, H&E.)

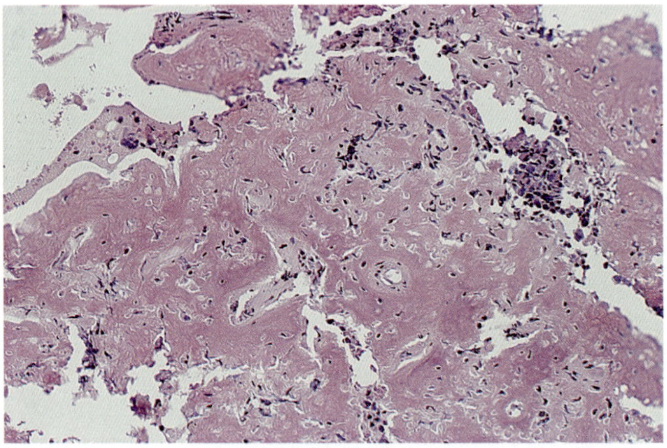

FIGURE 13.37 Nodules of amorphous, pinkish to brown material are characteristic of chondroid. Tinctorially, chondroid and osteoid may be virtually indistinguishable, but the former usually is laid down in plates, whereas the latter more often exhibits a lace-like pattern. (H&E.)

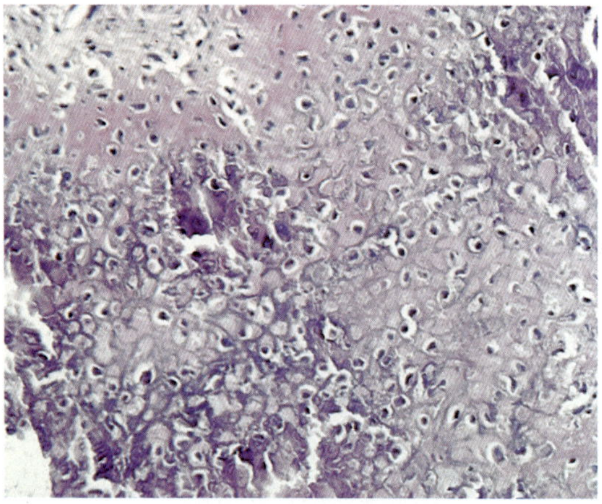

FIGURE 13.38 In the appropriate clinical setting, pericellular "chicken wire" calcifications are virtually pathognomonic of chondroblastoma. (H&E.)

documented.[46,47] These metastases are clinically nonprogressive, however, and often can be treated satisfactorily by surgical resection or simple observation.[47] There are no reliable histologic parameters capable of predicting more aggressive behavior. The existence of a true "malignant" variant of chondroblastoma is controversial, and many investigators propose that most of these tumors represent postradiation sarcomas or simply misdiagnoses.[38]

Chondromyxoid Fibroma

Clinical Features

Chondromyxoid fibroma occurs most commonly in patients between 10 and 30 years old with a slight male predominance. Chondromyxoid fibroma may arise in a variety of osseous sites but is observed most frequently around the knee. In decreasing order of frequency, the most commonly involved bones are the proximal tibia, distal femur, and ilium. The metatarsal bones of the feet are involved less frequently. Localized pain is the most common presenting complaint and may be of several years' duration.[48] Soft tissue swelling is noted most often in tumors arising in the digits.

Radiographically, chondromyxoid fibromas in the long bone usually form eccentric, metaphyseal, and sharply marginated lesions with thinning and expansion of the cortex (Fig. 13.40). Most appear lucent and surrounded by a sclerotic rim. Mineralization is seen in slightly more than 10% of cases.[48] Periosteal reaction and cortical destruction with extension into adjacent soft tissues are observed uncommonly.

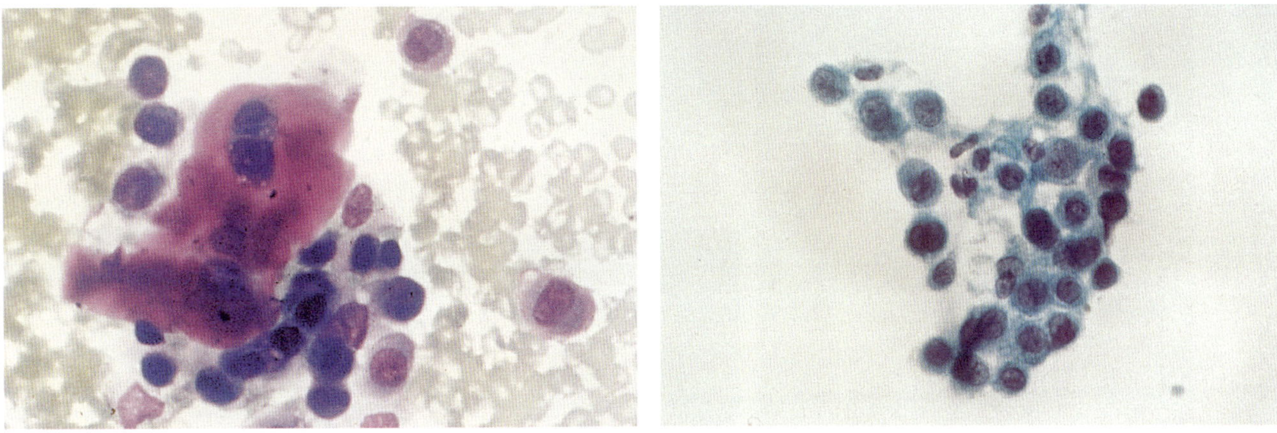

A B

FIGURE 13.39 Fine needle aspiration biopsy specimen of chondroblastoma with uniform-appearing, round to polygonal-shaped chondroblasts intimately associated with metachromatic matrix consistent with chondroid **(A)**. Individual chondroblasts exhibit round-to-ovoid nuclei that may show prominent grooves or folds **(B)**. **(A,** Diff-Quik; **B,** Papanicolaou.) (From Kilpatrick SE, Pike EJ, Geisinger KR, et al: Chondroblastoma of bone: Use of fine needle aspiration biopsy and potential diagnostic pitfalls. Diagn Cytopathol 1997;16:65.)

Pathologic Findings

Histology

A characteristic microscopic feature of chondromyxoid fibroma is a variably lobulated myxoid matrix, distinctly more cellular at the periphery than at the center of the lobules.[48] Individual tumor cells appear ovoid to spindled, often exhibiting atypical and pleomorphic nuclei, suggestive of malignancy (Fig. 13.41). Despite the atypia of the individual tumor cells, mitotic figures are uncommon, and atypical forms are never observed. Osteoclast-like giant cells usually are distributed in the more cellular zones at the periphery of the myxoid lobules (Fig. 13.42). Well-developed hyaline cartilage differentiation is present in fewer than 20% of cases (Fig. 13.43). Cystic changes within the myxoid matrix are infrequent and focal. For reasons that are unclear, coarse calcifications are more common in tumors removed from patients older than age 40 (Fig. 13.44).[49]

Fine Needle Aspiration Biopsy

Cytologic smears are usually moderately cellular with ill-defined fragments of background myxoid fibrillar matrix and mostly discohesive, variably sized, round to stellate-appearing cells. Although most tumor cells appear uninucleated, occasional binucleated and multinucleated cells also are observed (Fig. 13.45).[50] The nuclear chromatin ranges from fine to smudgy and condensed. Likewise, the cytoplasm is variable, ranging from foamy to dense and abundant. The amount of nuclear atypia in the neoplastic cells of chondromyxoid fibroma may be enough to cause diagnostic confusion with more ominous entities, such as chondrosarcoma. Particular attention to clinical and radiographic features helps avoid this diagnostic pitfall, however.

Ancillary Studies

Ultrastructurally the tumor cells of chondromyxoid fibroma may show features of chondroblasts, chondrocytes, or myofibroblasts, including numerous filopodia, dilated and nondilated rough endoplasmic reticulum, intermediate filaments, dense bodies, and abundant glycogen.[51] Immunohistochemically, the chondromyxoid areas appear variably positive for S-100 protein, whereas the peripheral, more cellular zones show diffuse positivity for smooth muscle actin but appear negative for S-100 protein. All areas appear negative for CD34 and desmin.[51] Cytogenetic analysis of a limited number of chondromyxoid fibromas has revealed recurrent structural rearrangements of 6q13 and 6q25.[52]

Prognosis and Therapy

Complete block resection, when possible, is recommended. Curettage usually also is successful but may be associated with local recurrence in 25% of patients.[48] Distant metastasis has not been documented.

Clear Cell Chondrosarcoma

Clear cell chondrosarcoma is an extraordinarily rare form of low-grade chondrosarcoma, most commonly observed involving the epiphyseal ends of the long bones of the extremities.

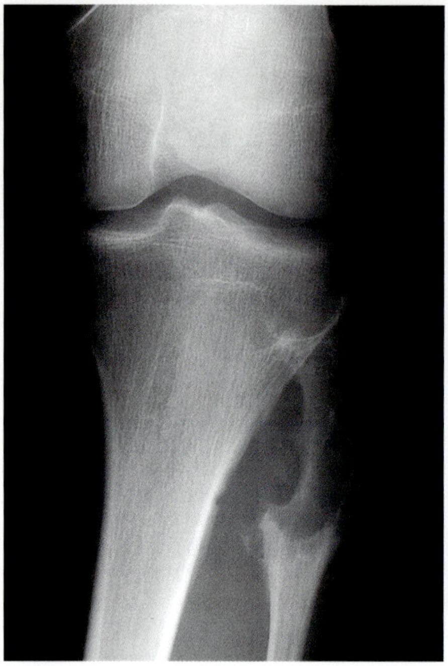

A

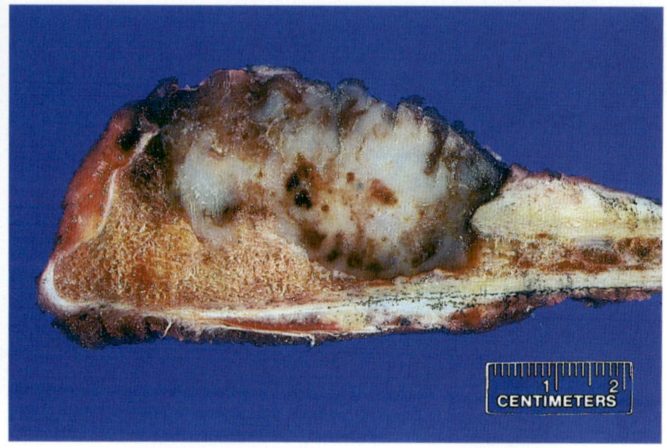

B

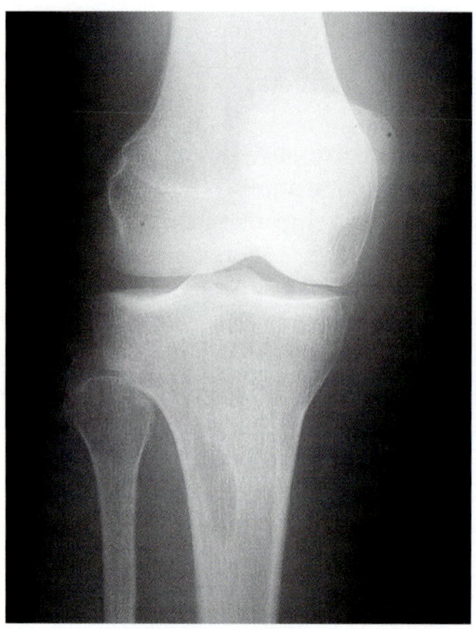

C

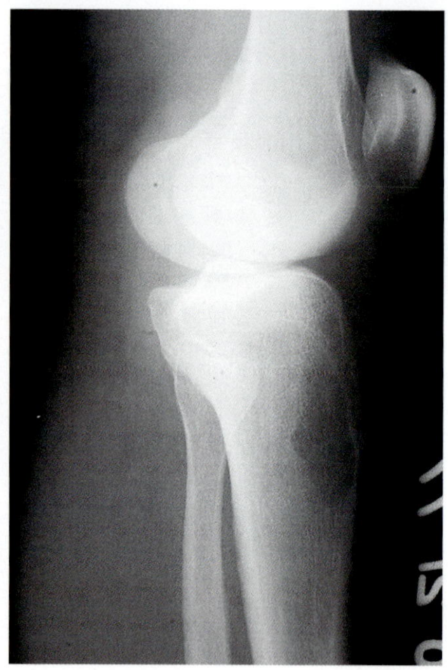

D

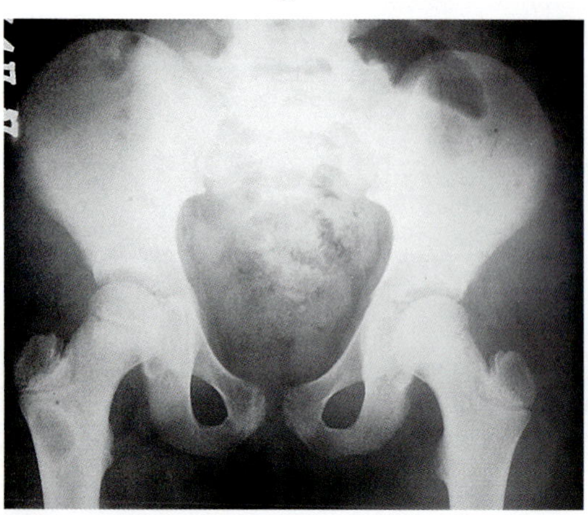

E

FIGURE 13.40 Chondromyxoid fibroma. An oblique radiograph of the proximal fibula **(A)** and the corresponding gross specimen **(B)** show a large, destructive lesion in the proximal fibula with destruction of the medial fibular cortex. In another patient, oblique **(C)** and lateral **(D)** views of the knee show an eccentric lytic lesion in the proximal tibia. The tumor is well demarcated and produces a mild degree of scalloping of the endosteal surface of the tibia, but no matrix calcification is evident. An anteroposterior view of the pelvis in another patient **(E)** reveals a sharply marginated lytic lesion in the proximal right femoral metaphysis. The lesion has sclerotic margins; smudgy density within the lesion indicates fibrous matrix calcification.

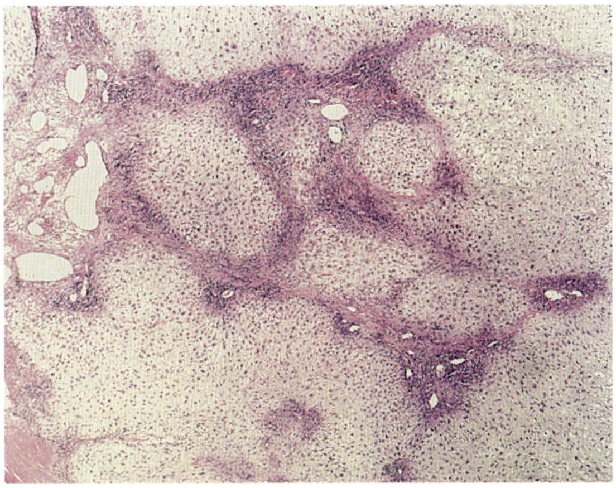

A

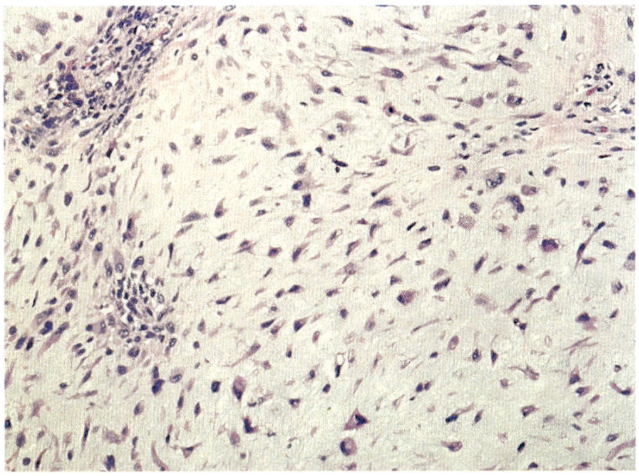

B

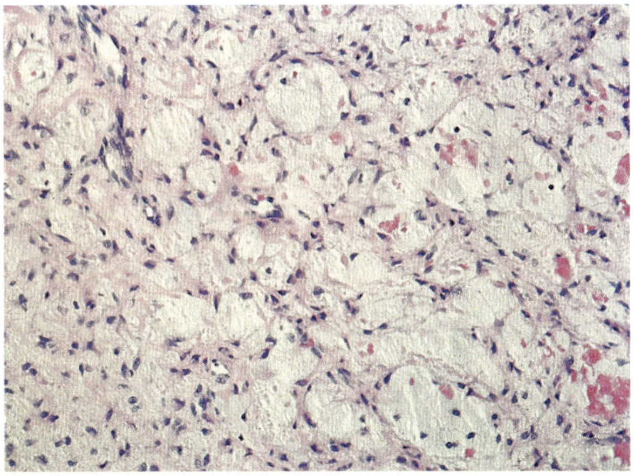

C

FIGURE 13.41 Chondromyxoid fibroma characteristically shows distinct lobulation with hypercellular areas at the edges of the lobules and less cellular myxoid regions centrally **(A)**. Individual tumor cells within the lobules range from stellate to spindled and may show significant nuclear atypia **(B)**. Less frequently the lobulation of chondromyxoid fibroma may be at the cellular level (microlobular pattern) **(C)**. (**A,** low power, H&E; **B,** high power, H&E; **C,** H&E.)

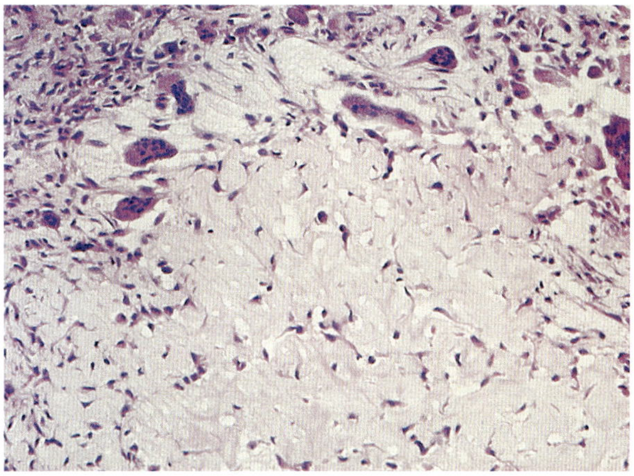

FIGURE 13.42 Chondromyxoid fibroma with numerous osteoclast-type giant cells at the edges of the myxoid nodules. (H&E.)

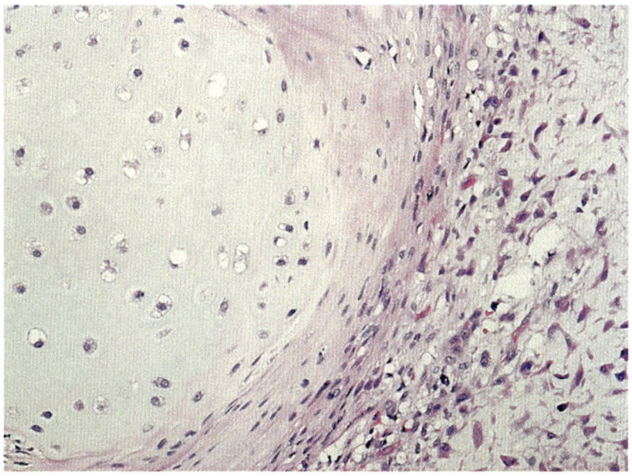

FIGURE 13.43 Despite the name, well-developed hyaline cartilage is seen in less than 20% of chondromyxoid fibromas. (H&E.)

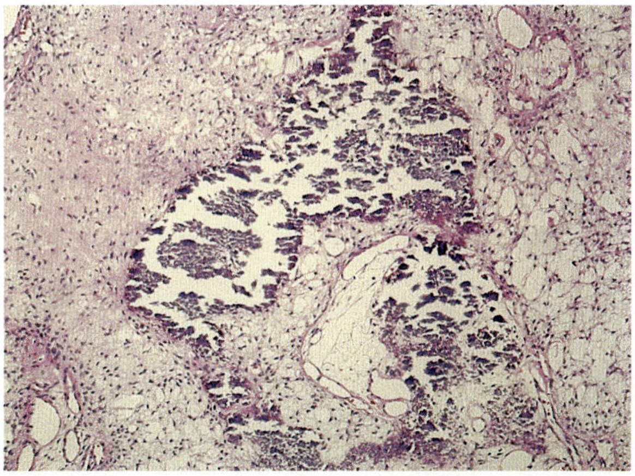

FIGURE 13.44 In contrast to the pericellular "chicken wire" calcifications of chondroblastoma, the calcifications in chondromyxoid fibroma appear more coarse and chunky. (H&E.)

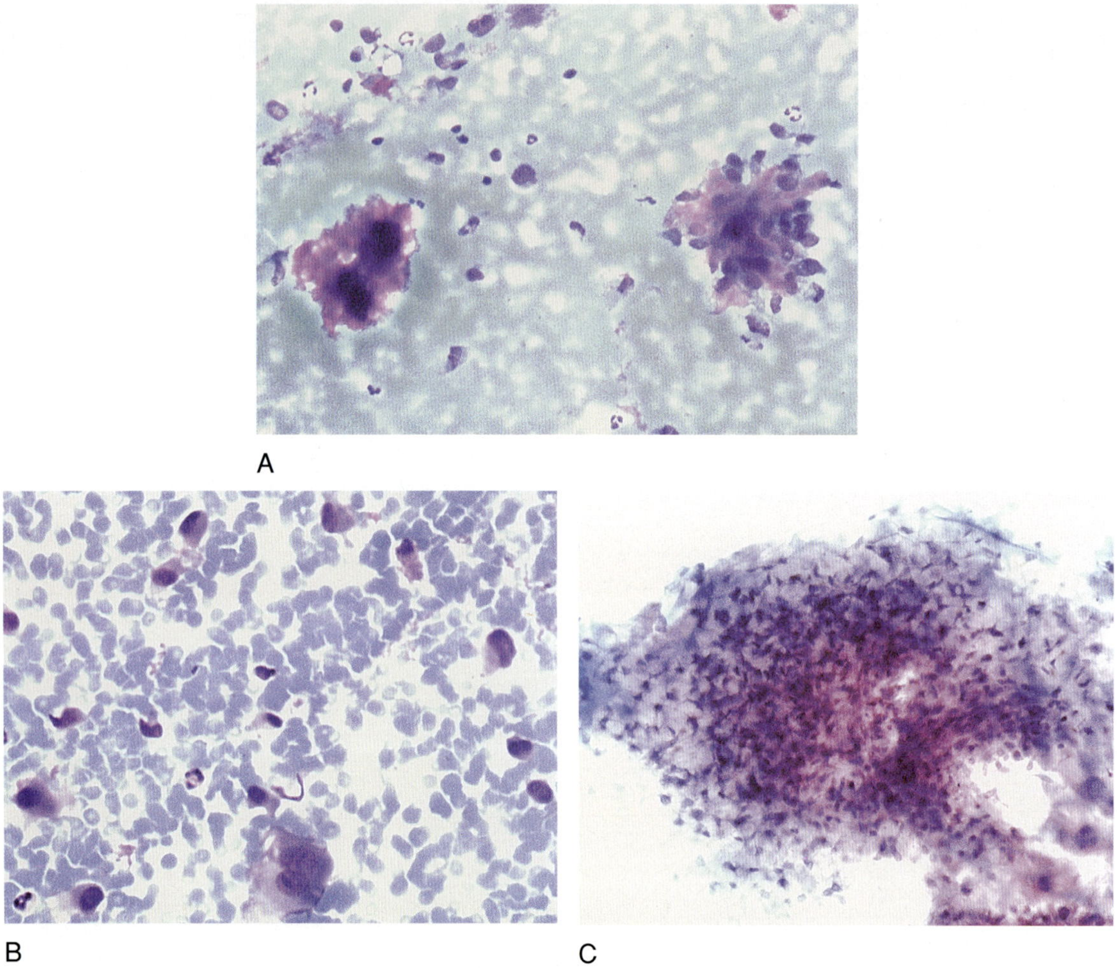

FIGURE 13.45 Fine needle aspiration biopsy of chondromyxoid fibroma yields hypercellular smears composed of aggregates of metachromatic matrix material. Individual tumor cells appear singly and within the stromal material. Cytologically, the tumor cells show significant variability and may be markedly pleomorphic. Correlation with clinical and radiographic features avoids an overdiagnosis of malignancy **(A-C)**. **(A, B,** Diff-Quik; **C,** Papanicolaou.)

Most patients are adults, but clear cell chondrosarcoma has been reported in children and the elderly; there is a male predominance. The most common anatomic sites are the humeral and femoral ends of bone (epiphyses).[53] Complaints of pain, often of long duration, are typical. Radiographically, clear cell chondrosarcoma usually presents with a sharply demarcated and lytic lesion of a long bone end, rarely associated with a sclerotic rim. The radiographic features may be indistinguishable from chondroblastoma (Fig. 13.46). The characteristic clear cells are observed as lobules and sheets infiltrating adjacent bone. They have a large, round-to-ovoid central nucleus with inconspicuous-to-small nucleoli and abundant clear cytoplasm. Occasional cells may have a more eosinophilic appearance, resembling chondroblasts. Osteoclast-like giant cells are distributed randomly throughout the lesion. Mitotic features tend to be rare. Variable amounts of hyaline cartilage, resembling low-grade conventional chondrosarcoma, may be present. Prominent osteoid or bone trabeculae may impart an osteoblastoma-like appearance (Figs. 13.47 through 13.49).[53] Immunohistochemically, individual tumor cells appear positive for vimentin and S-100 protein. Local recurrence invariably occurs after curettage or incomplete excision. En bloc resection generally results in cure. Metastases, when they occur, usually involve the lungs. High-grade dedifferentiation has been reported in three cases of clear cell chondrosarcoma.[54]

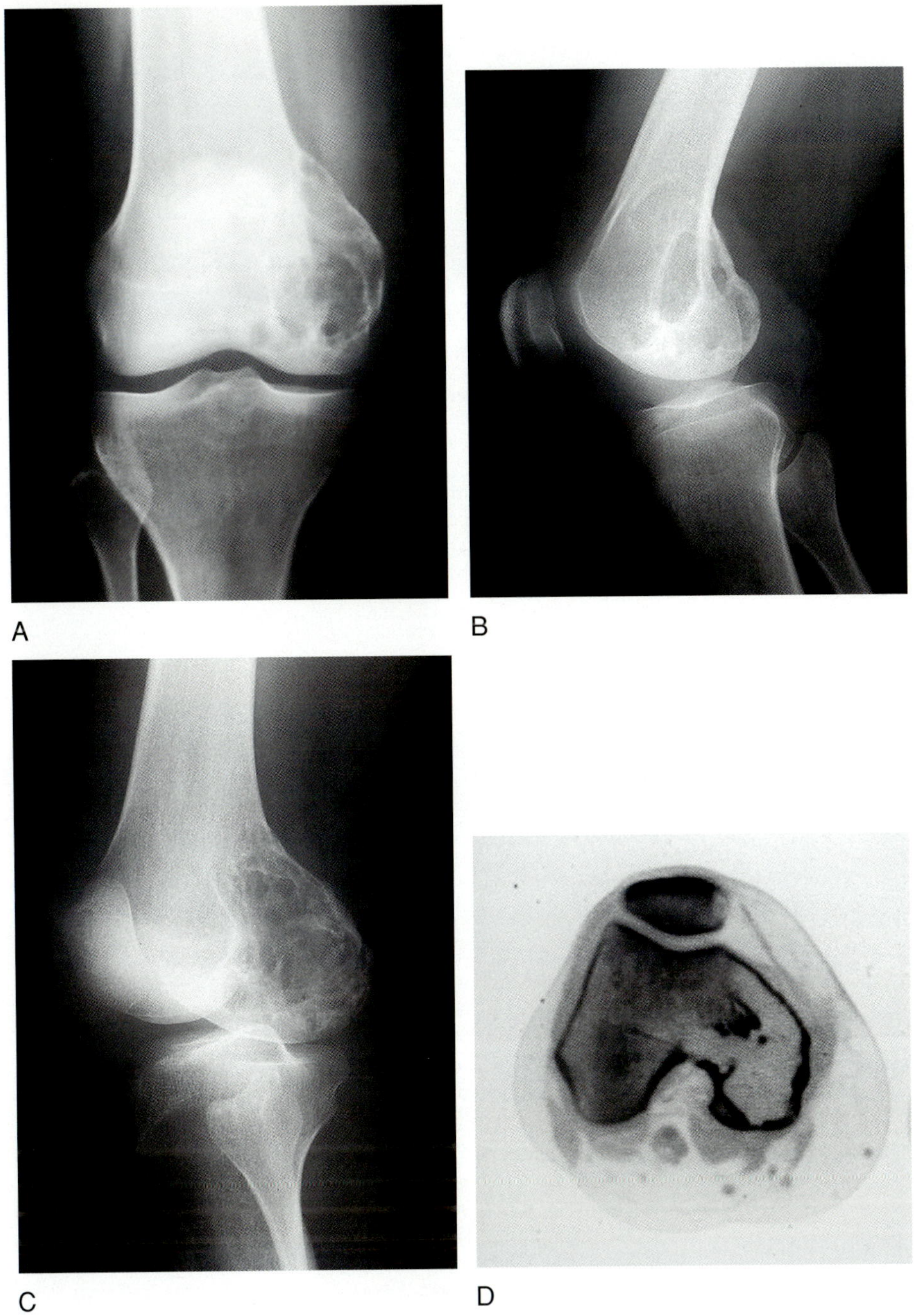

FIGURE 13.46 Clear cell chondrosarcoma. Anteroposterior **(A)**, lateral **(B)**, and oblique **(C)** radiographs of the knee show a lytic lesion in the medial aspect of the distal femur. In contrast to a giant cell tumor, this tumor does not extend radiographically to the subchondral bone of the involved bone. An axial computed tomographic scan **(D)** of the distal femur shows the lytic lesion in the distal femur. There is no intralesional calcification.

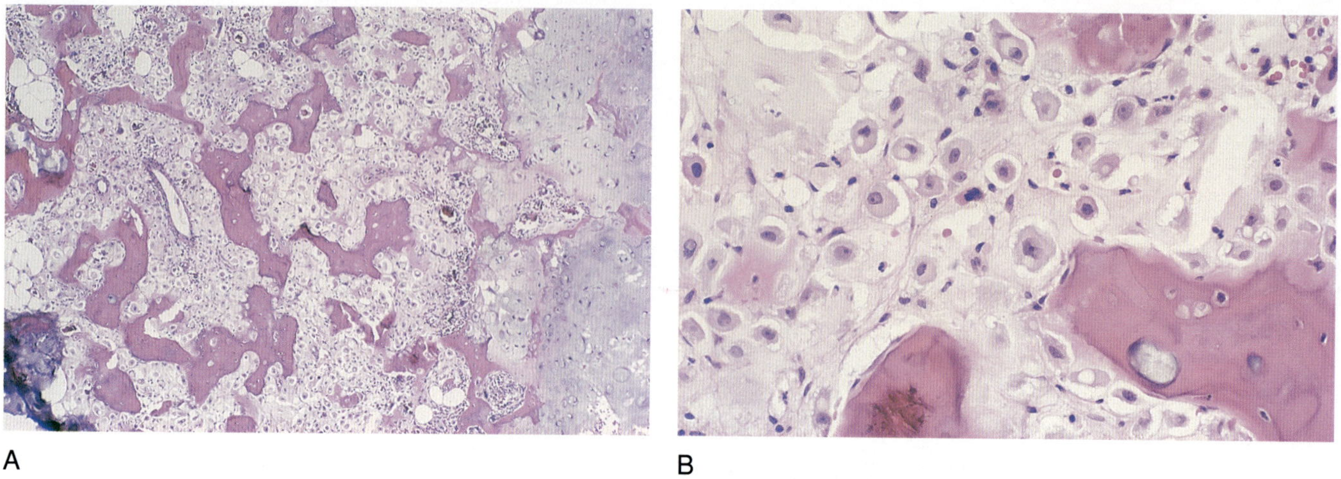

FIGURE 13.47 Clear cell chondrosarcoma. On low power, infiltrating tumor cells with abundant new bone formation and hyaline cartilage are seen **(A)**. On closer inspection, the polygonal-shaped tumor cells appear mostly uniform with round-to-ovoid nuclei and abundant pale to slightly eosinophilic cytoplasm **(B)**. (**A** and **B**, H&E.)

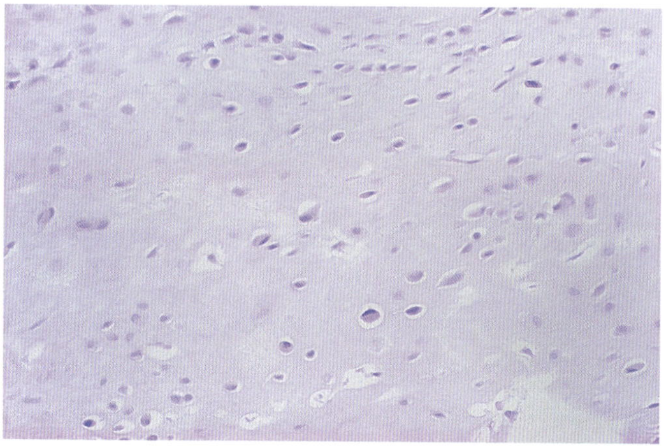

FIGURE 13.48 The hyaline cartilage of clear cell chondrosarcoma is generally indistinguishable from low-grade conventional chondrosarcoma. (H&E.)

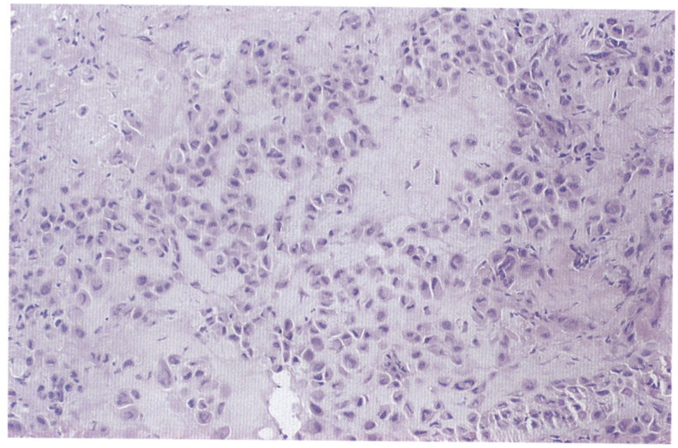

FIGURE 13.49 Occasional examples of clear cell chondrosarcoma may exhibit cords and sheets of tumor cells resembling chondroblastoma. (H&E.)

REFERENCES

Osteochondroma/Osteochondromatosis

1. Unni KK: Osteochondroma. In Dahlin's Bone Tumors: General Aspects and Data on 11,087 Cases, 5th ed. Philadelphia, Lippincott-Raven, 1996, p 11.
2. Schmale GA, Conrad EU, Raskind WH, et al: The natural history of hereditary exostosis. J Bone Joint Surg Am 1994;76:986.
3. Garrison RC, Unni KK, McLeod RA, et al: Chondrosarcoma arising in osteochondroma. Cancer 1982;49:1890.
4. Hudson TM, Springfield DS, Spanier SS, et al: Benign exostosis and exostotic chondrosarcomas: Evaluation of cartilage thickness by CT. Radiology 1984;152:595.
5. Kilpatrick SE, Pike EJ, Ward WG, et al: Dedifferentiated chondrosarcoma in patients with multiple osteochondromatosis: Report of a case and review of the literature. Skeletal Radiol 1997;26:370.
6. Bridge JA, Nelson M, Orndal C, et al: Clonal karyotypic abnormalities of the hereditary multiple exostosis chromosomal loci 8q24.1 (EXT1) and 11p11-12 (EXT2) in patients with sporadic and hereditary osteochondromas. Cancer 1998;82:1657.
7. Mertens F, Rydholm A, Kreicbergs A, et al: Loss of chromosome band 8q24 in sporadic osteocartilaginous exostoses. Genes Chromosomes Cancer 1994;9:8.

Enchondroma

8. Ostrowskit ML, Spjut HJ: Lesions of the bones of the hands and feet. Am J Surg Pathol 1997;21:676.
9. Unni KK: Chondroma. In Dahlin's Bone Tumors: General Aspects and Data on 11,087 cases, 5th ed. Philadelphia, Lippincott-Raven, 1996, p 25.
10. Mirra JM, Gold RG, Downs J, et al: A new histologic approach to the differentiation of enchondroma and chondrosarcoma of the bones: A clinicopathologic analysis of 51 cases. Clin Orthop 1985;201:214.
11. Ogose A, Unni KK, Swee RG, et al: Chondrosarcoma of the small bones of the hands and feet. Cancer 1997;80:50.
12. Walaas L, Kindblom LG, Gunterberg B, et al: Light and electron microscopic examination of fine-needle aspirates in the preoperative diagnosis of cartilaginous tumors. Diagn Cytopathol 1990;6:27.
13. Bridge JA, Persons DL, Neff JR, et al: Clonal karyotypic aberrations in enchondromas. Cancer Detect Prev 1992;16:215.
14. Gunawan B, Weber M, Bergmann F, et al: Clonal chromosome abnormalities in enchondromas and chondrosarcomas. Cancer Genet Cytogenet 2000;120:127.

Enchondromatosis

15. Fanburg JC, Meis-Kindblom JM, Rosenberg AE: Multiple enchondromas associated with spindle-cell hemangioendotheliomas: An overlooked variant of Maffucci's syndrome. Am J Surg Pathol 1995;19:1029.

16. Mertens F, Unni K: Enchondromatosis: Ollier disease and Maffucci syndrome. In Fletcher CDM, Unni KK, Mertens F (eds): Pathology and Genetics: Tumours of Soft Tissue and Bone. World Health Organization Classification of Tumours. Lyon, France, IARC Press, 2002, p 356.
17. Liu J, Hudkins PG, Swee RG, et al: Bone sarcomas associated with Ollier's disease. Cancer 1987;59:1376.
18. Sun BT, Swee RG, Shives TC, et al: Chondrosarcoma in Maffucci's syndrome. J Bone Joint Surg Am 1985;67:1214.

Chondrosarcoma

19. Bjornsson J, McLeod RA, Unni KK, et al: Primary chondrosarcoma of long bones and limb girdles. Cancer 1998;83:2105.
20. Young CL, Sim FH, Unni KK, et al: Chondrosarcoma of bone in children. Cancer 1990;66:1641.
21. Unni KK, Dahlin DC: Grading of bone tumors. Semin Diagn Pathol 1984;1:165.
22. Layfield LJ, Glasgow BJ, Anders KH, et al: Fine needle aspiration cytology of primary bone lesions. Acta Cytol 1987;31:177.
23. Rosenberg AE, Nielsen GP, Keel SB, et al: Chondrosarcoma of the base of the skull: A clinicopathologic study of 200 cases with emphasis on its distinction from chordoma. Am J Surg Pathol 1999;23:1370.
24. Sheth DS, Yasko AW, Johnson ME, et al: Chondrosarcoma of the pelvis: Prognostic factors for 67 patients treated with definitive surgery. Cancer 1996;78:745.
25. Bovee JV, van der Heul RO, Taminiau AHM, et al: Chondrosarcoma of the phalanx: A locally aggressive lesion with minimal metastatic potential: Report of 35 cases and a review of the literature. Cancer 1999;86:1724.

Periosteal Chondroma/Chondrosarcoma

26. Nojima T, Unni KK, McLeod RA, et al: Periosteal chondroma and periosteal chondrosarcoma. Am J Surg Pathol 1985;9:666.
27. Vanel D, De Paolis M, Monti C, et al: Radiological features of 24 periosteal chondrosarcomas. Skeletal Radiol 2001;30:208.
28. Mandahl N, Willen H, Rydholm A, et al: Rearrangement of band q13 on both chromosomes 12 in a periosteal chondroma. Genes Chromosomes Cancer 1993;6:121.
29. Mitchell A, Rudan JR, Fenton PV: Juxtacortical dedifferentiated chondrosarcoma from a primary periosteal chondrosarcoma. Mod Pathol 1996;9:279.

Synovial Chondromatosis/Chondrosarcoma

30. Villacin AB, Brigham LN, Bullough PG: Primary and secondary synovial chondrometaplasia: Histopathologic and clinicoradiologic differences. Hum Pathol 1979;10:439.
31. Bertoni F, Unni KK, Beabout JW, et al: Chondrosarcomas of the synovium. Cancer 1991;67:155.
32. Miller MV, King A, Mertens F: Synovial chondromatosis. In Fletcher CDM, Unni KK, Mertens F (eds): Pathology and Genetics: Tumours of Soft Tissue and Bone. World Health Organization Classification of Tumours. Lyon, France, IARC Press, 2002, p 246.

Soft Tissue Chondroma

33. Chung EB, Enzinger FM: Chondroma of soft parts. Cancer 1978;41:1414.
34. Dahlin DC, Salvador AH: Cartilaginous tumors of the soft tissues of the hands and feet. Mayo Clin Proc 1974;49:721.
35. Cates JM, Roseberg AE, O'Connell JX, et al: Chondroblastoma-like chondroma of soft tissue: An underrecognized variant and its differential diagnosis. Am J Surg Pathol 2001;25:661.
36. Nayler S, Helm S: Soft tissue chondroma. In Fletcher CDM, Unni KK, Mertens F (eds): Pathology and Genetics: Tumours of Soft Tissue and Bone. World Health Organization Classification of Tumours. Lyon, France, IARC Press, 2002, p 180.
37. Fletcher CD, Krause T: Cartilaginous tumours of soft tissue. Appl Pathol 1988;6:208.

Chondroblastoma

38. Turcotte RE, Kurt A-M, Sim FH, et al: Chondroblastoma. Hum Pathol 1993;24:944.
39. Bloem JL, Mulder JD: Chondroblastoma: A clinical and radiological study of 104 cases. Skeletal Radiol 1985;14:1.
40. Roberts PF, Taylor JG: Multifocal benign chondroblastomas: Report of a case. Hum Pathol 1990;11:296.
41. Bertoni F, Unni KK, Beabout JW, et al: Chondroblastoma of the skull and facial bones. Am J Clin Pathol 1987;88:1.
42. Kilpatrick SE, Pike EJ, Geisinger KR, et al: Chondroblastoma of bone: Use of fine needle aspiration biopsy and potential diagnostic pitfalls. Diagn Cytopathol 1997;16:65.
43. Steiner GC: Ultrastructure of benign cartilaginous tumors of intraosseous origin. Hum Pathol 1979;10:71.
44. Edel G, Ueda Y, Nakanishi J, et al: Chondroblastoma of bone: A clinical, radiological, light and immunohistochemical study. Virchows Arch A 1992;421:355.
45. Semmelink HJF, Pruszczynski M, Wiersma V, et al: Cytokeratin expression in chondroblastomas. Histopathology 1990;16:257.
46. Jambhekar NA, Desai PB, Chitale PB, et al: Benign metastasizing chondroblastoma: A case report. Cancer 1998;82:675.
47. Riddell RJ, Louis CJ, Bromberger NA: Pulmonary metastases from chondroblastoma of the tibia: Report of a case. J Bone Joint Surg Br 1973;55:848.

Chondromyxoid Fibroma

48. Wu CT, Inwards CY, O'Laughlin S, et al: Chondromyxoid fibroma of bone: A clinicopathologic review of 278 cases. Hum Pathol 1998;29:438.
49. Yamaguchi T, Dorfman HD: Radiographic and histologic patterns of calcification in chondromyxoid fibroma. Skeletal Radiol 1998;27:559.
50. Gupta S, Dev G, Marya S: Chondromyxoid fibroma: A fine-needle aspiration diagnosis. Diagn Cytopathol 1993;9:63.
51. Nielsen GP, Keel SB, Dickersin GR, et al: Chondromyxoid fibroma: A tumor showing myofibroblastic, myochondroblastic, and chondrocytic differentiation. Mod Pathol 1999;12:514.
52. Granter SR, Renshaw AA, Kozakewich HP, et al: The pericentromeric inversion, inv (6)(p25q13), is a novel diagnostic marker in chondromyxoid fibroma. Mod Pathol 1998;11:1071.

Clear Cell Chondrosarcoma

53. Unni KK, Dahlin DC, Beabout JW, et al: Chondrosarcoma: Clear-cell variant: Report of sixteen cases. J Bone Joint Surg Am 1976;58:676.
54. Kalil RK, Inwards CY, Unni KK, et al: Dedifferentiated clear cell chondrosarcoma. Am J Surg Pathol 2000;24:1079.

CHAPTER 14

Cysts of Bone and Soft Tissue

A variety of cysts may arise within bone and soft tissue (Table 14.1). Many neoplasms may undergo cystic changes, and adequate tissue sampling is essential. Table 14.2 summarizes benign and malignant lesions frequently associated with cystic changes. Included in this table are giant cell tumor, chondroblastoma, and fibrous dysplasia, which are commonly associated with engrafted aneurysmal bone cysts, accounting for most of their cystic features, when present. This chapter addresses the clinicoradiologic and pathologic features of ganglion cyst, solitary bone cyst, aneurysmal bone cyst, and subchondral bone cyst.

Solitary Bone Cyst

Solitary bone cyst is also known as *unicameral bone cyst* and *simple cyst*. Although the pathogenesis is unknown, there may be an association with prior trauma or bone infarct, as evidenced by increased frequency of these cysts observed in Navy deep-sea divers.

Clinical Features

Although virtually any age may be affected, most patients are younger than age 20.[1] There seems to be a slight male predominance. Clinical symptoms may include localized pain, soft tissue swelling, and joint stiffness.

Most patients are asymptomatic, and the presence of a solitary bone cyst usually represents an incidental finding. Greater than 80% of solitary bone cysts occur in the metaphyseal regions of the proximal humerus and proximal femur (Fig. 14.1). In adults, localization within the pelvic bones, especially the ilium, and the calcaneus is commonly observed (Fig. 14.2).[2]

Radiographically, solitary bone cysts typically form purely lytic, well-marginated, metaphyseal-centered lesions, often abutting the physis and arising within skeletally immature patients with an open physis. In most cases, the affected bone appears slightly expanded and generally exceeds the width of the adjacent physis. Although the overlying cortex may be thinned, it is not penetrated. In some cases, solitary bone cysts may become large but remain sharply marginated.

Pathologic Findings

Histology

Solitary bone cyst is characteristically a unilocular, intramedullary cavitary lesion containing clear to slightly yellow fluid. Despite the large size of some lesions, the amount of material generally obtained by curettage from a simple bone cyst rarely exceeds more than a single slide. The bone cyst lining ranges from thin, single-cell, fibroblastic strands to broader, benign-appearing fibrous tissue septa containing variable numbers of multinucleated osteoclast-type giant cells (Fig. 14.3). The cyst wall often appears at least focally myxoid (Fig. 14.4). Additionally, aggregates of eosinophilic fibrin-like debris, sometimes calcified, resembling dental cementum, frequently are observed (Fig. 14.5).[3]

TABLE 14.1 Cysts of Bone and Soft Tissue

Bone Origin	Soft Tissue Origin
Ganglion cyst	Ganglion cyst
Solitary (unicameral) bone cyst	Juxta-articular myxoma
Aneurysmal bone cyst	Aneurysmal bone cyst
Subchondral bone cyst	

TABLE 14.2 Benign and Malignant Lesions Commonly Associated with Cystic Changes

Bone Origin	Soft Tissue Origin
Giant cell tumor	Organizing hematoma
Chondroblastoma	Myositis ossificans
Fibrous dysplasia	Schwannoma
Metaphyseal fibrous defect	Synovial sarcoma
Chondromyxoid fibroma	
Telangiectatic osteosarcoma	

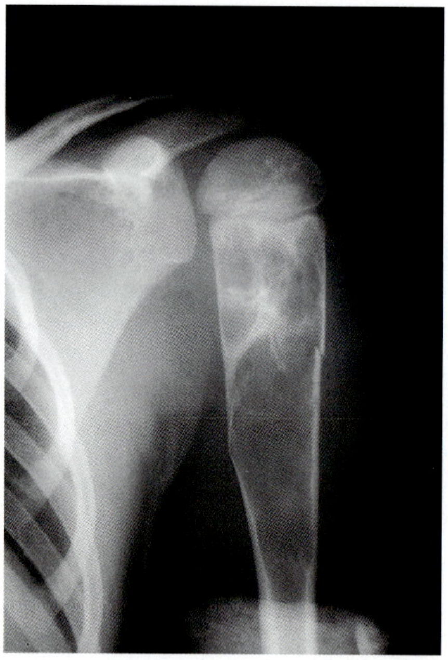

FIGURE 14.1 Solitary bone cyst. An anteroposterior radiograph of the proximal humerus shows a well-defined lytic lesion in the metaphysis. The lesion extends to the physis and slightly expands the metaphysis. A pathologic fracture has developed through the lateral aspect of the metaphysis.

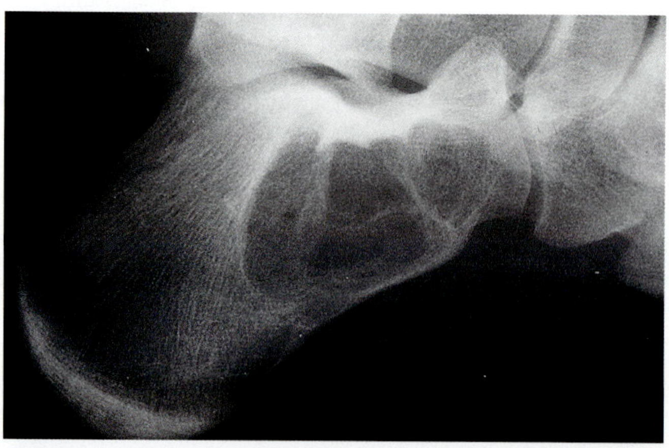

FIGURE 14.2 Solitary bone cyst. A lateral radiograph shows a well-defined lytic lesion in the body of the calcaneus. No periosteal reaction, cortical destruction, or soft tissue extension is observed.

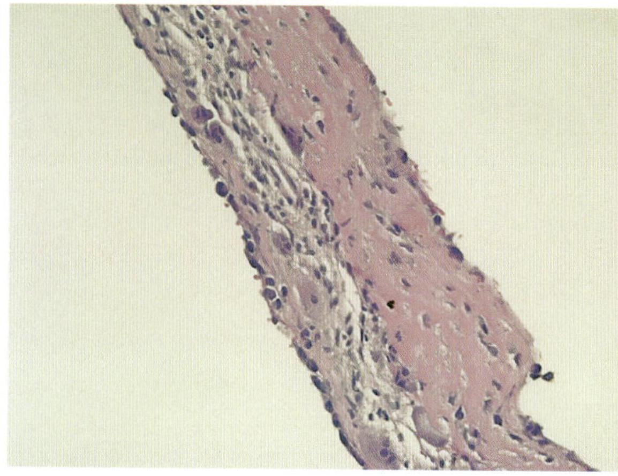

FIGURE 14.3 Solitary bone cyst exhibits a typical, thin fibrous cyst wall with benign-appearing fibroblasts, osteoclasts, and collagen deposition. (H&E.)

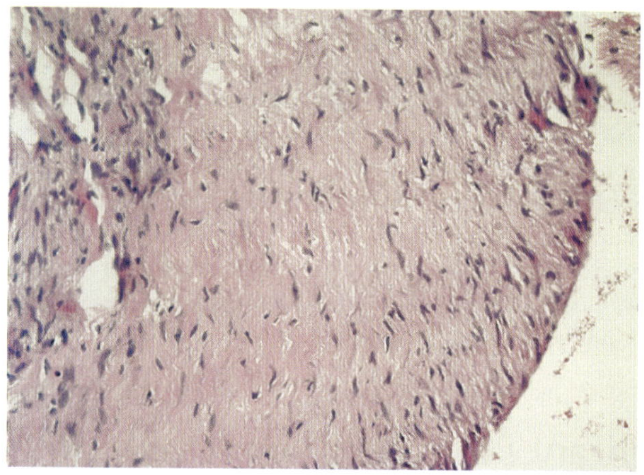

FIGURE 14.4 Solitary bone cyst with fibromyxoid changes. (H&E.)

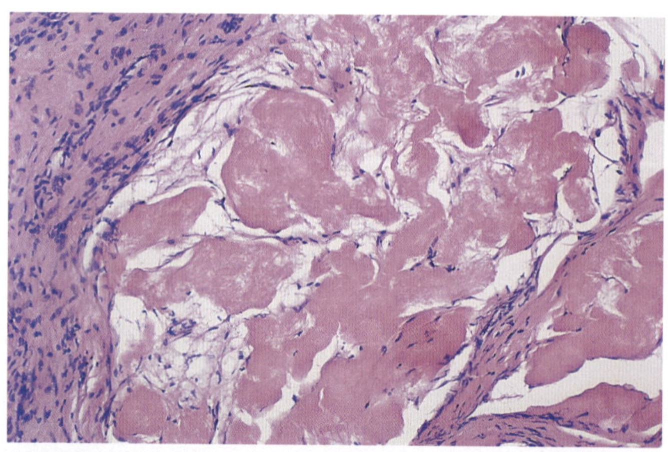

FIGURE 14.5 Fibrino-osteoid (cementum-like) material in a solitary bone cyst. (H&E.)

Even in the absence of fracture, reactive osteoid and bone may be evident within the cyst wall.

Fine Needle Aspiration Biopsy

Fine needle aspiration biopsy generally yields hypocellular-to-acellular, clear to slightly yellow fluid. Despite low-to-absent cellularity, the presence of this fluid coupled with classic radiographic features may be considered diagnostic for solitary bone cyst.

Therapy and Prognosis

The therapy of solitary bone cyst is controversial. Traditional treatment has included bone curettage and packing with bone chips. More recent therapy has employed aspiration and removal of cyst fluid followed by steroid injections. The overall local recurrence rate is similar for both types of therapy, ranging from 15% to 20%.[4] The rate of local recurrence seems to be greater among patients younger than 10 years old.

Aneurysmal Bone Cyst

Aneurysmal bone cyst generally is considered a reactive process, characteristically producing multiloculated, expansile lesions. Up to 50% of cases may be associated with other entities, primarily giant cell tumor, chondroblastoma, and fibrous dysplasia. Evidence suggests that "chromosome bands 16q22 and/or 17p11-13 are nonrandomly rearranged in aneurysmal bone cyst, irrespective of subtype (classic, solid, primary, secondary) and location (osseous or extraosseous)."[5] These findings raise the possibility that aneurysmal bone cyst may represent a neoplastic process.

Clinical Features

Aneurysmal bone cyst occurs predominantly before age 20 years but, similar to solitary bone cyst, may be observed at virtually any age. There seems to be a slight female predominance.[6,7] Complaints of pain and soft tissue swelling are frequently present. The metaphyseal regions of the long bones and vertebral column are the most common anatomic sites. Within the long bones, the distal femur and the proximal tibia commonly are affected. When aneurysmal bone cyst involves the vertebral column, the dorsal (posterior) arches and spinous processes typically are involved. Multiple bone involvement rarely may be seen with vertebral lesions. It has become apparent that aneurysmal bone cyst-like lesions also may occur in soft tissues, primarily involving the upper extremities.[8]

Radiographically, as expected, aneurysmal bone cyst produces an aneurysmal, lytic, metaphyseal-centered dilation of the affected long bone, generally well circumscribed with a sclerotic rim and often associated with periosteal new bone formation (Fig. 14.6). Involvement of the spine usually is seen as an expansile, lytic defect of the dorsal elements (Fig. 14.7). Less commonly, aneurysmal bone cyst may simulate a primary bone sarcoma with considerable cortical destruction.

Pathologic Findings

Histology

Cardinal morphologic features include the presence of numerous but variably-sized cavernous spaces filled with blood but lacking a definite endothelial lining, as observed in "true" vascular neoplasms. The cyst walls comprise randomly distributed fibroblasts, osteoclast-type giant cells, and variable amounts of osteoid and new bone formation (Fig. 14.8).[9] Less commonly, chondroid and hyaline cartilage may be observed (Fig. 14.9).[7] Within the fibroblastic areas, numerous mitotic figures may be present, but atypical forms are never seen. "Solid" lesions composed of similar-appearing collections of osteoclast-type giant cells, fibroblasts, and osteoid have been referred to as the *solid variant* of aneurysmal bone cyst (Fig. 14.10).[10] Regardless of anatomic location, all biopsy or curettage material from a suspected aneurysmal bone cyst should be sampled meticulously to exclude other pathologic entities, often associated with so-called secondary aneurysmal bone cyst, including but not limited to metaphyseal fibrous defect, fibrous dysplasia, chondroblastoma, chondromyxoid fibroma, osteoblastoma, and osteosarcoma. Additionally, cytologic atypia is not observed in

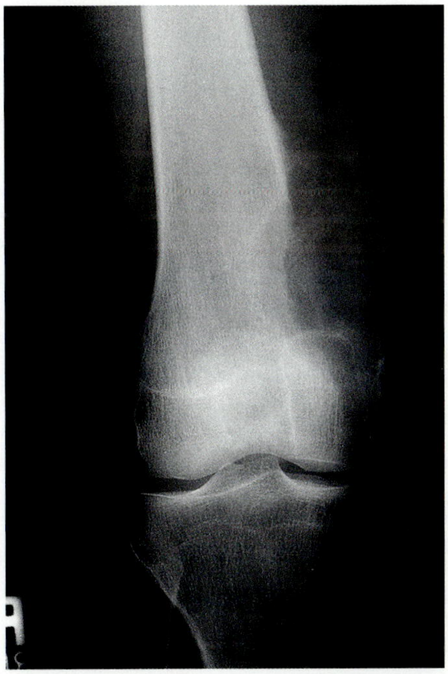

FIGURE 14.6 Aneurysmal bone cyst. An anteroposterior radiograph of the distal femur shows a lytic lesion in the metaphysis. The cortex is ballooned and expanded medially. A thin shell of periosteal new bone production is along the superior aspect of the lesion, but no matrix calcifications, suggesting a mesenchymal neoplasm, are observed.

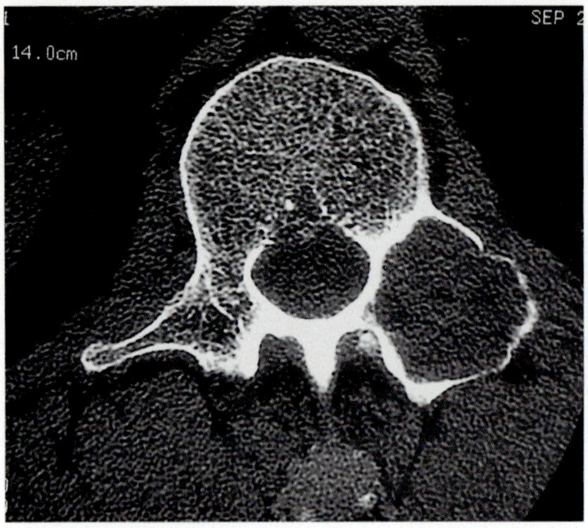

FIGURE 14.7 Aneurysmal bone cyst. A computed tomographic scan of a lumbar vertebral body shows an expansile lesion in the left articular pillar and pedicle. A thin shell of new bone production remains. The lesion spares the vertebral body centrum.

aneurysmal bone cysts and, if present, should raise the possibility of telangiectatic osteosarcoma.

Fine Needle Aspiration Biopsy

Fine needle aspiration biopsy generally yields scantly cellular smears with a few stromal fragments of benign-appearing fibroblasts, pigmented histiocytes, and individual osteoclast-type giant cells (Fig. 14.11). Because aneurysmal bone cysts may be engrafted onto other neoplasms, it may be impossible to exclude fully a pre-existing "precursor" lesion.

Therapy and Prognosis

Surgical intervention is often necessary and may include excision, curettage, and bone grafting.[7] Expendable bones, such as the fibula or rib, may be resected with a wide margin,

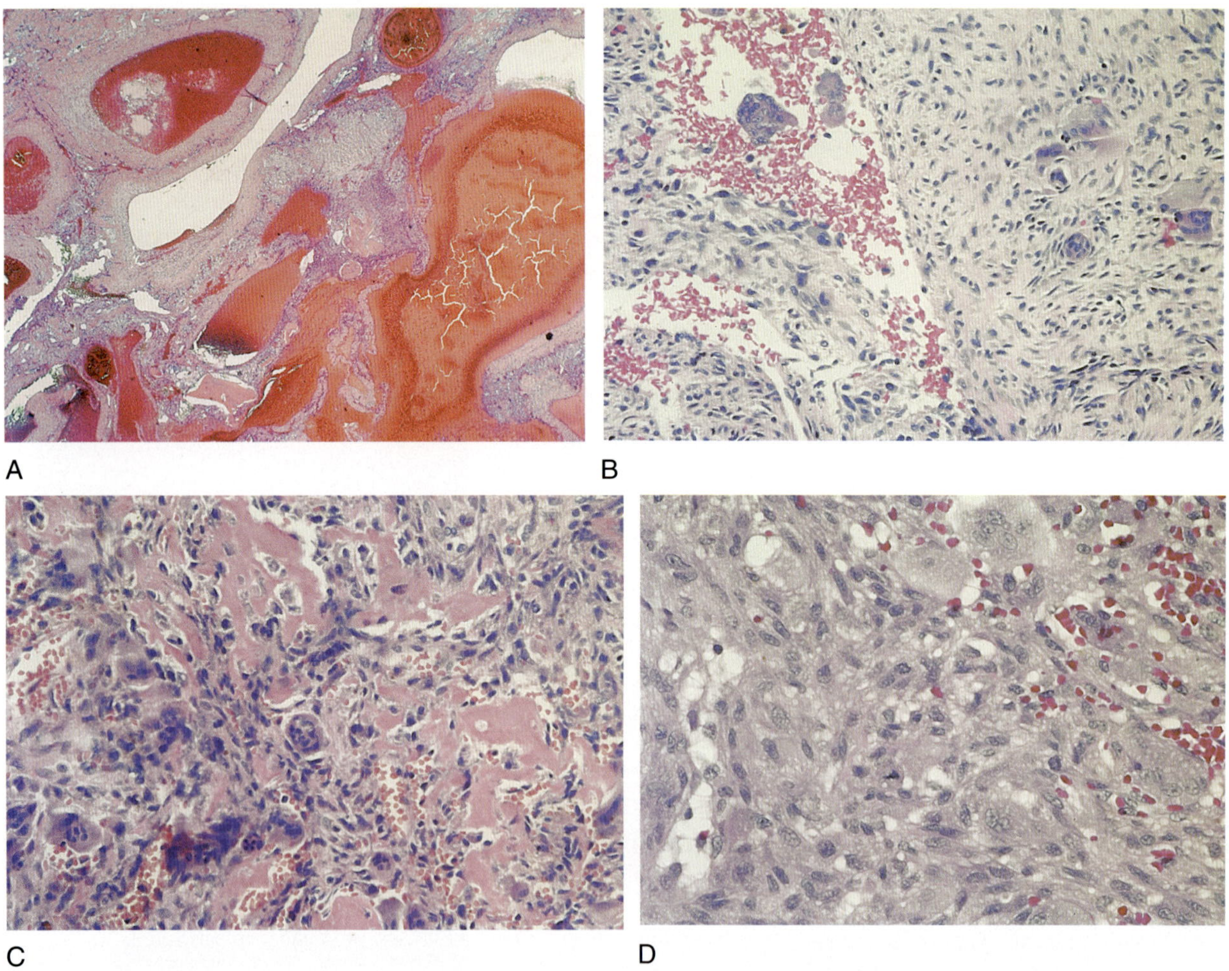

FIGURE 14.8 Aneurysmal bone cyst characterized by multilocular cystic spaces filled with blood **(A)**. The cyst walls are lined by mostly loose-appearing fibrous tissue with scattered osteoclasts **(B)**; osteoid or bone production usually is observed at least focally **(C)**. At high power, the individual fibroblasts (stromal cells) lack cytologic atypia, helping to distinguish aneurysmal bone cyst from telangiectatic osteosarcoma **(D)**. **(A-D,** H&E.)

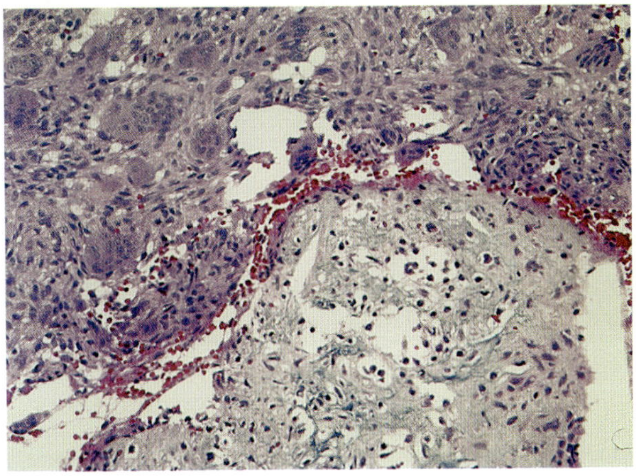

FIGURE 14.9 Infrequently, hyaline cartilage may be seen in aneurysmal bone cysts. (H&E.)

when necessary. Other less commonly used forms of therapy include low-dose radiation and cryotherapy. Local recurrence may occur in 19% of patients after curettage and seems to be more likely in younger patients (<20 years) and within the long bones.[7]

Subchondral Cyst

Subchondral cysts are arguably the most common form of bone cyst, occurring with degenerative joint disease in a variety of clinical settings, including osteoarthritis and rheumatoid arthritis. Although the pathogenesis is unclear, there is speculation that these cysts are the result of extravasation of synovial fluid through articular cartilage defects, secondary to a destructive arthritis.[11] Because of the typical clinical setting, most subchondral cysts are observed in older patients with a known history of degenerative joint disease. The hip bones, especially the proximal femur, are affected most commonly. Radiographically, subchondral bone cysts are lytic, sharply marginated lesions involving subchondral bone (Fig. 14.12).[11,12] Microscopically the cyst typically is surrounded by benign-appearing fibrous-to-fibromyxoid tissue without an obvious epithelial lining and may contain gelatinous-to-mucinous fluid (Fig. 14.13). No specific therapy is required.

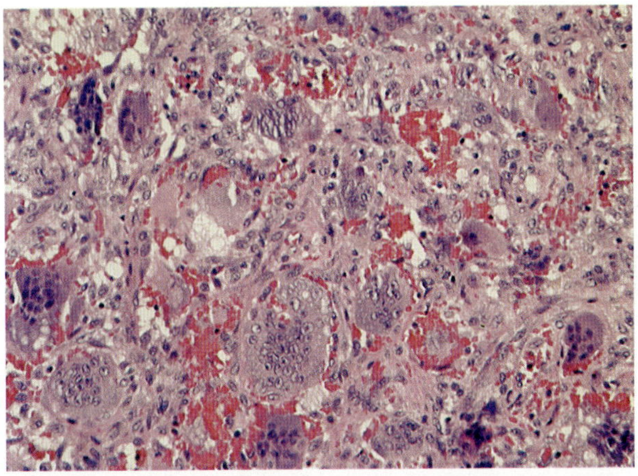

FIGURE 14.10 Solid aneurysmal bone cyst with loose-appearing, fibroblastic and hypervascular tissue and numerous, haphazardly arranged osteoclast-type giant cells. The appearance is remarkably similar to giant cell reparative granuloma and osseous lesions of hyperparathyroidism. (H&E.)

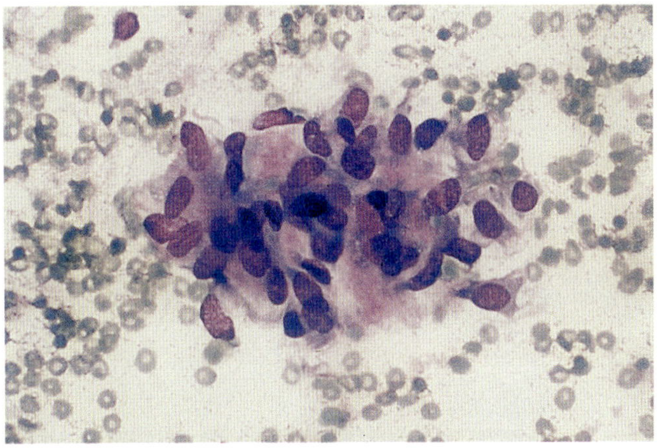

A

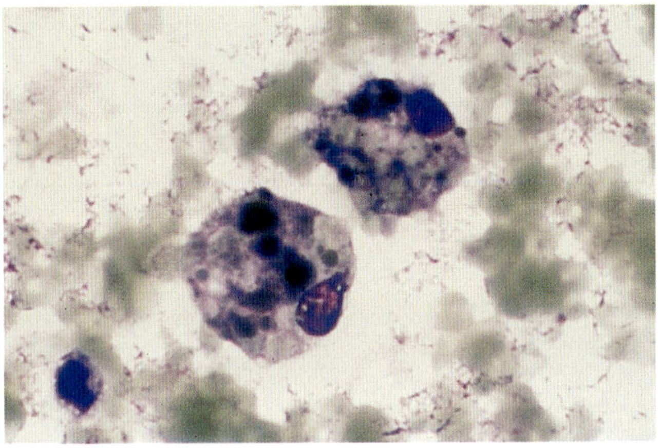

B

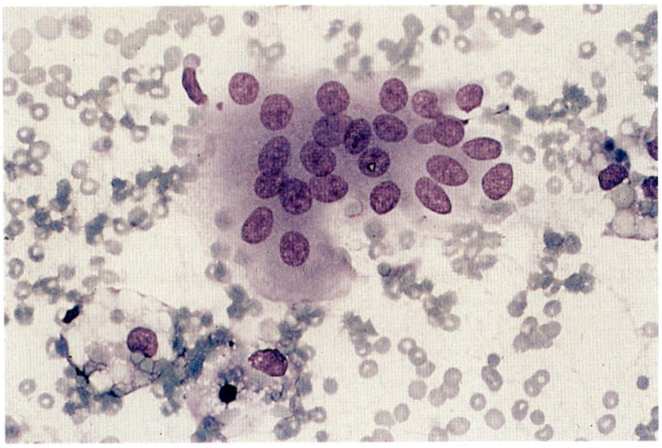

C

FIGURE 14.11 Fine needle aspiration biopsy of aneurysmal bone cyst with a few scattered aggregates of fibroblasts **(A)**, pigment-laden macrophages **(B)**, and osteoclasts **(C)**. **(A-C,** H&E.)

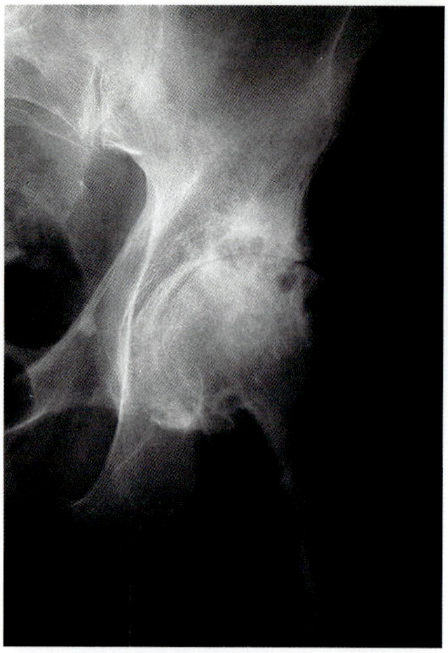

FIGURE 14.12 Subchondral bone cyst. An anteroposterior radiograph of the hip in a patient with severe primary osteoarthritis shows well-defined, lytic lesions in the subchondral bone of the femoral head and acetabulum. These subchondral cysts are not specific for osteoarthritis and may be seen in other degenerative conditions, including rheumatoid arthritis, hemophilic arthropathy, calcium pyrophosphate deposition disease, and osteonecrosis in subchondral bone.

Ganglion Cyst

Ganglion cysts may involve either soft tissue or bone. *Synovial cysts* and *juxta-articular bone cysts* refer to histologically identical lesions. As with most of the cysts discussed in this chapter, the pathogenesis of ganglion cyst is largely unknown.

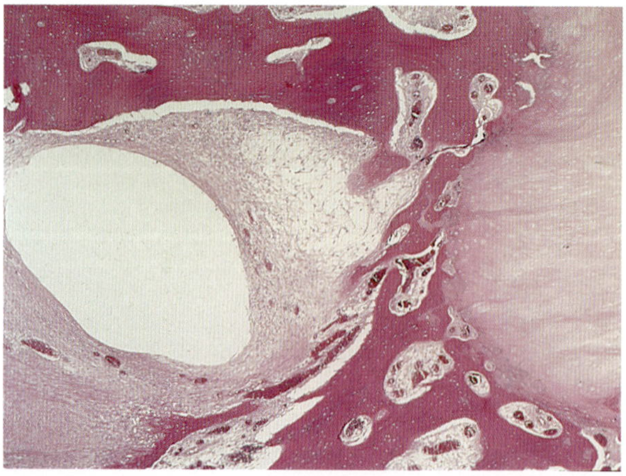

FIGURE 14.13 Subchondral bone cyst with fibromyxoid stroma and overlying degenerative articular cartilage. (H&E.)

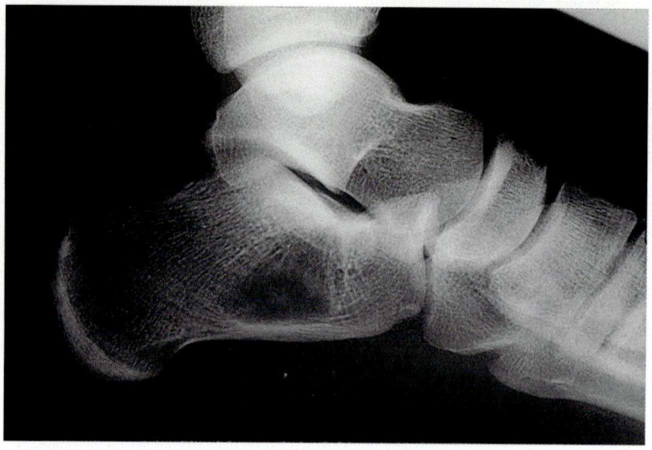

FIGURE 14.14 Ganglion cyst. A lateral radiograph shows a lytic lesion, closely resembling a solitary bone cyst, in the midcalcaneus. Although not observed in this case, computed tomography and magnetic resonance imaging may show communication of the ganglion cyst with an adjacent joint.

Clinical Features

Patients are usually between 30 and 50 years old, and men are affected slightly more commonly than women. Within soft tissues, most cases involve the dorsal aspects of the hand, often presenting as circumscribed and localized soft tissue swellings. Within bone, ganglion cysts localize to the following anatomic sites in decreasing order of frequency: distal tibia, proximal tibia, and proximal femur.[13,14] Less commonly, the small tubular bones of the hands and feet may be involved.

Radiographically, intraosseous ganglion cysts form eccentric, purely lytic lesions with sharply defined, sclerotic margins, exclusively localized to the epiphysis (Fig. 14.14). In contrast to subchondral bone cysts, the overlying articular surface shows no evidence of degenerative changes or destructive arthritis.

Pathologic Findings

Histology

Ganglion cysts consist of strands of variably thickened, fibrous-to-fibromyxoid tissue surrounding a gelatinous-to-mucinous, hypocellular-to-acellular fluid. A few randomly distributed histiocytes are often within the mucinous fluid (Fig. 14.15). Additionally, intraosseous ganglion cysts may be surrounded by reactive new bone formation.

Fine Needle Aspiration Biopsy

Fine needle aspiration biopsy may be used as a therapeutic approach for ganglion cysts and, in the appropriate clinical setting, is usually diagnostic. Cytologic smears from

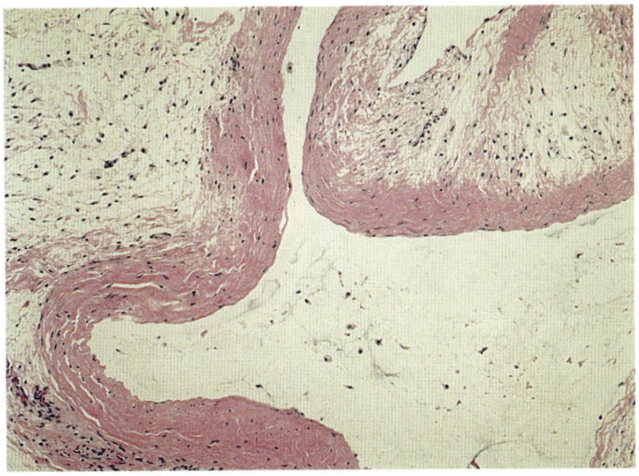

FIGURE 14.15 Ganglion cyst with benign-appearing fibromyxoid cyst wall and mucinous contents with a few histiocytes. (H&E.)

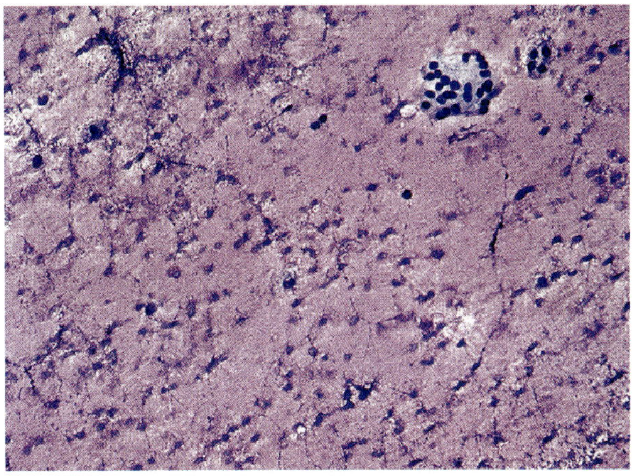

FIGURE 14.16 The mucinous contents of a ganglion cyst are observed best in Romanowsky preparations as a diffuse metachromatic film generally covering the entire slide. Scattered histiocytes are seen individually and in rare clusters. (Diff-Quik.)

either bone or soft tissue lesions are characteristically hypocellular and composed of a thick, mucinous, fluid film within which are scattered, benign-appearing histiocytes (Fig. 14.16).

Therapy and Prognosis

Therapy for soft tissue ganglion cyst may include aspiration or surgical excision. Curettage with bone grafting is generally curative for intraosseous lesions, although local recurrence occasionally occurs.[15]

REFERENCES

Solitary Bone Cyst

1. Norman A, Shiffman M: Simple bone cyst: Factors of age dependency. Radiology 1977;124:779.
2. Struhl S, Edelson C, Pritzker H, et al: Solitary (unicameral) bone cyst: The fallen fragment sign revisited. Skeletal Radiol 1989;18:261.
3. Mirra JM, Bernard CW, Bullough PG, et al: Cementum-like bone production in solitary bone cysts (so-called "cementoma" of long bones): Report of three cases: Electron microscopic observation supporting a synovial origin to the simple bone cyst. Clin Orthop 1978;135:295.
4. Capanna R, Albisinni U, Caroli GC, et al: Contrast examination as a prognostic factor in the treatment of solitary bone cyst by cortisone injection. Skeletal Radiol 1984;12:97.

Aneurysmal Bone Cyst

5. Sciot R, Dorfman HD, Brys P, et al: Cytogenetic-morphologic correlations in aneurysmal bone cyst, giant cell tumor of bone and combined lesions: A report from the CHAMP study group. Mod Pathol 2000;13:1206.
6. Tillman BP, Dahlin DC, Lipscomb PR, et al: Aneurysmal bone cyst: An analysis of ninety-five cases. Mayo Clin Proc 1968;43:478.
7. Vergel De Dios A, Bond JR, Shives TC: Aneurysmal bone cyst: A clinicopathologic study of 238 cases. Cancer 1992;69:2921.
8. Nielsen GP, Fletcher CDM, Smith MA, et al: Soft tissue aneurysmal bone cyst: A clinicopathologic study of five cases. Am J Surg Pathol 2002;26:64.
9. Dabska M, Buraczewski J: Aneurysmal bone cyst: Pathology, clinical course, and radiographic appearances. Cancer 1969;23:371.
10. Sanerkin NG, Mott MG, Roylance J: An unusual intraosseous lesion with fibroblastic, osteoclastic, osteoblastic, aneurysmal and fibromyxoid elements: "Solid" variant of aneurysmal bone cyst. Cancer 1983;51:2278.

Subchondral Cyst

11. Landells JW: The bone cysts of osteoarthritis. J Bone Joint Surg Br 1953;35:643.
12. Rahney K, Lamb DW: The cysts of osteoarthritis of the hip: A radiographic and pathological study. J Bone Joint Surg Br 1955;37:663.

Ganglion Cyst

13. Bauer TW, Dorfman HD: Intraosseous ganglion: A clinicopathologic study of 11 cases. Am J Surg Pathol 1982;6:207.
14. Pope TL Jr, Fechner RE, Keats TE: Intra-osseous ganglion: Report of four cases and review of the literature. Skeletal Radiol 1989;18:185.
15. Schajowicz F, Clavel Sainz M, Slullitel JA: Juxta-articular bone cysts (intra-osseous ganglia): A clinicopathologic study of eighty-eight cases. J Bone Joint Surg Br 1979;61:107.

CHAPTER 15

Nonmesenchymal Tumors of Bone and Soft Tissue

Although one usually associates mesenchymal lesions with bone and soft tissue tumors, nonmesenchymal tumors occur with relatively high frequency, especially involving the skeleton. Neoplasms of nonmesenchymal origin that secondarily may involve connective tissues are summarized in Table 15.1. Hematopoietic disorders are discussed in Chapter 3. This chapter concentrates mainly on metastatic carcinoma but also emphasizes malignant melanoma, especially the spindle cell (desmoplastic) variant, and spindle cell (sarcomatoid) carcinoma.

Metastatic Carcinoma

Metastatic disease may affect bone and extraskeletal soft tissues; however, involvement of the skeleton is much more common. It is well documented that cancer affecting the skeleton is more commonly metastatic than primary.[1,2] Overall the skeleton is the third most common site for metastases. Approximately 15% to 20% of cancer patients develop clinically evident skeletal metastases; however, large autopsy series show a much higher incidence, presumably owing to the ability to detect clinically silent or asymptomatic lesions.[3] In a series of patients with skeletal metastases reviewed by Katagiri and colleagues,[4] 30% had bone lesions as the initial manifestation of disease.

TABLE 15.1 Nonmesenchymal Tumors That May Involve Bone and Soft Tissues

Metastatic carcinoma
Malignant melanoma
Malignant lymphoma
Hodgkin's disease

Clinical Features

Clinically, patients with skeletal metastases may have pain, pathologic fractures, problems with local neuromuscular function, or disruption of bone marrow hematopoiesis.[2] Anatomically, the axial skeleton is involved in 70% of cases, followed, in decreasing order of frequency, by the appendicular skeleton and craniofacial regions; skeletal metastasis beyond or distal to the knee or elbow is rare.[5,6]

In adults, approximately 80% of metastases are from primary adenocarcinomas of the breast, prostate, lung, kidney, or thyroid.[7] In children, neuroblastoma, rhabdomyosarcoma, and retinoblastoma are the most common initiators of skeletal metastatic disease. Rare cases of virtually every malignant neoplasm have been observed, however, to metastasize to bone.

Radiographically, a wide variety of responses to metastatic tumor may be elicited. These associated non-neoplastic reactions are generally easy to distinguish from metastatic disease, but the importance of knowledge of the different possible patterns should not be underemphasized. Metastases are most often destructive and osteolytic (Fig. 15.1). The osteolytic process may result in pathologic fracture, a common clinical presentation of bony metastases.[2] The fracture in turn may elicit callus formation, causing various degrees of fibrocartilaginous proliferation that may mask metastatic disease or simulate a primary bone tumor. Less commonly, metastases may be osteoblastic, especially carcinomas arising from prostate or breast in adults (see Fig. 15.1). In children, osteoblastic examples include medulloblastoma, osteosarcoma, carcinoid tumors, and occasionally retinoblastoma. The osteoblastic response may be so pronounced as to obscure the underlying neoplasm. Additionally, periosteal reactions may be observed, with or without soft tissue extension.

In the examination of bone lesions, the fundamental role of the pathologist is to provide an accurate diagnosis. Consequently, several questions must be answered. Figure 15.2

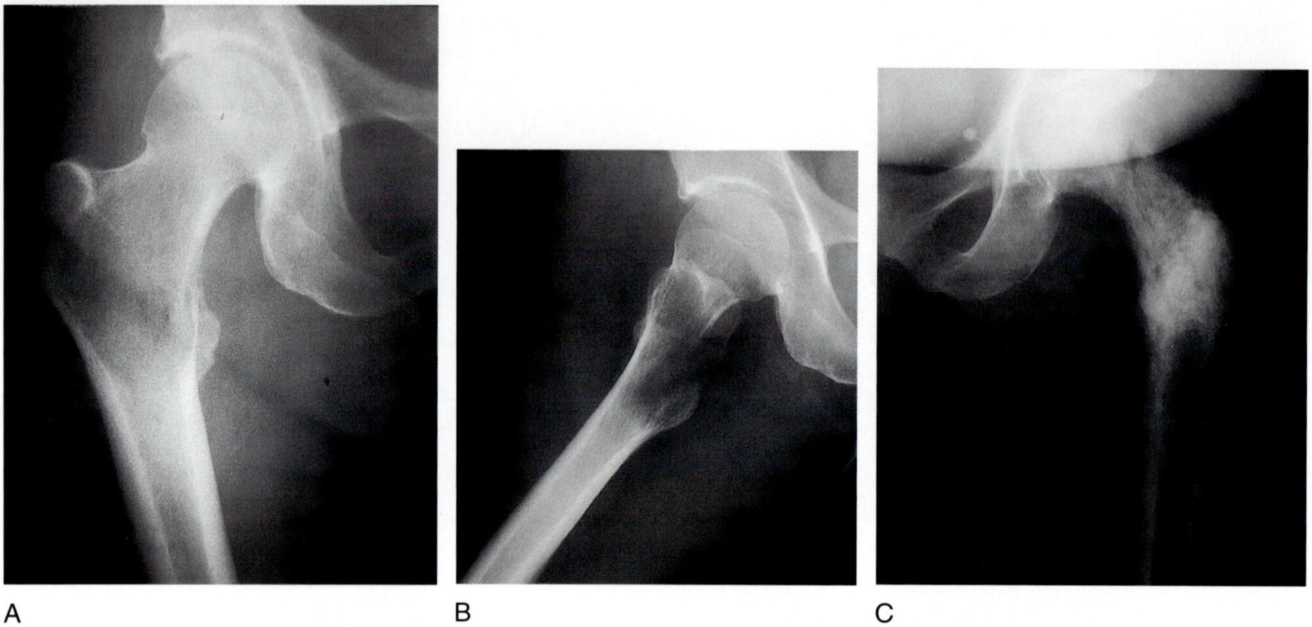

FIGURE 15.1 Metastatic hepatocellular carcinoma **(A** and **B)** and metastatic prostate carcinoma **(C)**. Anteroposterior **(A)** and lateral **(B)** radiographs of the proximal femur show an extensive, purely lytic tumor at the level of the lesser trochanter of the proximal femur. No blastic response is evident. The appearances are not specific for hepatocellular carcinoma metastases because a wide variety of other primary tumors may produce purely lytic metastatic disease in bone. An anteroposterior radiograph **(C)** of the left hip shows an extensive osteoblastic lesion in the proximal left femur, extending from the femoral neck to the subtrochanteric portion of the femur. The osteoblastic response should be distinguished from osteoid matrix calcification associated with primary mesenchymal neoplasm.

illustrates a useful algorithm. The first goal is the exclusion of a non-neoplastic process, such as an infectious, inflammatory, or metabolic lesion. When the lesion is proved to be neoplastic, a primary bone tumor must be excluded, at which point one can be relatively certain the lesion is metastatic. If a diagnosis of metastasis is rendered, the pathologist must categorize the tumor further. The clinical history is an invaluable resource, and comparison of the histology of the metastasis with that of the patient's known primary tumor often provides a definitive diagnosis; however, in other cases, tissue sections from the primary tumor may be unavailable for comparison. The pathologist must rely on other clues to aid in further classifying the tumor into one of several categories. The most common metastatic tumors are carcinomas,[2] but the possibility of a hematopoietic disorder (plasmacytoma, lymphoma, leukemia) or sarcoma also must be considered. If the lesion is a carcinoma, additional histologic classification may suggest common anatomic origins of the tumor type, as summarized in Table 15.2. Of patients with cancer, however, 3% to 4% have metastatic disease without a known primary.[8]

Pathologic Findings

Histology

The histopathologic appearance of metastatic bone lesions varies from obvious, well-differentiated tumors with distinctive features that readily suggest a specific primary site to more poorly differentiated examples, requiring ancillary studies for further classification. Rarely, neoplasms defy specific characterization. As previously stated, carcinoma, especially adenocarcinoma, is the most common histologic type of metastasis to bone in adults. Well-differentiated to

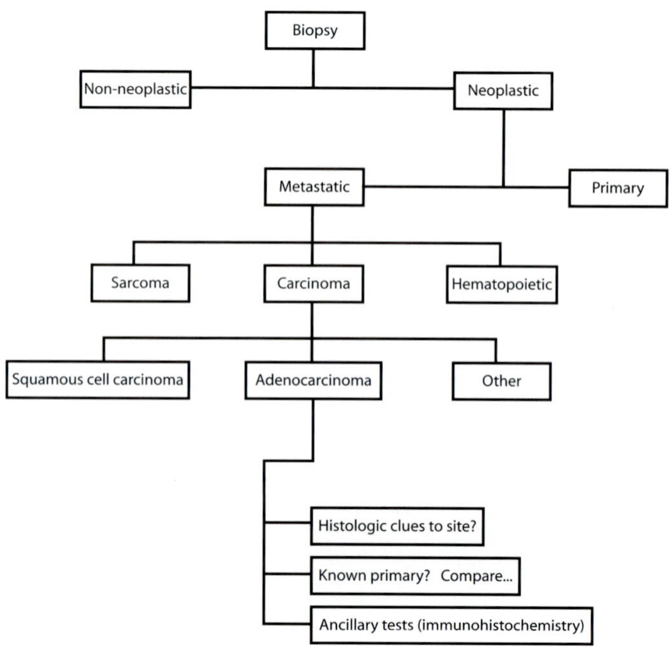

FIGURE 15.2 Algorithm for the work-up of a previously undiagnosed bone lesion.

TABLE 15.2 Relationship of Common Histologic Subtypes of Carcinoma to Anatomic Sites

Subtype	Anatomic Site
Adenocarcinoma	Breast
	Prostate
	Lung
	Kidney
	Thyroid
	Gastrointestinal tract
	Pancreas
	Gallbladder and biliary tract
	Endometrium/endocervix
Squamous cell carcinoma	Head and neck
	Lung
	Skin
	Ectocervix
Transitional cell carcinoma	Urinary bladder
	Ureters
	Renal pelvis
Small cell carcinoma	Lung

moderately differentiated carcinomas often have features specific for a particular type of carcinoma. Specific examples, well known to most pathologists, include adenocarcinoma (duct or glandular formation, mucin production, eccentric nuclei, prominent nucleoli), squamous cell carcinoma (keratin formation, densely eosinophilic cytoplasm, intercytoplasmic bridges), and small cell carcinoma (round-to-ovoid, hyperchromatic nuclei, high nuclear-to-cytoplasmic ratios with scant cytoplasm, nuclear molding) (Fig. 15.3). Examples of features that readily identify primary sites include colloid-filled follicles of well-differentiated follicular carcinoma of the thyroid and clusters of round to polygonal-shaped cells with clear cytoplasm amid a hypervascular stroma that suggest renal cell carcinoma (Fig. 15.4). Many examples of metastatic adenocarcinoma do not show site-specific morphologic characteristics, sometimes necessitating the use of ancillary studies. Complicating matters further, some carcinomas exhibit a predominant spindle cell population, such as spindled squamous cell carcinomas or sarcomatoid renal cell carcinomas. As a result, these tumors may mimic primary or metastatic sarcoma (Fig. 15.5). For this reason, we recommend excluding the diagnosis of metastatic carcinoma in any sarcomatoid lesion arising in the skeleton of older (>50 years old) patients. Occasionally, epithelioid sarcomas and malignant lymphomas, particularly large cell anaplastic lymphoma, may mimic poorly differentiated carcinomas and should be considered.

As previously mentioned, neuroblastoma, rhabdomyosarcoma, and retinoblastoma are the most common metastatic tumors to involve the skeleton in children. Clear cell sarcoma of the kidney, also known as bone-metastasizing renal tumor of childhood, is another rare tumor seen in children with a high propensity to cause multiple lytic bone lesions during the course of the disease.

Metastatic carcinomas sometimes elicit a prominent osteoblastic response, at times mimicking a primary bone tumor (Fig. 15.6). Inflammatory changes, including lymphoplasmacytic infiltrates, also may be seen. We have seen a case in which a granulomatous inflammatory response to a metastasis not only simulated an infectious process, but also masked the underlying malignancy. In these cases, histochemical stains for infectious organisms (Gomori's methenamine silver, acid-fast bacilli) should be negative, whereas immunohistochemical stains (i.e., cytokeratin) may be helpful in recognizing the occult tumor. Careful correlation with clinical and radiographic findings is imperative.

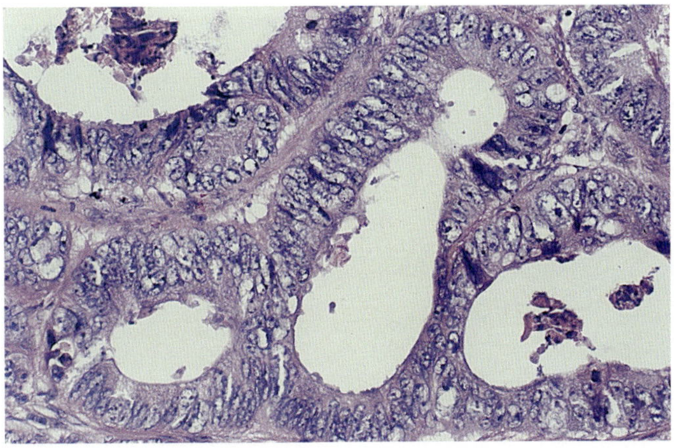

A

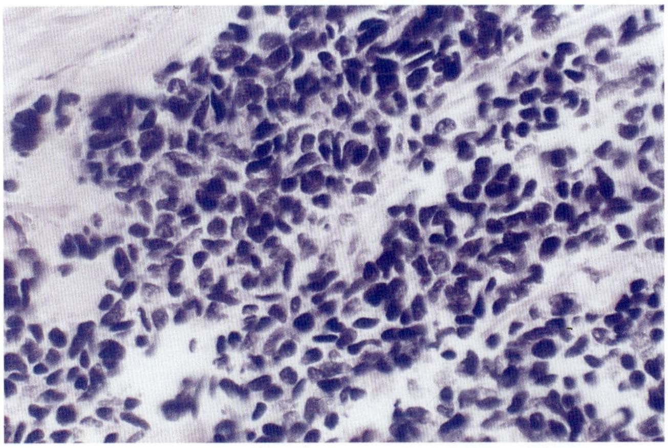

B

FIGURE 15.3 Colonic adenocarcinoma with well-formed glands and pseudostratification of nuclei **(A)**. Small cell carcinoma characterized by sheets of mostly uniform cells with hyperchromatic nuclei, high nuclear-to-cytoplasmic ratios, and nuclear molding **(B)**. (**A** and **B**, H&E.)

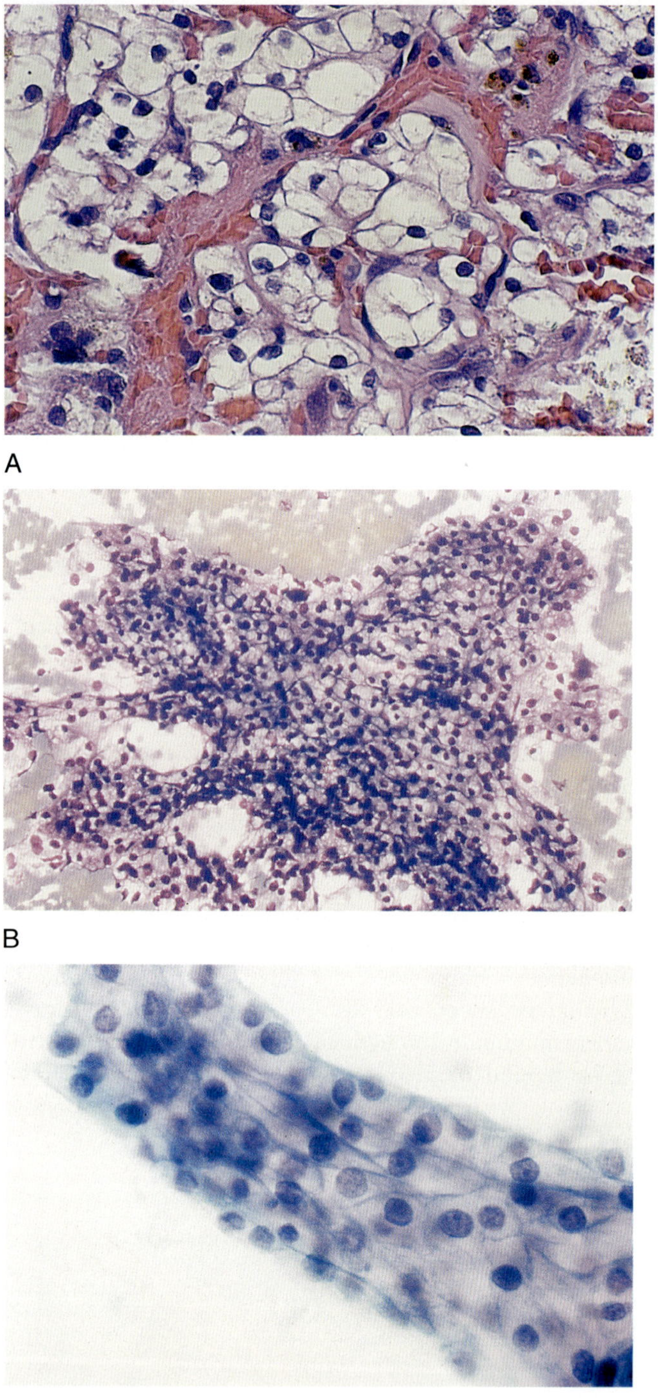

FIGURE 15.4 Metastatic renal cell carcinoma forming cohesive nests and aggregates of mostly uniform cells with abundant clear cytoplasm, as observed in histologic specimens **(A)** and cytologic specimens **(B** and **C)**. **(A,** H&E; **B,** Diff-Quik; **C,** Papanicolaou.)

Fine Needle Aspiration Biopsy

Cytologic smears from metastatic carcinomas are generally hypercellular and composed of cohesive aggregates of round-to-polygonal, epithelioid cells. Intracytoplasmic vacuoles, eccentrically located nuclei, and, rarely, glandular structures indicate adenocarcinoma (Fig. 15.7). Keratinization, best visualized in Papanicolaou preparations, is characteristic of squamous cell carcinoma (Fig. 15.8). A uniform cell population with high nuclear-to-cytoplasmic ratios and nuclear molding suggests small cell carcinoma.

For the evaluation of primary and metastatic tumors in bone, the diagnostic accuracy of fine needle aspiration biopsy approaches 95%, a relatively high degree of accuracy considering the size of the sample obtained with this technique.[9–11]

Ancillary Studies

The use of ancillary techniques, such as serum tumor markers, flow cytometry, immunohistochemistry, cytogenetics, and electron microscopy, greatly expands the data used to arrive at a correct diagnosis. It cannot be overemphasized that these studies must be considered in the clinical context, incorporating patient history, radiographs, and light microscopy. For most pathologic practices, immunohistochemistry has become the most commonly used ancillary test for the work-up of

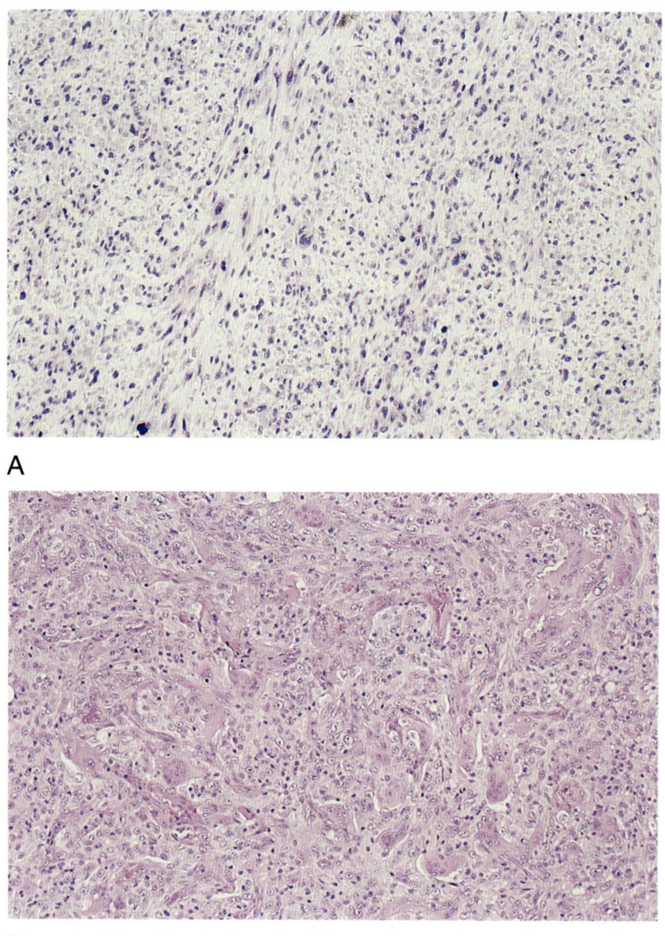

FIGURE 15.5 Sarcomatoid carcinoma may exhibit a wide variety of appearances, ranging from fascicles of tumor cells within a loose, myxoid stroma **(A)** to more solid, compact features. The presence of osteoclast-type giant cells also may confound the diagnosis **(B)**. **(A** and **B,** H&E.)

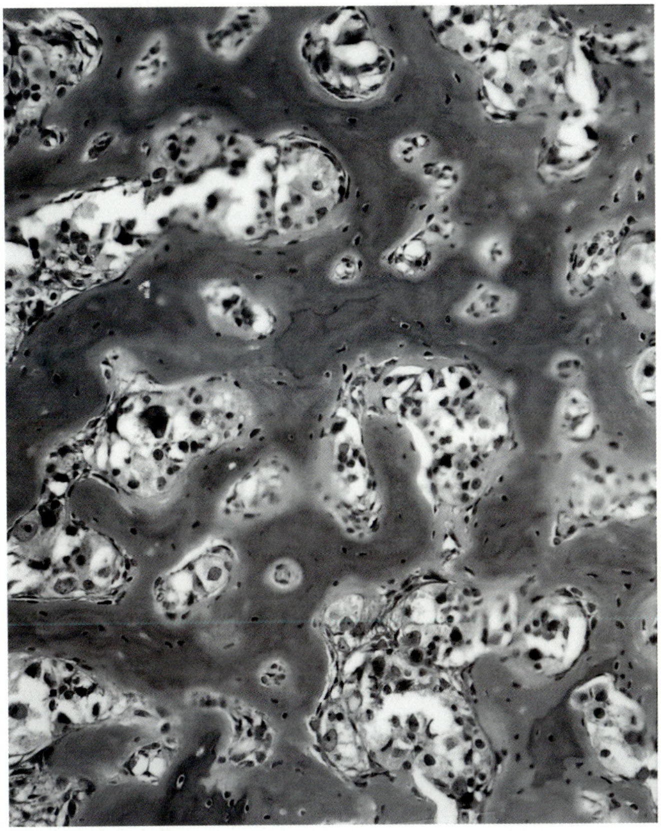

FIGURE 15.6 Metastatic prostatic carcinoma associated with an extensive osteoblastic response, obscuring the underlying carcinoma. (H&E.)

unknown tumors. Table 15.3 lists common immunohistochemical stains that may aid in characterization of metastatic tumors. For metastatic carcinomas arising in males, the most useful immunohistochemical marker is prostate-specific antigen because of its high sensitivity and specificity for prostate adenocarcinoma. Thyroglobulin is useful for papillary, follicular, and anaplastic carcinomas of the thyroid but is not expressed by medullary carcinomas. Helpful immunohistochemical markers in the latter include calcitonin and carcinoembryonic antigen (CEA). Among metastatic carcinomas arising in women, estrogen/progesterone receptors and CA-125 are especially useful, albeit not totally specific, for confirming breast and ovarian serous adenocarcinomas. In our experience, probably because of its low sensitivity, we have not found gross cystic disease fluid protein-15 particularly useful in confirming or excluding metastatic breast adenocarcinoma. CEA is generally positive in most adenocarcinomas, and its expression does not usually help in identifying a specific primary site. CEA is generally negative, however, in adrenal and renal cell carcinomas.

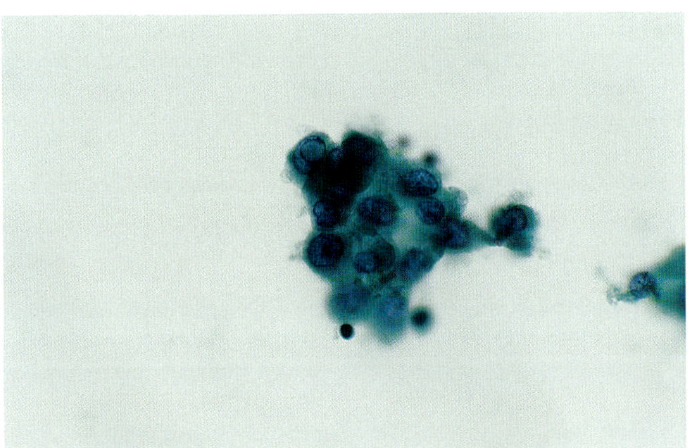

FIGURE 15.7 Metastatic adenocarcinoma with focal glandular differentiation. (Papanicolaou.)

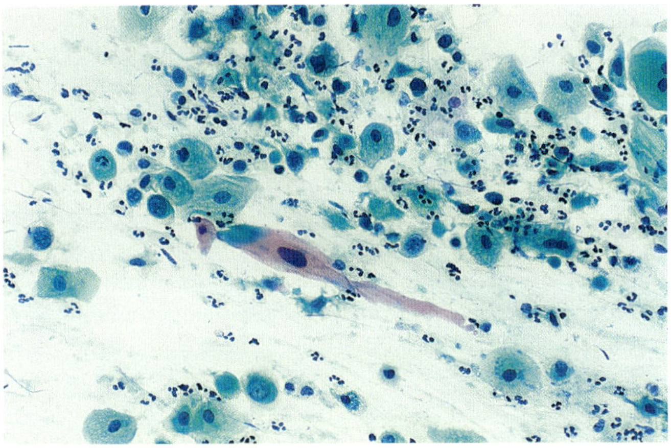

FIGURE 15.8 Squamous cell carcinoma with "tadpole"-shaped cell with keratinization. (Papanicolaou.)

TABLE 15.3 Immunohistochemical Stains for Evaluation of Metastases

Antigen	Associated Tumor Type
Cytokeratin	Carcinomas
CEA (carcinoembryonic antigen)	Adenocarcinomas, especially gastrointestinal tract
CA-125 (cancer antigen)	Serous adenocarcinomas of the female genital tract
Chromogranin	Neuroendocrine carcinomas, including small cell
Synaptophysin	Neuroendocrine carcinomas, including small cell
LCA (leukocyte common antigen)	Hematopoietic lesions (lymphoma)
ER (estrogen receptor)	Breast, ovary, endometrial tumors
PR (progesterone receptor)	Breast, ovary, endometrial tumors
GCDFP-15 (gross cystic disease fluid protein-15)	Breast, apocrine differentiation
Thyroglobulin	Thyroid carcinomas (excluding medullary)
PSA (prostate-specific antigen)	Prostatic adenocarcinoma
PAP (prostatic acid phosphatase)	Prostatic adenocarcinoma

Cytokeratins or keratins are intracellular proteins that are present in virtually all epithelia. Because most skeletal metastases are of epithelial origin, the presence of cytokeratin expression is not generally helpful. On the basis of their molecular weight, several subclasses of cytokeratin have been identified, however, and some of these seem to be more specific for certain epithelia than others. Consequently an especially popular and useful profile for carcinomas of unknown origin is cytokeratin 7 and cytokeratin 20. The relationship of this profile among various carcinoma subtypes and origins is summarized in Table 15.4.

Prognosis and Therapy

The overall prognosis in a patient with metastatic disease to the skeleton is generally dismal but ultimately depends, to a large extent, on the subtype and origin of the tumor. Survival rates for metastatic small cell carcinoma of the lung are generally worse than rates observed with metastatic breast carcinoma. If performed at all, surgical therapy and radiation therapy are usually palliative and generally focus on quality of life and functional issues. The role of chemotherapy, similar to prognosis, depends on the type and origin of the carcinoma in question.

Sarcomatoid (Spindle Cell) Carcinoma

For spindle cell malignancies arising in the skin, mucosa, or visceral organs, especially among adults older than age 50, one always must consider the diagnosis of sarcomatoid (spindle cell) carcinoma. Sarcomatoid carcinomas are observed most often in squamous cell carcinoma arising from the mucous membranes of the head and neck region, but also are a well-recognized phenomenon in the kidney.[13] Nevertheless, these tumors may arise in virtually any viscera, including the breast, lung, gastrointestinal tract, urinary bladder, and prostate gland.[14-18] Most clinicians consider sarcomatoid carcinomas to represent a form of metaplastic change.[15,18]

Morphologically, sarcomatoid carcinomas generally are arranged as fascicles of mostly uniform but moderately pleomorphic, frankly malignant tumor cells with ovoid-to-elongated vesicular nuclei, prominent nucleoli, and abundant eosinophilic cytoplasm. Marked nuclear pleomorphism, fascicles, and occasional storiform patterns, resembling malignant fibrous histiocytoma, sometimes are observed (see Fig. 15.5). The histologic findings are relatively nonspecific, however, and, in the clinical context of a mucosal-based or visceral tumor, should prompt a meticulous search for a mucosal in situ component or a more obvious epithelioid carcinomatous pattern (e.g., clear cell carcinoma of the kidney) or both. Less commonly, the sarcomatoid pattern may exhibit one or more heterologous elements, including osteosarcoma, chondrosarcoma, liposarcoma, leiomyosarcoma, and rhabdomyosarcoma. Depending on the anatomic site in which these tumors arise, a variety of designations have been applied to them. In the breast, these tumors are called *metaplastic carcinomas*[15]; in the lung and prostate, they are called *carcinosarcomas*[16,17]; and in the gynecologic organs, they are called *malignant mixed müllerian tumors*.[18] Regardless of anatomic site, it is most important therapeutically that sarcomatoid carcinomas be recognized as *carcinomas* and not diagnosed as primary sarcomas.

Rarely an epithelioid component or, if applicable, overlying mucosal carcinoma in situ is not readily identifiable, necessitating the use of ancillary studies. In most cases, if a

TABLE 15.4 Relationship of Cytokeratin 7 and Cytokeratin 20 Profiles to Carcinoma Subtypes and Origins

Result	Usually	Sometimes	Virtually Never
CK 7+, CK 20+	Urothelial (transitional), pancreatic, ovarian (mucinous)	Gastric, lung (adenocarcinoma), gallbladder and bile duct, breast, colorectal, thyroid, prostate, endometrial, small intestine, hepatoma	Lung (squamous and small cell), ovarian (nonmucinous), renal cell
CK 7+, CK 20−	Ovarian (nonmucinous), breast, gallbladder and bile duct, thyroid, endometrium, small intestine, lung (adenocarcinoma)	Pancreatic, urothelial (transitional), gastric, renal cell, lung (small cell)	Lung (squamous cell), colorectal
CK 7−, CK 20+	Colorectal	Gastric, prostate, pancreas, breast (ductal), lung (squamous)	Lung (adenocarcinoma and small cell), urothelial (transitional), breast (lobular), ovarian, endometrial
CK 7−, CK 20−	Lung (squamous and small cell), hepatoma, prostate, renal cell	Colorectal, gastric, lung (adenocarcinoma), endometrial	Urothelial (transitional), pancreas, ovarian (nonmucinous), breast

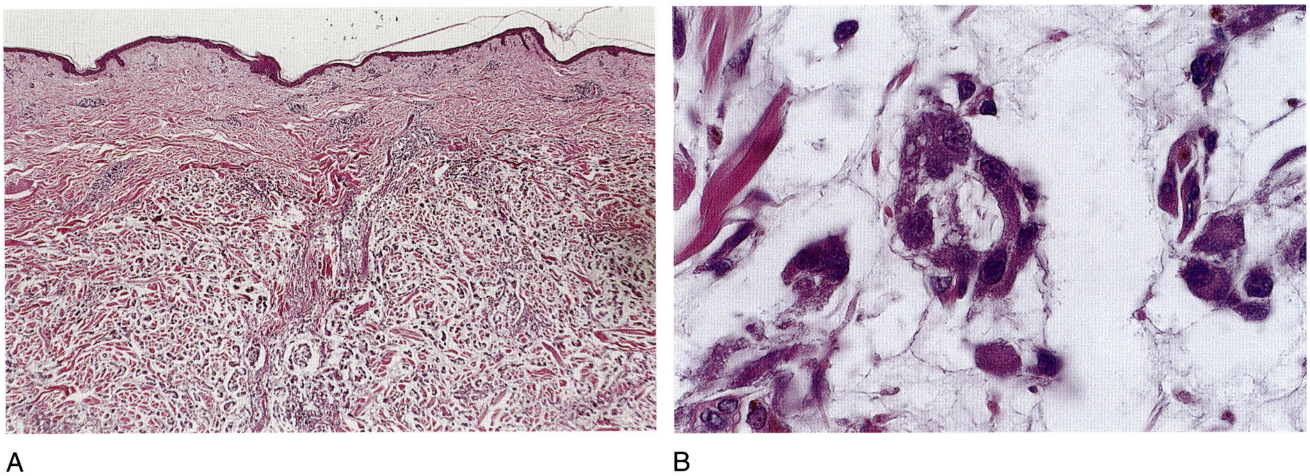

FIGURE 15.9 Myxoid melanoma resembling a primary myxofibrosarcoma (**A** and **B**). (**A**, Low power; H&E; **B**, high power, H&E.) (Courtesy of Dr. Michael Hitchcock.)

panel of keratin subsets is used, expression of one or more keratins is observed in the sarcomatoid component. With rare exception, definite keratin immunoexpression in a fibrosarcomatous or malignant fibrous histiocytoma-like neoplasm arising in skin, mucosal-based lesions, or visceral organs confirms the diagnosis of sarcomatoid carcinoma.

Malignant Melanoma

No discussion of mesenchymal mimics is complete without mentioning the differential diagnosis of melanoma. As with sarcomatoid carcinoma, the recognition and separation of melanoma from primary sarcoma is essential for proper therapy and follow-up. A small (1 cm) superficial sarcoma that is excised completely likely represents a cure, even if the tumor is high grade. Conversely, a small (1 cm) but level 5 melanoma often is associated with metastatic disease and death. For this reason, the diagnosis of melanoma always should be entertained in any epithelioid or spindle cell lesion arising from skin or a mucosal surface.

From a morphologic perspective, no neoplasm shows the range of histologic patterns and cell types as does melanoma (Figs. 15.9 to 15.11).[19] In less common clinical settings, only a high index of suspicion results in the recognition of melanoma. The overlying skin or mucosal surface always must be inspected carefully for the characteristic dermoepidermal junctional component (Fig. 15.12). This diagnostic junctional component may be absent, especially in metastatic melanoma. In our experience, the finding of melanin pigment is not sufficiently present in most cases to warrant its usefulness as a reliable diagnostic criterion. Most melanomas appear as variably-sized nests of mostly uniform, epithelioid-appearing tumor cells with vesicular nuclei; prominent and large nucleoli; and abundant, clear-to-eosinophilic, eccentrically placed cytoplasm. Binucleated forms, especially in cytologic preparations, frequently are observed. Most pathologists are familiar with the aforementioned features. Less often, but

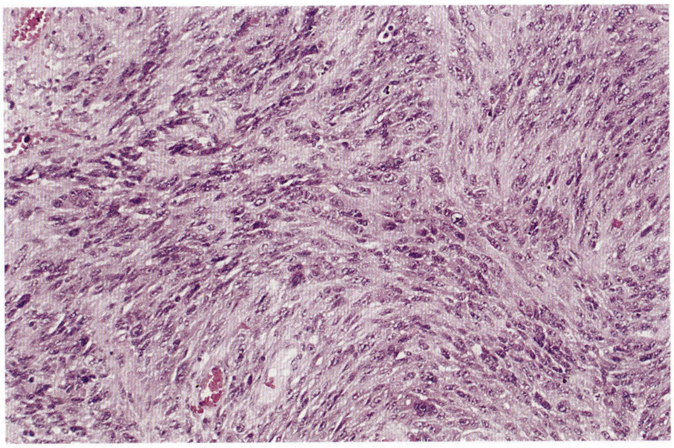

FIGURE 15.10 Fascicles of spindle cell melanoma with vague storiform patterns, resembling malignant fibrous histiocytoma. (H&E.)

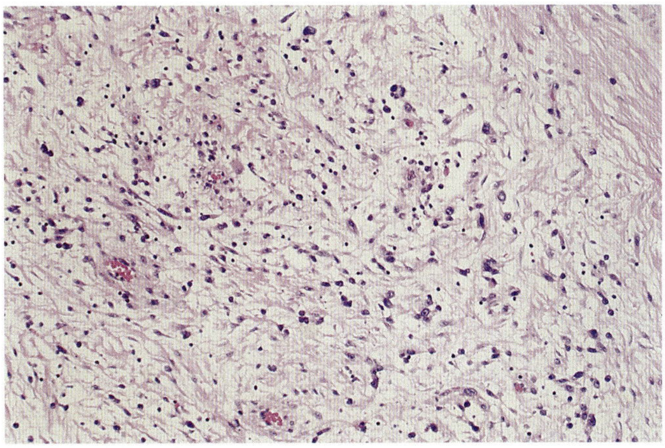

FIGURE 15.11 Spindle cell melanoma with ill-defined, loose fascicles of spindle-shaped tumor cells. Note the multinucleated tumor giant cells. (H&E.)

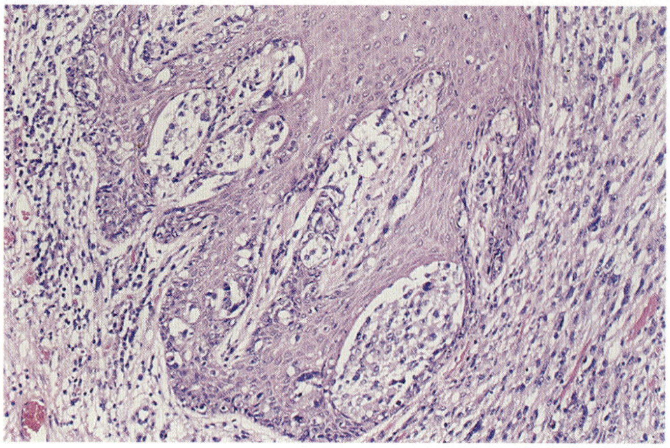

FIGURE 15.12 The finding of a junctional component in this desmoplastic spindle cell melanoma of the oral mucosa helps confirm the diagnosis. (H&E.)

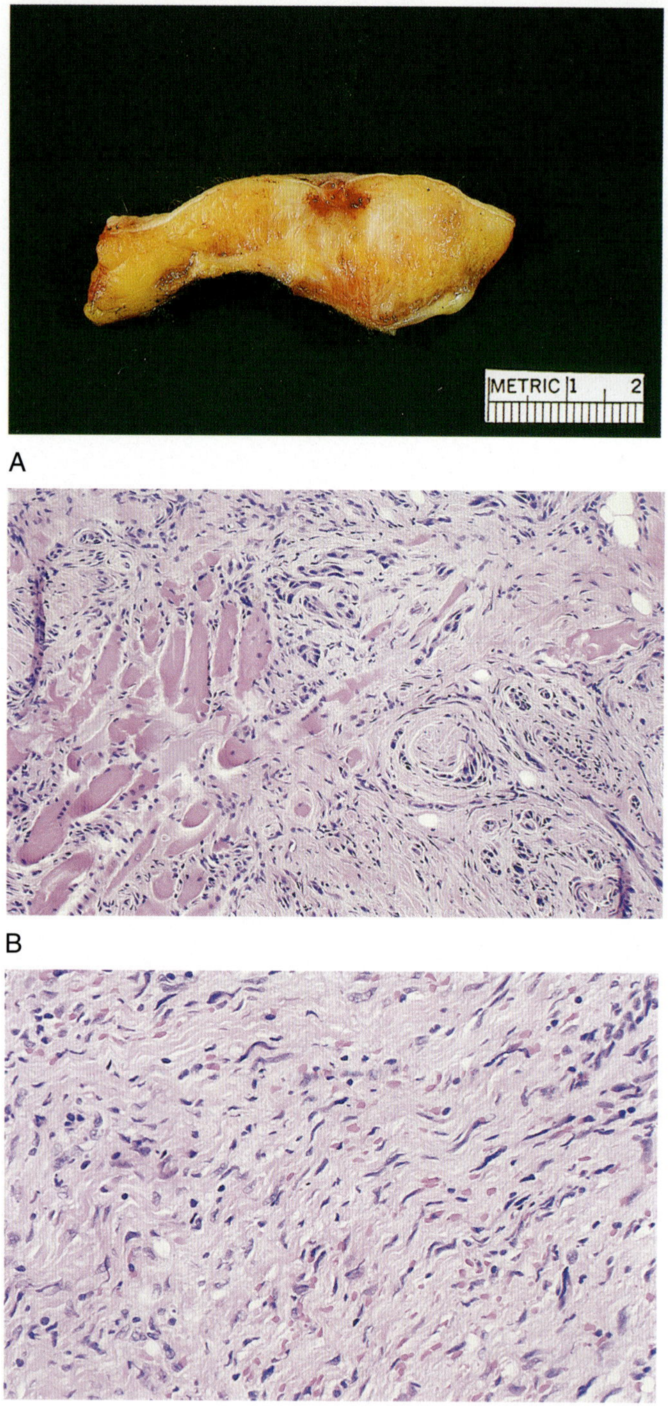

A

B

C

FIGURE 15.13 Resection specimen from the skin of the chin in an elderly man with desmoplastic melanoma. Note the scar-like appearance of the tumor within the dermis **(A)**. Perineural invasion is a common feature **(B)**, and the neoplasm may appear deceptively benign, exhibiting "wavy" and bland nuclei resembling neurofibroma **(C)**. (**B** and **C**, H&E.)

of greater diagnostic difficulty, are cases that are predominantly spindled. Such tumors commonly are misdiagnosed as desmoid tumor, fibrosarcoma, neurofibrosarcoma, traumatic neuroma, neurofibroma, malignant fibrous histiocytoma, and carcinoma.[20,21]

Spindled melanoma subtypes may be referred to as *desmoplastic* and *neurotropic* because of their tendency to exhibit an intense fibroblastic desmoplastic reaction and prominent perineural invasion (Fig. 15.13). Desmoplastic or neurotropic melanomas most commonly arise as nonpigmented lesions from the sun-exposed skin of the head and neck in elderly patients but also may be seen arising from oral mucosa.[20-22] The histologic appearance of spindle cell melanomas is highly variable, ranging from streaks of ill-defined spindle cells separated by strands of fibrous tissue to more cellular compact zones with well-defined fascicles or storiform patterns (see Fig. 15.10). Nuclei are generally uniform but binucleated and multinucleated giant cells sometimes are observed, mimicking malignant fibrous histiocytoma (see Fig. 15.11).[20-23]

Fine needle aspiration biopsy of malignant melanoma yields highly cellular smears and, most commonly, a population of discohesive, epithelioid-to-polygonal tumor cells with abundant, eccentrically placed cytoplasm; a mostly round nucleus; and prominent nucleoli. Less frequently, intracytoplasmic melanin pigment and intranuclear pseudoinclusions may be observed (Fig. 15.14).

Immunhistochemically, almost all melanomas coexpress S-100 protein and vimentin in a diffuse, strong pattern. An obviously malignant tumor, whether spindled or epithelioid, that shows diffuse and strong immunopositivity for S-100 protein should be considered melanoma until proved otherwise. Malignant peripheral nerve sheath tumors are generally deep-seated lesions, often associated with large nerve trunks or pre-existing benign nerve sheath tumors, and usually express S-100 protein in a focal and patchy fashion. Furthermore, up to 50% may be negative for S-100 protein. HMB-45 positivity is more specific for melanoma than is S-100 protein but tends to be less sensitive, especially among spindle cell variants.[24] Most cases of desmoplastic melanoma do not show immunoexpression for HMB-45.[25,26] The finding of melanosomes by ultrastructural examination is a helpful clue for the diagnosis of melanoma; however, as with HMB-45 positivity, melanosomes may not be obvious, and their absence does not exclude the diagnosis of melanoma.

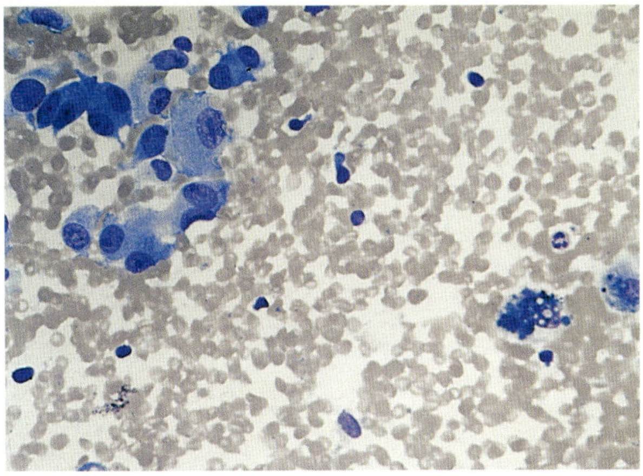

A

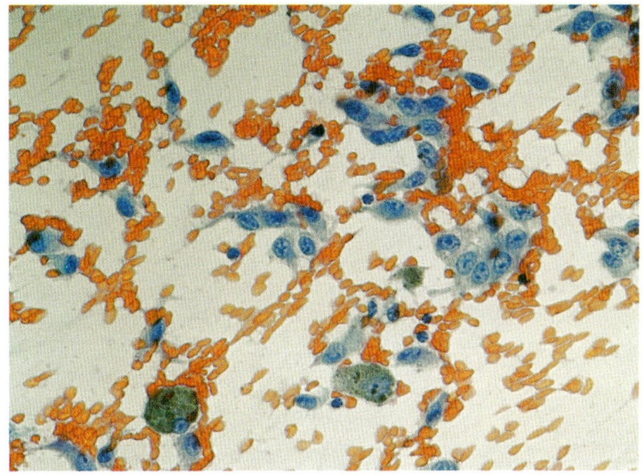

B

FIGURE 15.14 Fine needle aspiration biopsy specimen shows findings typical of malignant melanoma, including cellular smears with epithelioid to polygonal-shaped tumor cells, eccentrically placed nuclei and prominent nucleoli, and intracytoplasmic melanin pigment **(A** and **B)**. The presence of nuclear pseudoinclusions is also a helpful diagnostic clue **(C)**. **(A,** Diff-Quik; **B,** Papanicolaou; **C,** Diff-Quik.)

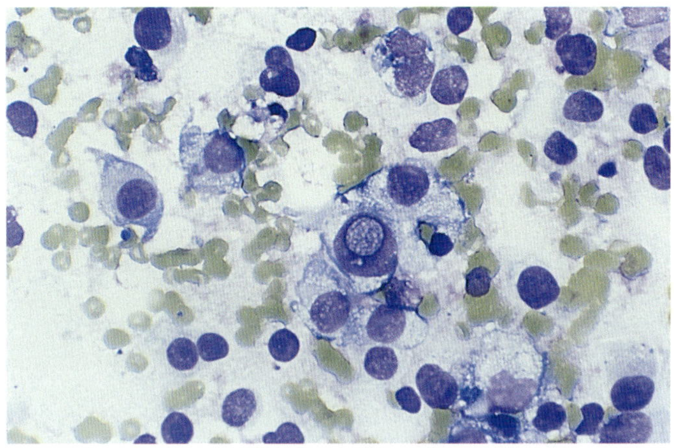

C

REFERENCES

Metastatic Carcinoma

1. Simon MA, Bartucci EJ: The search for the primary tumor in patients with skeletal metastases of unknown origin. Cancer 1986;58:1088.
2. Berrettoni BA, Carter JR: Current concept review: Mechanisms of cancer metastasis to bone. J Bone Joint Surg Am 1986;68:308.
3. Fechner RE, Mills SE: Metastatic tumors involving bone. In Rosai J, Sobin LH (eds): Atlas of Tumor Pathology: Tumors of the Bones and Joints. Washington, DC: Armed Forces Institute of Pathology, 1993, pp 245-252.
4. Katagiri H, Takahashi M, Inagaki J, et al: Determining the site of primary cancer in patients with skeletal metastasis of unknown origin. Cancer 1999;89:533.
5. Leeson MC, Makley JT, Carter JR: Metastatic skeletal disease distal to the elbow and knee. Clin Orthop 1986;206:94.
6. Unni KK: Conditions that commonly simulate primary neoplasms of bone. In Dahlin's Bone Tumors, General Aspects and Data on 11,087 Cases, 5th ed. Philadelphia: Lippincott-Raven, 1996, pp 355-432.
7. Cramer SF, Fried L, Carter KJ: The cellular basis of metastatic bone disease in patients with lung cancer. Cancer 1981;48:2649.
8. Holmes FF, Fouts TL: Metastatic cancer of unknown primary site. Cancer 1970;26:816.
9. Bommer KK, Ramzy I, Mody D: Fine-needle aspiration biopsy in the diagnosis and management of bone lesions: A study of 450 cases. Cancer (Cancer Cytopathol) 1997;81:148.
10. Kilpatrick SE, Ward WG, Chauvenet AR, et al: The role of fine-needle aspiration biopsy in the initial diagnosis of pediatric bone and soft tissue tumors: An institutional experience. Mod Pathol 1998;11:923.
11. Papanicolaou Society of Cytopathology Task Force on Standards of Practice: Guidelines of the Papanicolaou Society of Cytopathology for fine-needle aspiration procedure and reporting. Mod Pathol 1997;10:739.
12. Agarwal PK, Goel MM, Chandra T, et al: Predictive value of fine needle aspiration cytology of bone lesions. Acta Cytol 1997;41:659.

Sarcomatoid Carcinoma

13. de Peralta-Venturina M, Moch H, Amin M, et al: Sarcomatoid differentiation in renal cell carcinoma: A study of 101 cases. Am J Surg Pathol 2001;25:275.
14. Torenbeek R, Blomjous CEM, de Bruin PC, et al: Sarcomatoid carcinoma of the bladder: Clinicopathologic analysis of 18 cases with immunohistochemical and electron microscopic findings. Am J Surg Pathol 1994;18:241.
15. Wargotz ES, Norris HJ: Metaplastic carcinomas of the breast: III. Carcinosarcoma. Cancer 1989;64:1490.
16. Koss MN, Hochholzer L, Frommelt RA: Carcinosarcomas of the lung: A clinicopathologic study of 66 patients. Am J Surg Pathol 1999;23:1514.
17. Dundore PA, Cheville JC, Nascimento AG, et al: Carcinosarcoma of the prostate: Report of 21 cases. Cancer 1995;76:1035.
18. Sreenan JJ, Hart WR: Carcinosarcomas of the female genital tract: A pathologic study of 29 metastatic tumors: Further evidence for the dominant role of the epithelial component and the conversion theory of histogenesis. Am J Surg Pathol 1995;19:666.

Malignant Melanoma

19. Nakhleh RE, Wick MR, Rocamora A, et al: Morphologic diversity in malignant melanomas. Am J Clin Pathol 1990;93:731.

20. Jain S, Allen PW: Desmoplastic malignant melanoma and its variants: A study of 45 cases. Am J Surg Pathol 1989;13:358.
21. Kilpatrick SE, White WL, Browne JD: Desmoplastic malignant melanoma of the oral mucosa: An underrecognized diagnostic pitfall. Cancer 1996;78:383.
22. Reiman HM, Goellner JR, Woods JE, et al: Desmoplastic melanoma of the head and neck. Cancer 1984;54:907.
23. Egbert B, Kempson R, Sagebiel R: Desmoplastic malignant melanoma: A clinicopathologic study of 25 cases. Cancer 1988;62:2033.
24. Gown AM, Vogel AM, Hoak D, et al: Monoclonal antibodies specific for melanocytic tumors distinguishing subpopulations of melanocytes. Am J Pathol 1986;123:195.
25. Carlson JA, Dickersin GR, Sober AJ, et al: Desmoplastic neurotropic melanoma: A clinicopathologic analysis of 28 cases. Cancer 1995;75:478.
26. Anstey A, Cerio R, Ramnarain N, et al: Desmoplastic malignant melanoma: An immunocytochemical study of 25 cases. Am J Dermatopathol 1994;16:14.

CHAPTER 16

Infectious, Metabolic, and Arthritic Diseases of the Musculoskeletal System

Osteomyelitis

The term *osteomyelitis* almost always implies an infection of bone. Although virtually any microorganism may cause osteomyelitis, most cases are of bacterial origin. Access to bone generally occurs either through the bloodstream (hematogenous osteomyelitis) or by direct extension (secondary osteomyelitis) through pre-existing decubiti or open fractures. The initial infection and the resulting clinical features represent acute osteomyelitis. Failure to eradicate the microorganism completely may result in continued microorganism growth and reactive bone formation, a process called *chronic osteomyelitis*. Less commonly, the symptoms of osteomyelitis may not be clinically evident (subclinical); this clinical presentation is called *subacute osteomyelitis*.

Clinical Features

Acute hematogenous osteomyelitis is observed at virtually any age, but most patients are younger than 15 years old at presentation. *Staphylococcus aureus* is the offending organism in more than 80% of cases. Among patients younger than 3 years old, *Haemophilus influenzae* is the most common bacterial agent. For unknown reasons, 50% of affected patients lack an obvious distant site of infection. Symptoms generally include fever, localized pain, soft tissue swelling, and loss of function of the involved limb. In this clinical context, the physical finding of marked bone tenderness is highly suggestive of osteomyelitis. Laboratory studies usually reveal an elevated erythrocyte sedimentation rate and white blood cell count, principally neutrophils.

Certain diseases may predispose to the development of osteomyelitis. Patients with chronic renal failure on hemodialysis are at increased risk of osteomyelitis, most commonly involving the spine and ribs.[1] These infections are presumably a result of bacterial seeding from an infected catheter site. Intravenous drug abusers may develop osteomyelitis in unusual anatomic locations, including the sternoclavicular joints and the symphysis pubis (osteitis pubis), most commonly resulting from *Pseudomonas aeruginosa*. Patients with sickle cell anemia are at increased risk for developing osteomyelitis, often from *Salmonella* infections. As expected, patients with acquired immunodeficiency syndrome are at increased risk for the development of osteomyelitis that may be secondary to a wide range of bacterial and fungal agents.[2]

The radiographic findings are often not apparent early in the onset of the disease but may include ill-defined lucent areas within the metaphyseal region of a long bone (Fig. 16.1). Although nonspecific, bone scans generally are considered more sensitive than conventional radiographs early in the course of acute osteomyelitis.[3] In infants, because of transphyseal blood vessels, the epiphysis also may be involved.[4] With progression and more extensive intramedullary bone destruction, periosteal reactions develop and may be associated with soft tissue extension (abscess), mimicking a primary sarcoma. Occasionally a portion of necrotic bone (sequestrum) may be observed as a radiodense area within the lytic defect (Fig. 16.2).

Primary and secondary osteomyelitis have similar clinical symptoms, but the latter generally is associated with an adjacent soft tissue infection, implantation from a puncture wound, or an obviously contaminated open fracture wound. Consequently, this process may affect any bone. Secondary

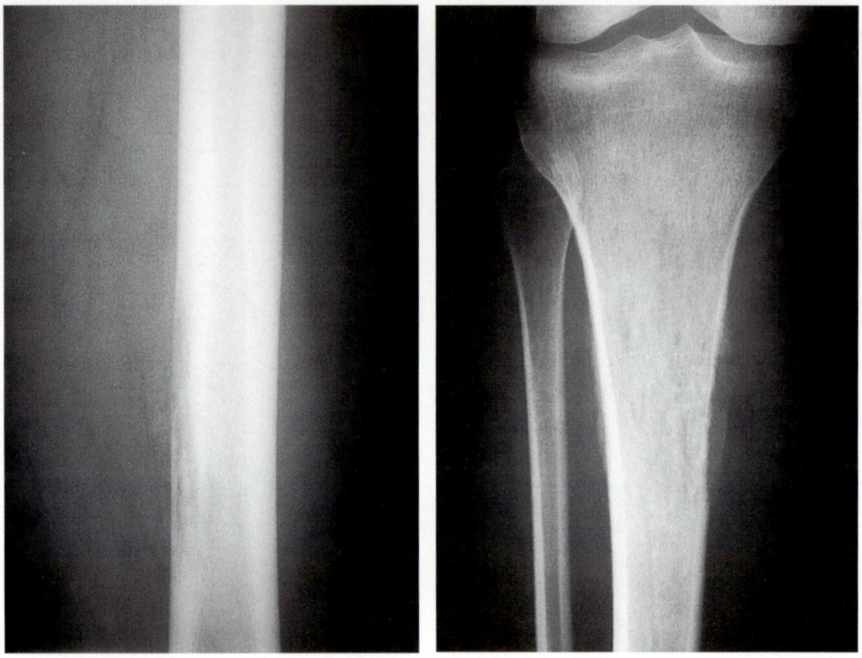

A B

FIGURE 16.1 Acute osteomyelitis. An anteroposterior radiograph of the midfemoral shaft shows cortical permeation with faint periosteal new bone production **(A)**. An anteroposterior radiograph of the proximal tibia in another patient shows extensive permeative bone destruction affecting the metaphyseal portion of the tibia **(B)**. Prominent immature periosteal new bone production is seen, especially medially.

osteomyelitis most commonly is the result of direct extension of an infection from a decubitus or diabetic ulcer (Fig. 16.3).

If the infection is contained but not completely eradicated, the result may be subacute osteomyelitis (Brodie's abscess). The radiographic findings are generally more characteristic than those observed in acute osteomyelitis (Fig. 16.4). Most commonly, a metaphyseal-centered, lucent area appears well circumscribed and at least partially surrounded by a sclerotic rim. The most common anatomic location is the tibia.

Failure to eradicate acute osteomyelitis completely, regardless of cause, can result in long-term sequelae, including chronic osteomyelitis. Clinical symptoms include nonspecific complaints of malaise and intermittent pain. The development of sinus tracts extending from bone to skin may complicate the clinical picture. Malignancy, especially squamous cell carcinoma and, less commonly, fibrosarcoma, develops in these sinus tracts in fewer than 1% of patients with chronic osteomyelitis.[5] Radiographically the bone has a

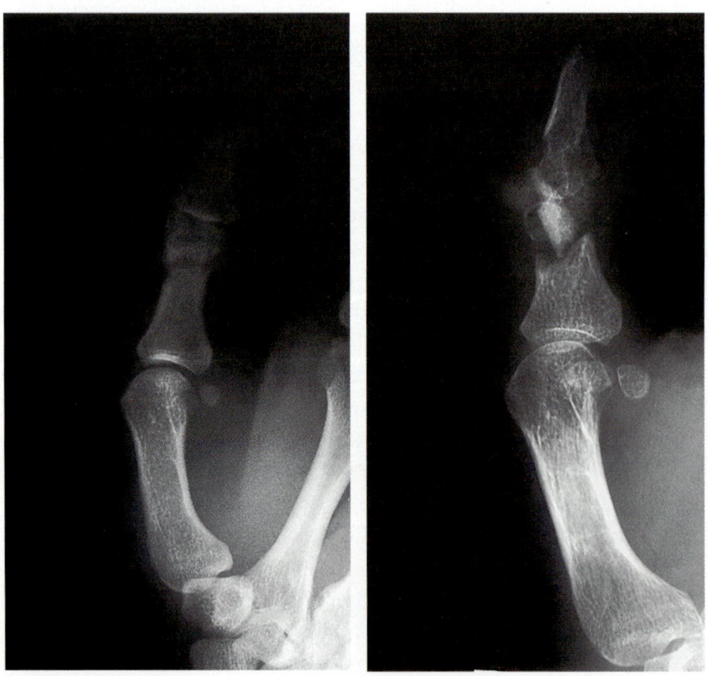

A B

FIGURE 16.2 Osteomyelitis with sequestrum. A permeative lesion in the distal end of the proximal phalanx of the thumb represents acute osteomyelitis developing after a human bite and complicated by a pathologic fracture **(A)**. Eight months later, a radiodense, sclerotic fragment of bone at the site of the previous fracture represents a sequestrum **(B)**.

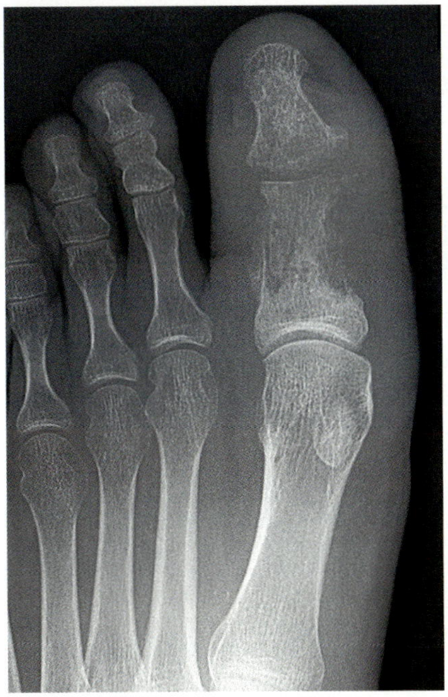

FIGURE 16.3 Secondary osteomyelitis. An anteroposterior radiograph of the foot in a man with diabetes mellitus and skin ulceration reveals marked bone destruction affecting most of the proximal phalanx and the base of the distal phalanx of the great toe. Erosion of the articular surfaces of both bones indicates septic arthritis in the interphalangeal joint of the great toe.

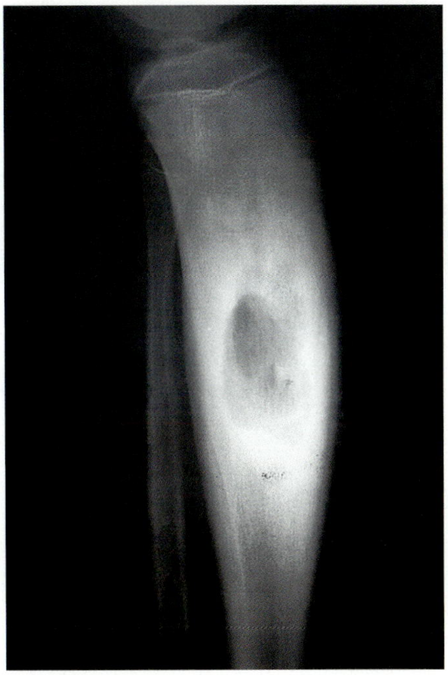

FIGURE 16.4 Brodie's abscess. A lateral radiograph of the proximal tibia shows a lytic lesion in the proximal tibial metaphysis surrounded by a well-defined, sclerotic margin that fades gradually into the adjacent medullary bone. Enlargement of the tibial shaft about the abscess reflects chronic remodeling.

mottled appearance with alternating radiolucent and radiodense areas (Fig. 16.5). Significant periosteal bone reaction may be present.

Chronic multifocal osteomyelitis is a relatively recently described entity. Most patients are children or young adults and present with symptoms of low-grade fever, localized pain and soft tissue swelling, and multiple sites of bony involvement. Virtually any site may be affected, but it is observed most commonly in the metaphyses of the long bones and clavicles. Chronic multifocal osteomyelitis may be observed as part of the SAPHO (synovitis, acne, pustulosis, hyperostosis, osteitis) syndrome, emphasizing the rare link between cutaneous and osteoarticular infections.[6] Some patients also have inflammatory bowel disease. Pathologic examination is nonspecific, generally revealing evidence of subacute or chronic osteomyelitis, often associated with necrotic bone. Although a few patients may have persistent disease, long-term clinical outcome appears favorable.[7]

Pathologic Findings

Histology

As with all pathologic diagnoses, correlation with clinical and radiographic findings is essential to establishing the diagnosis of osteomyelitis. Regardless of stage (e.g., acute versus chronic), osteomyelitis generally consists of an inflammatory infiltrate and bone destruction. Later stages may include reactive bone formation. The histologic hallmarks of acute osteomyelitis are the replacement of bone marrow by neutrophils, extensive bone resorption, and osteonecrosis (Fig. 16.6). Subacute osteomyelitis tends to show an admixture of neutrophils, plasma cells, and lymphocytes occupying loose-appearing granulation tissue. The inflammatory infiltrate in subacute osteomyelitis is usually less cellular (Fig. 16.7). Chronic osteomyelitis is characterized by the presence of chronic inflammation, principally lymphocytes and plasma cells, and marrow fibrosis. Necrotic bony trabeculae may be observed in any stage of osteomyelitis but are seen most commonly in the chronic form (Fig. 16.8). Acute inflammation may be present at least focally in acute, subacute, and chronic osteomyelitis. When squamous cell carcinoma complicates a sinus tract, the morphologic features are often those of a well to moderately differentiated carcinoma (Fig. 16.9).

Fine Needle Aspiration Biopsy

Fine needle aspiration biopsy usually is performed in cases associated with significant bone destruction or soft tissue extension. Most cases represent acute hematogenous osteomyelitis. Cytologic smears tend to be highly cellular and composed of innumerable neutrophils, cellular debris, and necrosis (Fig. 16.10). Randomly distributed histiocytes also may be present.

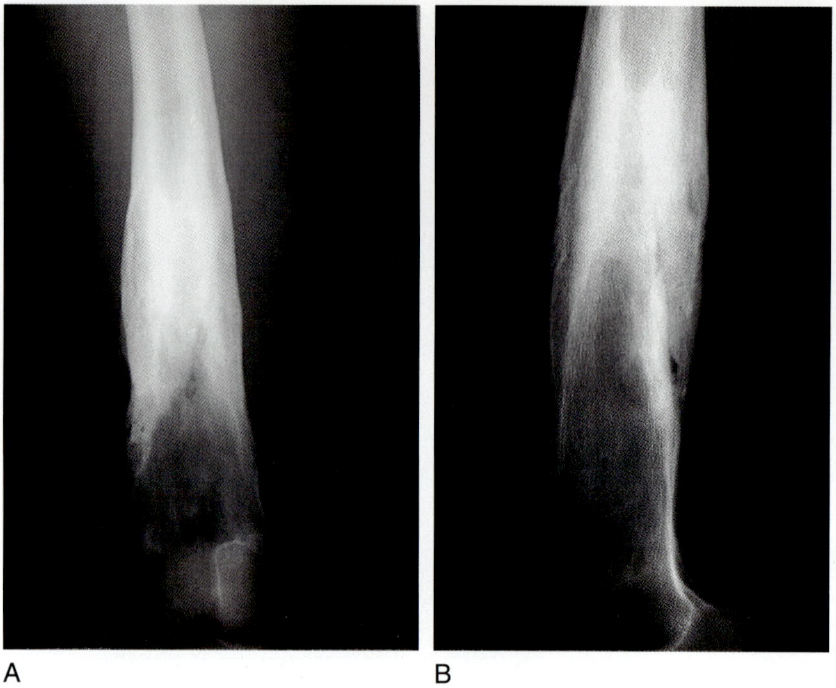

FIGURE 16.5 Chronic osteomyelitis. Anteroposterior **(A)** and lateral **(B)** radiographs of the distal femur show prominent zones of mixed bone lysis and sclerosis. The degree of sclerosis obscures the normal corticomedullary junction along the endosteal surface of the bone. Extensive, thick, and mature periosteal new bone formation surrounds the femoral shaft.

Prognosis and Therapy

Therapy for acute bacterial osteomyelitis consists of antibiotic treatment for several weeks. Although controversial, incision and drainage are recommended sometimes. Conversely, chronic osteomyelitis usually requires extensive surgical therapy, including débridement of lesional tissue and reconstruction. The ultimate prognosis depends on several factors, including the age of the patient, anatomic location (e.g., vertebra versus long bone), and extensiveness of bone destruction.

Tuberculous Osteomyelitis

Tuberculosis infections of the bones and joints are virtually always the result of hematogenous spread from the lungs.[8] Although any bone may be affected, the spine (Pott's disease) is the most common site of involvement followed by the knees and hips. Complaints of pain, tenderness, night sweats, and weight loss are common. Radiographically, erosive changes are observed on the articular bony surfaces of both sides of the joint and are associated with subsequent

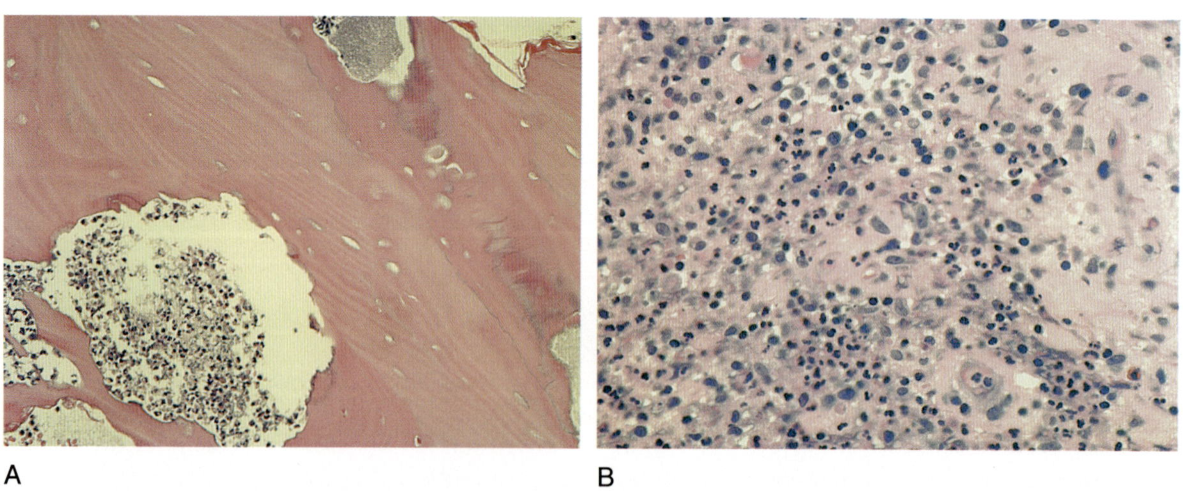

FIGURE 16.6 Acute osteomyelitis characterized by bone resorption, bone necrosis, and a neutrophilic infiltration **(A** and **B)**. **(A,** Low power; **B,** high power, H&E.)

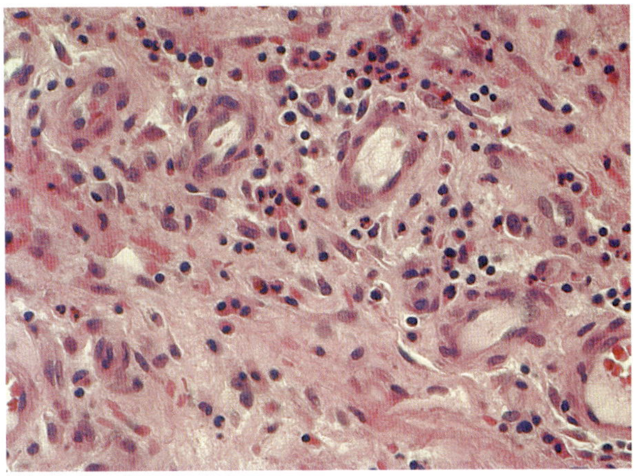

FIGURE 16.7 Subacute osteomyelitis characterized by a mixture of inflammatory cells, including neutrophils, plasma cells, and lymphocytes, within granulation tissue. (H&E.)

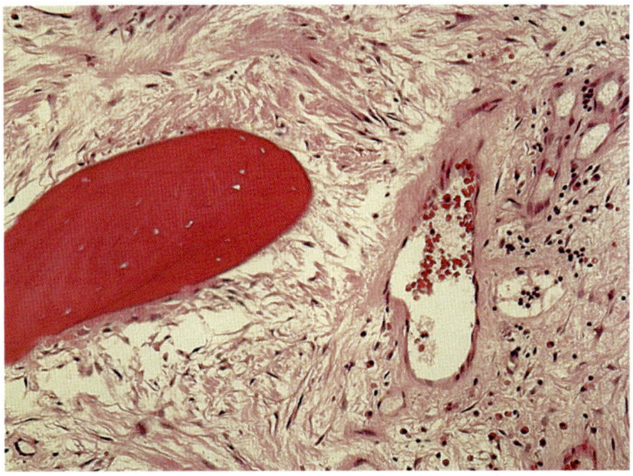

FIGURE 16.8 Chronic osteomyelitis with marrow fibrosis and a fragment of necrotic bone. (H&E.)

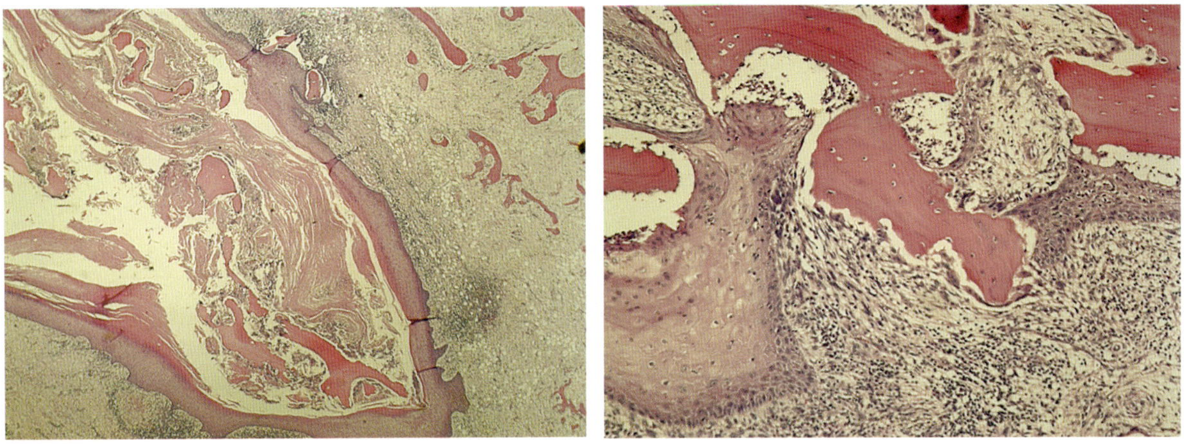

A B

FIGURE 16.9 Well-differentiated squamous cell carcinoma arising in an osteomyelitis sinus tract **(A** and **B)**. **(A,** Low power; **B,** high power, H&E.)

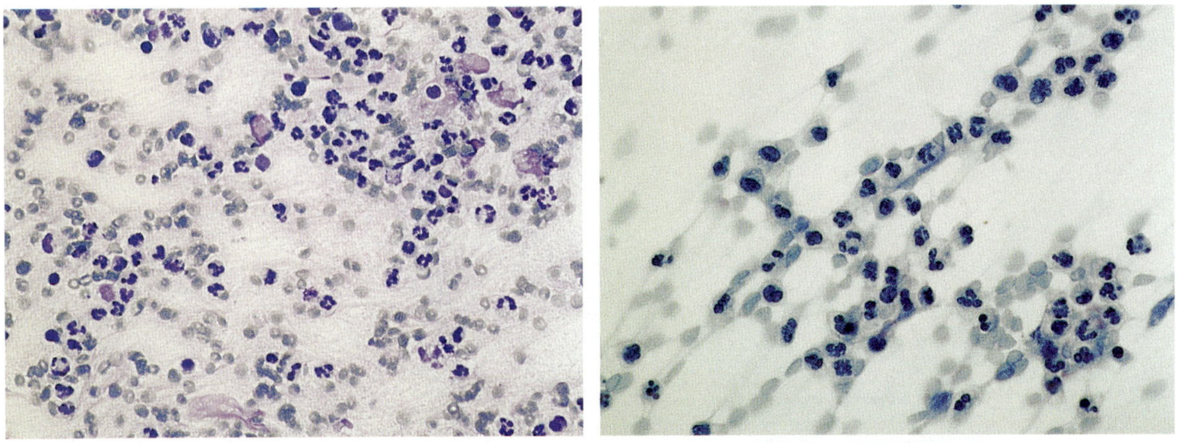

A B

FIGURE 16.10 Fine needle aspiration biopsy of acute osteomyelitis typically shows sheets of neutrophils **(A** and **B)**. **(A,** Diff-Quik; **B,** Papanicolaou.)

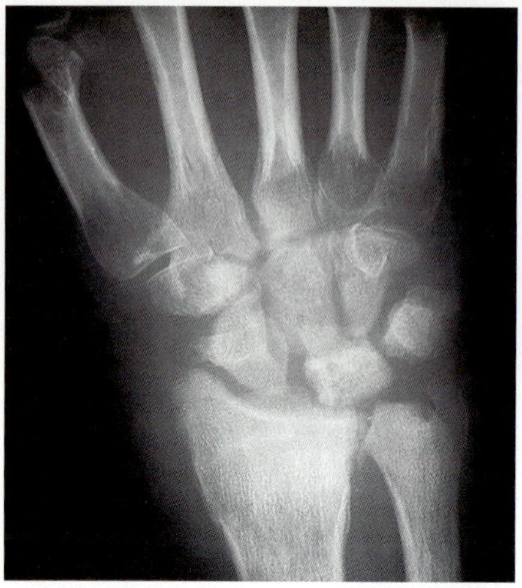

FIGURE 16.11 Tuberculous osteomyelitis and arthritis. A posteroanterior radiograph of the wrist reveals severe osteoporosis affecting the carpus and metacarpal bases. Marked erosion of articular surfaces is evident throughout the wrist, and there is joint widening, particularly at the scapholunate and triquetrohamate joints. The degree of osteoporosis is characteristic of a chronic, indolent infection and is greater than would be expected in an acute pyogenic arthritis.

narrowing and loss of the joint space (Fig. 16.11). Within the spine, tuberculosis often involves multiple vertebrae and intervertebral disks with compression fractures and paraspinal abscesses (Fig. 16.12). Destruction of vertebrae may lead to permanent spinal deformities, nerve compression, and neurologic deficits. Pathologic examination of affected tissue reveals the characteristic necrotizing granulomas (Fig. 16.13). It may be difficult, however, to show the tuberculosis mycobacteria, even with acid-fast bacilli stains, and culture is often necessary to establish the diagnosis. Patients who are immunosuppressed (e.g., human immunodeficiency virus) may not show classic granulomas but instead may exhibit an inflammatory infiltrate of histiocytes and neutrophils. It is important to exclude other potential causes of infectious granulomatous inflammation, especially fungal infections. Appropriate therapy includes antituberculosis drugs, and, occasionally, surgery is required for correction of severe skeletal abnormalities.

Septic Arthritis

Septic arthritis refers to inflammation, usually from bacterial infection, of the joint cavity in the absence of bone involvement (osteomyelitis). Microorganisms gain access to the synovial membrane and joint cavity typically through hematogenous spread and, less commonly, through direct extension (e.g., puncture wound). Similar to osteomyelitis, septic arthritis generally affects children and is most commonly the result of *S. aureus* infection.[9] Clinical symptoms and signs include fever, soft tissue swelling, pain localized to the joint, and elevated white blood cell count (Fig. 16.14). The most common anatomic location is the knee. In young adults, *Neisseria gonorrhoeae* is the most common causative agent, usually the complication of a more disseminated infection. Because the inflammatory process rapidly destroys overlying articular cartilage, accurate diagnosis and appropriate antibiotic therapy are necessary to avoid permanent joint morbidity.

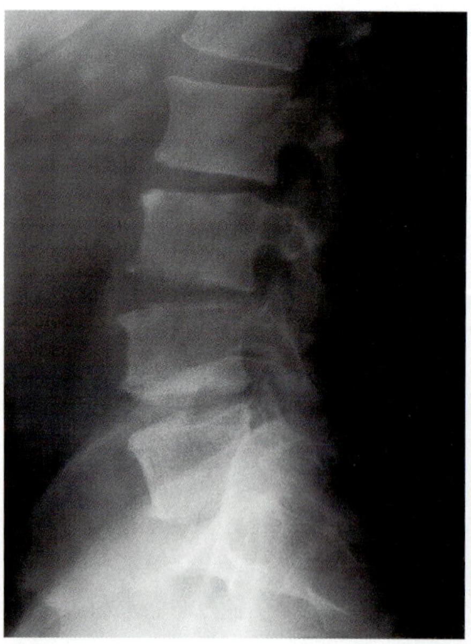

A

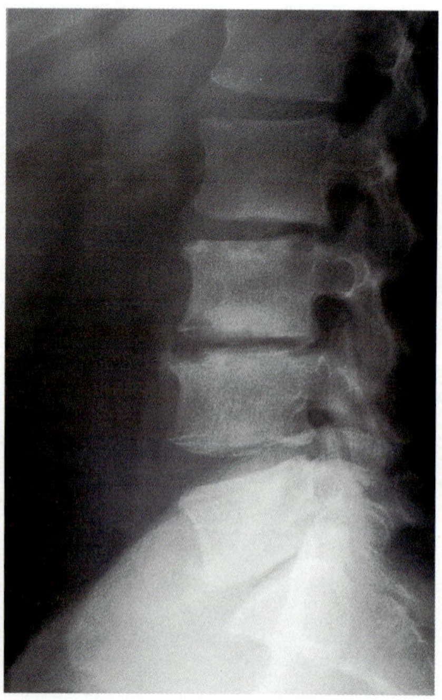

B

FIGURE 16.12 Tuberculous spondylitis (Pott's disease). A lateral radiograph of the lumbar spine shows erosion of the inferior L3 end plate and the superior L4 end plate **(A)**. The features indicate infectious diskitis but are not specific for a tuberculous infection. Six months later, the erosion is accompanied by increasing sclerosis and disk space narrowing **(B)**. Progressive erosion of the superior L3 end plate reflects subligamentous spread of the infection from the lower disk space, common in tuberculous spondylitis but not usually seen in bacterial diskitis.

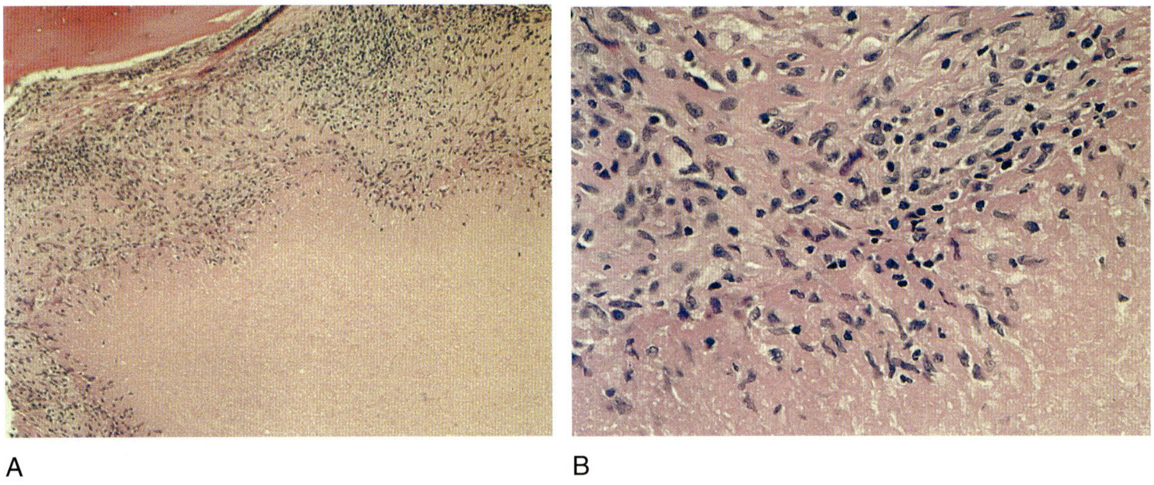

FIGURE 16.13 Necrotizing granulomatous inflammation is characteristic of tuberculosis infection of bone (**A** and **B**). (**A,** Low power; **B,** high power, H&E.)

Fractures

Fractures may occur in normal bone or a previously diseased, abnormal bone, so-called pathologic fracture. *Closed (simple) fractures* are fractures associated with an uninvolved, intact overlying skin; conversely, *open (compound) fractures* communicate with the skin surface. A fracture with both cortices displaced is considered a *complete fracture;* if one cortex is fractured but the opposing cortex is simply bent, the process is called an *incomplete (greenstick) fracture*. Slowly developing *stress fractures* are the result of increased and sustained physical activity to an affected bone. The histologic findings of a fracture depend largely on the age at which it is observed. Initially the fracture site consists simply of a hematoma that, over the next several days, begins the process of organization and healing, beginning with ingrowth of granulation tissue. Within the soft tissues adjacent to a fracture site, mesenchymal cells begin to form fibrocartilage and hyaline cartilage plates that ultimately undergo enchondral ossification. Concurrently, activated osteoblasts within the periosteum deposit woven bone trabeculae within the medullary cavity and perpendicular to the cortex. This process of bridging together the fractured ends of the bone with a mixture of fibrous tissue, woven bone, and cartilage is called *fracture callus* formation (Fig. 16.15). The healing and remodeling process ultimately results in mature medullary and cortical bone, often indistinguishable from the previously undamaged areas. Proper maturation of the callus requires adequate immobilization and union of the fracture site, however. Consequently, the pathologic features of nonunion (failed immobilization) generally consist of persistence and lack of maturation of the fracture callus. If too much motion is allowed to occur, the central portion of the callus may undergo cystic degeneration, resulting in a pseudarthrosis. A synovial-lined membrane that secretes synovial fluid may envelop the latter. Most important for the surgical pathologist, meticulous examination of any bone removed from a fracture site should exclude an underlying disease process (e.g., metastatic carcinoma) (Fig. 16.16).

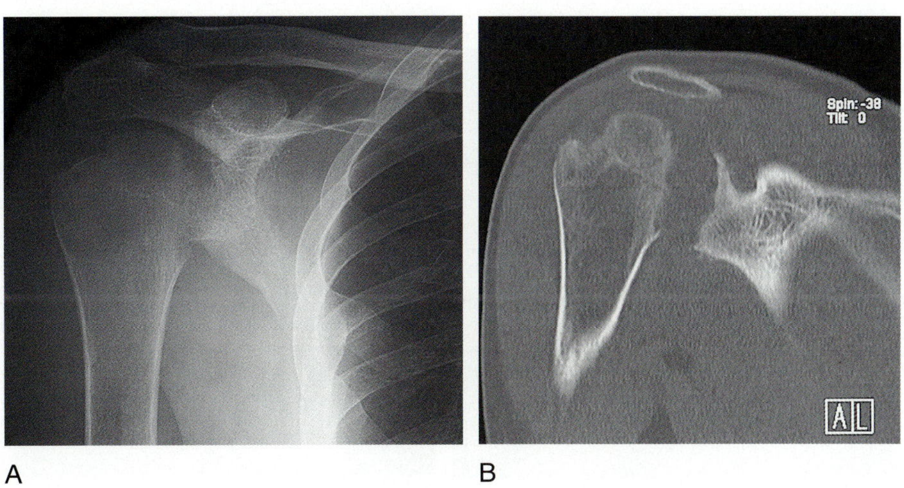

FIGURE 16.14 Septic arthritis. An anteroposterior radiograph of the shoulder shows erosion of bone along the articular surface of the humeral head medially, the superior surface of the humeral head laterally, and the glenoid fossa (**A**). A coronal reconstruction from a computed tomographic study shows the erosion of bone along the humeral head and adjacent glenoid fossa (**B**).

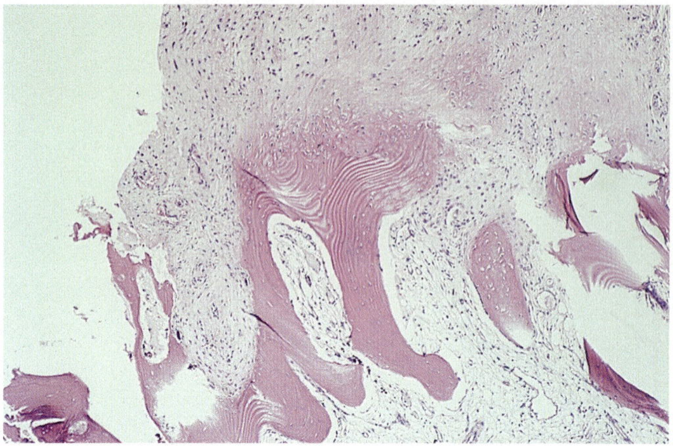

FIGURE 16.15 Fracture callus with woven bone and osteoid gradually being remodeled toward lamellar bone. (H&E.)

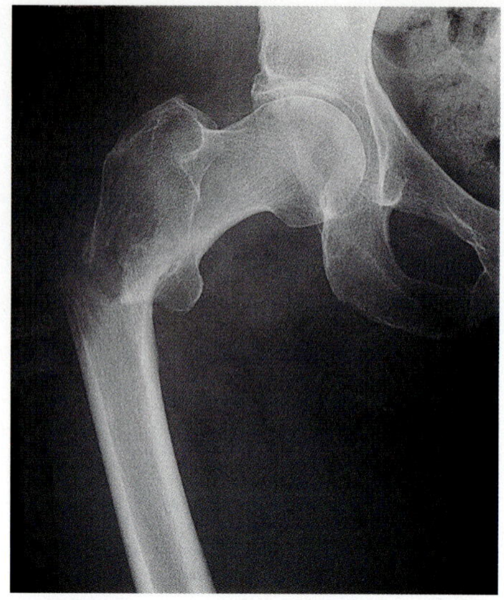

FIGURE 16.16 Metastatic breast carcinoma with pathologic fracture. An anteroposterior radiograph of the proximal femur shows a permeative, lytic lesion in the proximal femur. A pathologic fracture has developed through the lesion at the level of the lesser trochanter. The fracture is slightly displaced laterally and is in slight varus angulation.

Osteonecrosis

Osteonecrosis, also known as *bone infarction,* is a relatively common disorder. Regardless of cause, osteonecrosis is the result of ischemia, but it may be secondary to a variety of mechanisms, including fracture, thromboembolus, vasculitis, and radiation therapy or drug abuse. In many cases, the underlying cause is unclear.

Clinical Features

The clinical symptoms of osteonecrosis vary depending on the anatomic location and the extent of the infarction. Although virtually any bone may be affected, the subchondral regions, possibly because of limited collateral circulation, are affected most commonly, especially the femoral head. Less frequently, the metaphyseal and diaphyseal medullary canals of the long bones develop infarcts. Patients who develop intramedullary osteonecrosis usually have one or more underlying medical problems. Predisposing medical conditions include alcohol abuse, sickle cell disease, steroid therapy or abuse, dysbarism (decompression sickness caused by nitrogen bubbles), and Gaucher's disease.[10,11] When the underlying medical disease is not known, the osteonecrotic process may be referred to as *idiopathic* or *avascular necrosis*.

Patients presenting with the more common subchondral infarcts generally complain of chronic pain, initially associated only with activity but gradually progressing to pain at rest. Conversely, intramedullary infarcts associated with the shaft of the long bone are often subclinical and frequently represent incidental findings.

The radiographic findings in subchondral necrosis depend on the stage at which the abnormality is identified. Early in the process, subchondral osteonecrosis may exhibit nonspecific mottled radiolucencies or radiodensities. With progression, a "crescent" develops between the subchondral plate and underlying bone (Fig. 16.17). Later stages include narrowing of the joint space and the development of subchondral

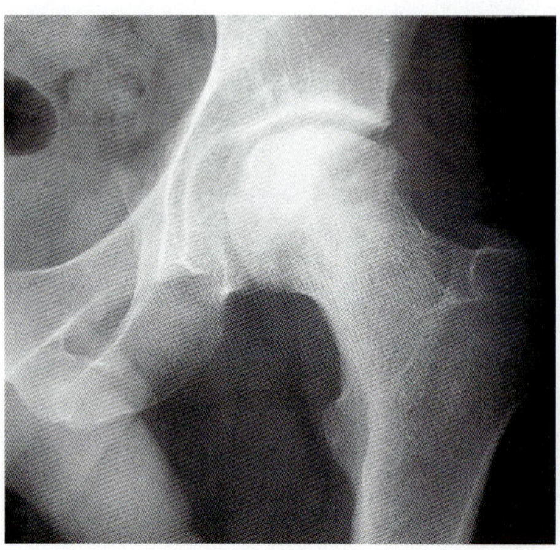

A

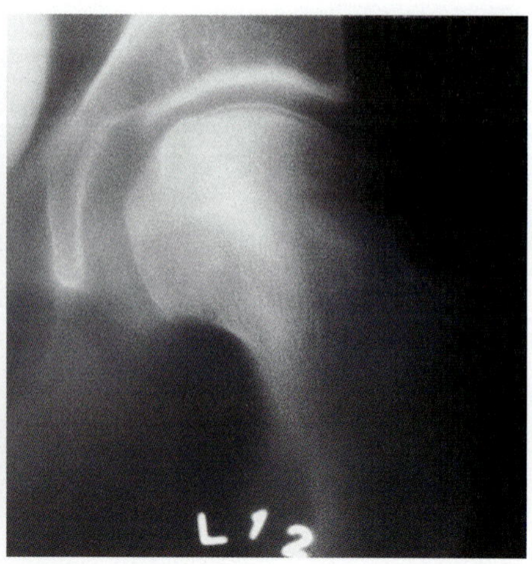

B

FIGURE 16.17 Subchondral osteonecrosis (avascular necrosis) of the femoral head. An anteroposterior radiograph of the femoral head reveals mixed areas of sclerosis and lucency **(A)**. Slight flattening of the femoral head is present superolaterally. A conventional tomogram shows the subchondral radiolucent crescent sign indicating collapse of the subchondral bone **(B)**.

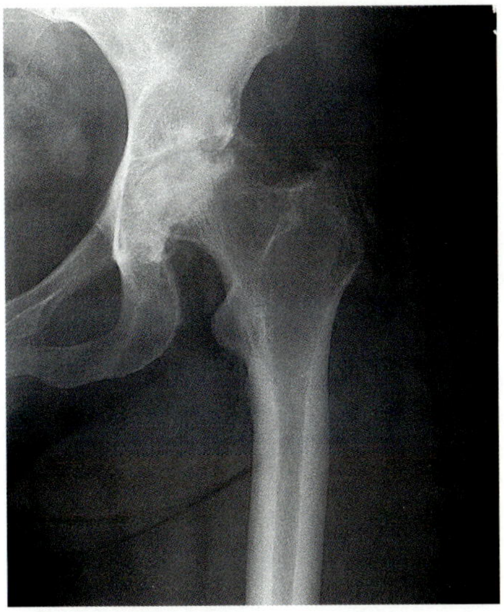

FIGURE 16.18 Subchondral osteonecrosis (avascular necrosis) with secondary joint disease. An anteroposterior radiograph of the femoral head reveals areas of mixed femoral head sclerosis and lucency with flattening of the femoral head, acetabular sclerosis, medial joint narrowing, and acetabular osteophytosis.

cysts and osteophytes, complications of degenerative joint disease (Fig. 16.18).[12] Intramedullary infarcts occurring within the metaphyseal and diaphyseal regions of a long bone usually present as well-circumscribed areas of calcification and radiodensity (Fig. 16.19).

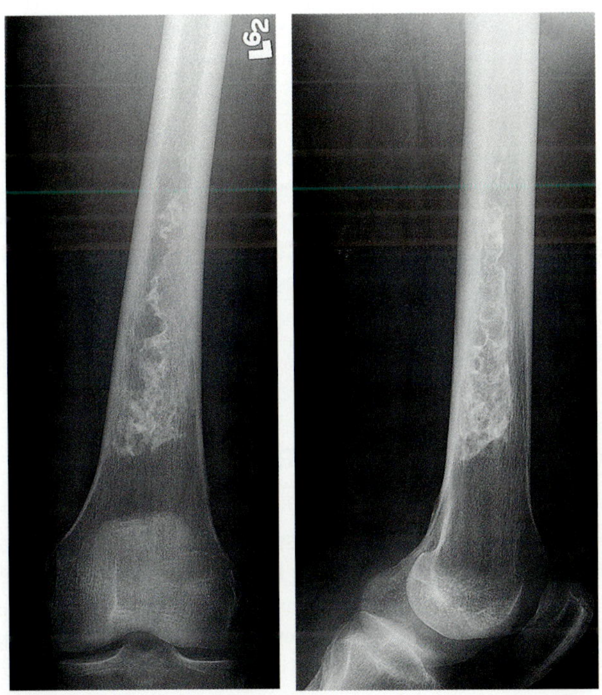

A B

FIGURE 16.19 Intramedullary osteonecrosis (infarction). Anteroposterior **(A)** and lateral **(B)** radiographs of the femoral shaft show serpentine areas of calcification within the medullary canal of the metadiaphyseal portion of the femur.

Pathologic Findings

Histology

The pathologic features of osteonecrosis are similar, regardless of cause. Histologic hallmarks include the presence of marrow fat necrosis and empty osteocyte lacunae. Because of collateral blood flow, the cortical bone is usually not affected. Additionally, some subchondral infarcts are associated with a wedge-shaped area of necrosis extending from the subchondral bone plate toward the center of the epiphyseal medullary cavity (Fig. 16.20). The hematopoietic bone marrow cells and marrow fat are the most sensitive indicators of early osteonecrosis, generally exhibiting changes within a few days of infarction and occurring before osteocyte dropout (empty lacunae) is evident. Over time, calcification of the necrotic marrow frequently develops. A reparative process usually begins after several weeks, replacing necrotic bone marrow with scar-like fibrous tissue (Fig. 16.21).

Histologic features of degenerative joint disease, such as loss of the articular cartilage surface, exposure and eburnation of subchondral bone, and intramedullary cysts, frequently accompany subchondral necrosis. In some cases, the degenerative changes precede the osteonecrosis, whereas in other circumstances, they seem to follow it.[12]

Decompression core biopsies, often used in the therapy of osteonecrosis, are therapeutic procedures, not diagnostic ones. Generally, these biopsies comprise fragments of bone and bone dust that may or may not be obviously necrotic.

Prognosis and Therapy

In the early stages of femoral head subchondral osteonecrosis, decompression core biopsy may help maintain the integrity of the articular surface, delaying extensive surgery.[13] Decompression core biopsy is thought to decrease intraosseous pressure, improving perfusion and providing a pathway for

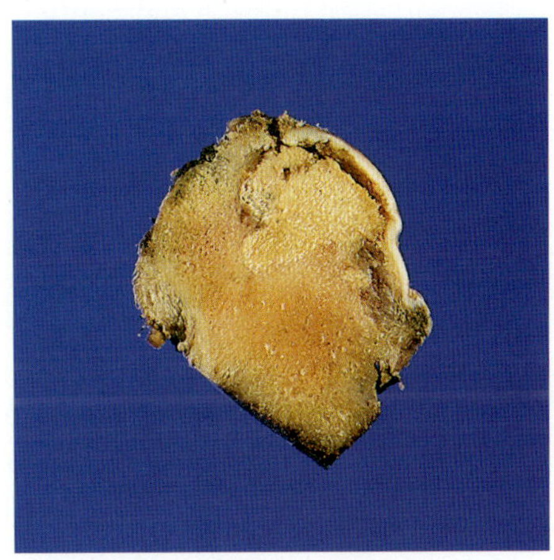

FIGURE 16.20 A femoral head with a wedge-shaped area of subchondral osteonecrosis. Also note the cleft between the subchondral bone and overlying articular cartilage.

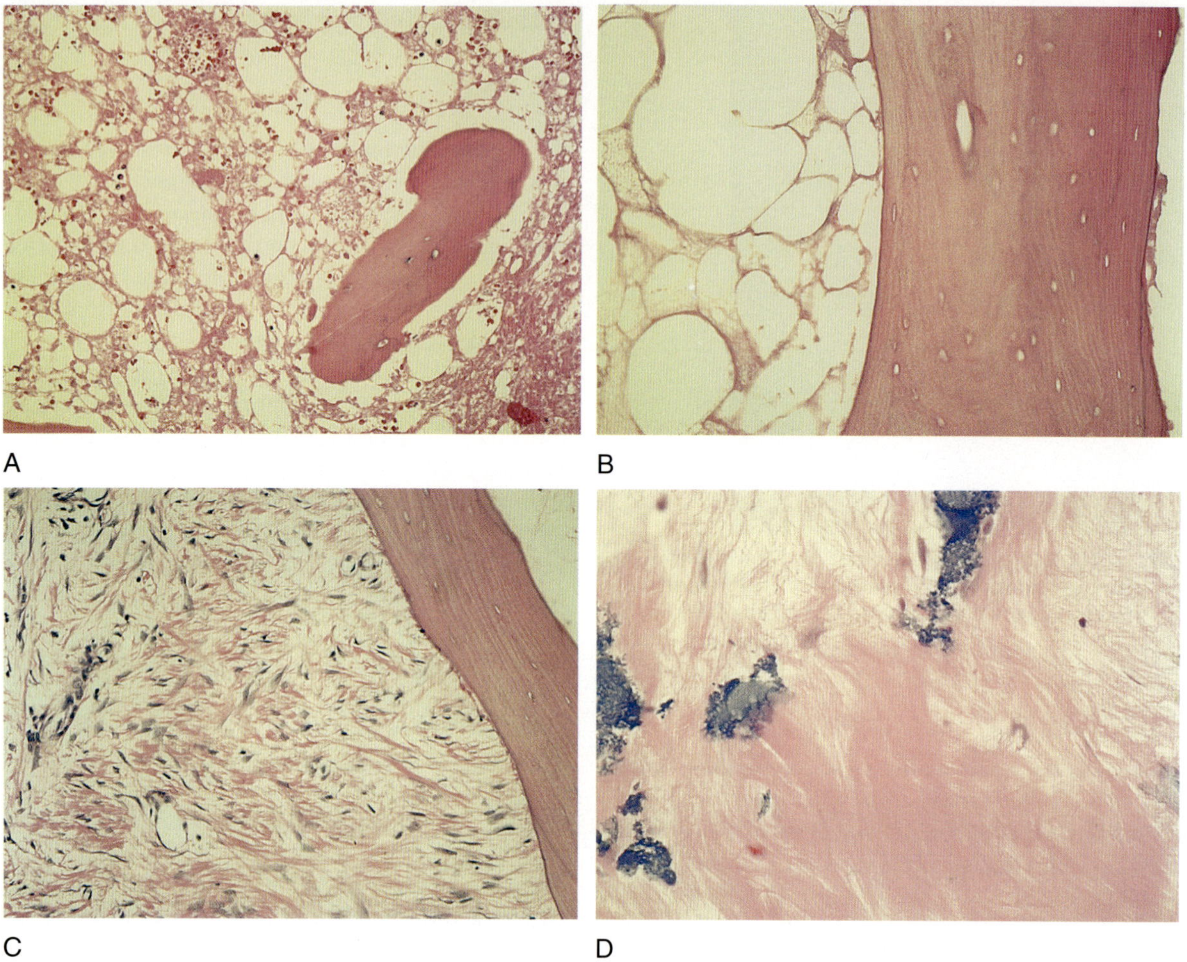

A B C D

FIGURE 16.21 The earliest indicator of osteonecrosis is necrosis of the marrow fat and cellular elements **(A)**, followed by osteocyte dropout (empty lacunae) **(B)**. The later stages of osteonecrosis include replacement of the necrotic marrow with reparative fibrous tissue **(C)**. Dystrophic calcifications may be observed within the fibrous tissue **(D)**. **(A-D,** H&E.)

reparative tissue to grow. The development of the radiographic crescent sign indicates, however, the necessity for total hip surgery to prevent progressive collapse and severe secondary degenerative joint disease. Because intramedullary long bone infarcts are generally asymptomatic, incidental findings, simple observation is usually sufficient. A small proportion (<1%) of these infarcts develop sarcomatous transformation, most often histologically representing an osteosarcoma or malignant fibrous histiocytoma.[14]

Osteochondritis Dissecans

Osteochondritis dissecans is a special form of osteonecrosis, the result of joint trauma with shearing of a segment of articular cartilage and underlying bone, with or without detachment. It is observed most commonly in adolescents, and the medial femoral condyle is the most common affected site.[15] Patients may complain of joint pain and limitation of movement. Radiographically, osteochronditis dissecans is characterized by a radiolucent defect involving the articular surface, usually the lateral aspect of the medial femoral condyle of the knee (Fig. 16.22). The histologic specimen consists of a portion of articular cartilage with underlying bone that may be necrotic. Therapy for osteochondritis dissecans consists of either reattachment of the segment of cartilage or its complete removal.

Hyperparathyroidism

Hyperparathyroidism is a common endocrine disorder, but because of early detection, involvement of the skeleton by hyperparathyroidism is observed only rarely. Hyperparathyroidism may exist as a primary disorder, may be secondary to autonomous secretion by the parathyroid gland, or may be secondary to underlying renal disease (renal osteodystrophy).[16] Regardless of cause, the skeletal changes appear similar but tend to be more pronounced in secondary hyperparathyroidism.

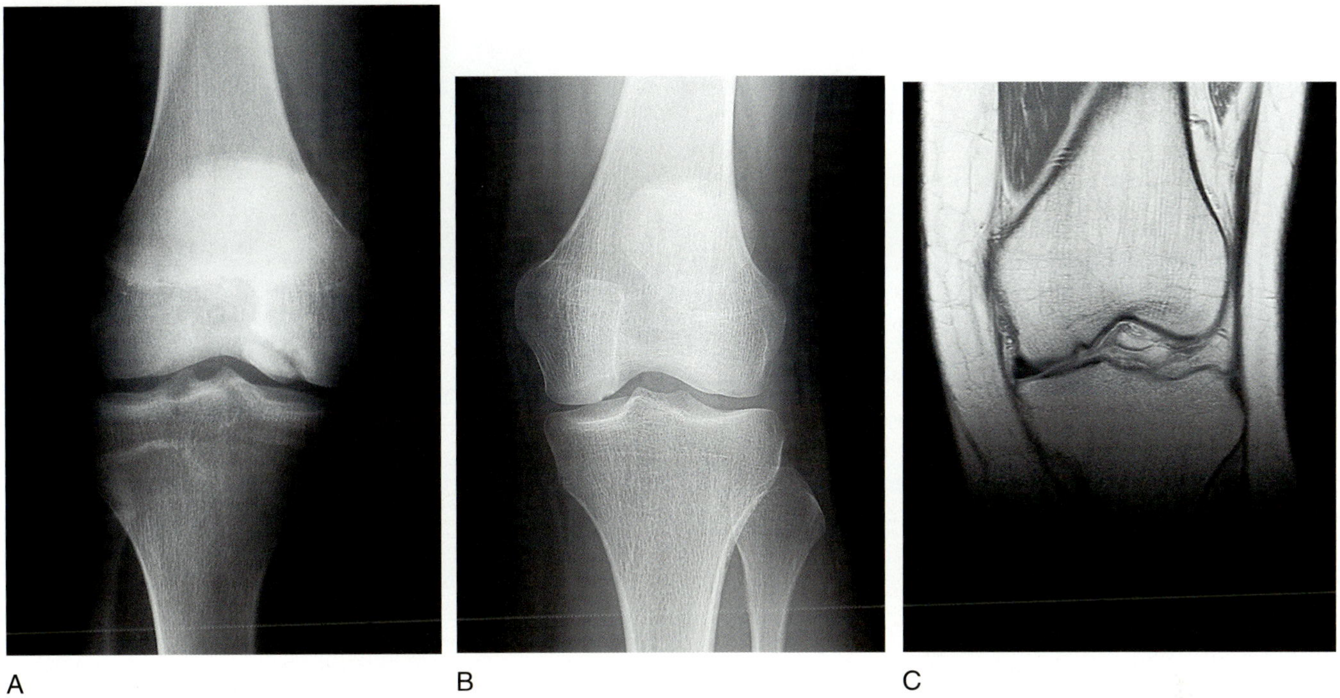

FIGURE 16.22 Osteochondritis dissecans. An anteroposterior radiograph of the knee shows a fragment of bone along the lateral aspect of the medial femoral condyle, typical in appearance for osteochondritis dissecans **(A)**. In another patient, a smaller defect is seen on the lateral surface of the medial femoral condyle **(B)**. A coronal magnetic resonance image from the patient in **B** shows the defect in the articular cartilage and underlying cortical and subchondral bone **(C)**.

Clinical Features

Primary hyperparathyroidism is observed most commonly in young to middle-aged adults, and women tend to be affected more frequently than men. Today, the most common presenting abnormality is asymptomatic hypercalcemia, often accompanied by hypophosphatemia. An elevated serum parathyroid hormone level confirms the diagnosis. Less commonly, patients complain of nausea and vomiting, headaches, muscular weakness, and fatigue. A history of recurrent kidney stones or peptic ulcer disease may suggest the diagnosis of hyperparathyroidism.[17]

Secondary hyperparathyroidism almost always is seen in the setting of chronic renal failure. Patients often complain of bone pain and weakness. Serum calcium levels tend to be low, whereas phosphorus levels often are elevated, opposite to that observed in primary hyperparathyroidism.

In primary and secondary hyperparathyroidism, the most common radiographic abnormalities are subperiosteal and subchondral bone resorption (Fig. 16.23). Early in the course of the disease, these changes are limited to or most obvious in the distal phalanges and clavicle, but in more advanced stages, similar changes may be seen in other skeletal sites as well (Fig. 16.24). Well-defined, lytic lesions, sometimes called *brown tumors* (owing to their color), are seen more commonly in the secondary form of the disease (Fig. 16.25); this may reflect the fact that secondary hyperparathyroidism is more common than the primary form. Brown tumors are usually metaphyseal and may be multiple (osteitis fibrosa cystica).

Pathologic Findings

Histology

Hyperparathyroidism causes increased osteoclastic activity resulting in resorption cavities (tunnels) of trabecular bone, which, early in the course of the disease, are not visualized easily on conventional hematoxylin and eosin slides. These abnormalities are analyzed best by histomorphometry techniques, typically beyond the scope of most surgical pathologists. More advanced cases of hyperparathyroidism exhibit paratrabecular fibrosis and an increase in bone formation.

The abnormality of hyperparathyroidism most likely to be encountered by the surgical pathologist is the brown tumor. Morphologically, brown tumors are typically well-circumscribed lesions composed of randomly distributed, osteoclast-type giant cells within a hypervascular background stroma containing bland-appearing, proliferating fibroblasts and hemosiderin deposition. The histologic appearance is virtually identical to that observed with giant cell reparative granuloma of the jaw and giant cell reaction in the digits (Fig. 16.26). Clinical and radiographic correlation is essential to distinguish these entities. Brown tumor also is discussed in Chapter 7.

Prognosis and Therapy

Because most examples of primary hyperparathyroidism result from a localized parathyroid adenoma, surgical excision of the involved gland usually results in cure and restoration of normal serum calcium levels. Similarly, in more advanced cases of secondary hyperparathyroidism, removal of the hyperplastic glands helps resolve the clinical symptoms. After medical or surgical management of hyperparathyroidism, brown tumors usually regress or heal, leaving behind only an area of sclerosis.[18]

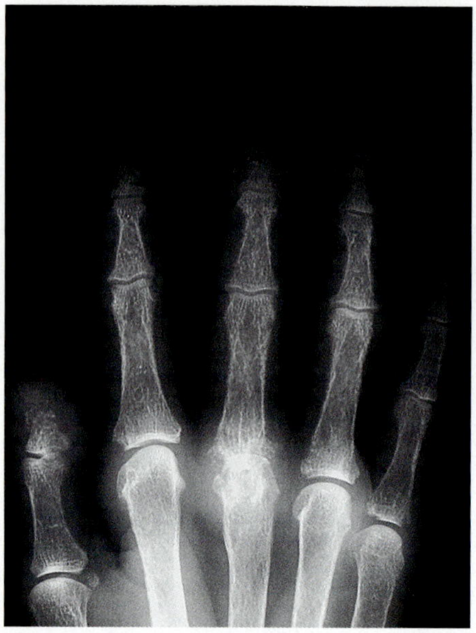

FIGURE 16.23 Secondary hyperparathyroidism. In a patient with chronic renal failure and secondary hyperparathyroidism, a posteroanterior radiograph of the hand reveals marked bone resorption along the subperiosteal surfaces of the phalanges. There is prominent resorption of the terminal tufts and subchondral bone, especially at the third metacarpophalangeal joint.

Paget's Disease

Paget's disease of bone is a chronic condition associated with solitary-to-multifocal bone remodeling. The initial bone resorption phase is followed by disorganized and haphazard bone formation that, over several years, frequently results in bone pain and predisposition to fractures.

Clinical Features

Paget's disease generally affects patients older than age 50. Patients who have family members with the disease are most likely to develop it themselves. Paget's disease is seen more commonly in northern Europeans and Americans and is rare in Asians and Africans. Most cases are monostotic and discovered incidentally; rarely, Paget's disease involves multiple (polyostotic) bones. Although Paget's disease may involve any bone, it is observed most commonly in the axial skeleton (pelvis, spine, and skull) and is virtually never seen within the digits. Although frequently asymptomatic, patients, especially those with polyostotic disease, may complain of pain, possibly the result of microfractures. Radiographically, Paget's disease begins as a radiolucent process (Fig. 16.27), gradually progressing, in the late stages, to a more radiodense picture with loss of clear demarcation between cortex and medulla (Fig. 16.28). The differential diagnosis may include metastatic disease. Although the number of disease foci present initially does not tend to increase, each individual focus usually progresses at a similar rate.

In the spine, Paget's disease usually involves the lumbar vertebrae, and compression fractures are relatively common. With progression, the vertebral body gradually

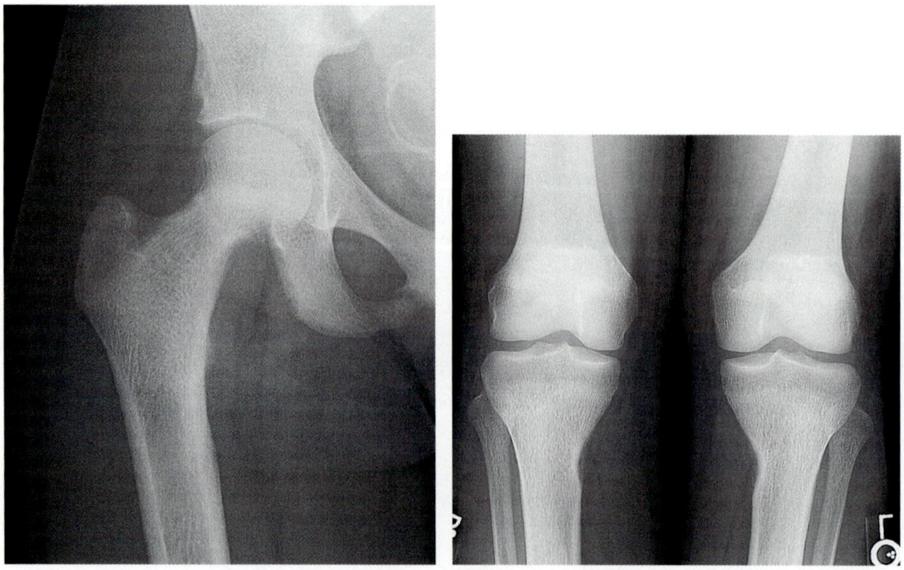

A B

FIGURE 16.24 Secondary hyperparathyroidism. In a patient with chronic renal failure, an anteroposterior radiograph of the hip shows bone resorption along the medial femoral neck, pubis, and sacroiliac joint **(A)**. A peritoneal dialysis catheter lies coiled in the pelvis. An anteroposterior radiograph of the knees in the same patient shows subperiosteal bone resorption along the proximal tibial metaphysis **(B)**.

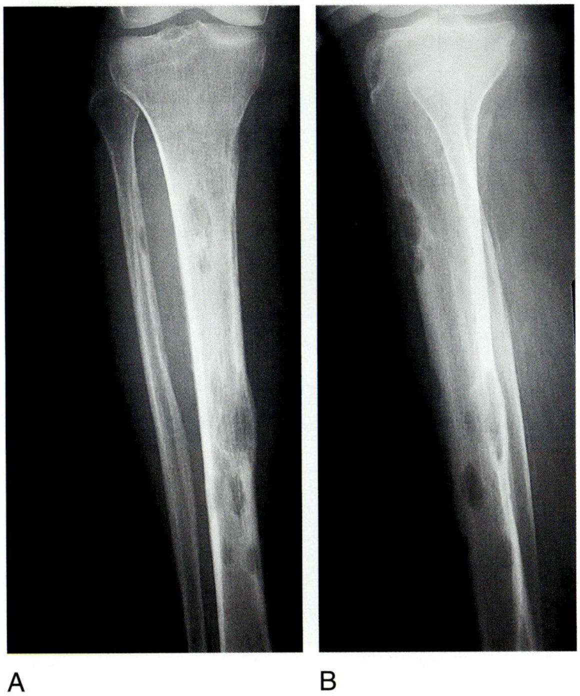

FIGURE 16.25 Primary hyperparathyroidism. Anteroposterior (A) and lateral (B) radiographs of the tibia in a patient with a parathyroid adenoma and resulting primary hyperparathyroidism show multiple, well-defined lytic lesions centered in the medullary canal of the tibia and producing cortical erosion.

enlarges, and sclerosis is observed below the subchondral plate. Clinical symptoms may include cord or nerve root compression. When Paget's disease affects the skull, lytic areas often develop in the frontal and occipital regions; these areas gradually may enlarge to involve the entire skull. Serum alkaline phosphatase often is markedly elevated, despite normal calcium and phosphorus levels, and tends to correlate with the degree of skeletal involvement.

Pathologic Findings

Histology

The histologic findings in Paget's disease vary depending on the phase at which the bone is biopsied. Initially, marked bone resorption is observed and is characterized by abundant and enlarged osteoclasts and marrow fibrosis. This phase is followed by an increase in woven bone formation and osteoblastic activity. This bone is distinctly abnormal, disorganized, and characterized by irregular and intersecting cement lines, imparting a "mosaic pattern" (Fig. 16.29). Ultimately the woven bone is converted to more mature-appearing lamellar bone.

Prognosis and Therapy

The medical treatment of Paget's disease includes drugs that inhibit osteoclastic resorption, particularly calcitonin and bisphosphonates. Untreated, Paget's disease renders bones susceptible to fracture. Despite an increase in total bone density, pagetoid bone tends to be inflexible and unable to handle the usual stresses of everyday life. Additionally, when fracture does occur, the healing process usually is impaired. Degenerative joint disease may develop when Paget's disease involves the articular ends of bones. Surgery, such as total joint arthroplasty, sometimes is needed to correct this complication. The hypervascularity and increased blood flow create demands on the heart, and rarely high-output cardiac failure may result. Nevertheless, the most serious complication of Paget's disease is the development of a secondary sarcoma.[19,20] Although difficult to determine, the incidence is reportedly about 1% but is likely much lower, especially if asymptomatic, monostotic cases are included. These secondary sarcomas, generally

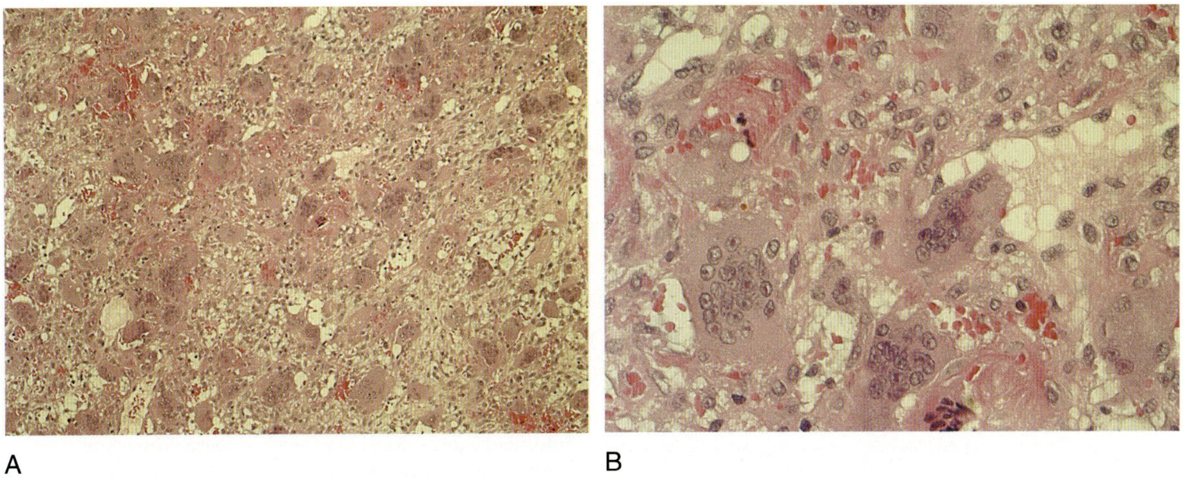

FIGURE 16.26 The histologic features of brown tumor of hyperparathyroidism are identical to features observed in giant cell reparative granuloma. Randomly distributed, benign-appearing, osteoclast-type giant cells are within a hypervascular-to-fibrotic, bland-appearing stroma (A and B). (A, Low power; B, high power, H&E.)

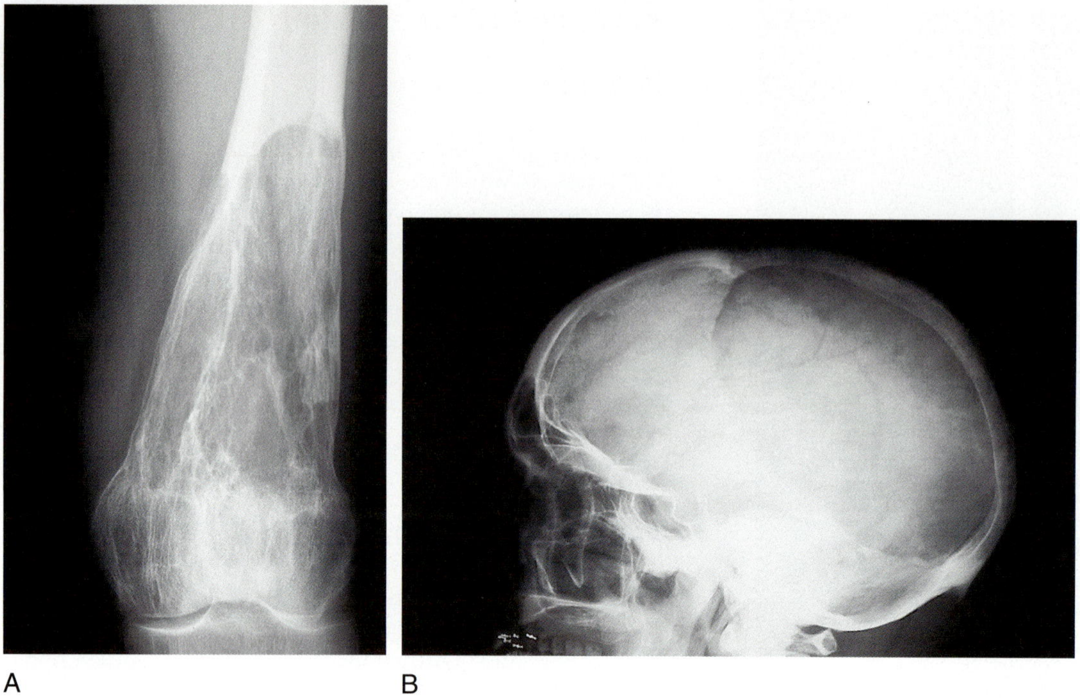

FIGURE 16.27 Lytic Paget's disease. An anteroposterior radiograph of the distal femur shows a well-demarcated lytic process in the distal femur **(A)**. In the more distal portion of the lesion, bone lysis is being replaced by reparative bone with thickened, disordered trabeculae. A lateral skull radiograph in another patient reveals extensive bone lysis in most of the posterior calvaria **(B)**. Such calvarial bone lysis in Paget's disease is referred to as *osteoporosis circumscripta*.

osteosarcomas or malignant fibrous histiocytomas, arise within bones most commonly affected by Paget's disease, typically the axial skeleton. Sarcomas arising in Paget's disease are often poorly responsive to conventional sarcoma therapy and almost always fatal (Fig. 16.30). In addition to sarcomatous transformation, patients with Paget's disease have an increased tendency to develop giant cell lesions of the skull.[21]

Amyloidosis

Amyloid deposition in bone is a rare phenomenon, and most cases seem to be secondary to multiple myeloma. At present, amyloidosis is classified based on the protein subtype found in the deposits. Most systemic forms may be classified into one of three categories—AL or myeloma-associated amyloid (immunoglobulin light chains), AA or inflammation-associated amyloid (liver proteins, nonimmunoglobulin), and β_2-microglobulin or hemodialysis-associated amyloid.[22,23] All of these forms of amyloid may be deposited in bone; however, the AL form is seen most commonly. Although amyloid deposition in bone generally reflects widespread systemic disease, isolated, solitary deposition (amyloidoma) occurs rarely and, similar to the systemic form, is usually secondary to a plasma cell dyscrasia.[22] The radiographic features of amyloidosis are variable, but most cases appear lytic and often show aggressive features (Fig. 16.31). Virtually any bone may be involved, and most patients are older adults, reflecting an association with multiple myeloma. Morphologically, amyloid usually is deposited as amorphous, eosinophilic masses with an associated giant cell histiocytic response. A lymphoplasmacytic infiltrate is generally also present (Fig. 16.32). Less commonly, the amyloid deposits may form more organized corpora amylacea–like patterns.[22] Calcification and osseous metaplasia of amyloid deposits may confound the diagnosis. Congo red staining and the characteristic apple-green birefringence by polarizing microscopy confirm the diagnosis. The prognosis of amyloidosis of bone is generally poor. Even patients presenting with solitary disease usually develop additional tumors, and most die of complications related to amyloidosis within 5 years of the initial diagnosis.

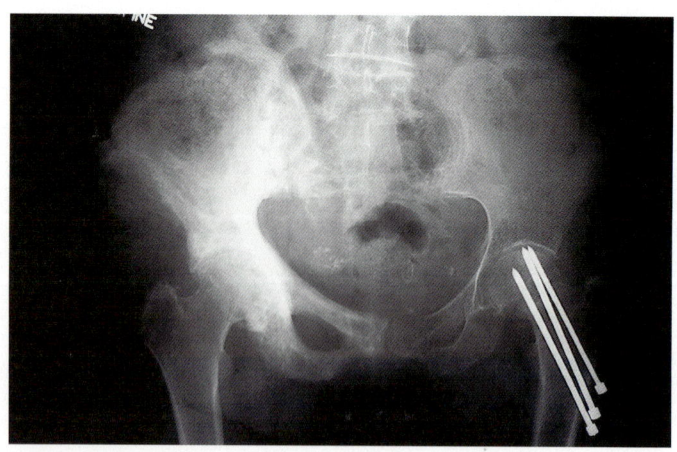

FIGURE 16.28 Late-stage Paget's disease. The entire right hemipelvis is involved in this patient with long-standing Paget's disease. The ilium, pubis, and ischium are enlarged and have thickened cortex and coarsened trabeculae. These radiographic features are characteristic of long-standing Paget's disease. Surgical pins traverse a left femoral neck fracture.

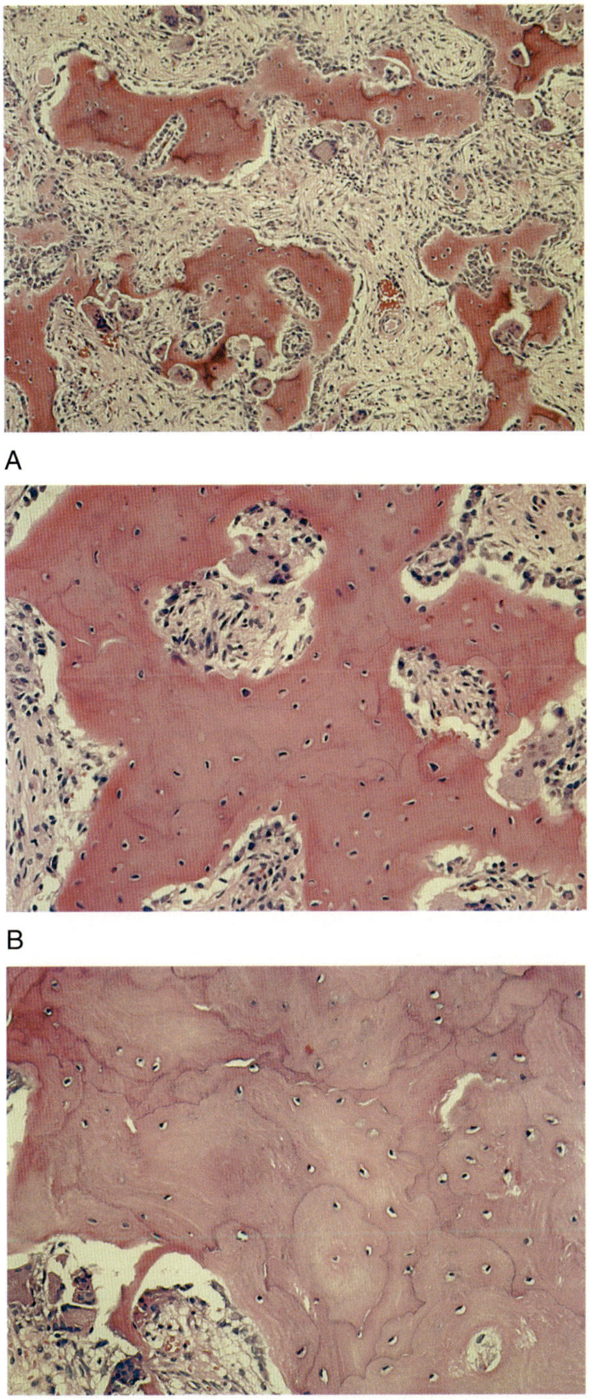

A

B

C

FIGURE 16.29 Paget's disease with anastomosing woven bone trabeculae lined by osteoblasts and osteoclasts; the intervening marrow consists of benign-appearing fibrovascular tissue **(A** and **B)**. Note the characteristic intersecting, "mosaic" pattern to the cement lines **(C)**. **(A,** Low power; **B,** high power, H&E; **C,** H&E.)

Arthritides

The arthritides, or joint disorders, may be one of the most common medical problems. Although many diseases may affect the joint (some of these are discussed in other chapters), in this chapter, we concentrate on more common forms of arthritis likely to be encountered by the surgical pathologist.

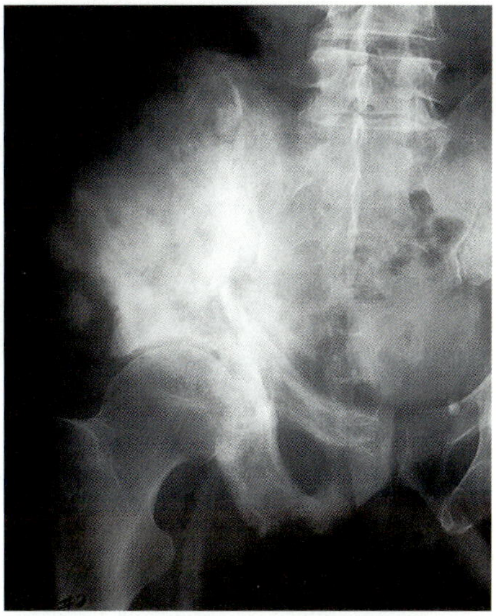

FIGURE 16.30 Paget's disease and secondary sarcoma. Typical features of Paget's disease are evident in the right hemipelvis. Ill-defined soft tissue calcification is seen lateral to the ilium and extending into the pelvis and represents a secondary osteosarcoma.

To understand the pathologic findings and clinical features of the various joint disorders, one first must acquire an appreciation for the normal anatomy of the joint space. Most joints are diarthrodial joints, characterized by a joint space partially lined by synovial membrane. The synovial membrane is lined by rows of cuboidal-appearing cells (synoviocytes), usually two to three cell layers thick.[24] Within the synovial space, a clear, viscous fluid rich in hyaluronic acid acts as a lubricant and provides nutrition for the articular cartilage surfaces. The two bones associated with the joint are covered by an articular cartilage surface. This articular cartilage serves as a "shock absorber." Because a source of blood supply is lacking, nutrients are obtained from the synovial fluid secreted by the synoviocytes. Similar to the osteoblasts and osteocytes of bone, chondrocytes associated with the articular cartilage matrix are involved in the synthesis and degradation of hyaline cartilage. Under normal circumstances, these processes are considered to be in equilibrium but may be disrupted by a variety of factors, including trauma, inflammation, and many of the disorders discussed next.

Degenerative Joint Disease

Degenerative joint disease, also known as *osteoarthritis* or *osteoarthrosis*, is the most common form of joint disease in the United States. Degenerative joint disease is a disease of articular cartilage, characterized by progressive erosion of the articular surface with secondary changes to the underlying subchondral bone. The term *degenerative joint disease* or *osteoarthrosis* is preferred to *osteoarthritis* because, in general,

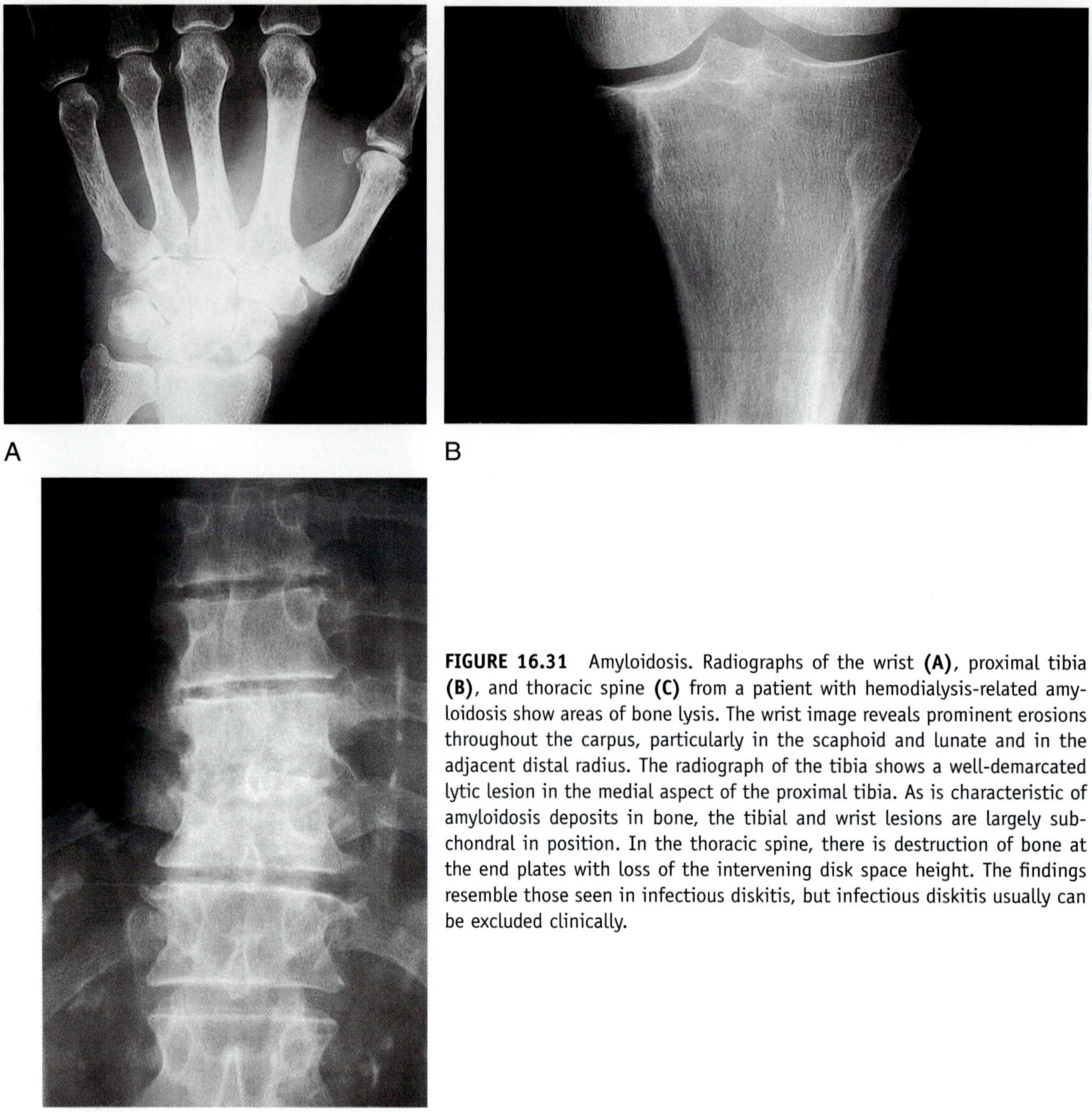

A B C

FIGURE 16.31 Amyloidosis. Radiographs of the wrist **(A)**, proximal tibia **(B)**, and thoracic spine **(C)** from a patient with hemodialysis-related amyloidosis show areas of bone lysis. The wrist image reveals prominent erosions throughout the carpus, particularly in the scaphoid and lunate and in the adjacent distal radius. The radiograph of the tibia shows a well-demarcated lytic lesion in the medial aspect of the proximal tibia. As is characteristic of amyloidosis deposits in bone, the tibial and wrist lesions are largely subchondral in position. In the thoracic spine, there is destruction of bone at the end plates with loss of the intervening disk space height. The findings resemble those seen in infectious diskitis, but infectious diskitis usually can be excluded clinically.

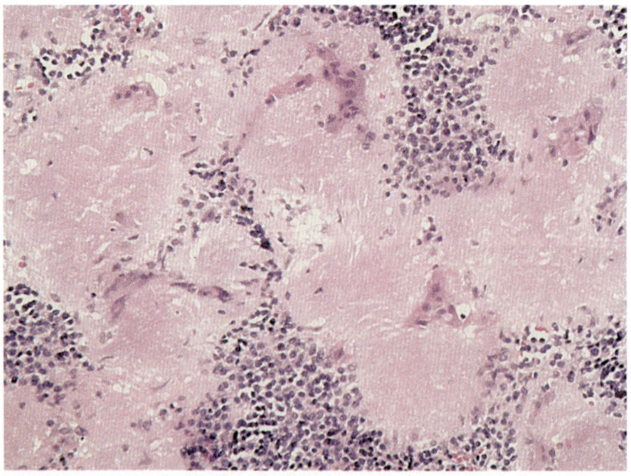

FIGURE 16.32 Amorphous aggregates of eosinophilic amyloid associated with a lymphoplasmacytic infiltrate are characteristic of amyloidosis of bone. (H&E.)

degenerative joint disease is not associated with a significant inflammatory component. Degenerative joint disease may be a primary (without a predisposing factor or disease) disorder or may occur secondary to other conditions, including trauma, inflammation, gouty arthritis, osteonecrosis, and congenital abnormalities.

Clinical Features

Most examples of degenerative joint disease arise as a primary condition, possibly related to aging. Most patients are older than age 50 at presentation. In general, degenerative joint disease is seen more commonly in women than in men. Although any joint may be affected, degenerative joint disease most commonly involves the knees and hands in women and the hips in men. Clinical symptoms include joint pain, often worse in the morning, and stiffness. Range of motion typically is reduced. Patients with secondary degenerative joint disease report similar symptoms but often present at an earlier age.

Radiographically, in the initial stages of degenerative joint disease, joint space narrowing typically is observed. With progression, erosion and loss of articular cartilage, sclerosis of subchondral bone, and cyst formation may become evident. Osteophytes frequently develop and may contribute to displacement of the joint space (Fig. 16.33). The patient's symptoms often do not correlate with the radiographic changes. In other words, severe radiographic findings do not necessarily indicate severe clinical symptoms.

Pathologic Findings

Histology

The earliest stages of degenerative joint disease are characterized by vertical and horizontal tears and fissures of the hyaline articular cartilage matrix associated with "cloning" (discrete nests of chondrocytes) of the proliferating chondrocytes. As the articular cartilage erosion progresses, the surface ultimately is sloughed, exposing the underlying bone plate. Portions of sloughed cartilage and subchondral bone may remain within the joint space, forming so-called loose bodies. The exposed subchondral bone is forced to counter the frictional forces of the joint, normally reserved for the articular cartilage surface, and consequently, it becomes polished and eburnated. Below the subchondral bone, the intratrabecular layer becomes progressively fibrotic and may develop focal myxomatous degeneration with subchondral cyst formation. Focal aggregates of lymphocytes and plasma cells may be present. Rarely, subchondral acute inflammation is seen, often associated with cyst formation, and likely represents a form of noninfectious sterile inflammation.[25] At the periphery, away from the weight-bearing surface of the joint, fibrocartilage and hyaline cartilage osteophytes often develop (Fig. 16.34).

In general, the changes within the synovium of degenerative joint disease are minimal, consisting of a slight lymphoplasmacytic infiltrate, occasionally accompanied by mild synovial cell hyperplasia. Fragments of sloughed articular cartilage and subchondral bone may become embedded within the synovial fronds, a process called *detritic synovitis*. These changes may progress to a secondary synovial chondromatosis.

Prognosis and Therapy

In the initial stages of degenerative joint disease, medical therapy is employed, generally consisting of nonsteroidal anti-inflammatory drugs (NSAIDs) and exercise. When necessary, total joint arthroplasty may be performed.

Neuropathic (Charcot) Osteoarthropathy

Neuropathic osteoarthropathy (neuropathic joint) is a severe form of joint destruction resulting from denervation. Because the disease originally was described as a complication of

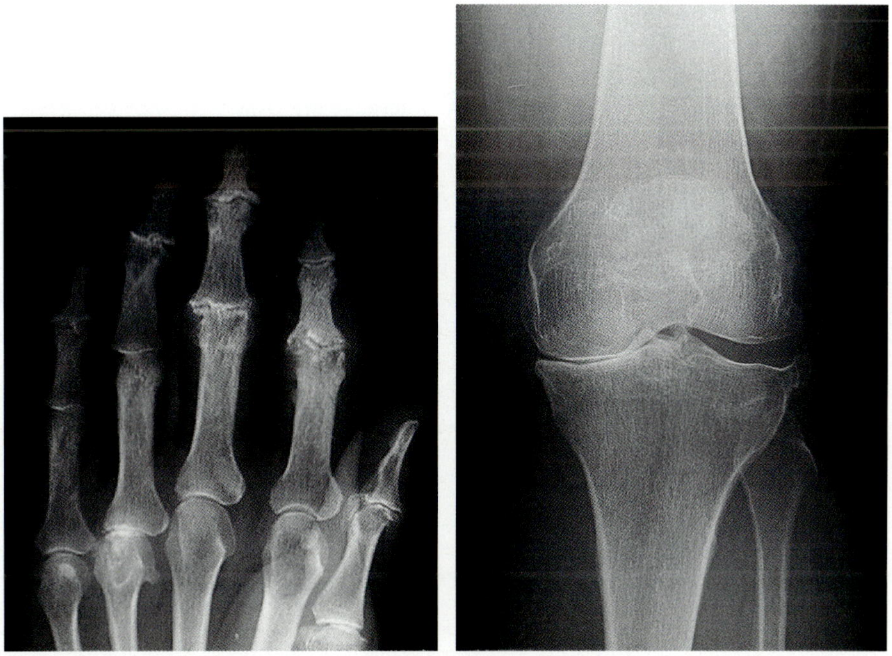

A B

FIGURE 16.33 Degenerative joint disease. A posteroanterior radiograph of the hand shows marked narrowing of multiple interphalangeal joints associated with sclerosis, subchondral cysts, and osteophytes **(A)**. Central joint erosion is evident in the distal interphalangeal joint of the fifth digit, suggesting inflammatory osteoarthrosis. Metacarpophalangeal joint narrowing and osteophytosis are also present. An anteroposterior radiograph of the knee shows marked medial femorotibial narrowing, subchondral sclerosis, and osteophytosis **(B)**.

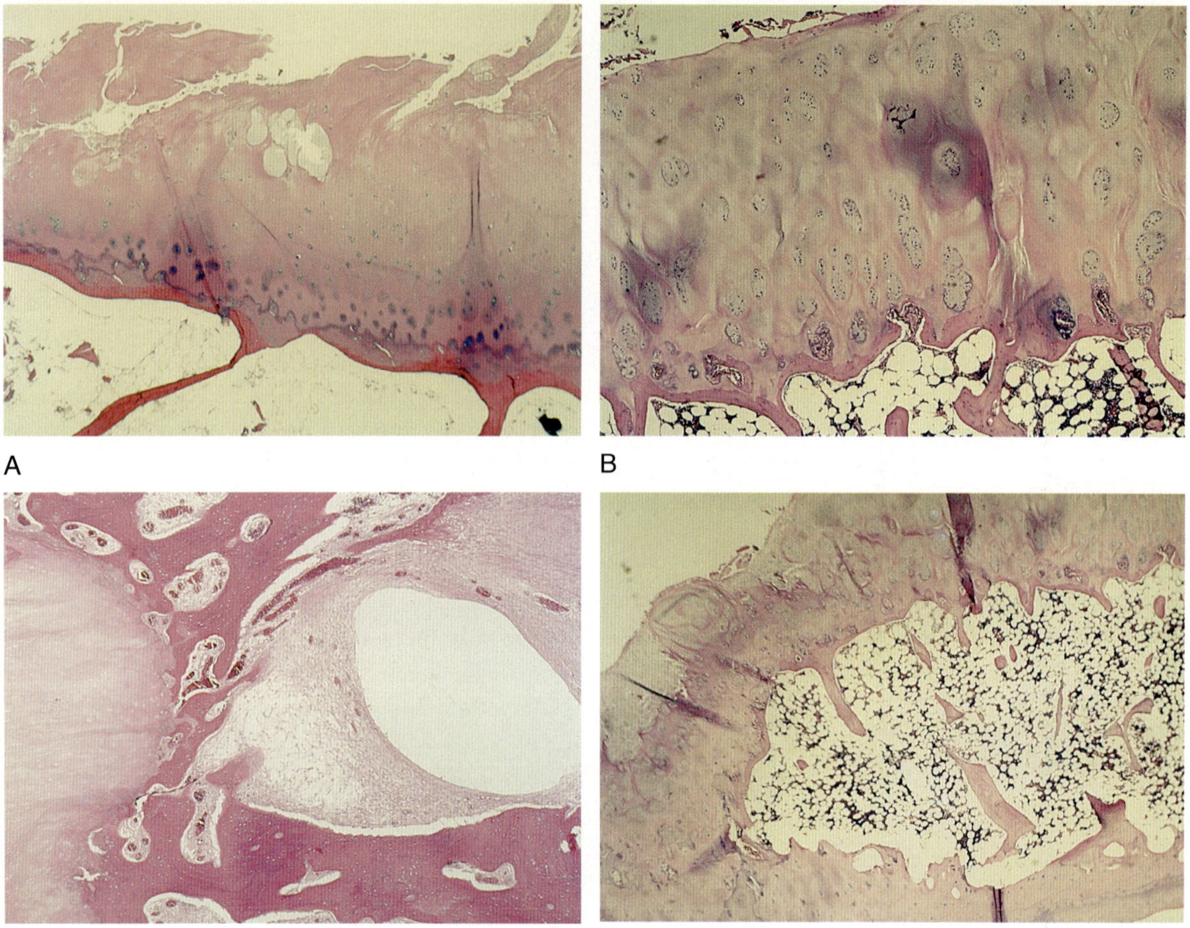

A B C D

FIGURE 16.34 Degenerative joint disease in the early stages reveals erosion and tears of the articular cartilage surface associated with a "cloning" proliferation of chondrocytes **(A** and **B)**. Later stages may result in sloughing of the articular cartilage and the formation of subchondral bone cysts **(C)**. Away from the weight-bearing surfaces of the joint, osteophytes may develop **(D)**. **(A** to **D,** H&E.)

syphilis, it also is known as *Charcot joint*. At present, the most common cause of neuropathic joint in the United States is diabetes mellitus. Other potential causes include alcoholism, amyloidosis, and demyelinating nerve disorders. Virtually any joint within the body may develop neuropathic changes. In diabetes, the foot bones are involved most commonly. Radiographically, evidence of severe, rapidly destructive degenerative joint disease is observed, with severe erosion and subluxation, multiple loose bodies, and massively enlarged osteophytes (Fig. 16.35). The pathologic changes reveal severe degenerative joint disease with marked deformities of the articular surface and numerous shards (detritus) of articular cartilage and subchondral bone embedded within the synovial membrane.

Rheumatoid Arthritis

In contrast to degenerative joint disease, rheumatoid arthritis is a systemic disorder. It may involve sites other than the joints, including the skin, heart valves, and lungs and has a significant inflammatory component. Most evidence suggests an autoimmune cause, possibly related to an infectious agent.

Clinical Features

Rheumatoid arthritis is observed more commonly in women and typically affects patients 30 to 50 years old. Clinical complaints include fatigue, weakness, and joint pain and stiffness. Although virtually any joint may be affected, the earliest changes are observed in the metacarpophalangeal and proximal interphalangeal joints of the hands. Swelling and tenderness is usually present. Severe involvement of the metacarpophalangeal joints with subsequent subluxation leads to characteristic ulnar deviation. Other joints commonly affected by rheumatoid arthritis include the elbows, wrists, and feet.

The finding of serum rheumatoid factor, a circulating IgM immunoglobulin directed against the Fc portion of autologous circulating IgG antibody, supports the diagnosis of rheumatoid arthritis. Patients with rheumatoid arthritis also frequently have an elevated white blood cell count and erythrocyte sedimentation rate.

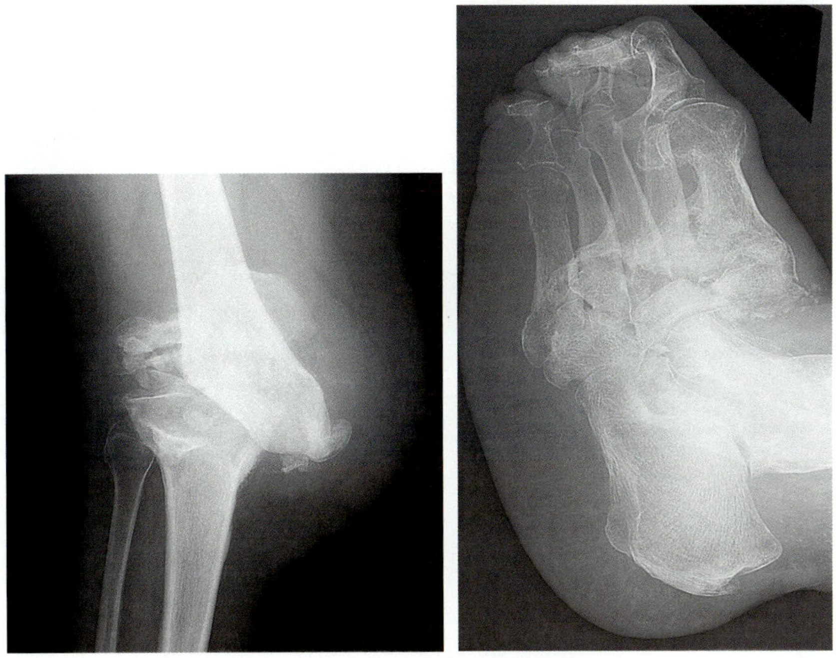

FIGURE 16.35 Neuropathic osteoarthropathy. An anteroposterior radiograph of the knee shows gross destruction and fragmentation of the articular surfaces of the femur and tibia **(A)**. The tibia is displaced laterally. Despite the degree of bone fragmentation, bone density is preserved. An oblique radiograph of the foot in another patient shows gross fragmentation of bone with medial displacement of the remnants of the first metatarsal and medial cuneiform **(B)**. As in **A,** the bone density is preserved despite the destruction of bone and articular surfaces.

Classic rheumatoid nodules occur in one fourth of patients, most commonly involving the subcutaneous tissues, but also seen in other tissues and organ systems. Rheumatoid nodules typically arise in areas subjected to increased pressure, especially the extensor aspects of the forearm and elbow.

Radiographically, symmetric joint space narrowing and marginal erosions, best observed in the small bones of the digits, characterize rheumatoid arthritis. Because these erosions often disrupt supporting ligaments of the joint, subluxations and dislocations are observed frequently. Bone loss (osteopenia) also is seen. In contrast to degenerative joint disease, however, cartilage proliferation and osteophytes are uncommon (Fig. 16.36).

Pathologic Findings

Histology

Morphologically, rheumatoid arthritis is characterized by a nonsuppurative, chronic proliferative synovitis. The proliferating synovium may be several cell layers thick and frequently contains multinucleated giant cells. Lymphoid aggregates with germinal centers often accompany a significant plasma cell infiltrate, occupying the superficial synovium. Neutrophils are less commonly present. A characteristic histologic feature of rheumatoid arthritis is the presence of a fibrinoid exudate on the synovial frond surface (Fig. 16.37). With progression, the chronically inflamed synovium (pannus) extends over the articular surface, causing erosion and destruction of the articular cartilage, presumably by blocking chondrocyte nutrition (Fig. 16.38). Ultimately the entire cartilaginous surface may be destroyed with exposure of the underlying subchondral bone.

The diagnosis of rheumatoid arthritis may be established easily by the finding of a classic rheumatoid nodule. These nodules are characterized histologically by a proliferation of epithelioid-appearing histiocytes and chronic inflammatory cells surrounding a central core of fibrinoid necrosis (Fig. 16.39). The main differential diagnosis includes epithelioid sarcoma, but correlation with clinical and radiographic findings is usually sufficient to exclude this diagnosis. In difficult cases, immunohistochemical stains for cytokeratin, positive in epithelioid sarcoma but negative in rheumatoid nodules, may be necessary.

Fine Needle Aspiration Biopsy

Fine needle aspiration biopsy of joint effusions often reveals histiocytes and histiocytic giant cells, lymphocytes, and necrotic debris.[26,27] Early in the course of the disease, the joint fluid may contain numerous neutrophils, resembling a septic arthritis. Rheumatoid nodules often show similar features with background necrotic debris and scattered histiocytes, lymphocytes, and plasma cells.

Prognosis and Therapy

Rheumatoid arthritis typically is managed medically. Virtually all patients receive steroids and NSAIDs. Additional drug treatment may include methotrexate and gold injections. Physical therapy and exercise are essential for maintaining range of motion and muscle strength. Most

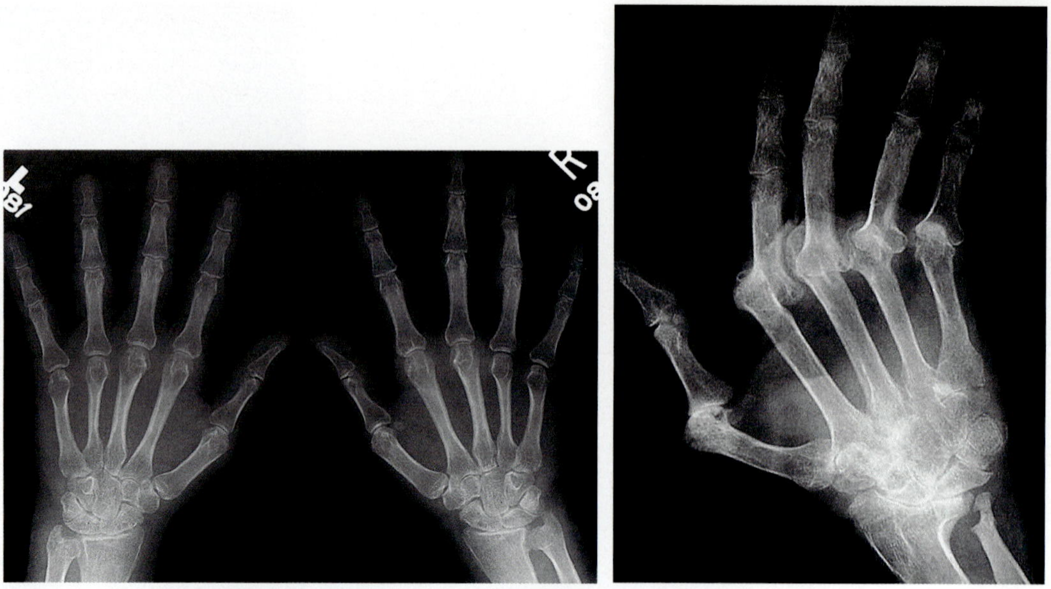

A B

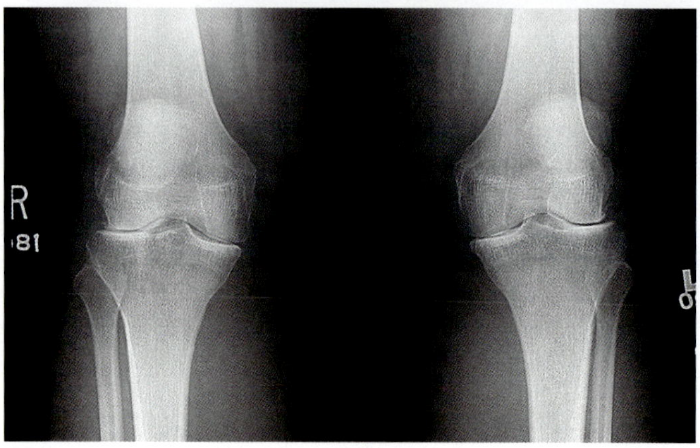

C

FIGURE 16.36 Rheumatoid arthritis. A posteroanterior radiograph of the hands reveals periarticular osteoporosis with narrowing and soft tissue swelling at multiple metacarpophalangeal joints **(A)**. Ulnar styloid process erosions are evident bilaterally, and there are multiple carpal and metacarpal head erosions. In another patient with more advanced disease, there is severe erosion at multiple metacarpophalangeal joints and at the distal radioulnar joint **(B)**. These joints and the carpus show marked joint narrowing. Ulnar angulation at the metacarpophalangeal joints and radial angulation at the wrist are characteristic of rheumatoid arthritis. An anteroposterior radiograph of the knees shows medial and lateral femorotibial narrowing with only minimal osteophyte formation and sclerosis **(C)**.

complications, such as peptic ulcer disease or infections, are secondary to long-standing steroid therapy. Surgery, including synovectomy and total joint arthroplasty, are reserved for more advanced stages of the disease.

Juvenile Rheumatoid Arthritis

Juvenile rheumatoid arthritis also is known as *Still's disease* and is the most common form of arthritis seen in children. Despite similarities to rheumatoid arthritis, most children lack serum rheumatoid factor. Juvenile rheumatoid arthritis shows a varied presentation, ranging from disease limited to the joints to generalized lymphadenopathy and hepatosplenomegaly. Nevertheless, in contrast to the adult form of the disease, patients with juvenile rheumatoid arthritis usually recover completely. A few have disability, and rarely death may occur. The pathologic features are similar to those observed with adult rheumatoid arthritis.

Ankylosing Spondyloarthritis

Ankylosing spondyloarthritis, also called *Marie-Strumpell disease* or *rheumatoid spondylitis*, is a chronic inflammatory synovitis predominantly affecting the axial skeleton, especially the sacroiliac joints. In contrast to degenerative joint disease, it usually manifests in adolescence or young adults, especially males who are HLA-B27 positive. Patients typically complain of low back pain that, with progression, may result in severe spinal immobility. Radiographically, the process begins in the sacroiliac joints as bony surface erosions progressing to total fusion of the joint. In a few patients, ankylosing spondyloarthritis may involve the entire spine, resulting in complete fusion ("bamboo spine") (Fig. 16.40). Extraskeletal manifestations include uveitis, which occurs in about one quarter of patients. Microscopic examination reveals a chronic "inflammatory" synovitis associated with erosion and destruction of articular cartilage. The inflammation may extend into tendons and ligaments, resulting in

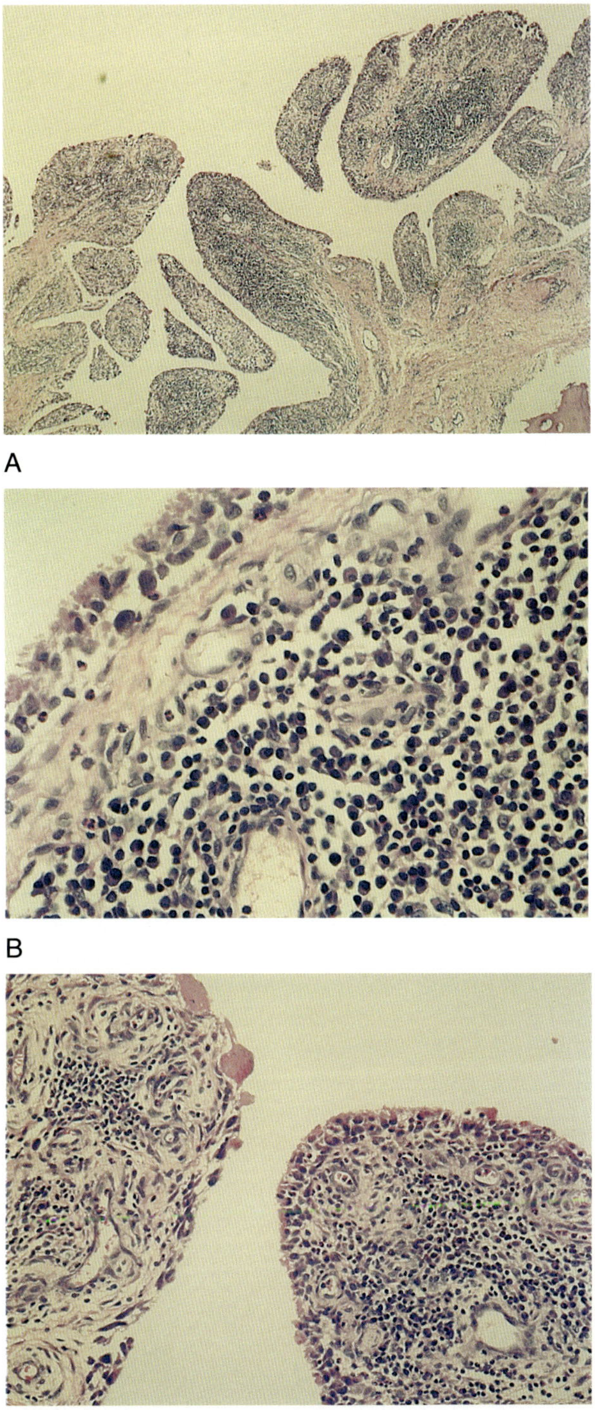

FIGURE 16.37 Rheumatoid arthritis characterized by expansion of the synovial fronds by a marked lymphoplasmacytic infiltrate **(A** and **B)**. Note the pink eosinophilic deposits of fibrin on the surface of the synovial fronds, a common finding in rheumatoid arthritis **(C)**. **(A,** Low power; **B,** high power, H&E; **C,** H&E.)

bony outgrowths or spurs. In contrast to rheumatoid arthritis, ankylosing spondyloarthritis is a seronegative arthropathy. Physical therapy, exercise, and NSAIDs are the mainstays of therapy. Surgery is rarely necessary.

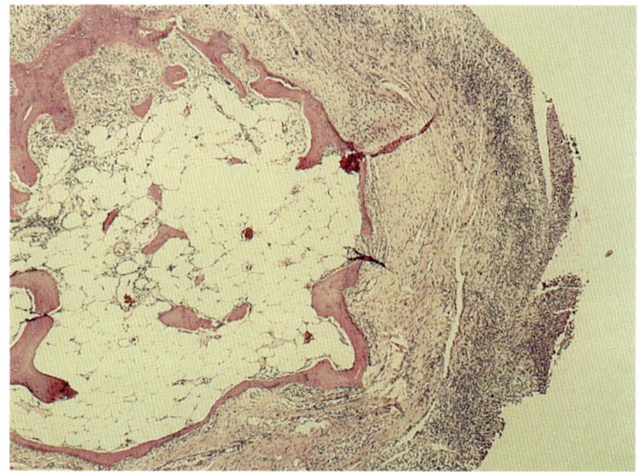

FIGURE 16.38 Rheumatoid arthritis. Growth of the inflamed synovium (pannus) over the articular surface ultimately causes its destruction. (H&E.)

Alkaptonuria (Ochronosis)

Alkaptonuria is an autosomal recessive disorder associated with a genetic lack of the enzyme homogentisic acid oxidase. This enzyme allows for the metabolism of homogentisic acid within the phenylalanine-tyrosine pathway. Consequently, homogentisic acid accumulates in various sites throughout the body. The disorder often first is manifested in childhood by the black color of an affected patient's urine after oxidation. The more severe arthropathy is not usually seen until adulthood.[28] Homogentisic acid has a predilection for connective tissue collagen and tends to deposit in collagen-rich areas, imparting a blue-black pigmentation (Fig. 16.41). Deposits of homogentisic acid on the heart valves and blood vessel walls may lead to premature atherosclerosis. Similar deposits in joints result in premature destruction of the articular cartilage surface. The axial skeleton is the most commonly affected anatomic site. Pathologically the findings are those of severely destructive degenerative joint disease with fragments of bone and cartilage embedded within the underlying bone or

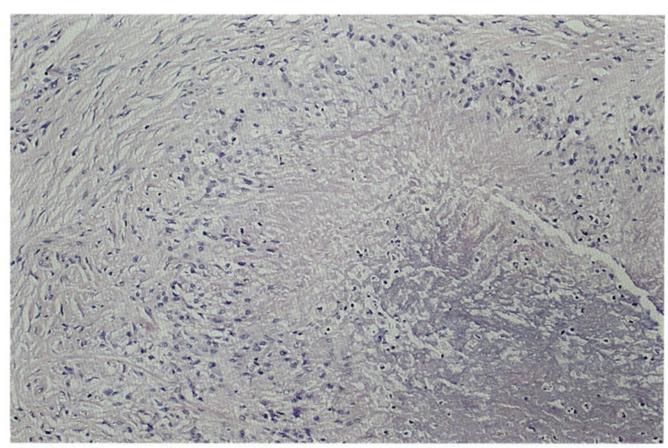

FIGURE 16.39 Rheumatoid arthritis. Classic rheumatoid nodules show a peripheral zone of proliferating histiocytes surrounding a central area of geographic necrosis. (H&E.)

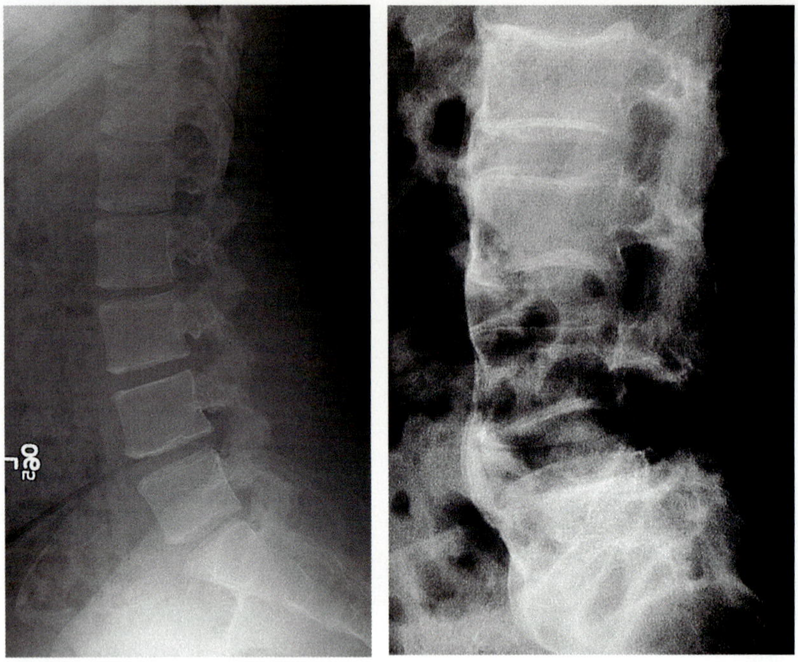

A B

FIGURE 16.40 Ankylosing spondylitis. A lateral radiograph of a young man with early ankylosing spondylitis reveals small foci of sclerosis at multiple vertebral body corners, known radiologically as the "shiny corner sign" and reflecting new bone formation at erosions at the margins of the annulus fibrosus **(A)**. In another patient with more advanced ankylosing spondylitis, smooth, flowing bony excrescences extend from end plate to end plate, represent syndesmophytes, and result in the "bamboo spine" appearance **(B)**. The facet joints are solidly ankylosed posteriorly.

surrounding synovial tissues, resulting in multiple loose bodies (Fig. 16.42).

Gout

Clinical Features

Gout, one of the several crystal arthritides, is caused by persistent chronic hyperuricemia. Table 16.1 summarizes three common crystal deposition diseases. In its primary form, hyperuricemia is the result of an inborn error of purine metabolism or diminished renal excretion of uric acid. Secondary hyperuricemia, resulting from pre-existing disease, is generally the result of either extensive cell turnover (e.g., myeloproliferative disorders or drug therapy) or acquired renal diseases that decrease the urinary excretion of uric acid. Regardless of whether hyperuricemia occurs as a primary or secondary form, the clinical manifestations of gouty arthritis encompass four distinct syndromes—asymptomatic hyperuricemia, acute gouty arthritis, chronic tophaceous gout, and nephrolithiasis. Symptomatic gout more commonly strikes men than women and typically occurs in patients older than age 30. Among

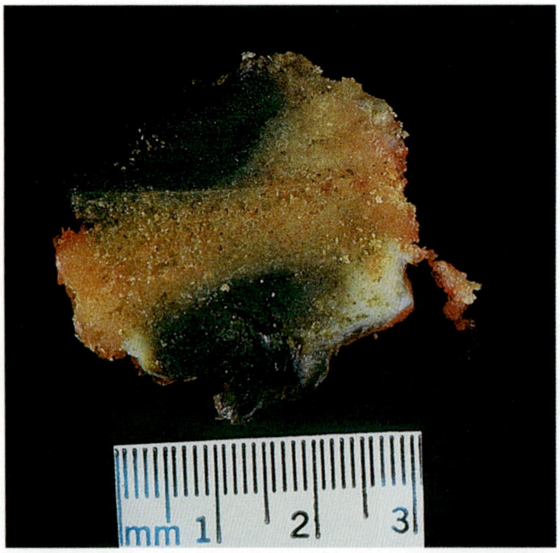

FIGURE 16.41 Alkaptonuria. A fragment of diseased cartilage and subchondral bone has the characteristic blue-black pigmentation of homogentisic acid.

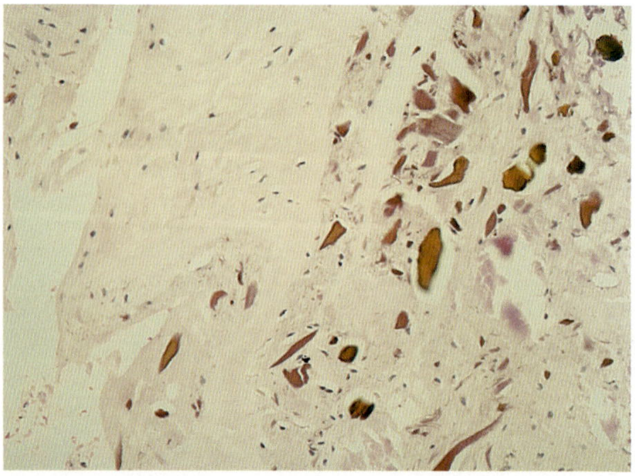

FIGURE 16.42 Alkaptonuria. Numerous, pigmented shards of bone and cartilage are embedded in the surrounding synovial tissues, resulting in a "detritic synovitis." (H&E.)

TABLE 16.1 Clinicopathologic Features of Gout, Pseudogout, and Tumoral Calcinosis

	Gout	Pseudogout	Tumoral Calcinosis
Age (yr)*	30-50	>50	10-40
Sites†	First MTP joint	Knee	Hips
Crystal Morphology	Needle-shaped	Rhomboid-shaped	Amorphous, plates
Polarizing Features	Strong negative birefringence	Weak positive birefringence	No birefringence
Cartilage Metaplasia	No	Sometimes	No
Histiocytic Reaction‡	Usually prominent	Often not present and less prominent	Usually prominent

*Most common ages at presentation.
†Most common anatomic site for deposits.
‡Histiocytic inflammatory reaction with giant cells surrounding the crystal deposits.
MTP joint, metatarsophalangeal joint.

these clinical syndromes, the most common manifestation is a painful arthritis, frequently monarticular and most often affecting the extremities. In more than half of patients, the first attack of gout involves the first metatarsophalangeal joint (the great toe). These attacks generally resolve within a couple of days to weeks only to recur at a later time. Repeated attacks over years lead to chronic gout. Tophi, soft tissue masses consisting of urate crystals, are seen most commonly in this setting. Rarely, tophi may be the initial manifestation of the disease.

Radiographic findings tend to be minimal in the early course of the disease, consisting simply of soft tissue swelling. With progression, tophi accompany bony erosions on both sides of the joints, most commonly observed in the digits of the hands and feet (Fig. 16.43). With the exception of the tophi, the radiographic findings may be similar to findings observed with rheumatoid arthritis. Osteopenia, characteristic of rheumatoid arthritis, is not observed in gout.

Pathologic Findings

Histology

The histologic features of gout vary depending on the stage at which it is diagnosed. Early in the course of the disease, a mixture of numerous inflammatory cells, including neutrophils, lymphocytes, and histiocytes, infiltrates the synovial membranes. Diagnostic urate crystals may be difficult to identify and tend to be seen more easily within the synovial fluid. Using compensated polarizing microscopy, these crystals usually appear needle-shaped and show strong negative birefringence (Fig. 16.44).[29] The typical tophus is composed of amorphous, chalky, white, acellular material surrounded by a prominent histiocytic giant cell reaction (Fig. 16.45). Within the amorphous material, diagnostic urate crystals generally are observed easily but may be lost with tissue processing.

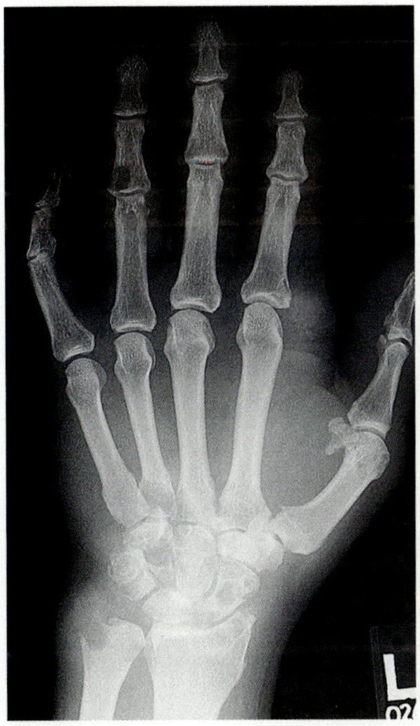
A

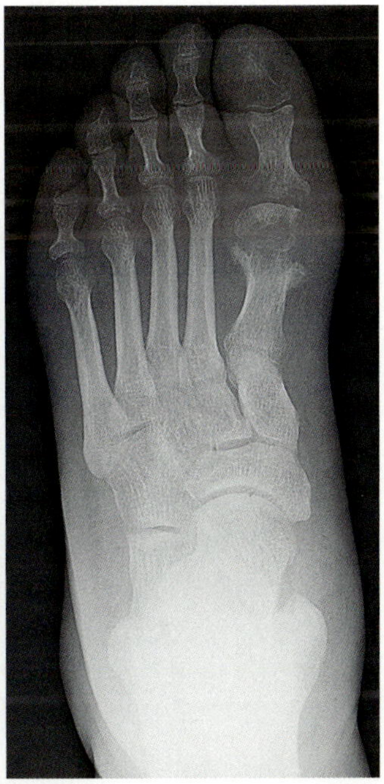
B

FIGURE 16.43 Gout. An anteroposterior radiograph of the hand shows multiple, well-defined erosions **(A)**. Bulky soft tissue masses with faint calcification represent tophi, particularly evident adjacent to the second metacarpophalangeal joint and the eroded ulnar styloid process. In contrast to the findings of rheumatoid arthritis noted earlier, bone density and joint width are preserved. In another patient, severe erosions are present at the first metatarsophalangeal joint, a favored site for gout **(B)**. There is also an erosion at the base of the distal phalanx of the great toe, and joint width remains relatively preserved, despite the extent of erosion.

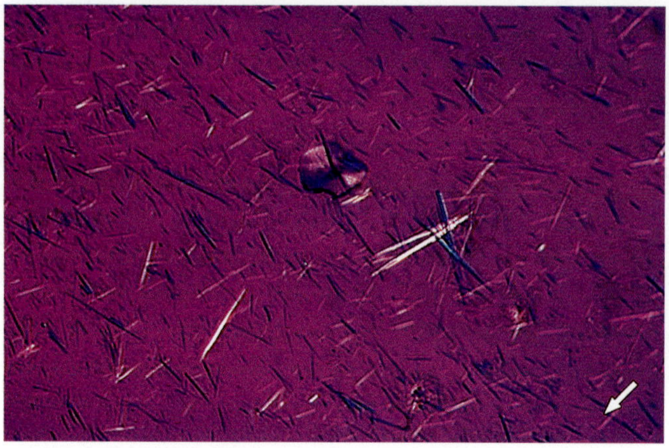

FIGURE 16.44 Gout. When visualized with compensated polarizing microscopy, needle-shaped crystals of urate show strong negative birefringence. The arrow signifies the direction of the compensating filter line. Parallel and yellow equates to negative birefringence. (H&E.)

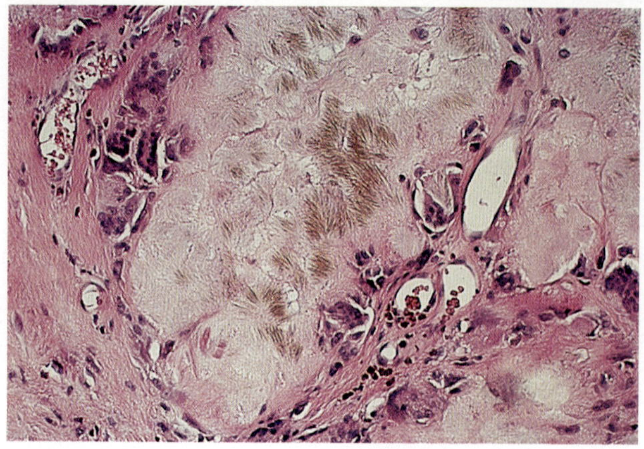

FIGURE 16.45 Gout. Amorphous, white-tan deposits of urate crystals and debris with surrounding histiocytic giant cell reaction are the characteristic findings of gouty tophi. Note the needle-shaped crystals. (H&E.)

Fine Needle Aspiration Biopsy

Fine needle aspiration biopsy of gouty tophi easily establishes the diagnosis of gout. We have observed several patients who presented with "chronic gout" and a gouty tophus without a pre-existing history or diagnosis of gouty arthritis. In some of these cases, soft tissue sarcoma was suspected. Fine needle aspiration biopsy generally yields abundant, needle-shaped, negatively birefringent crystals accompanied by scattered histiocytes, foreign body–type giant cells, neutrophils, and amorphous debris (Fig. 16.46).[30]

Prognosis and Therapy

Medical drug therapy is the principal form of gout therapy. Overall, therapy involves relieving the pain of acute gout, using NSAIDs, and preventing future attacks with colchicine or allopurinol or both. Serum urate levels also tend to decrease with low-protein diets and abstinence from alcohol. Surgical therapy is reserved for more severe cases and may include removal of infected tophi.

Calcium Pyrophosphate Dihydrate Deposition Disease (Pseudogout)

Similar to gouty arthritis, calcium pyrophosphate dihydrate deposition disease is a form of arthritis characterized by crystal deposition within the joints. Instead of urate, calcium pyrophosphate dihydrate deposition disease involves calcium deposits.

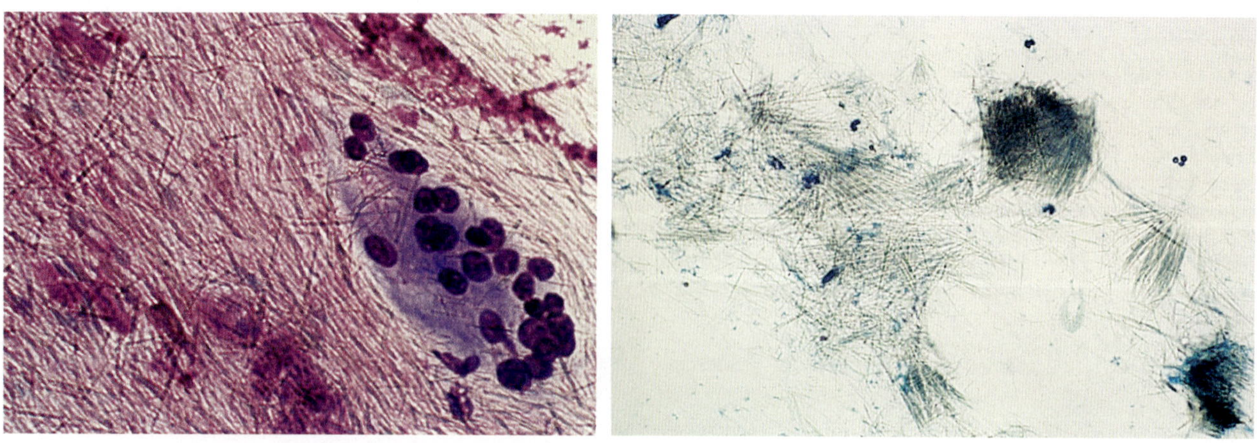

A B

FIGURE 16.46 Fine needle aspiration biopsy specimen of tophi reveals abundant needle-shaped crystals and occasional multinucleated histiocytes **(A** and **B)**. **(A,** Diff-Quik; **B,** Papanicolaou.)

Clinical Features

The clinical features of calcium pyrophosphate dihydrate deposition disease vary considerably, ranging from asymptomatic, incidental joint calcifications (chondrocalcinosis) to an acute arthritis, closely resembling gout (pseudogout). Some forms of the disease resemble degenerative joint disease, whereas others may mimic acute rheumatoid arthritis. Most patients are middle-aged to older adults; the most common anatomic location is the knee. Other sites, including the wrist and vertebrae, may be affected, however, and multiple joints are often involved. Consequently, pathologists may encounter calcium pyrophosphate dihydrate deposition disease in a variety of clinical settings, ranging from incidental findings in herniated intervertebral disk material to total joint replacement specimens for degenerative joint disease.

Radiographic features are variable, ranging from tumorlike deposition of calcium pyrophosphate within joints, including synovial membrane, menisci, and articular cartilage, to osteoarthritis with joint space narrowing and subchondral sclerosis (Fig. 16.47).

Pathologic Findings

Histology

The histologic hallmark is the presence of deeply basophilic fragments of calcification deposited within articular cartilage, synovial fronds, or menisci. In contrast to the needle-shaped profiles of urate crystals, calcium pyrophosphate dihydrate crystals generally have a more rhomboid-type configuration and show weak positive birefringence with compensated polarizing microscopy.[29,31] Paradoxically the crystals may not be associated with an inflammatory/histiocytic response, especially when deposited in articular cartilage; however, an inflammatory reaction is observed more frequently when the calcium deposits localize to the synovial membrane (Fig. 16.48). Chondroid metaplasia, a feature not seen with tumoral calcinosis, is sometimes present with calcium pyrophospate dihydrate deposition disease, especially in the digits.

Fine Needle Aspiration Biopsy

At present, there have been only rare descriptions of the cytologic findings in pseudogout.[32] Cytologic findings are similar to gout with the exception that the crystals are more rhomboid-shaped with blunted or squared ends.

Prognosis and Therapy

The therapy of calcium pyrophosphate dihydrate disease is generally conservative. Complaints of pain are relieved by the use of NSAIDs. In contrast to gouty arthritis, the tendency to form crystals cannot be prevented with medical therapy. Surgery is reserved for more severe and advanced cases and may include total joint arthroplasty.

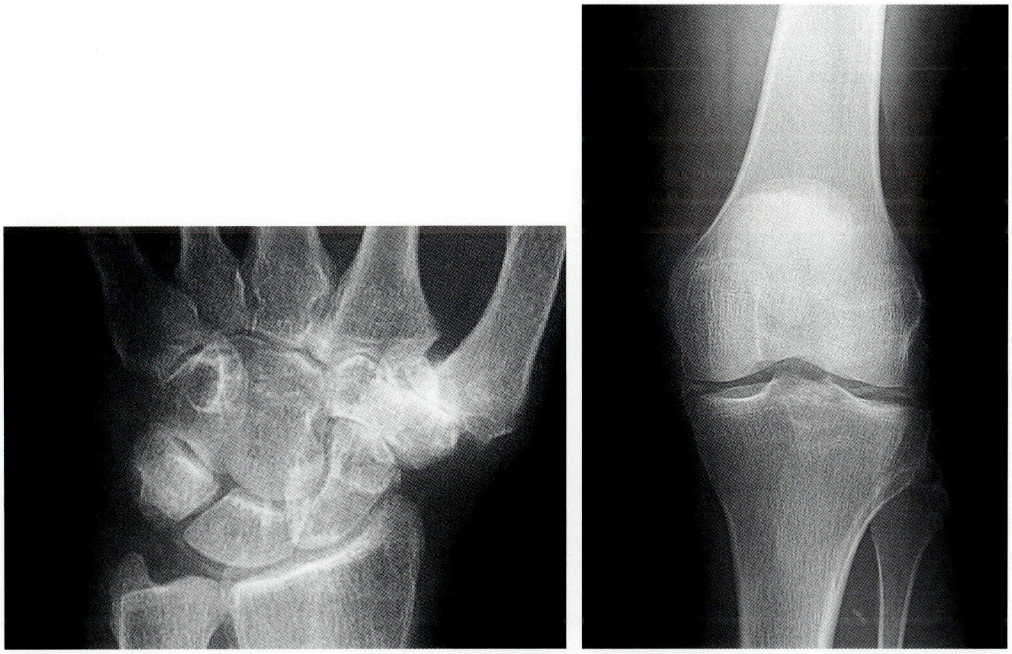

A B

FIGURE 16.47 Calcium pyrophosphate dihydrate deposition disease. A posteroanterior radiograph of the wrist reveals chondrocalcinosis throughout the carpus, particularly at the triangular fibrocartilage complex adjacent to the proximal aspect of the lunate **(A)**. Degenerative narrowing and sclerosis are present at the thumb carpometacarpal joint. In another patient, a radiograph of the knee shows marked calcification of the menisci and articular cartilage **(B)**.

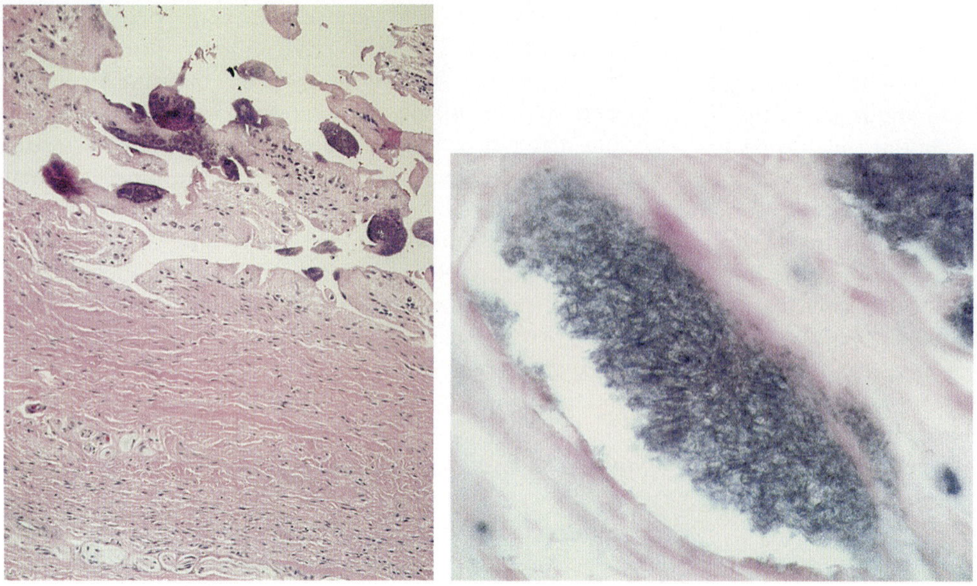

A B

FIGURE 16.48 Calcium pyrophosphate dihydrate deposition disease characterized by multifocal deposits of closely packed, rhomboid-shaped calcium crystals. Note the absence of a significant inflammatory response surrounding the calcium crystals **(A** and **B)**. **(A,** Low power; **B,** high power, H&E.)

Tumoral Calcinosis

Tumoral calcinosis is localized deposits of calcium crystals, usually calcium hydroxyapatite, within soft tissues, often adjacent to joints. When presenting within tendons, the process sometimes is referred to as *calcific tendinitis*. Tumoral calcinosis most commonly occurs sporadically, possibly resulting from local trauma, but may be the result of a metabolic abnormality of calcium metabolism. Most patients range in age from the teens to the 40s at presentation, and painless periarticular, soft tissue swelling, involving one or more joints, is the most frequent complaint. Patients with chronic renal failure may develop multifocal deposits of calcium hydroxyapatite. Radiographically, tumoral calcinosis presents as multiple, soft tissue calcifications often localized around a joint (Fig. 16.49). The most frequent periarticular sites are the hips (57%), followed by the elbows and shoulders.[33] Pathologic examination reveals nodules and plates of nonbirefringent, basophilic calcifications.[29] Surrounding the cartilaginous plates and nodules are numerous histiocytes and multinucleated giant cells (Fig. 16.50). Cytologic smears from fine needle aspiration biopsy specimens generally show amorphous, refractile crystalline material with scattered histiocytic giant cells and lymphocytes.[34] Occasional examples of "tumoral calcinosis," especially involving the temporomandibular joint and digits,

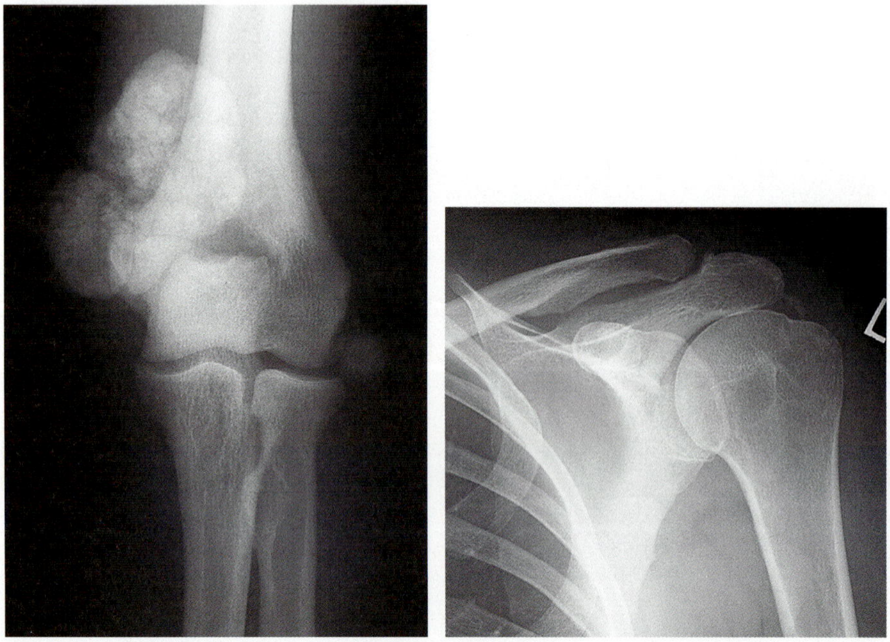

A B

FIGURE 16.49 Tumoral calcinosis. A large, amorphous mass of calcification is present overlying and medial to the distal humerus in a patient with chronic renal failure **(A)**. Calcareous masses developing in this setting are known radiologically as *metastatic calcification*. An anteroposterior radiograph of the shoulder in another patient shows amorphous calcification superior to the humeral head, in the supraspinatus tendon, representing calcific tendonitis **(B)**. In contrast to masses of metastatic calcification, these deposits of calcific tendinitis are often quite painful.

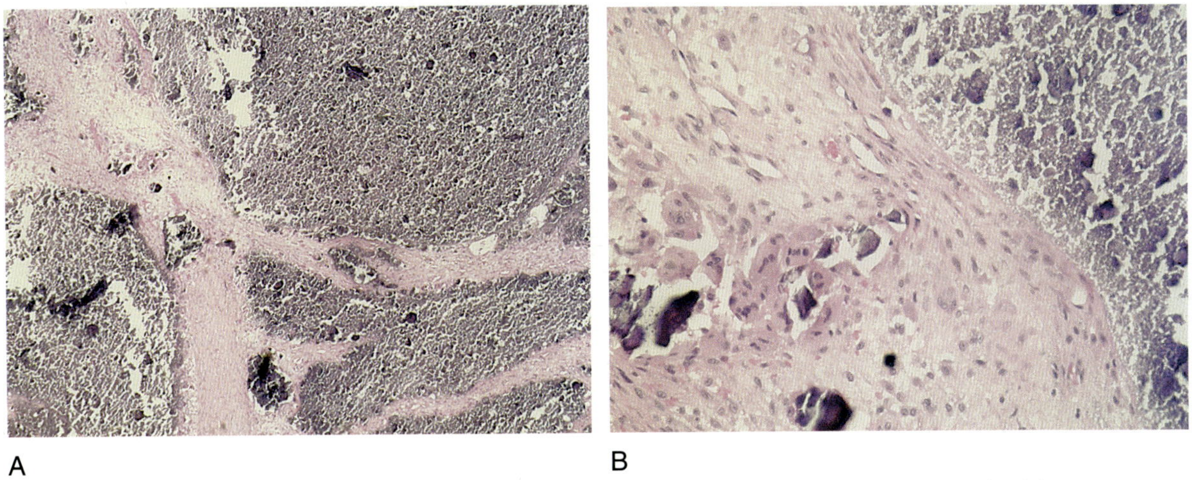

FIGURE 16.50 Tumoral calcinosis characterized by deposits of amorphous plates of calcium crystals with a surrounding histiocytic giant cell reaction **(A** and **B)**. **(A,** Low power; **B,** high power, H&E.)

represent deposits of calcium pyrophosphate that show positive birefringence with polarizing light microscopy. Therapy generally consists of surgical excision, but medical therapy with oral aluminum hydroxide (phosphate binder) also has been used successfully in a few cases.[35]

A similar lesion, calcifying pseudotumor of the neural axis (crudoma), occurs adjacent to the skull base and spine and is seen most commonly in middle-aged adults. The cause of these unusual calcific deposits is unknown.

Role of the Pathologist in Failed Joint Arthroplasty

Total large joint arthroplasty or replacement is one of the most common surgical procedures performed in the United States. Consequently, surgical pathologists frequently are required to examine bone and soft tissue obtained from the original replacement and from tissue removed surrounding the subsequently failed joint implant. Failed joint replacements are generally the result of either mechanical wear (aseptic loosening) or infection. This distinction has clinical consequences because the orthopedic surgeon must decide, based on all available information, whether to resect the joint or implant a new prosthesis in one or two stages. The latter appears to result in an improved clinical outcome in cases of septic loosening.

The histologic findings in tissue from large joint revision arthroplasty include abundant mechanical wear debris—polyethylene, metal, and methyl methacrylate. Polyethylene debris almost always is observed, usually abundant, and consists of fine granular to thread-like particles generally present within histiocytes. Larger fragments of polyethylene may be seen in multinucleated giant cells (Fig. 16.51). With compensated polarizing microscopy, polyethylene debris shows strong birefringence. In contrast, methyl methacrylate (cement) is dissolved during processing and is not usually

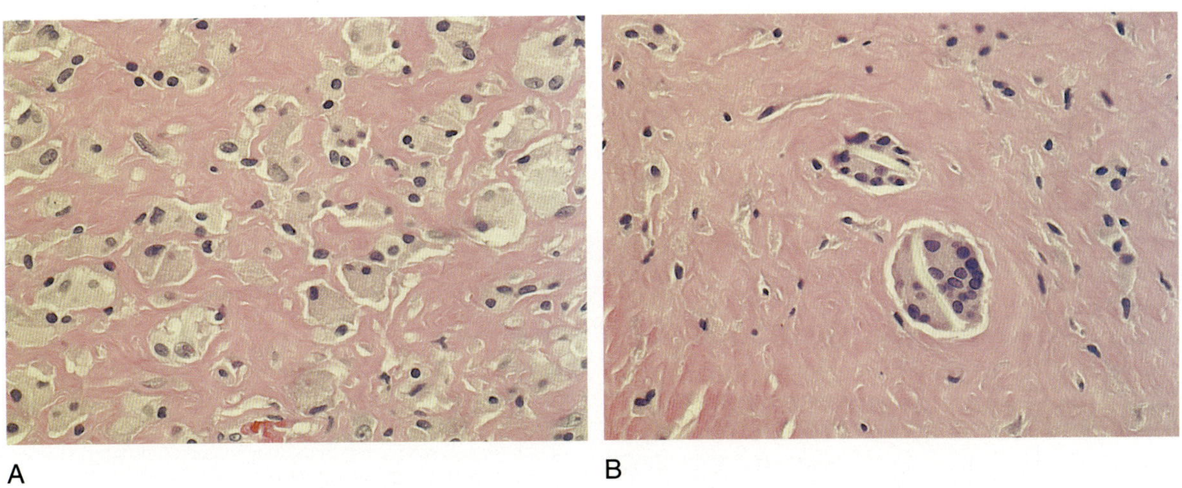

FIGURE 16.51 Polyethylene debris generally consists of small, finely granular material within histiocytes (arthroplasty effect) **(A)**. Less commonly, larger fragments or shards of polyethylene debris may be observed in multinucleated histiocytes **(B)**. **(A** and **B,** H&E.)

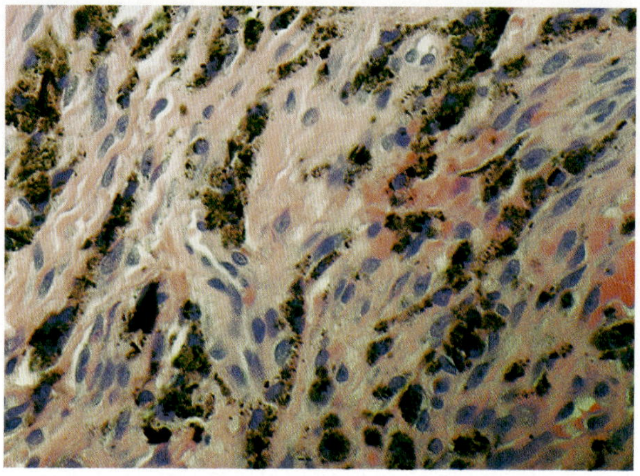

FIGURE 16.52 Titanium debris is characterized by multiple small particles of black discoloration primarily within histiocytes. (H&E.)

apparent in hematoxylin and eosin–stained sections. Only the spaces, usually within giant cells, where the cement once localized, are seen. Metallic debris, especially titanium, manifests as small particles of black discoloration most often within histiocytes (Fig. 16.52). Although chronic inflammation (lymphocytes and plasma cells) is frequently present, neutrophils generally should not be seen outside of infection. There is no foolproof method for diagnosing infection. Several studies have shown that histologic examination of periprosthetic tissues in revision arthroplasty may be highly predictive of infection.[36-38] At our institution, if septic loosening is suspected intraoperatively, frozen section is requested. Defining the exact parameters of what constitutes "acute inflammation" is difficult and controversial, however. In the literature, the range of significant neutrophilic infiltration predictive of infection has varied from one to five neutrophils per high-power field.[36-38] All pathologists recognize the fact that acute inflammation may be a focal phenomenon and may not be sampled initially. The absence of neutrophils at frozen section does not mean that no infection is present; likewise, the presence of neutrophils does not imply the presence of infection. Other potential causes of a neutrophilic infiltrate include a previously undocumented inflammatory arthritis, fracture, or tissue samples obtained late in the course of the operating room case. We believe it is more important to report accurate information than to decide arbitrarily on the significance of the information. As a result, we typically report simply the presence or absence of neutrophils and the number observed per high-power field. The finding of neutrophils within fibrin should not be considered "positive"; only neutrophils localized in extravascular soft tissues should be documented.

Less commonly, prostheses, different from those used with large joints, are used to replace smaller joints, such as the hands or feet. Most small joint prostheses are composed of silicone polymers and are usually solid Silastic. The same problems that may plague large joint prostheses, including mechanical failure and infection, may be observed in small joint silicone prostheses.[39,40] Histologically the synovial membrane shows a histiocytic giant cell reaction associated with yellow-green fragments of silicone material. The latter is not birefringent with polarizing microscopy. Lymphocytes and plasma cells also may be present, but neutrophils should not be seen and indicate potential infection.

REFERENCES

Osteomyelitis and Septic Arthritis

1. Leonard A, Comty CM, Shapiro FL, et al: Osteomyelitis in hemodialysis patients. Ann Intern Med 1973;78:651.
2. Hughes R, Rowe I, Shanson D, et al: Septic bone, joint and muscle lesions associated with human immunodeficiency virus infection. Br J Rheumatol 1992;31:381.
3. Merkel KD, Fitzgerald RH, Brown ML: Scintigraphic evaluation in musculoskeletal sepsis. Orthop Clin North Am 1984;15:401.
4. Sorenson TS, Hedeboe J, Christensen ER: Primary epiphyseal osteomyelitis in children. J Bone Joint Surg Br 1988:70:818.
5. Morris JM, Lucas DB: Fibrosarcoma within a sinus tract of chronic draining osteomyelitis: Case report and review of the literature. J Bone Joint Surg Am 1964;46:853.
6. Beretta-Piccoli BC, Sauvain MJ, Schibler GI, et al: Synovitis, acne, pustulosis, hyperostosis, osteitis (SAPHO) syndrome in childhood: A report of ten cases and review of the literature. Eur J Pediatr 2000;159:594.
7. Huber AM , Lam PY, Duffy CM, et al: Chronic recurrent multifocal osteomyelitis: Clinical outcomes after more than five years of follow-up. J Pediatr 2002;141:198.
8. Davidson PT, Horowitz I: Skeletal tuberculosis: A review with patient presentations and discussion. Am J Med 1970;48:77.
9. Alderson M, Speers D, Emslie K, et al: Acute hematogenous osteomyelitis and septic arthritis—a single disease. J Bone Joint Surg Br 1986;68:268.

Osteonecrosis and Osteochondritis Dissecans

10. Mont MA, Hungerford DS: Current concepts review: Nontraumatic avascular necrosis of the femoral head. J Bone Joint Surg Am 1995;77:459.
11. Keeley K, Buchanan G: Acute infarction of long bones in children with sickle cell anemia. J Pediatr 1982;101:170.
12. Ilardi CF, Sokoloff L: Secondary osteonecrosis in osteoarthritis of the femoral head. Hum Pathol 1984;15:79.
13. Smith S, Febring T, Griffin W, et al: Core decompression of the osteonecrotic femoral head. J Bone Joint Surg Am 1995;77:674.
14. Jacobs B, Huvos AG: Malignant fibrous histiocytoma and osteosarcoma in association with bone infarcts: Report of four cases, two in caisson workers. J Bone Joint Surg Am 1974;56:932.
15. Milgram JW: Radiological and pathological manifestations of osteochondritis dissecans of the distal femur: A study of 50 cases. Radiology 1978;126:305.

Hyperparathyroidism

16. Heath HH, Hodgson SF, Kennedy MA: Primary hyperparathyroidism: Incidence, morbidity, and potential economic impact in a community. N Engl J Med 1980;302:189.
17. Silverberg SJ, Shane E, Jacobs TP, et al: Nephrolithiasis and bone involvement in primary hyperparathyroidism. Am J Med 1990;89:327.
18. Singhal S, Johnson CA, Udelsman R: Primary hyperparathyroidism: What every orthopedic surgeon should know. Orthopedics 2001;24:1003.

Paget's Disease

19. Huvos AG, Butler A, Bretsky SS: Osteogenic sarcoma associated with Paget's disease of bone: A clinicopathologic study of 65 patients. Cancer 1983;52:1489.
20. Smith J, Botet JF, Yeh SDJ: Bone sarcomas in Paget's disease: A study of 85 patients. Radiology 1984;152:583.
21. Magitsky S, Lipton JF, Reidy J, et al: Ultrastructural features of giant cell tumors in Paget's disease. Clin Orthop 2002;402:213.

Amyloidosis

22. Pambuccian SE, Horyd ID, Cawte T, et al: Amyloidoma of bone, a plasma cell/plasmacytoid neoplasm: Report of three cases and review of the literature. Am J Surg Pathol 1997;21:179.
23. Casey TT, Stone WJ, DiRaimondo CR, et al: Tumoral amyloidosis of bone of beta2-microglobulin origin in association with long-term hemodialysis: A new type of amyloid disease. Hum Pathol 1986;17:731.

Arthritides

24. O'Connell JX: Pathology of the synovium. Am J Clin Pathol 2000;114:773.
25. O'Connell JX, Nielsen GP, Rosenberg AE: Subchondral acute inflammation in severe arthritis: A sterile osteomyelitis? Am J Surg Pathol 1999;23:192.
26. Dodd LG, Major NM: Fine-needle aspiration cytology of articular and periarticular lesions. Cancer (Cancer Cytopathol) 2002;96:157.
27. Bjelle A, Norberg B, Sjogren G: The cytology of joint exudates in rheumatoid arthritis: Morphology and preparation techniques. Scand J Rheumatol 1982;11:124.
28. Laskar FH, Sargison KD: Ochronotic arthropathy: A review with four case reports. J Bone Joint Surg Br 1970;52:653.
29. Shidam V, Chivukula M, Basir Z, et al: Evaluation of crystals in formalin-fixed paraffin-embedded tissue sections for the differential diagnosis of pseudogout, gout, and tumoral calcinosis. Mod Pathol 2001;14:806.
30. Nicol KK, Ward WG, Pike EJ, et al: Fine needle aspiration biopsy of gouty tophi: Lessons in cost-effective patient management. Diagn Cytopathol 1997;17:30.
31. Ishida T, Dorfman HD, Bullough PG: Tophaceous pseudogout (tumoral calcium pyrophosphate dihydrate crystal deposition disease). Hum Pathol 1995;26:587.
32. Allen EA, Ali SZ, Erozan YS: Tumoral calcium pyrophosphate dihydrate deposition disease: Cytopathologic findings on fine-needle aspiration. Diagn Cytopathol 1996;15:349.
33. Pakasa NM, Kalengayi RM: Tumoral calcinosis: A clinicopathologic study of 111 cases with emphasis on the earliest changes. Histopathology 1997;31:18.
34. Saran RK, Gupta SK, Radotra BD, et al: Fine needle aspiration of tumoral calcinosis. Acta Cytol 2001;45:1086.
35. Gregosiewicz A, Warda E: Tumoral calcinosis: Successful medical treatment. J Bone Joint Surg Am 1989;71:1244.
36. Abdul-Karim FW, McGinnis MG, Kraay M, et al: Frozen section biopsy assessment for the presence of polymorphonuclear leukocytes in patients undergoing revision of arthroplasties. Mod Pathol 1998;11:427.
37. Athanasou NA, Padney R, Steiger R, et al: Diagnosis of infection by frozen section during revision arthroplasty. J Bone Joint Surg Br 1995;77:28.
38. Fehring TK, McAlister JA: Frozen histologic section as a guide to sepsis in revision joint arthroplasty. Clin Orthop 1994:304:229.
39. Christie AJ, Pierret G, Levitan J: Silicone synovitis. Semin Arthritis Rheum 1989;19:166.
40. Gordon M, Bullough PG: Synovial and osseous inflammation in failed silicone-rubber prostheses: Report of six cases. J Bone Joint Surg Am 1982;64:574.

INDEX

Note: Page numbers followed by f indicate figures; those followed by t indicate tables.